BSAVA Manual of Canine and Feline
Surgical Principles
A Foundation Manual

T0261052

Editors:

Stephen J. Baines
MA VetMB PhD CertVR CertSAS DipECVS MRCVS
RCVS and European Specialist in Small Animal Surgery

Willows Veterinary Centre and Referral Service, Highlands Road, Shirley, Solihull B90 4NH

Vicky Lipscomb
MA VetMB CertSAS FHEA DipECVS MRCVS
European Specialist in Small Animal Surgery

Department of Veterinary Clinical Sciences, Royal Veterinary College, Hawkshead Lane, North Mymms, Hertfordshire AL9 7TA

and

Tim Hutchinson
BVSc CertSAS MRCVS

Larkmead Veterinary Group, 111–113 Park Road, Didcot, Oxfordshire OX11 8QT

Published by:

British Small Animal Veterinary Association
Woodrow House, 1 Telford Way, Waterwells
Business Park, Quedgeley, Gloucester GL2 2AB

A Company Limited by Guarantee in England.
Registered Company No. 2837793.
Registered as a Charity.

A catalogue record for this book is available from the British Library.

ISBN 978 1 905319 25 1

The publishers, editors and contributors cannot take responsibility for information provided on dosages and methods of application of drugs mentioned or referred to in this publication. Details of this kind must be verified in each case by individual users from up to date literature published by the manufacturers or suppliers of those drugs. Veterinary surgeons are reminded that in each case they must follow all appropriate national legislation and regulations (for example, in the United Kingdom, the prescribing cascade) from time to time in force.

Printed in the UK by Severn, Gloucester GL2 5EU – a carbon neutral printer
Printed on ECF paper made from sustainable forests

18529PUBS23

Titles in the BSAVA Manuals series:

For further information on these and all BSAVA publications, please visit our website: **www.bsava.com**

Contents

Contributors

Sophie Adamantos BVSc CertVA DipACVECC FHEA MRCVS
RCVS Specialist in Emergency and Critical Care
Department of Veterinary Clinical Sciences, Royal Veterinary College, Hawkshead Lane,
North Mymms, Hertfordshire AL9 7TA

Davina Anderson MA VetMB PhD DSAS(ST) DipECVS MRCVS
RCVS and European Specialist in Small Animal Surgery
Anderson Sturgess Veterinary Specialists, The Granary, Bunstead Barns, Poles Lane, Hursley,
Winchester, Hampshire SO21 2LL

Elizabeth Armitage-Chan MA VetMB FHEA DipACVA MRCVS
RCVS and American Specialist in Veterinary Anaesthesia
Davies Veterinary Specialists, Manor Farm Business Park, Higham Gobion, Hertfordshire SG5 3HR

Nicholas J. Bacon MA VetMB DipECVS DipACVS MRCVS
Department of Small Animal Clinical Sciences, College of Veterinary Medicine, University of Florida,
Gainesville, Florida FL 32610-0126, USA

Stephen J. Baines MA VetMB PhD CertVR CertSAS DipECVS MRCVS
RCVS and European Specialist in Small Animal Surgery
Willows Veterinary Centre and Referral Service, Highlands Road, Shirley, Solihull B90 4NH

Noel Berger DVM MS DABLS
Animal Hospital and Laser Center of South Carolina, 13057 Ocean Hwy, Suite D, Pawleys Island,
South Carolina SC 29585, USA

Andrew J. Brown[†] MA VetMB DipACVECC MRCVS
Vets Now Referral Hospital, 123–145 North Street, Glasgow G3 7DA, Scotland

Daniel L. Chan DVM DipACVECC DipACVN FHEA MRCVS
RCVS Specialist in Emergency and Critical Care
Department of Veterinary Clinical Sciences, Royal Veterinary College, Hawkshead Lane,
North Mymms, Hertfordshire AL9 7TA

Peter H. Eeg BSc DVM CVLF
Poolesville Veterinary Clinic, 19621 Fisher Avenue, Poolesville, Maryland MD 20837, USA

Terry Emmerson MA VetMB CertSAS DipECVS MRCVS
RCVS and European Specialist in Small Animal Surgery
North Downs Specialist Referrals, The Friesian Buildings 3 and 4, Brewerstreet Dairy Business Park,
Brewer Street, Bletchingley, Surrey RH1 4QP

Gillian R. Gibson VMD DipACVIM MRCVS
Axiom Veterinary Laboratories, The Manor House, Brunel Road, Newton Abbot, Devon TQ12 4PB

Robert Goggs BVSc DipACVECC MRCVS
School of Physiology and Pharmacology, Faculty of Medical and Veterinary Sciences,
University of Bristol, University Walk, Bristol BS8 1TD

Michael H. Hamilton BVM&S CertSAS DipECVS MRCVS
European Specialist in Small Animal Surgery
Fitzpatrick Referrals Ltd, Halfway Lane, Eashing, Surrey GU7 2QQ

David Holt BVSc DipACVS
School of Veterinary Medicine, University of Pennsylvania, 3900 Delancey Street,
Philadelphia PA 19104, USA

Arthur House BSc BVMS PhD CertSAS DipECVS
Melbourne Veterinary Specialist Centre, 70 Blackburn Road, Glen Waverley, Victoria 3150, Australia

Karen Humm MA VetMB CertVA DipACVECC FHEA MRCVS
Department of Veterinary Clinical Sciences, Royal Veterinary College, Hawkshead Lane,
North Mymms, Hertfordshire AL9 7TA

Geraldine B. Hunt BVSC MVetClinStud PhD FACVSc
Department of Veterinary Surgical and Radiological Sciences, School of Veterinary Medicine,
University of California Davis, Davis, California CA 95616-8745, USA

Tim Hutchinson BVSc CertSAS MRCVS
Larkmead Veterinary Group, 111–113 Park Road, Didcot, Oxfordshire OX11 8QT

John Lapish BSc BVetMed MRCVS
Veterinary Instrumentation, Broadfield Road, Sheffield S8 0XL

Elizabeth A. Leece BVSc CVA DipECVAA MRCVS
Department of Veterinary Medicine, University of Cambridge, Madingley Road, Cambridge CB3 0ES

Vicky Lipscomb MA VetMB CertSAS FHEA DipECVS MRCVS
European Specialist in Small Animal Surgery
Department of Veterinary Clinical Sciences, Royal Veterinary College, Hawkshead Lane,
North Mymms, Hertfordshire AL9 7TA

Anette Loeffler DrMedVet PhD DVD DipECVD MRCVS
Department of Veterinary Clinical Sciences, Royal Veterinary College, Hawkshead Lane,
North Mymms, Hertfordshire AL9 7TA

Kathryn M. Pratschke MVB MVM CertSAS DipECVS MRCVS
School of Veterinary Medicine, College of Medical, Veterinary and Life Sciences,
University of Glasgow, Bearsden, Glasgow G61 1QH

Verónica Salazar LV MSc PhD DipACVA
Hospital Clinico Veterinario, Universidad Alfonso X El Sabio, Villanueva de la Cañada, Madrid

Chris Shales MA VetMB CertSAS DipECVS MRCVS
European Specialist in Small Animal Surgery
Willows Veterinary Centre and Referral Service, Highlands Road, Shirley, Solihull B90 4NH

Thomas Sissener MS DVM CertSAS DipECVS MRCVS
Oslo Dyreklinikk, Ensjoveien 14, 0655 Oslo, Norway

Jeffrey Wilson DVM DipACVA
School of Veterinary Medicine, University of Pennsylvania, 3900 Delancey Street,
Philadelphia PA 19104, USA

Foreword

The *BSAVA Manual of Canine and Feline Surgical Principles: A Foundation Manual* covers those key topics required for surgical success that are often overshadowed in larger textbooks of veterinary surgery and which are relevant to all members of the veterinary team.

The Manual is divided into three main sections: surgical facilities and equipment; perioperative considerations for the surgical patient; and surgical biology and techniques. The first section contains chapters dedicated to theatre design, equipment, sterilization and personnel. The chapter on surgical instruments doesn't just contain lists of equipment, but provides a well illustrated review of the instruments seen in surgical kits and, most importantly, when and how to use them.

The second section is central to the Manual and provides guidelines for the preoperative and postoperative management of the surgical patient: essential for the successful outcome of surgery. Preoperative assessment and stabilization, fluid therapy and shock are covered in this section. In addition, there are also chapters dedicated to the immune response to anaesthesia and surgery, analgesia, postoperative management and clinical nutrition.

The final section of the Manual is devoted to surgical biology and surgical techniques. The chapters in this section provide information on aseptic technique, wound healing and how to minimize surgical site infections. In addition, a useful summary on the control of hospital-acquired infections, providing practical guidelines to this very emotive subject, is included here. This section concludes with chapters on haemostasis, operative techniques, suture patterns and knots.

I am sure that the *BSAVA Manual of Canine and Feline Surgical Principles* will be a must read for veterinary surgeons studying for the RCVS Certificate in Advanced Veterinary Surgery, veterinary nurses with an interest in surgery, and practice managers. Well done to the editorial team for their enjoyable and practical covering of this essential subject.

Karla Lee MA VetMB PhD CertSAS DipECVS MRCVS
Royal Veterinary College

Preface

The aim of this new BSAVA Foundation Manual is to bring together all the basic principles of veterinary surgery that are usually relegated to the introductory chapter or paragraph of other surgical textbooks. Meticulous attention to the basic principles of surgery is critical if we are to achieve a good surgical outcome. Good surgeons are not those who are simply skilled at surgery, but those who ensure that every aspect of the care of their patient is performed to the highest standard, from the initial physical examination, preoperative investigation and stabilization, right through to the anaesthesia, analgesia and postoperative care. Complications that arise following surgery are often attributable to a lack of understanding or appreciation of the importance of these basic principles. These complications may be avoided by adhering to a set of basic principles, and this should be our aim.

This manual provides a solid grounding in best practice for the basic principles of veterinary surgery, which will be particularly helpful for veterinary nurses, veterinary students and new graduates, but will also be useful to any veterinary surgeon wishing to update their knowledge of these topics. We have attempted to relate specific recommendations that are made in the text to evidence in the veterinary literature and provide further reading where necessary. We have also endeavoured to concentrate on practical aspects of perioperative and intraoperative patient care and management to help the reader translate these principles into practice. Several chapters, including the innate immune/inflammatory response to anaesthesia and surgery, surgical staplers, lasers and hospital-acquired infections, provide particularly new or topical information for veterinary surgeons. Veterinary critical care has grown enormously due to the availability of advanced monitoring and specialist training in this discipline, and the chapters covering fluid therapy, shock, SIRS and postoperative care have the benefit of up to date recommendations for our surgical patients from such specialists.

We hope that this manual will spread knowledge and information about the fundamental principles of veterinary surgery. We would like it to be a useful resource that individuals will turn to for reference, as well as a stimulus to initiate discussion, reflection and review of current practices amongst veterinary colleagues with a view to establishing routines based on current knowledge and practice. Our ultimate aim is to improve the outcome for our surgical patients and reduce the incidence of complications and resulting morbidity and mortality.

Stephen Baines
Vicky Lipscomb
Tim Hutchinson

Surgical facilities – design, management, equipment and personnel

1

Terry Emmerson

Introduction

The basic aims of good theatre design and practice are to create a flexible work space, efficient work flow and as clean an environment as possible to minimize contamination of the surgical patient. Minimizing patient contamination will, in turn, reduce the number of surgical infections. Surgical infections have significant cost to the patient, owner and practice. Although surgical infections will occur in even the best designed and managed theatres, a good understanding of basic principles of design and management will keep them to a minimum.

Surgical facility design

In modern veterinary practice, operating facilities vary from single rooms to large multiple-theatre surgical suites. Although some of the design elements are not feasible due to lack of space or finance, the basic principles can be applied to even the smallest practices.

General design

Traffic flow

The surgical areas should be located in an area within the practice where there is low general traffic flow, as people and animal traffic increase the levels of contamination in the environment. To minimize traffic, there should be only one entrance to the surgical areas, but a second exit may be required where fire regulations dictate. This should be marked 'For emergency use only'.

Clean *versus* contaminated areas

The surgical facilities are divided into clean and contaminated areas:

- **Clean areas** include the operating theatres, scrub area and sterile stores
- **Contaminated areas** include the patient preparation area and changing rooms.

There should be a clear divide between the clean and contaminated areas, with closed doors to minimize the risk of contamination entering the clean areas. Staff should don surgical attire when entering the clean area. Ideally they should enter via a changing room located between the clean and contaminated areas. If this is not possible, surgical attire should be covered by a clean coat when in the contaminated areas and surgical footwear should only be worn in the clean areas (see Chapter 16).

Radiography

In planning the surgical area, allowance should also be made for easy access to radiography to enable simple transfer of patients for preoperative and post-operative radiographs.

Anaesthesia induction and patient preparation room

This area is where anaesthesia is induced and patients are prepared for surgery (Figure 1.1).

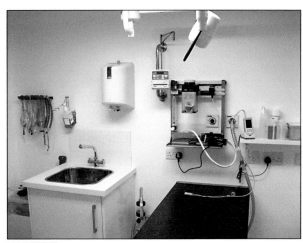

1.1 Anaesthesia and patient preparation area.

- Appropriate materials and equipment should be available for inducing and maintaining anaesthesia.
- For patient preparation this area should also be equipped with: clippers; a vacuum cleaner for removing loose hair after clipping; and skin preparation materials.
- Good lighting is important and movable spotlights can be useful for closer examination of the patient.

- Tables can be fixed or mobile. Fixed sinks/tubs or scrub tables are useful for performing dirty procedures and for preparing patients where copious cleaning or lavage is required.
- Mobile trolleys that can be raised and lowered are ideal when dealing with large and recumbent patients.
- Trolleys should be available for moving patients to theatre. To avoid carrying in dirt, dust and hair on the wheels, these trolleys should not cross into the clean areas. A separate trolley to transfer the patient into the clean area should be available (Figure 1.2).
- The point of transition from contaminated to clean areas should be clearly marked, e.g. by a clear line on the floor, or a change in floor colour.

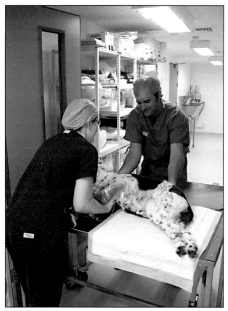

1.2 Transferring a patient from the contaminated area to the clean area of the surgical facility. Separate trolleys are used in each area.

Changing area

The changing area is located next to the clean area of the surgical suite. This allows staff to change into theatre attire **before** entering the clean area. Where this is not possible, staff should cover their theatre scrubs and wear outside shoes when in any area other than the clean areas of the theatre suite.

Nurses' station

Where there is a separate clean area in the surgical facility, a nurses' station should be provided. This acts as a point of contact for staff in the clean area from elsewhere in the practice and allows certain administrative functions to be performed. Both help to minimize the amount of traffic into and out of the clean area of the theatre. The station houses a computer and telephone, with storage for manuals relating to theatre equipment and contact details for suppliers.

Sterile store

Storage space needs to be provided for sterilized surgical instruments and sterile consumables used in theatre. An adequate amount of shelving needs to be provided to allow a logical arrangement to assist in locating items and in stock taking.

Sterile instruments should be stored in closed cabinets to extend the period of sterility following sterilization. Shelves and doors should be constructed of glass to allow for easy cleaning and visualization of the sterile packs. Pass-through cabinets between the sterile corridor and theatres (Figure 1.3) help to minimize traffic into and out of the theatre, and provide easy access to extra instruments required during surgery.

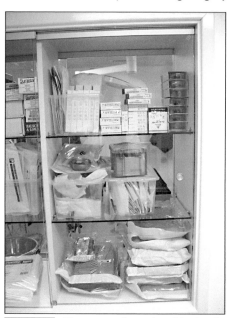

1.3 Glass pass-through cabinets allow storage of sterile items between the theatre and the sterile corridor.

Surgeon preparation area

The scrub area is located close to operating theatres, but is separate from them and the sterile stores to avoid contamination from water droplets produced whilst scrubbing. A deep stainless steel sink is provided (Figure 1.4) with taps operated by foot, knee, elbow or infrared to allow for appropriate aseptic scrubbing technique. The sink should be set at waist height to minimize splashing when scrubbing. An infra-red or elbow-operated soap dispenser and a supply of sterile scrub brushes should also be located at the sink.

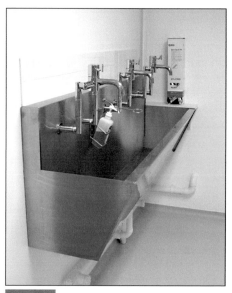

1.4 Sinks in the surgeon scrub area.

It is particularly important that flooring in this area is non-slip. Rubber mats can be placed by the sink to reduce the slip hazard, but it is essential that these are moved and cleaned regularly.

Gowning and gloving area

The pack containing the gown and hand towel should be opened on a surface away from the surgical field. Gowning should not be performed using the instrument trolley, due to the risk of droplets of water contaminating the sterile field during the hand-drying process.

A separate area for gloving and gowning can be provided outside the theatre. This area requires only a clean surface on which to lay out sterile gowns and gloves.

PRACTICAL TIP

The reason for providing an area **outside** the theatre is that there is less risk there of contaminating gloves and gowns compared to gloving and gowning inside the theatre. This is because there is more movement of people and equipment in the theatre, particularly in small theatres. However, there is no definitive evidence that a separate area reduces contamination compared with gloving and gowning in the operating theatre, so this is a design feature of low priority for practices with constraints on space.

Operating theatres

General design

Operating theatres should be large enough to accommodate the necessary surgical equipment and staff whilst allowing for easy movement around the theatre when it is in use. Theatres with larger equipment, such as operating microscopes, will need to be more spacious.

The general design should be simple, with minimal clutter or ledges and other areas that form dust traps and are difficult to clean. The surfaces of walls, floors and ceilings should be non-porous and easy to clean and should be able to withstand regular wet cleaning. Options for wall surfaces include waterproof paints, ceramic tiles and PVC sheets. PVC is probably the best finish as it produces the smoothest, most knock-resistant surface and with welded joins is easily cleaned. Coving should be used where the floor meets the wall (Figure 1.5) and at wall corners, to allow for easy cleaning.

- Theatre doors should be wide enough to move patients through easily and should swing both ways to allow a scrubbed surgeon to move through without touching the door with their hands.
- If windows are present in the operating theatre they should be sealed so that they cannot be opened, to prevent contamination from outside.
- The theatre should contain no taps, as these will produce water droplets that could contaminate the patient.
- There should be no sinks, drains or gullies in the floor, as these could act as a source of contamination and a reservoir for bacteria.

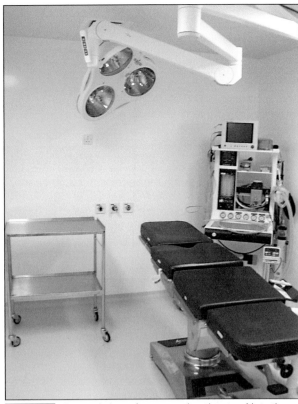

1.5 General view of an operating theatre. Note the PVC-lined walls and coved flooring.

- There should be enough power outlets for all equipment required (both surgical and anaesthetic).
- Piped anaesthetic gases, piped compressed surgical air and active scavenging systems are ideal, as they help to minimize the equipment in the theatre (Figure 1.6). Piped gases also minimize traffic into and out of theatre to change cylinders and they minimize the need to bring cylinders from contaminated areas into the clean areas.
- An anaesthetic trolley is preferable to wall-mounted machinery, as it allows more flexibility in how the theatre is organized. This can be useful for certain procedures, such as head, neck and ophthalmic surgery, where ideally the anaesthetist is moved away from the head of the patient to allow the surgeon maximum access. One disadvantage of anaesthetic trolleys is the increased space requirement, which may make them inappropriate in smaller theatres.
- A clock should be mounted on the wall to allow for timing of certain procedures, particularly vascular occlusion.
- Facilities for either digital or conventional radiographic image viewing should be provided.

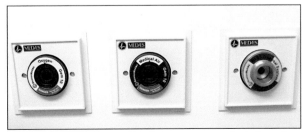

1.6 Piped gas outlets for oxygen, surgical air and active scavenging.

Ventilation

Operating theatres should be ventilated using a positive pressure ventilation (PPV) system, producing approximately 20 air changes per hour. The aim of the system is to reduce the airborne contamination in the theatre as the air becomes laden with skin squames and respiratory droplets from staff. Each air change reduces this contamination to approximately 37% of its former level.

> ### PRACTICAL TIP
>
> The air coming through the ventilation system can be filtered to remove bacteria, but this is not essential as the main source of airborne contamination comes from the staff within the theatre and not from the outside environment.
>
> Filtering to prevent more gross contaminants such as dust and insects entering the theatre is essential.

As well as providing air changes, PPV prevents contaminated air from entering the operating theatre by setting up a pressure gradient between the clean and contaminated areas of the theatre suite. Higher air pressure in the theatre forces air towards the contaminated areas, which are at lower pressure.

Heating and humidity

Ideal ambient theatre temperature is 20–21°C, which produces a comfortable working temperature whilst helping to minimize patient hypothermia. Higher temperatures up to 24°C may be more appropriate for paediatric patients who are more prone to hypothermia. Ideally the theatres are heated using warm air through the PPV system. If this type of system is not installed, radiators can be used but care should be taken not to create dust traps with the radiators and pipes.

Humidity of 40–60% maximizes staff comfort as well as reducing the multiplication of environmental bacteria.

Lighting

Lighting in the operating theatres should be good, with background light provided by fluorescent lights. The surgical site is illuminated by one, or preferably two, sets of theatre lights (Figure 1.7). Two sets of lights directed from different angles give maximum illumination of the surgical site (see Chapter 21).

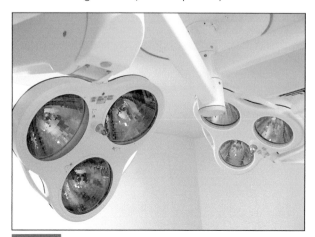

1.7 A pair of ceiling-mounted theatre lights.

Floor-standing and ceiling-mounted theatre lights are available. Ceiling-mounted lights are preferred, as they avoid clutter in the theatre and are more easily repositioned. Ceiling lights should have hinged arms to allow maximum manoeuvrability.

Ideally it should be possible to focus surgical lights and they should also be equipped with removable sterile handles to allow the surgeon to adjust their position during procedures.

Operating theatre equipment

The equipment required for an operating theatre is listed in Figure 1.8.

For a basic operating theatre
■ Height-adjustable operating table.
■ Positioning aids.
■ Basic anaesthetic monitoring equipment.
■ Stainless steel instrument trolleys.
■ Stainless steel kick buckets.

Additional equipment to be considered where there is sufficient surgical caseload
■ Patient-warming facility.
■ Surgical suction.
■ Diathermy.
■ More advanced anaesthetic monitoring equipment.

1.8 Operating theatre equipment.

■ The height of the operating table should be adjustable and the ability to tilt the table can be useful for some procedures (Figure 1.9). Fastenings to tie patients and attach certain equipment to the table can be useful. Instrument trays, anaesthetic monitoring and patient-warming devices can be attached to certain tables.

■ A variety of aids may be used to position patients for surgery, including cradles, sandbags, ties and vacuum bean bags (Figure 1.10). As well as positioning the patient, these are used to prevent

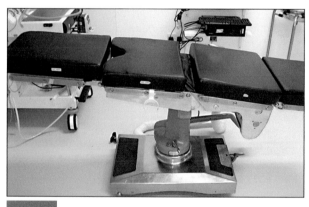

1.9 Height-adjustable operating table.

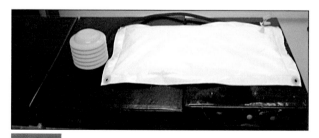

1.10 Vacuum theatre positioning aids.

injuries to the patient due to poor support or cushioning. To minimize contamination from other areas of the practice, the positioning aids should only be used in the theatre.

■ A patient warming system in theatre will help to reduce patient hypothermia. It should preferably be either a circulating warm-water bed or a warm-air blanket such as a Bair Hugger (Figure 1.11). Electric heat pads are less desirable and should be used with care, as there is a higher risk of thermal burns to an immobile patient.

■ The amount and types of anaesthetic monitoring equipment (Figure 1.12) are numerous. What is required will depend on the types of procedures to be performed.

■ Surgical suction is extremely useful and has many applications, including removing effusions, lavage, and clearing the surgical field of blood. A model with the appropriate suction rate and suitable reservoir capacity (e.g. 1 litre) should be selected.

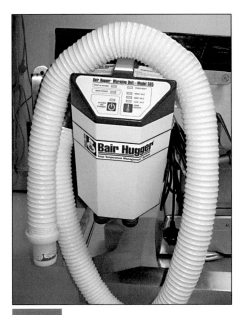

1.11 A Bair Hugger patient warming system.

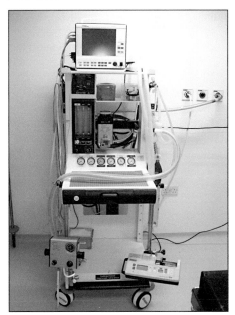

1.12 Anaesthetic machine, demonstrating extensive monitoring, ventilation and fluid delivery systems.

Recovery area

An area is provided adjacent to the clean areas of the surgical suite where animals can be carefully monitored until they are fully recovered from anaesthesia. Thereafter, patients are returned to normal wards or an intensive care facility.

■ To help reduce postoperative hypothermia, the recovery area should be warmer than the wards. Temperatures of 22–24°C are usually appropriate.

■ Facilities should be available to warm patients and deal with emergencies during recovery.

■ A well stocked crash cart and oxygen supply should be available.

■ There needs to be a high ratio of nurses to patients in this area to allow for intensive monitoring.

> **PRACTICAL TIP**
>
> For many practices a separate recovery area is not practical, but the basic principles of close monitoring, prevention of hypothermia and easy access to oxygen and crash supplies should still be maintained.

Personnel and responsibilities

In larger teaching and referral hospitals a number of staff may be involved in routine cases.

■ The **veterinary surgeon** is ultimately responsible for the patient, performing the surgery and directing the procedures in theatre.

■ The **sterile scrub nurse** is scrubbed in to assist, provide retraction and pass sterile instruments.

■ The **circulating nurse** organizes theatre, helps with gowning and gloving, passes instruments to sterile staff, records use of consumables and controls non-sterile equipment such as diathermy and suction.

■ The veterinary **anaesthetist** in larger hospitals allows the surgeon to concentrate solely on the surgery, but must liaise with the surgeon when the surgery affects patient physiology or if anaesthetic complications occur.

For routine procedures in smaller practices, a veterinary nurse may monitor the anaesthetic (under the direction of the veterinary surgeon) and act as the circulating nurse at the same time. Other roles may only be filled during more complex cases.

> **WARNING**
>
> In smaller practices a veterinary nurse may monitor the anaesthetic, but changes to it must be made *under the direction of the veterinary surgeon.*

Theatre coordinator

Whatever the size of the practice, one person should be responsible for the overall management of the theatres and theatre staff. This role includes organizing surgical lists, ensuring that cleaning protocols are followed, maintaining stocks of sterile consumables and maintaining theatre equipment.

Good theatre practice

In combination with good theatre design, good theatre practice and management are essential to minimize surgical contamination and maximize efficiency of workflow. Good theatre management requires a thorough understanding of the roles of the various staff, promoting good theatre practice (Figure 1.13), arranging appropriate theatre lists and setting and monitoring an effective cleaning programme.

DOs

- Wear appropriate theatre clothing and either change or cover theatre clothing when leaving the operating theatre.
- Wear theatre hats and masks.
- Maintain good personal hygiene.
- Limit access to theatre to surgical staff.
- Keep movement to a minimum, particularly staff entering and leaving the theatre during procedures.
- Keep staff numbers in the operating theatre to the minimum required.
- Keep talking in the operating theatre to a minimum.
- Maintain good hand-washing policy between patients.
- Maintain a theatre log of all patients and procedures. This can be useful in identifying trends in infection related to specific surgeons, theatres or procedures.

DON'Ts

- Do not wear jewellery or false nails.
- Non-sterile staff should not lean over the sterile field.
- Non-sterile staff should not pass between the instrument trolley and surgical site.

1.13   General good theatre practice.

Designation of theatres

Where there are multiple theatres, each can be designated for clean procedures or for contaminated procedures. The aim is to maintain the lowest level of contamination in the clean theatre, where clean procedures such as orthopaedics and neurosurgery are performed. This is particularly important for procedures involving implants, such as joint replacement.

'Dirty' procedures should be performed in a separate designated theatre where available or, more practically, in the preparation room.

WARNING

Dirty procedures involving body cavities (e.g. pyothorax) require an operating theatre. Use of the patient preparation room is not appropriate in such cases.

Arranging a surgical list

To maintain the highest level of surgical asepsis, the surgical list should be arranged relative to the greatest risk of contamination of the surgical environment. This is best achieved by classifying the procedures as clean, clean–contaminated, contaminated or dirty (Figure 1.14) and then starting with the clean procedures and progressing through, finishing with the dirty procedures.

WARNING

Patients with known hospital-acquired infections such as *Pseudomonas* and MRSA should be at the end of the surgical list.

Classification	Description
Clean	Non-traumatic wound Respiratory, genitourinary or gastrointestinal tract not entered
Clean–contaminated	Respiratory, genitourinary or gastrointestinal tract entered but no gross spillage Minor break in aseptic technique
Contaminated	Traumatic wound <4 hours old Major break in aseptic technique Major spillage of gastrointestinal contents, or encountering infected urine or bile
Dirty	Established bacterial infection in tissue Traumatic wounds with devitalized tissue, gross contamination or >4 hours old

1.14   Classification of surgical procedures.

Due to individual patient needs, such as stability or urgency, it is not always possible to maintain this order; for example, a gastric dilatation–volvulus may take priority over an elective orthopaedic surgery. Where there is such a break in the order, more thorough cleaning of the theatre between patients may be required. Breaks in order are less of an issue where a PPV system is in place, as the airborne bacterial numbers decrease rapidly due to air changes. However, cleaning the surfaces with which the patient has been in contact is still critical.

Cleaning the surgical facility

Thorough cleaning is essential to maintain optimum aseptic technique in the surgical facility. A cleaning protocol should be established and its implementation closely monitored by the theatre supervisor.

PRACTICAL TIP

Regular microbiological testing of surfaces in theatres is probably of limited value but should be performed in the event of an increase in postsurgical infections.

- Decontamination should always precede disinfection, as large particles of organic matter impede the action of the chemical agents used for disinfection.
- Gross matter should be removed with disposable towels that can then be discarded.
- Cleaning should be performed with a broad-spectrum surface disinfectant, used at appropriate dilutions and allowed the necessary contact time.
- Mops and buckets used for floor cleaning should be designated 'Theatre only' (Figure 1.15) and should not be used in any other areas of the practice. Colour coding of buckets and mops for different areas in the practice can help to make this clearer.
- Mop heads act as reservoirs for bacteria and should therefore be hot-washed daily.
- Buckets should be emptied and stored dry to reduce bacterial multiplication.
- Surfaces should be cleaned using paper towels and single-use cloths to stop them acting as bacterial reservoirs.

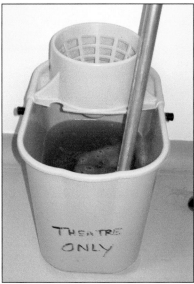

1.15 Colour-coded and labelled theatre cleaning bucket.

Figures 1.16 and 1.17 suggest regular cleaning schedules for the scrub area and operating theatre. For other areas:

- Clean floors and walls as for operating theatres
- Clean any phones and computers weekly, as they will harbour bacteria from human contact
- On a regular basis, ideally every 2–3 months, clear all shelving and clean with an appropriate surface disinfectant.

Written cleaning schedules should be created and should be signed and dated to create accountability and allow audit of the cleaning process.

Between scrubbing sessions

- Remove from the sink any packaging from pre-packed sterile scrub brushes.
- Clean any water spilled on the floor, to reduce the risk of slipping.

End of day

- Remove all packaging.
- Clean and disinfect the sink.
- Clean and refill surgical scrub dispenser and restock scrub brushes.
- Clean the floor area.

1.16 Cleaning protocol for a scrub area.

Start of day

- Wipe down all surfaces with an appropriate disinfectant to remove dust that has settled overnight.

Between patients

- Remove all used surgical equipment and instruments from the theatre.
- Wipe down the operating table and instrument trolleys with disinfectant.
- Spot-clean any gross blood or body fluid contamination on floors, walls and furniture.
- Clean any items that have come into contact with the patient, such as water blankets, blood pressure cuffs, oesophageal thermometers and stethoscopes.
- Remove any clinical waste and rubbish generated by the procedure.

End of day

- Remove all furniture from the theatre.
- Clean and disinfect all tables and trolleys, ensuring that joints and undersides are also checked.
- Clean and disinfect the anaesthetic machine and vaporizer.
- Clean theatre lights.
- Roll wheeled equipment through a small amount of disinfectant on the floor.
- Clean and disinfect the floors.
- Clean and disinfect the door handles.
- Close the theatre doors.

Weekly – in addition to daily cleaning schedule

- Clean and disinfect walls and ceilings.
- Scrub floors or clean them with a rotary cleaner.
- Thoroughly clean and disinfect the operating table.
- Vacuum ventilation grilles to remove accumulated dust.
- Change or clean filters in warm-air heating systems.
- Check maintenance of all equipment.
- Thoroughly clean and disinfect the suction unit.

1.17 Cleaning protocol for an operating theatre.

References and further reading

Dean A (2004) Strategies for infection control in the operating theatre. In: *Fundamentals of Operating Department Practice, 2nd edn*, ed. A Davey and C Ince, pp. 37–42. Cambridge University Press, Cambridge

Fortunato N (2000) Physical facilities and care of the perioperative environment. In: *Berry & Kohn's Operating Room Technique, 9th edn*, ed. N Phillips, pp. 147–160. Mosby, St. Louis

Fortunato N (2000) Care of the perioperative environment. In: *Berry & Kohn's Operating Room Technique, 9th edn*, ed. N Phillips, pp. 169–182. Mosby, St. Louis

Hobson P (2003) Surgical facilities and equipment. In: *Textbook of Small Animal Surgery, 3rd edn*, ed. D Slater, pp. 179–184. WB Saunders, Philadelphia

Sterilization and disinfection

2

Michael H. Hamilton

Introduction

Terminology

The terms sterilization, disinfection, asepsis and antisepsis are often used interchangeably and frequently incorrectly.

Sterilization

Sterilization is the process of **destruction of all forms of microbial life**. This includes bacteria, viruses, fungi, algae and protozoans. The term also implies the complete elimination of dormant bacterial spores, which are highly resistant to environmental changes and can survive within the environment for many years. One of the most well known spore-forming bacteria is *Bacillus anthracis*, the causative agent of anthrax, which can survive extremely hostile conditions for decades or even centuries. Of recent public health importance is the eradication of prions, the smallest known infectious agents, which are associated with spongiform encephalopathies.

Following the process of sterilization an item is deemed to be **sterile**. Sterilization is an absolute phenomenon: an item is either sterile or non-sterile; there is no such thing as partially sterile.

Disinfection

Disinfection is the process of **removal of microbes that may result in infection**. It does not imply the elimination of all microorganisms, as some viruses and bacterial spores are not inactivated by disinfection. Sterilization may or may not be achieved during the process of disinfection, depending on the process used and the number and resilience of any microorganisms present.

- A **disinfectant** is an agent used in the process of disinfection. The term is most commonly associated with chemicals that are applied to inanimate objects such as floors or items of equipment. These chemicals are usually too caustic to be used on living tissue without causing cellular damage.
- A **high-level disinfectant** is a disinfectant that has the capacity to achieve sterilization if an increased exposure time is used.

Antisepsis

Antisepsis is the process of **removal of pathogenic organisms from the skin or mucous membranes**, but with some resident flora remaining. Bacterial numbers are decreased to a level that can be controlled by the patient's local defences, should there be a breach in the normal protective barrier of the patient's body. Antisepsis may also describe the removal of particularly virulent microbes that even in small numbers may result in infection.

- An **antiseptic** is an agent used in the process of antisepsis.
- Strictly speaking, any agent that inhibits bacterial growth may be referred to as an antiseptic, whereas the terms **biocide** and **germicide** are given to agents that kill bacteria and other microorganisms outright.

Asepsis

Asepsis is the **absence of pathogenic microbes on living tissue**. It is important to understand that this term is not synonymous with sterilization, as only inanimate objects can be rendered completely sterile.

All surgical wounds are contaminated with bacteria, but usually to a level where clinical infection does not result; the wound is thus described as being in a state of asepsis, or **aseptic**. Asepsis describes a degree of contamination of living tissue that does not result in clinical infection or disease and **aseptic surgical technique** describes the general principles employed to minimize the degree of contamination of a surgical wound.

Cleaning

Cleaning is the **physical removal of surface contaminants**. Such contaminants include dust, soil and organic matter such as blood, faeces and vomit. Inadequate removal of surface debris may impact on the effectiveness of subsequent disinfection and sterilization, by acting as a physical barrier that protects microorganisms or by inactivating the disinfectant or sterilant being used. In addition to routine cleaning with detergent and water, enzyme solutions and ultrasonic cleaners may be used to dislodge material from objects that cannot be adequately cleaned manually. Cleaning is discussed in more detail in Chapters 1, 3 and 16.

Sanitation

Sanitation relates to measures employed to remove microbes that pose a threat to public health. Isolation of infective animals and avoiding faecal and urinary contamination of food and water are examples of sanitation procedures. This is not a term usually associated with surgery.

Sterility assurance level

The effectiveness of any sterilization or disinfection procedure depends on a number of factors. Some of these are intrinsic qualities of the microorganism, whereas others depend on the external environment. All sterilization strategies in terms of exposure times and concentration levels are designed to destroy the most resistant microorganisms. When describing a sterilization process it is acceptable if the sterility assurance level results in the chances of a single microbe surviving the process as one in a million, i.e. 10^{-6}.

Spaulding's classification

In 1968 Earle Spaulding devised a rational approach to sterilization and disinfection based on the level of risk associated with the intended use of an item of medical equipment. This has been refined over the years and is now referred to as Spaulding's classification, with instruments and equipment divided into three categories (Figure 2.1).

High risk (critical)

Items that will be placed into an aseptic region, as is the case for the majority of surgical instruments, are deemed to have a high level of risk with regard to potential development of infection. There is no acceptable alternative to sterilization for these items.

Intermediate risk (semi-critical)

Intermediate-risk items are those that come into contact with, but do not penetrate, mucosal surfaces. The term is particularly relevant to flexible endoscopes. Ideally, endoscopic equipment should be sterilized but because of the fragility and complexity of the instruments they cannot withstand the temperatures and pressures of steam sterilization. Unless there is penetration of the mucosa, the risk of infection is deemed as intermediate and thus high-level disinfection is deemed appropriate.

WARNING
Endoscopic instruments that **do** enter tissue must be sterile.

In human surgery, single-use instruments are frequently employed for some surgical procedures, where there is concern that the re-sterilization process may not be completely effective. This may be due to the dimensions or complexity of the instrument precluding effective sterilization, or due to potential presence of highly resistant microbes. A recent example is the use of disposable forceps during tonsillectomy procedures due to concern regarding the potential presence of prion proteins responsible for transmissible spongiform encephalopathies.

Low risk (non-critical)

Low-risk items are those that come into contact with intact skin only. Cleaning with water and a detergent is all that is required.

Disinfection

Although Spaulding's classification is related to items of surgical equipment, it can be extrapolated to include the hospital environment and it should be borne in mind that an effective infection control regime does not start and end with sterility of the surgical instruments. The environment *per se* may be thought of as low risk, but over time microbial numbers may increase to the point whereby the environment does in fact pose a significant risk with regard to the potential for development of infection (Figure 2.2). Disinfection protocols should be formulated accordingly (see Chapter 1).

Disinfectants

The most common liquid disinfectants used for environmental decontamination include those containing quaternary ammonium compounds, chlorine compounds, phenols or iodine compounds.

Quaternary ammonium compounds

Organically substituted ammonium compounds, such as cetrimide and benzalkonium chloride, act as cationic detergents and their biocidal activity is due to their ability to dissolve lipids in microbial cell walls. These compounds are non-toxic to tissue and have a pleasant smell, making them a popular choice of disinfectant for domestic use and in hospitals. They are not effective against viruses or spores, and bacteria such as *Pseudomonas* can metabolize these compounds, using them as an energy source. Cetrimide agar is in fact used as a selective medium for laboratory isolation of pseudomonad bacteria.

Level of risk	Items concerned	Examples of items	Process required
High (critical)	Items that penetrate the skin or come into direct contact with aseptically prepared tissue or the bloodstream	Surgical instruments Needles Urinary and other catheters	Sterilization
Intermediate (semi-critical)	Items that come into contact with, but do not penetrate, mucous membranes	Flexible endoscopes Endotracheal tubes Laryngoscope blades	Ideally sterilization, but high-level disinfection satisfactory
Low (non-critical)	Items that contact intact skin	Stethoscopes Washing bowls	Cleaning with detergent

2.1 Spaulding's classification.

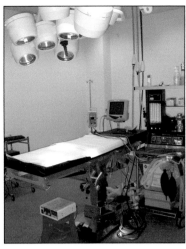
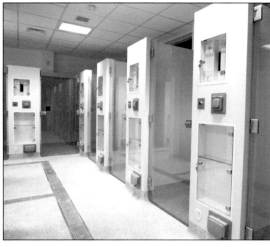

2.2 Regular disinfection is mandatory in operating theatres and kennel areas to minimize the risk of infection.

Modern disinfectants overcome these problems by using a synergistic blend of compounds. Probably the most commonly used disinfectant in veterinary hospitals today is Trigene™ (Medichem), which includes various active ingredients such as alkyl dimethyl benzyl ammonium chloride and dodecylamine sulphamate. These chemicals cause microbial cell death by destruction of cell walls, with a second proposed action of cell death via inactivation of energy-producing enzymes. They are not inactivated by organic debris and are highly effective against *Pseudomonas* species. The formulation of Trigene™ is viricidal, bactericidal, fungicidal, sporicidal, tuberculocidal and biodegradable and it may be used on virtually any surface. It is non-toxic, non-corrosive and non-irritant, with drying of the skin as the only potential side effect.

Chlorine compounds

The most commonly used chlorine compound is sodium hypochlorite, which is the chlorine preparation used in household bleach. Like other chlorine compounds, such as those used to prevent microbial growth in swimming pools or water supplies, the antimicrobial effect is due to the release of free chlorine atoms, which kill microbes by means of oxidation. Sodium hypochlorite is most commonly used as a domestic bleaching agent at a concentration of approximately 5%. At this concentration, it has a pH of around 11 and is extremely irritating to skin. At concentrations of 10–15% it has a pH of around 13, at which level it burns skin and is corrosive to metals. These compounds are therefore not used as antiseptics.

Phenols

Phenol, also known as carbolic acid, was the first disinfectant to be used in clinical practice. It is highly corrosive and toxic to humans and animals. Surgeons first wore rubber gloves not to prevent wound infection but to protect their hands from the phenol that was sprayed over wounds during surgical procedures. Many new derivatives have subsequently been developed, one of the most notable being chlorhexidine, which is commonly used for skin antisepsis. Soluble phenol products are commonly used for environmental disinfection. Phenol derivatives are very effective for killing most bacteria, including *Mycobacterium tuberculosis*, but they have limited activity against spores and viruses. They are not adversely affected by organic matter.

Iodine compounds

Like chlorine, iodine is a halogen and microbial destruction occurs due to oxidation secondary to the release of free iodine. Inorganic iodine is extremely irritant and may also result in the corrosion of instruments and fabric staining. It is now common to use iodophors, which comprise iodine in organic polymers such as detergents. These compounds are associated with fewer complications than inorganic iodine. The best known iodophor is povidone–iodine, which is used as an antiseptic. Iodine compounds are very good general disinfectants, with good activity against bacteria and viruses, but they have poor sporicidal activity and are inactivated by organic matter.

Methods of sterilization

There are various methods by which surgical equipment and materials can be sterilized, each having advantages and disadvantages. The rationale of which method is chosen is based on a variety of different factors:

- Efficacy
- Speed of the process
- Instrument compatibility
- Ease of use
- Cost of equipment
- Staff safety
- Ease of monitoring process.

By far the most common method of sterilization employed in veterinary medicine is steam sterilization in an autoclave, which produces an environment of saturated steam under high pressure. Steam sterilization is an example of a *physical* method of sterilization, as opposed to *chemical* sterilization, which refers to the use of liquid or gaseous chemicals.

Physical sterilization

Methods of physical sterilization are compared in Figure 2.3.

Steam sterilization

Heat kills microbes by coagulation of cellular proteins. Microbes can be destroyed either by dry heat (e.g. in an oven or over a flame) or by moist heat (e.g. steam). Death occurs more quickly and at a lower temperature

Method	Advantages	Disadvantages	Other comments
Dry heat	No packaging required Inexpensive	Time-consuming	May be helpful for delicate sharp instruments that may be blunted by steam
Steam (wet heat)	Economical Non-toxic Reliable sterilization	High temperature and pressure may damage delicate items	Appropriate autoclave packing required to ensure adequate sterilization. Pre-vacuum autoclaves permit emergency 'flashing' of instruments
Ionizing radiation	Very large quantities of objects can be sterilized simultaneously	Concrete chamber 2 m thick required to store isotope and protect handlers; therefore restricted to industrial use	Gamma X-rays produced by cobalt-60 most commonly used method
Filtration	Used to separate particles in solution or emulsion	Not useful for surgical disinfection and sterilization	Used most frequently in food industry and in biological research

2.3   Physical methods of sterilization.

with wet heat, as moisture catalyses the chemical re-actions of denaturation.

Provided that the volume of the sterilizing chamber remains the same, increasing the pressure of steam results in an increase in temperature, using the same principles as a domestic pressure cooker. The steam subsequently heats and kills microbes by the process of condensation. The steam penetrates porous surfaces and heat energy is imparted to the condensation surface as the steam condenses back to water, releasing the latent heat.

As well as being very economical and non-toxic, steam is the most reliable form of sterilization: if an item of equipment can be sterilized using steam sterilization, this is the method that should be used. Some delicate items of medical equipment such as endoscopic instruments are not suitable for steam sterilization, as irreparable damage may occur if they are exposed to either the pressures or temperatures involved in the autoclave process.

Steam sterilizers are usually referred to as autoclaves. The term **autoclave** means self-closing, which refers to the fact that during the process the chamber door is prevented from opening due to the high pressure inside the chamber. An autoclave consists of a thin outer chamber and a large inner chamber where items are placed to be sterilized. They work by replacing air within the sterilization chamber with steam.

Gravity-displacement autoclaves: Gravity- or downward-displacement autoclaves work on the principle that steam is lighter than air. Steam enters the top of the inner sterilizing chamber from the narrow outer chamber and displaces the heavier air downwards. One of the major problems with this type of autoclave is that air can become trapped within hollow objects, preventing exposure of an object's entire surface area to the steam, with the potential for inadequate sterilization. Air trapping reduces the effectiveness of sterilization, as the steam must displace this air to enable condensation to occur on all surfaces. The air is released via a thermostatic valve at the bottom of the chamber and discharged to the environment. Steam continues to be introduced under pressure and as more air is removed and the pressure continues to rise, the temperature also continues to increase.

The safe minimum standards for time and temperature for a gravity-displacement autoclave are 13 minutes at 120°C (250°F).

Pre-vacuum sterilization: Pre-vacuum sterilizers (Figure 2.4) are now most commonplace in veterinary practice and work by actively removing air from the sterilizing chamber prior to the introduction of steam. By creating a vacuum in the inner chamber, when the steam is introduced it penetrates the entire chamber very quickly and more effectively than in a gravity-displacement system. The time taken for the air to be displaced is eliminated and there are fewer problems with air bubbles being trapped within the chamber. These devices permit emergency flashing of surgical equipment, whereby an unwrapped non-sterile item is placed in a perforated metal container and subjected to the sterilization process. The tray is then carried directly to the operating theatre.

The safe minimum standards for time and temperature for a pre-vacuum sterilizer are 3 minutes at 131°C (270°F).

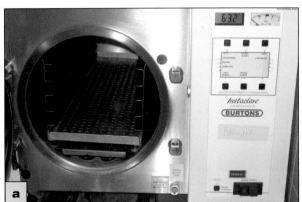
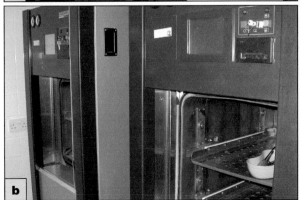

2.4   Pre-vacuum autoclaves. **(a)** A medium-sized tabletop unit. **(b)** Larger autoclaves are required for hospitals with a high surgical caseload.

Dry heat

With dry heat, energy is absorbed directly and micro-organisms are killed primarily by oxidation. This process occurs much more slowly than with moist heat and is becoming less frequently used in the clinical setting. It may be used for fine delicate instruments, particularly those with a sharp edge (e.g. ophthalmic instruments), since the edge may be dulled by steam. No packaging is required for dry heat sterilization.

The proper time and temperature for dry heat sterilization is 160°C (320°F) for 2 hours or 170°C (340°F) for 1 hour. Instruments must be allowed to cool before use.

Ionizing radiation

Sterilization of items by means of ionizing radiation is restricted to commercial use, due to the expense associated with such a facility and the safety measures that must be adhered to with radioactive materials. This form of sterilization is not dependent on humidity, temperature, vacuum or pressure. The only variables are source strength and exposure time.

Gamma irradiation: Ionizing radiation is distinguished from lower-energy radiation, such as infrared, in that the radiation has enough energy to displace electrons within atoms. Within microbial cells, this results in cellular dysfunction and death of the microorganism. Probably the most common application is the use of gamma radiation, with cobalt-60 as one of the most common sources. Gamma rays are very penetrating and thus the irradiation chamber is constructed of reinforced concrete 2 metres thick for the safety of the operators and for storage of the radioactive isotope. Due to the penetration of gamma rays, very large quantities of items can be sterilized at the same time and multiple packaging layers can be used with consistently good results. A perspex dosimeter is used to measure the received dose.

Many items are commonly sterilized using this method, including suture material, cannulas, sterile dressings and non-metallic implants. If re-sterilization of these items is required, the manufacturer's recommendations should be checked before any alternative sterilization process is used as this may affect the integrity of the item.

Sterile filtration

Liquids, particularly foodstuffs such as milk and other dairy products that may be damaged by other methods, can be sterilized by a mechanical filtration technique that is also frequently used in biological research, where it may be necessary to remove particles and microorganisms from solutions and emulsions. A filter pore size of 0.2 μm will remove bacteria, but a pore size of around 20 nm would be required to remove viruses. The filtration equipment is purchased as a pre-sterilized disposable unit. Filters that attach to a syringe are available and may be used clinically prior to injection of compounds such as methylene blue.

Chemical sterilization

Chemical sterilization may use liquid or gaseous sterilizing agents (Figure 2.5). Gaseous chemical sterilants are generally used to sterilize items that are sensitive to heat and/or moisture, such as endoscopes, plastics, cameras and power or light cables. Some liquid chemical agents are capable of sterilization, and soaking instruments in such a solution is termed cold sterilization (see below). The same agents used for shorter time periods more commonly form part of a disinfection protocol, as there is an exponential relationship between the number of organisms killed and the time taken to kill them.

- Solutions capable of sterilization are termed high-level disinfectants.
- Intermediate and low-level disinfectants should only be used where the level of risk is deemed as low (e.g. for cleaning floors and work surfaces).

Method	Advantages	Disadvantages	Other comments
Ethylene oxide	Diffuses rapidly and penetrates most packaged items easily. Effective sterilizing agent at room temperature. Useful for delicate items such as cameras and endoscopes	Toxic and highly inflammable. Time-consuming. Sterilized items must be aerated prior to use	Mechanical aeration decreases aeration time. Micro-dose method is used in a practice setting
Hydrogen peroxide	No toxic byproducts	Not suitable for linen, gauze swabs or paper	Radio waves are transmitted through hydrogen peroxide vapour to produce gas plasma
Quaternary ammonium compounds (QACs)	Modern halogenated tertiary amines are non-toxic, biodegradable and effective sterilants within 30 minutes	Standard QACs are corrosive, inactivated by organic debris and ineffective against *Pseudomonas* species	Effective due to a variety of mechanisms and also have added corrosion inhibitors
Glutaraldehyde	Non-corrosive to metals, rubbers and plastics	Irritating to skin and mucous membranes	Glycolated solutions are stable for long periods
Formaldehyde	Formaldehyde 'bombs' may be used periodically to disinfect theatres or kennel buildings	Extremely irritating to skin and mucosal membranes	Not commonly used
Ortho-phthalaldehyde (OPA)	Effective against glutaraldehyde-resistant spores. Decreased contact time. Not irritating to skin or eyes	Expensive. Will stain proteins (including skin) grey	Similar to glutaraldehyde but used in lower concentrations with fewer toxic side effects

2.5   Chemical methods of sterilization.

Ethylene oxide

Ethylene oxide (EtO) is used to sterilize objects that are sensitive to temperatures >60°C, such as optics, electrical items and plastics.

Ethylene oxide is a colourless gas that kills microorganisms by the process of alkylation. Alkylating agents contain molecules with highly reactive alkyl groups that readily combine with other molecules. In the context of sterilization these alkyl groups act on hydroxyl, carboxyl and amino groups, altering microbial RNA and DNA. Essential metabolic reactions are blocked and protein synthesis is altered, which subsequently leads to death of the microorganism.

EtO is mixed with carbon dioxide or fluorocarbons, as it is flammable and explosive at concentrations >3%. It diffuses rapidly, is an effective sterilizing agent at room temperature and enters the gaseous phase at 10.5°C. It penetrates most packaged items easily, but some plastics (e.g. nylon and polyester) are impermeable to ethylene oxide.

Historically, ethylene oxide sterilization was carried out by the 'gas chamber' method. This entailed flooding a large chamber with a combination of EtO and other diluent gases, such as carbon dioxide or CFCs. Due to environmental concerns and the logistical and safety issues inherent with the use of large quantities of ethylene oxide, the **micro-dose** method was developed. In this method gas is released within a specially designed bag, requiring much smaller doses of gas (Figure 2.6).

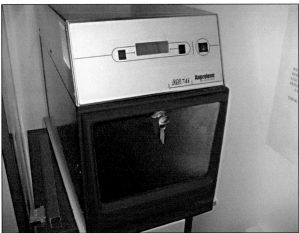

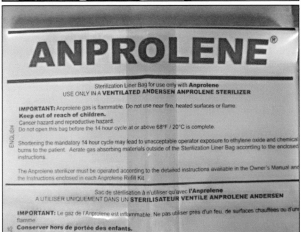

2.6 Micro-dose ethylene oxide sterilization machines use small doses of gas and are much safer to use than the earlier machines, where the entire sterilization chamber was flooded with EtO. A sterilizer liner bag is used.

As with other forms of sterilization, all items to be sterilized should be surgically cleaned and then left to air dry. Hot air should not be used to dry equipment as this may further desiccate bacterial spores, making them more resistant to the gas. Additionally, any water left on the instruments may react with the ethylene oxide, decreasing the efficiency of the sterilization process.

Sterilization time: The time required to achieve sterilization with ethylene oxide is dependent on temperature, gas concentration, humidity and the type of material being sterilized (Figure 2.7).

Temperature
■ The optimum temperature range is from 49°C to 60°C (120–140°F).
■ Most items are sterilized at 55°C for approximately 3 hours, with more heat-sensitive equipment sterilized at 38°C for 5–6 hours.
■ Sterilization at room temperature takes approximately 12 hours.
■ As a rough guide, increasing the temperature by 10°C doubles the effectiveness of ethylene oxide, thus halving the required exposure time.

Gas concentration
■ Ethylene oxide is effective in concentrations between 200 and 800 mg/l.
■ Most sterilizers use concentrations of approximately 600 mg/l.
■ Doubling the concentration decreases the exposure time required by half.

Humidity level
■ Moisture is essential for the effective germicidal activity of ethylene oxide; and rehydration of vegetative bacteria and desiccated spores is essential for effective sterilization.
■ Optimal humidity is approximately 40%.
■ It is extremely important that all water is removed from articles to be sterilized, as ethylene oxide will dissolve in the free water, lowering the local concentration of the ethylene oxide and decreasing its effectiveness.
■ Any organic debris left behind after inadequate cleaning may react with the gas to form toxic residues.
■ If an item cannot be disassembled and cleaned, it is not suitable for sterilization by ethylene oxide.

Type of material being sterilized
■ The manufacturer's guidelines for ethylene oxide exposure times should be strictly adhered to. For example, it is more difficult for the gas to penetrate an item with a long narrow lumen and thus many systems have the facility to increase the length of the cycle when sterilizing such equipment.
■ Items with a lumen longer than 1 metre usually require a cycle length of approximately twice the standard time.

2.7 Ethylene oxide sterilization: variables affecting sterilization time.

Gas elution:

> **WARNING**
>
> The biggest drawback to the use of ethylene oxide is the fact that the gas is extremely irritating to eyes and respiratory mucosa, and can cause serious pulmonary oedema. It may also cause depression of the central nervous system and there is some concern that it may be carcinogenic.

It is vital, therefore, that following sterilization with ethylene oxide sufficient elution time is allowed for all residual ethylene gas to diffuse from the sterilized items. The aeration may be achieved by allowing a minimum time to elapse at room temperature or may be aided by means of mechanical aeration, which employs a high vacuum and elevated temperatures to speed up the process of removing all traces of ethylene oxide from the sterilized items. The gas elution time varies depending on the material being sterilized. Metals, glass and certain plastics resist deep penetration of gas and thus have shorter aeration times. Rubber and some other plastics bind the gas more tightly and thus require more lengthy aeration times.

WARNING

Ethylene oxide should not be used to sterilize any object previously sterilized by irradiation, particularly those made from PVC, because this may result in the formation of highly toxic ethylene chlorhydrin, which is difficult to elute.

Hydrogen peroxide gas plasma

Hydrogen peroxide (H_2O_2) sterilization kills microorganisms by means of the generation of free radicals and ultraviolet (UV) photons, which react with cellular components essential for microbial metabolism.

PRACTICAL TIPS

- Hydrogen peroxide can be used to sterilize most items but is not suitable for linen, gauze swabs or paper. Instruments must therefore be wrapped in non-woven (non-cellulose) polypropylene fabric or special plastic pouches.
- Special adapters called H_2O_2 boosters are required for use with items with a lumen to ensure that the sterilant gains access to these areas.
- Items with a very long narrow lumen and those closed at one end are unsuitable for sterilization by this method.

Following initial cleaning, items are placed in a specially designed chamber from which the air is then evacuated by means of a vacuum pump. Sterilization proceeds as follows:

1. Aqueous hydrogen peroxide is introduced into the chamber and subsequently vaporized.
2. A vapour concentration of 6 mg/ml is maintained for approximately 50 minutes; this is called the **diffusion phase**.
3. Gas plasma is subsequently produced by transmitting radio waves through the chamber; this is known as the **gas phase**. The energy generates an electric field, which further excites the gas molecules to produce a fourth state of matter, distinguished from solid, liquid and gas, known as plasma. The ions and molecules in the plasma collide to produce free radicals, which damage microbial DNA. This state is held for a specified length of time, usually approximately 20 minutes, until all microorganisms have been killed.

The major advantage of plasma sterilization is that there are no toxic byproducts. Although hydrogen peroxide itself is an irritant, there is no direct human contact during the entire process. The liquid used initially

is sealed in a cassette and at the end of the procedure all vapour is removed via a filter that breaks down any excess hydrogen peroxide into water and oxygen. Similarly, hydrogen peroxide is continually depleted during the process as the components of the plasma recombine to form water and oxygen.

Cold sterilization

The complexity and fragility of some items of surgical equipment, namely endoscopic and arthroscopic equipment (Figure 2.8), preclude the use of heat sterilization. Ethylene oxide is a viable alternative but is not routinely available in the practice setting.

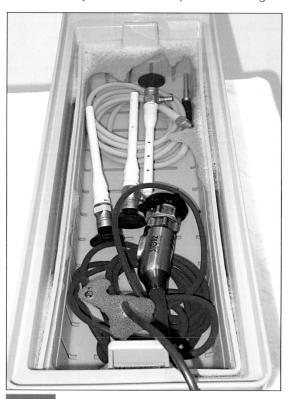

2.8 Cold sterilization of arthroscopic equipment.

The ideal chemical for cold sterilization should have high efficacy and rapid activity, have good material compatibility and be non-toxic. Unfortunately the ideal high-level disinfectant does not exist, as all products have some limitations. Oxidizing agents such as peracetic acid and chlorine-based agents have better 'cidal' activity than alkylating agents, but are more likely to corrode instruments. Alkylating agents such as glutaraldehyde and formaldehyde are generally not as effective a biocide as the oxidizing agents but have better material compatibility.

In modern surgical practice the most commonly used cold sterilants are a mix of various compounds that act synergistically to overcome the shortfalls of the more traditional chemical sterilants. Over time the minimum effective concentration (MEC) will be affected due to dilution and contamination, and thus either the solution must be changed regularly, or the MEC must be checked regularly to ensure effectiveness. The MEC can be monitored easily; the most common method is by the use of specific indicator strips that are dipped into the sterilant solution. The strips usually indicate a positive or negative result, the lack of a specific colour change indicating that the concentration of the solution has decreased below the MEC. Some glutaraldehyde solutions actually change colour themselves to indicate that the concentration has decreased below the MEC.

> **WARNING**
>
> The majority of chemicals used in cold sterilization are irritating to skin and mucous membranes. Any equipment sterilized by this method should be lavaged with sterile water prior to contact with the patient to ensure removal of all chemical residues.

Quaternary ammonium compounds: Although commonly used products such as MedDis™ (MediChem) contain powerful quaternary compounds such as didecyl dimethyl ammonium chloride, they also contain various other chemicals that are not inactivated by organic debris and are highly effective against *Pseudomonas* species (the major drawbacks of standard QACs, as described above under Disinfectants). These modern halogenated tertiary amines are nontoxic and safe to use as well as being biodegradable. They are effective due to a variety of mechanisms that cause cell wall destruction and damage to microbial DNA and also have added corrosion inhibitors. These compounds can achieve sterilization within 30 minutes, which is of obvious benefit in a busy practice environment.

Glutaraldehyde: This saturated dialdehyde has a wide acceptance as an effective high-level disinfectant and chemical sterilant. The biocidal activity of glutaraldehyde is due to alkylation of nucleic acids and proteins. Glutaraldehyde has good 'cidal' activity and is non-corrosive to metals, rubbers and plastics. Immersion for 10 hours at room temperature provides effective sterilization, whereas high-level disinfection is achieved at the same temperature within 10 minutes. Glycolated solutions are stable for longer periods.

> **WARNING**
>
> The main disadvantage of glutaraldehyde is that it is irritating to skin and mucous membranes; it is therefore imperative that exposure is kept to a minimum and relevant health and safety protocols are strictly observed.

Formaldehyde: Formalin is a 37% solution of formaldehyde in water. It is extremely irritating to skin and mucosal membranes and thus has limited application as a cold sterilizing agent. It may, however, be used as a vapour to disinfect or sterilize very bulky or inaccessible items of equipment. Formaldehyde 'bombs' may be used periodically to disinfect theatres or kennel buildings or to kill potentially dangerous pathogens prior to essential maintenance work.

Ortho-phthalaldehyde: OPA is a new alkylating agent that has increased 'cidal' activity against mycobacteria and is also effective against glutaraldehyde-resistant spores. Additional advantages include decreased contact time and increased stability, and it does not irritate skin or eyes. Disadvantages are that it is expensive and stains proteins (including skin) grey.

Peracetic acid: This oxidizing agent is more commonly used in large automated sterilization processors in human hospitals. It acts by oxidizing sulphur bonds in proteins, leading to disruption of cell wall permeability and protein denaturation.

Sterilization indicators

Failure of sterilization may occur for a variety of reasons, such as inadequate cleaning of instruments, inappropriate wrapping material or improper loading of the sterilization chamber. Although human error can only be controlled by appropriate training and supervision of personnel, sterilization indicators are used to ensure that appropriate sterilization conditions have been met and that mechanical failure has not occurred.

It is important to understand that complete microbial cell death does not occur instantaneously once certain conditions are met, as there is vast variability in the ability of microorganisms to survive hostile environments. The process of sterilization is also largely dependent on the length of time for which the appropriate conditions are maintained and therefore the fact that certain conditions have been achieved does not ensure that sterilization has occurred.

> **PRACTICAL TIP**
>
> An effective quality assurance programme relies on the use of multiple monitoring methods to ensure that the highest standards of surgical sterility are maintained. Records should be kept for each sterilization load as an audit and to help to identify the source of a problem should sterilization failure occur.

Sterilization indicators are classified as either chemical indicators or biological indicators, both of which should be used in conjunction with a routine sterilizer maintenance programme and physical monitoring with temperature, pressure and humidity probes.

Chemical indicators

Chemical indicators (CIs) are defined as sterilization process monitoring devices designed to respond with a physical or chemical change to one or more of the physical conditions within the sterilization chamber. They are used to detect sterilization failures that may arise due to improper loading of the chamber, incorrect packaging, deficiencies of the sterilizing agent or malfunction of the sterilizer itself. The indicators are usually either paper strips impregnated with a chemical or glass vials containing a liquid, which undergo a colour change when a certain predetermined variable, or set of variables, has been reached (Figure 2.9).

The Association for the Advancement of Medical Instrumentation (AAMI) has defined five classes of chemical indicators, as defined in Figure 2.10.

Chemical indicators are available for the majority of sterilization processes and are useful in that they provide a visible indication that the particular item has been subjected to the sterilization process, but this does not in any way reflect the duration of exposure. Indicators have been designed specifically to react to a variety of physical conditions such as temperature,

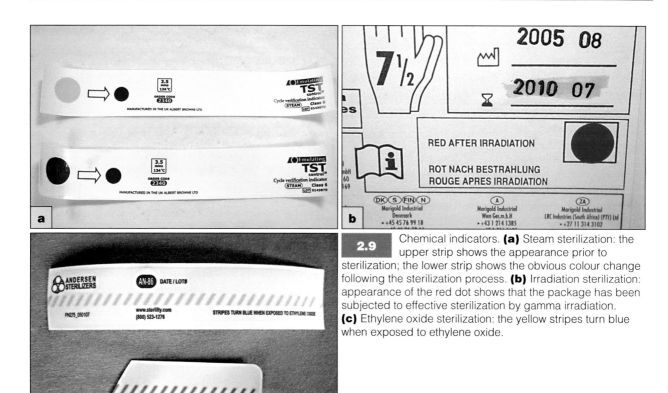

2.9 Chemical indicators. **(a)** Steam sterilization: the upper strip shows the appearance prior to sterilization; the lower strip shows the obvious colour change following the sterilization process. **(b)** Irradiation sterilization: appearance of the red dot shows that the package has been subjected to effective sterilization by gamma irradiation. **(c)** Ethylene oxide sterilization: the yellow stripes turn blue when exposed to ethylene oxide.

Class	Type	Description
1	Process indicators	Most basic of chemical indicators (e.g. autoclave tape and other indicators found on sterilization pouches), used with individual items to be sterilized and distinguish between processed and non-processed items
2	Specific test indicators	For use in specific test procedures (e.g. Bowie–Dick tape and Dart products used in autoclaves, which test for presence of air within the chamber)
3	Single parameter indicators	React to one of the critical parameters of the sterilization cycle (e.g. particular temperature or pressure)
4	Multi-parameter indicators	React to two or more critical parameters of the sterilization cycle (e.g. time and temperature for steam; or time and concentration for ethylene oxide)
5	Integrating indicators	React to all critical parameters required for sterilization to occur and may be used in place of biological indicators in many applications

2.10 AAMI classification of chemical indicators.

humidity and irradiation, as well as to concentrations of the various gaseous sterilants.

- A class 1 indicator is usually placed on the outside of the pack to show that the pack has been exposed to a sterilization process.
- A class 3, 4 or 5 indicator is placed inside the pack in a region that is deemed to be least accessible to the sterilant, which may not necessarily be in the centre of the pack. Ideally, indicators are placed in the centre of each packaged item but it is acceptable to place a single strip in the centre of a test pack located in the centre of the sterilization chamber.

WARNING

It should be remembered that a positive indicator test does NOT ensure sterility of a surgical item, merely that the condition that the indicator was designed to measure has been met.

Biological indicators

Biological indicators are in the form of extremely resistant organisms contained in a glass vial or within a paper strip, which are subjected to the sterilization process. The vials or strips are recovered and incubated for 24–48 hours. The presence of bacteria may be indicated by a variety of methods, often a colour change brought about by a change in pH due to bacterial metabolism. Other more sophisticated methods include indicating the presence of fluorescence given off by a particular microbial enzyme that is highly resistant to the particular sterilization method being used. If bacterial growth is documented, sterilization has been unsuccessful. Different organisms are used for different protocols, but the bacteria must be non-pathogenic, spore-forming and many times more resistant to the sterilization than the most likely naturally occurring contaminants (Figure 2.11).

The major disadvantage of biological indicators is that results are not immediately available, due to the time taken to perform the bacteriological cultures. They

Sterilization process	Biological indicator
Steam	Spore of *Geobacillus stearothermophillus* [a]
Ethylene oxide	Spore of *Bacillus atrophaeus* [b]
H_2O_2 gas plasma	Spore of *Bacillus subtilis* var. *niger*
Gamma irradiation	Spore of *Bacillus pumilus*

2.11 Biological indicators used for common sterilization protocols. [a] Reclassified from *Bacillus stearothermophillus;* [b] reclassified from *Bacillus subtilis* var. *globigii.*

are used periodically, ideally at least once a week, as part of an overall regime to ensure that high standards of sterility and asepsis are maintained at all times. A positive culture should instigate an immediate investigation as to why the sterilization process has failed.

Preparation and handling of surgical packs

A sound understanding of all steps involved in the sterilization process is essential. Failure of sterilization may be as a result of inadequate cleaning of instruments, poor packaging of surgical packs, poor loading of the sterilization chamber, or an inappropriate choice of sterilization technique.

Regardless of the process employed, meticulous preparation of surgical packs is mandatory to enhance the efficacy of the sterilization procedure.

Cleaning

Instruments should be cleaned *as soon as possible after they have been used*, as dried blood and debris are difficult to remove. Any linen or cotton drapes should be laundered and dried prior to packaging.

PRACTICAL TIPS

- Immediately following surgery, instruments should be rinsed with cold water to prevent coagulation of the plasma proteins, which makes removal of blood more difficult. If this is not possible and the blood has already become adherent, soaking in a warm water bath with an effective detergent makes subsequent cleaning much easier.
- It is absolutely essential that all complex instruments are disassembled for cleaning and processing, and all items are allowed to dry completely before being packaged and loaded into the sterilization chamber.
- Immediately prior to steam sterilization, items with a lumen should be flushed with a small amount of water as the water is vaporized during the process, forcing air out of the lumen.
- Conversely, when gas sterilization is used, any moisture left within the lumen may decrease the effectiveness of the gas.

Pack wrapping

Before loading instruments into the sterilization chamber, most are packaged together according to their intended use. Various surgical packs are made available containing the most frequently used instruments

for particular surgical procedures, such as ovariohysterectomy or stabilization of the cruciate-deficient stifle.

Wrapping materials

An appropriate wrapping material (Figure 2.12) must be used that, first and foremost, is a barrier to microbes in order to prevent contamination of the items within the pack. Additionally, for the sterilization process to be effective, the material must be sufficiently permeable to allow the sterilant to reach the contents within and must not react with the sterilization agent, which would potentially compromise the process. The ideal packaging material should also be easy to handle, durable and non-linting (Figure 2.13).

Sterilization method	Suitable wrapping materials
Steam	Cotton muslin; paper; polypropylene fabric; paper/Mylar
Ethylene oxide	Cotton muslin; paper; polypropylene fabric; polyethylene; paper/Mylar; Tyvek/Mylar
H_2O_2 gas plasma	Tyvek/Mylar; polypropylene

2.12 Packaging materials suitable for various sterilization protocols.

Wrapping material	Advantages	Disadvantages
Cotton muslin	Can be reused; easily handled	Requires double wrapping; not waterproof
Paper	Inexpensive	Requires double wrapping; not waterproof
Polypropylene fabric	Very durable; damage-resistant	Single use; requires double wrapping
Paper/Mylar and Tyvek/Mylar	Water-resistant; single wrap; long shelf life	Instruments may puncture pouch

2.13 Advantages and disadvantages of various packaging materials.

Cotton muslin and paper: Cotton muslin drapes and paper are still used most commonly, due to their ability to withstand the high temperatures of steam sterilization. They are inexpensive and can also be used with ethylene oxide, but are not recommended for use with plasma gas sterilization techniques as this causes damage to the cellulose within these materials, potentially affecting performance.

Plastic pouches: Newer materials such as Tyvek, which is a brand of flash-spun high-density polyethylene fibres, offer advantages such as being more resistant to microbial penetration, transparent so that the items inside may be viewed directly, extremely strong and repellent to liquid water and yet still permeable to gas sterilants. Many of these new plastic pouches incorporate one side of permeable material with the other side comprising a non-permeable material such as PVC or polyester (Figure 2.14). These plastic pouches are commonly used for individual items or small collections of instruments, whereas paper and cotton drapes are still preferred for large surgical packs and trays containing large numbers of surgical instruments such as may be used in a complex procedure (e.g. total hip replacement).

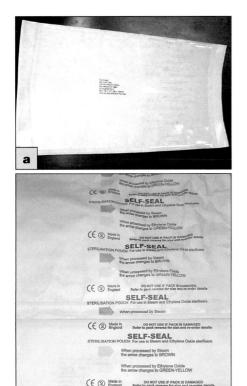

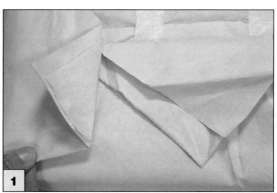

2.14	**(a)** Plastic pouch used for sterilization of small items of equipment. These pouches are sealed by means of an adhesive strip once the item to be sterilized has been placed inside. **(b)** Chemical indicator incorporated into the packing of a plastic pouch.

Safe storage times

The choice of wrapping material influences the degree of protection provided to the sterile content of the package, with woven materials such as cotton drapes providing a less effective barrier to moisture and particulate matter than the modern non-woven material now available. The term non-woven refers to any textile produced by unconventional methods and includes all engineered fabrics not classified as knitted or woven. Figure 2.15 provides a rough guideline to the safe storage times of surgical packs wrapped in various materials.

Packaging material	Shelf life
Single-wrapped cotton muslin (2 layers)	1 week
Double-wrapped cotton muslin (4 layers)	6 weeks
Single-wrapped cotton muslin over single layer crepe paper (3 layers)	8 weeks
Double-wrapped muslin tape-sealed in waterproof dust covers	12 weeks
Double-wrapped muslin heat-sealed in waterproof dust covers	8 months
Double-wrapped non-woven material (e.g. polypropylene)	9 months
Heat-sealed plastic pouches (e.g. Tyvek)	>12 months

2.15	Safe storage times for sterilized surgical items.

Wrapping technique

Items should be wrapped in such a way that they can be unwrapped easily without any break in sterile technique. Packaging materials are folded with small flaps folded outwards, so that these can be easily grasped during unwrapping of the package without contamination of the inner layer. The package is then taped closed with autoclave tape and is ready for sterilization (Figure 2.16). Likewise, surgical gowns should be packaged so that they may be donned without any compromise to sterility.

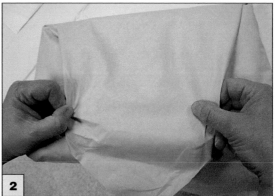

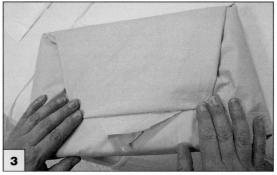

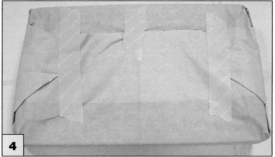

2.16	Surgical packs should be wrapped with each corner folded away from the centre of the pack.

Small flaps should be incorporated into the wrap so that they can be grasped and the packaging removed without contaminating the inner layer. Once folded, the pack is sealed with autoclave tape.

Excessive handling increases the risk of perforation of the wrapping material, particularly if a surgical instrument has sharp or pointed edges. To decrease the risk of perforation, equipment with sharp points or edges should have these sharp surfaces wrapped in a swab or protected with small plastic covers prior to sterilization (Figure 2.17). Any covers must be compatible with the sterilization process being used. Special metal boxes are available for use with orthopaedic pins and wires, which as well as preventing damage to the packaging also facilitate the efficient storage of multiple pins and wires of different sizes.

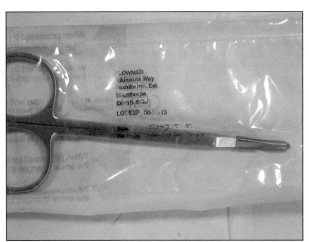

2.17 A small plastic protective covering has been placed over the tips of these sharp-pointed scissors. The covering must be compatible with the sterilization process being used.

Loading the chamber

Several specific guidelines should be considered with regard to loading the sterilization chamber:

- All hinged instruments should be sterilized with their box lock fully open
- Complex items must be disassembled
- The chamber should not be overloaded, as this prevents adequate circulation of steam or gas; packs should be separated by 3–5 cm and away from surrounding walls
- Instruments within each pack should ideally be separated by at least 3 mm.

Consideration should be given to the sterilization method. For example, surgical bowls should be placed horizontally or with the open end up to ensure appropriate steam penetration when using a gravity displacement autoclave, as steam is pushed from the top to the bottom of the chamber. This is of less importance with vacuum-assisted machines.

PRACTICAL TIP

Linen packs containing drapes, towels and gowns are very compact and difficult to sterilize and should not be stacked within the sterilization chamber. These bulky items may result in inadequate penetration of the sterilant to all areas of the autoclave and they should not be sterilized along with surgical instruments.

Preparation for storage

Following steam sterilization, all contents of the autoclave are slightly damp due to condensation of steam during the sterilization process.

This can be a particular problem when small bench-top autoclaves designed to sterilize small loads of surgical instruments are overloaded with absorbent items such as cloth gowns and drapes. In addition, these items are often placed inside autoclave pouches, which become heat-sealed before all of the moisture evaporates from these absorbent items. Large porous-load autoclaves are still relatively uncommon in general practice.

PRACTICAL TIPS

- All instruments and surgical packs should be allowed to cool and dry before being stored away for later use.
- Ensuring that the items are dry is critical with regard to maintaining sterility; moisture also increases the incidence of corrosion of instruments (see Chapter 3).
- Packs that have been wrapped in cotton drapes can then be placed in a sterile plastic pouch, which is subsequently heat-sealed. This waterproof post-sterilization wrap greatly increases the shelf life of the surgical pack.
- Small packs containing only a few smaller items can be wrapped and sterilized in plastic pouches and subsequently stored directly.

Storage

The concept of the loss of sterilization being related to a particular event rather than a defined length of time is referred to as **event-related expiration**. This suggests that if a pack is packaged and processed correctly, it remains sterile unless it gets wet or is damaged.

The safest method with regard to preserving sterility is to ensure that strict protocols are adhered to with regard to package handling and storage.

WARNING

If there is any concern that an item may have been damaged or handled inappropriately, or if there is any evidence that the environment has been 'contaminated', the item should be considered non-sterile.

PRACTICAL TIPS

- Ideally all packages should be stored in closed cabinets (Figure 2.18), rather than on open shelves.
- The shelves should be clean and dry, in an area of low humidity and away from any turbulent airflow.
- Items should be dated with either the date of sterilization or a proposed date of expiration.
- They should be stored in a logical manner and clearly labelled to avoid repeat handing of packages when a particular item needs to be located.

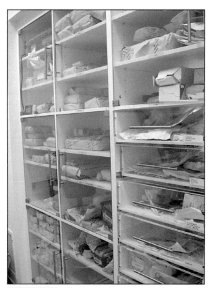

2.18 Sterile items should be stored in closed cabinets, which are labelled so that items can be found easily when required.

Transfer to the surgical team

The physical delivery of a sterile item from its packaging to the surgical team is of critical importance with regard to maintaining strict aseptic technique. Contamination of an item at this stage is of no less consequence than if sterility were lost at an earlier stage in the process.

Generally speaking, items are transferred to the sterile operating team in one of two ways. Items that are not cumbersome and can be easily held are opened by a member of the surgical theatre staff and offered to the surgical team whilst being held within the outer packaging. The item within is then grasped by a sterile member of the operating team (Figure 2.19). For larger items, the easiest method of transfer is to place the item in the centre of a separate table and remove the packaging with the item still on the table. The item is then collected and taken directly from the table by a member of the operating team.

If an item is double wrapped: either the outer layer only is removed and the item is taken still wrapped in the first layer of sterile packaging; or both layers are removed and the item is taken devoid of all packaging. Removal of only one layer of packaging prevents

contamination of the sterile item, but there is an increased risk that the inner layer may become contaminated by dust and debris from the outside of the outer layer. There are no significant differences in the incidence of contamination with either method as long as good technique is employed as the packaging is being removed.

PRACTICAL TIPS

The most important points to remember when unwrapping and transferring sterile packages are as follows:

- As the packaging is being removed, the edges should be folded away from the centre of the package one side at a time.
- Each fold that is unfolded should be secured so that it does not recoil and contaminate the item (Figure 2.20).
- Arms should never be held over the sterile package as the packaging is being removed.

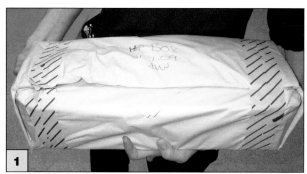

1

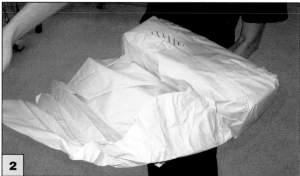

2

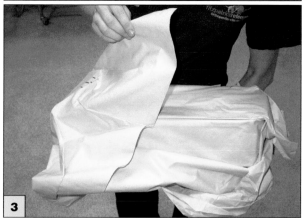

3

2.20 Unwrapping a sterile item. The outer packaging is unwrapped one corner at a time and the free ends collected and held with the non-free hand. The package is then offered whilst being held within the wrapping. (continues) ▶

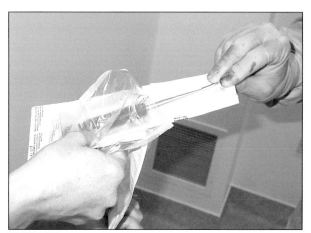

2.19 Transferring a small sterile item. The item is passed to the surgeon whilst being held in the outer packaging. This transfer should not be performed over the sterile field.

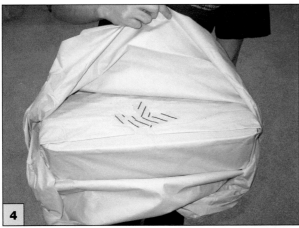

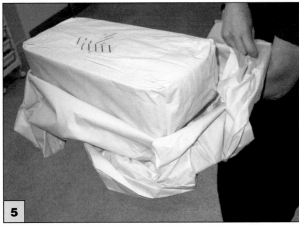

2.20 (continued) Unwrapping a sterile item. The outer packaging is unwrapped one corner at a time and the free ends collected and held with the non-free hand. The package is then offered whilst being held within the wrapping.

If an instrument has been sterilized in a plastic pouch, it is important that it does not come into contact with the outer packaging as it is transferred to the operating team. The edges should be pulled back sufficiently to ensure that the surgeon does not contaminate their gloves on the packaging when grasping the instrument.

WARNINGS

- Regardless of which wrapping has been used, items should never be dropped directly on to the sterile surgical table. This could result in a break in sterility due to perforation or damage to the table drapes, or from the direct shedding of dust and debris from the outer surface of the packaging or from hands.
- In addition, dropping may damage fragile instruments and may also result in the production of air currents that could carry environmental contaminants toward the sterile field.

References and further reading

Lemarie RJ and Hosgood G (1995) Antiseptics and disinfectants in small animal practice. *Compendium on Continuing Education for the Practicing Veterinarian* **17**, 1339–1349

Mitchell SL and Berg J (2003) Sterilization. In: *Textbook of Small Animal Surgery, 3rd edn*, ed. DH Slatter, pp. 155–162. WB Saunders, Philadelphia

Rutala WA (1996) APIC guidelines for selection and use of disinfectants. *American Journal of Infection Control* **24**, 313–342

Seim HB III (2002) Principles of surgical asepsis, sterilisation and disinfection. In: *Small Animal Surgery, 2nd edn*, ed. TW Fossum, pp. 1–10. Mosby, St. Louis

Spaulding EH (1939) Studies on chemical sterilization of surgical instruments. *Surgery, Gynaecology & Obstetrics* **69**, 738–744

Steelman V (1992) Ethylene oxide: the importance of aeration. *AORN Journal* **55**, 773–787

Surgical instruments – materials, manufacture and care

John Lapish

Introduction

Instruments have been designed and manufactured specifically for surgery since at least 3000 BC when Sumerians (in present-day Iraq) created small copper knives as surgical scalpels. Relatively sophisticated instruments, including bone-holding forceps, were found in the ruins of Pompeii (Vesuvius eruption AD 79). The requirement for special materials in instrument manufacture was recognized by the Roman surgeon philosopher Galen, who specified that his instruments should be made exclusively from iron ore found only in a quarry in the Celtic kingdom of Noricum (present-day Austria). The production of today's specialized surgical instruments relies on a long history of manufacturing skills and sophisticated metallurgy.

Materials

The manufacture of an instrument begins with the selection of the correct material. The majority of surgical instruments are manufactured from stainless steel and a smaller number use non-ferric materials such as titanium and alloys of copper.

Stainless steel

Stainless steels are a group of steel alloys, over 200 in number, all of which have the property of high corrosion resistance brought about by the inclusion of chromium in the alloy mix. The term stainless steel is, however, something of an oxymoron in that all types of stainless steel will stain and corrode in certain conditions. It is important to remember that even the most corrosion-resistant stainless steels contain at least 50% iron and the grades of stainless steel used in the manufacture of surgical instruments contain at least 80% iron. Preventing the iron from rusting is a challenge.

The iron within the steel is protected from oxidizing (rusting) by an envelope of chromium oxide that develops on the surface of stainless steel. In a high oxygen environment the layer of chromium oxide is passive, tenacious, self-renewing and self-repairing. Should the layer become scratched or cut, the newly exposed steel will form another protective film. The layer is very thin, approximately 300 Angstroms (an illustration of

just how thin this is in relation to an instrument is a layer of tissue paper on the top of the Empire State Building). The chromium oxide forms a physical barrier over the ferric elements. In less than optimum conditions, such as in the presence of chloride ions as a consequence of poor cleaning, the chromium oxide is no longer self-renewing or self-repairing; this leads to exposure of the ferric elements, which oxidize, creating staining and rust.

During the manufacturing process the layer is encouraged to grow by use of appropriate heat treatment and passivation in nitric acid. Within the veterinary environment certain activities have an influence on instrument corrosion (Figure 3.1).

Factors that encourage corrosion (i.e. removal of chromium oxide layer)
■ Moist environment. ■ Reducing agents, including chlorine solutions resulting from biological residues (standing instruments in a saline solution is a standard test for corrosion resistance). ■ Mixing of metals (e.g. carbon steel blades) during cleaning.

Factors that discourage corrosion (i.e. encourage build-up of chromium oxide layer)
■ Time (old instruments are less likely to rust than new ones). ■ Oxidizing agents. ■ Dry storage.

3.1 Factors affecting corrosion.

The addition of different elements significantly changes the properties of the resulting steel. Different alloys are used for instruments that have different functions. For example:

■ Hollow-ware such as bowls and kidney dishes must be made from a ductile alloy, as they are pressed from a thin sheet. They do not require great strength
■ Scissors are required to take and hold an edge and are therefore produced from a different steel from forceps, which do not need an edge but must be springy without breaking.

The level of carbon within the stainless steel is critical. High levels of carbon allow the steel to be heat-treated to a level of hardness that will allow a surface to be ground to a sharp edge. This degree of hardness unfortunately results in a relatively brittle product that is prone to fracture. Stainless steels containing high levels of carbon are also more prone to corrosion than lower-carbon steels. Thus, scissors are more likely to corrode and break than are dissecting forceps and bowls. Figure 3.2 illustrates how changing the composition of the steel affects its usefulness for instrument manufacture.

In some situations there is a requirement for even harder materials, such as certain pin cutters and needle-holder tips. Where a hardness of >70 HRC (see Figure 3.2 for explanation of HRC) is required, an insert of tungsten carbide, which has a hardness of 80 HRC, is usually added. Although tungsten carbide is very hard, it is also very brittle and requires the support of the surrounding steel to protect it from bending and breaking. This has implications for how it must be used, as will be seen later.

Manufacture of surgical instruments

The manufacture of a surgical hand instrument such as a pair of scissors involves over 30 different quality-controlled processes. As an example, the production of a pair of 16.5 cm Straight Mayo Scissors with tungsten carbide inserts is described here in detail.

Each half of the scissors begins as a sheet of AISI 420 stainless steel. A relatively crude outline is cut out of the sheet to create the blank (Figure 3.3). At this stage the steel is far from stainless, as surface impurities from the rolling process have stained it badly. The blank is heated to between 800 and 1100°C and pressed into a die having the shape of the scissor, using a hammer forge. Some excess steel is squeezed out around the edge, which is removed to leave the stamping. Further heating and stamping of the metal brings impurities to the surface, which will be removed at a later stage. At this point the stamping is relatively soft and may be worked on using hard metal tools.

The area that will become the joint is created using a spinning metal cutter known as a miller. The joint is then drilled for the screw. It is hardened and tempered at this stage by vacuum heat treatment. The scissor is brought to 1040°C and carefully cooled to give the metal a hardness of between 50 and 58 HRC. This process increases the instrument's resistance to corrosion. The ferric elements become more tightly bound up in the metal than in the soft unhardened state.

Early tungsten carbide scissors required that a sliver of tungsten carbide be soldered into position along the edge of the scissor. Most tungsten carbide scissors today have the tungsten carbide welded directly along the edge for greater support and security (Figure 3.4). At this stage the metal is too hard to be worked on using metal tools. Subsequent operations require the use of carbide wheels (Figure 3.5) and/or carbide abrasive belts. The excess tungsten carbide is ground back and the two halves are now ready for assembly.

Grade of stainless steel (AISI)	Chromium (%)	Carbon (%)	Nickel (%)	Rockwell C hardness	Qualities	Uses
316LVM	17.5	<0.025	13.5		Highly corrosion resistant	Orthopaedic implants
304	17–19	0.07	8–11		Ductile, corrosion resistant	Hollow-ware
410	11.5–113.5	0.09–0.15	1.0	40–42	Can be hardened	General instruments (e.g. forceps)
420	12–14	0.16–0.25	1.0	42–58	Can be hardened to take and keep an edge	Scissors
420X	13	0.39	0.2	58–60	Can be hardened to cut stainless implants	Pin and wire cutters

3.2 Qualities and uses of different grades of steel. AISI = American Iron and Steel Institute. The Rockwell C hardness (HRC) scale is a comparison of hardness of materials (tested by forcing a diamond into the surface of the material, under a specified load, and measuring the indentation produced); the higher the number, the harder the material.

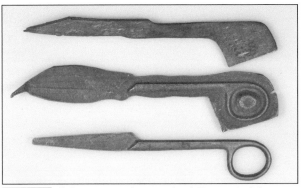

3.3 Scissors manufacture. (top) Raw material stainless steel AISI 420. (middle) After initial forging. (bottom) The forged blank.

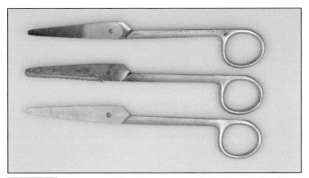

3.4 Scissors with a tungsten carbide insert. (top) After machining. (middle) After welding in the tungsten carbide. (bottom) After grinding back the tungsten carbide insert.

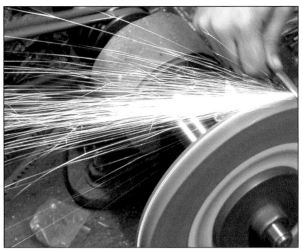

3.5 Grinding back the tungsten carbide on the scissor blade, using an abrasive wheel.

Once assembled, the instrument resembles the final scissors but there are still a number of important process that it must undergo before it will function properly. The scissors are 'set' so that the two blades come together at the edge along the full length of the blade (Figure 3.6). The set involves giving the blades just the correct amount of spring to keep the blades together as they shear. This part of the process is critical and is usually performed by a specialist senior craftsman known as a scissor putter-togetherer.

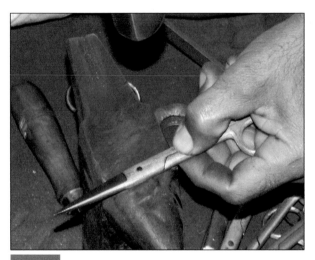

3.6 Setting the scissors.

As the scissors move toward the final stages, they are subjected to the polishing process. Polishing stainless steel involves rubbing the metal with finer and finer abrasives. Use of the finest abrasive powder creates a mirror finish (Figure 3.7). If a matt finish is required, the steel surface is blasted by small glass beads under high-pressure air to roughen the surface, reducing reflection and glare. Matt finishes have implications for corrosion and instrument care (see below). To indicate that the blades have tungsten carbide edges, the handles are electroplated with gold.

If the instrument is a pair of supercut scissors with much slimmer blades than standard tungsten carbide scissors, the edge of one blade is very finely serrated. A grooved steel wheel is used to add microserrations

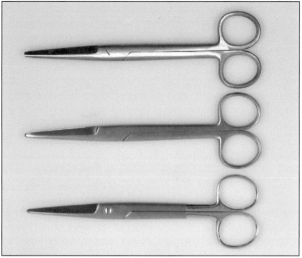

3.7 Polishing stage. (top) Scissors after assembly and setting. (middle) After blade sharpening and polishing. (bottom) After gold plating of the scissor rings 'bows'.

to the supercut blade (Figure 3.8). Without these fine serrations the tissues being cut tend to slide away from the shearing action.

Microscopically, the edges of even sharp stainless steel scissors are quite rough, enabling them to grip the tissues as they cut. Various scissor cutting edges are shown in Figure 3.9.

Passivation involves soaking the instrument in a solution of nitric acid to remove surface ferric elements that might cause staining.

The finished scissors are subjected to rigorous inspection and testing prior to marking and packing.

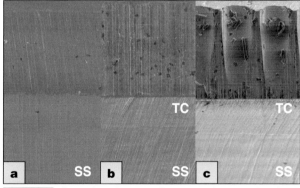

3.8 Adding microserrations to a supercut blade using a grooved steel wheel.

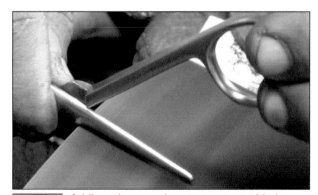

3.9 Scanning electron microscope images showing different blade types. **(a)** Standard cut stainless steel. **(b)** Standard cut tungsten carbide. **(c)** Supercut tungsten carbide. SS= Stainless steel; TC=Tungsten carbide.

Matt *versus* mirror finish

Stainless steel instruments are typically available in either a highly reflective mirror finish or in a dull matt finish (Figure 3.10). The matt finish is created by roughening the surface of the metal using pressurized glass beads or scouring brushes. The roughened surface scatters the light that lands on it, rather than reflecting it back to the surgeon. Matt-finish instruments are becoming increasingly common, partly through surgeon choice and partly because of cost. The mirror finish is largely a hand process and therefore expensive.

From a metallurgical perspective, the best stainless steel finish to minimize corrosion is one as smooth as possible. Any surface cavitation increases the surface of alloy exposed to corrosive conditions. In addition, the surface cavitation of matt finishes greatly increases water retention. Whereas water typically runs off a mirror finish, it tends to be retained by a matt finish and the retained moisture is the most common cause of corrosion (Figure 3.11).

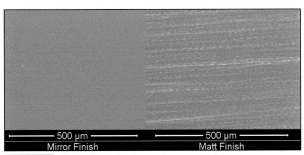

| 500 µm | 500 µm |
| Mirror Finish | Matt Finish |

3.10 Scanning electron microscope images contrasting mirror finish (left) with matt (brushed) finish (right).

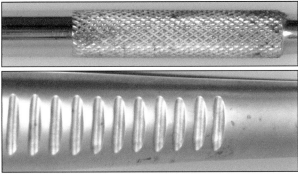

3.11 Corrosion due to retained moisture on matt-finish instruments. There are stained corroded areas on the matt knurled area of the scaler and the matt finish of the cutters, especially the grooved grip area. Water accumulates and is retained in these areas.

Instrument care

The failure to clean, lubricate and dry instruments adequately is the greatest cause of instrument failure. These problems are best avoided by the implementation of an effective instrument care protocol. Surgical instruments represent a significant investment and it is therefore important to consider investing in equipment to care for them. The protocol in Figure 3.12 will maintain instruments in good condition and extend their life. Longer times and repeated passes through certain stages, especially ultrasonic cleaning, will be required to bring neglected instruments up to the 'gold' standard.

1. Rinse soiled instruments in warm water and detergent. Removal of contaminants at this stage will extend the life of more expensive cleaning agents used later. Dismantle instruments to their constituent parts at this stage. Use soft nylon brushes to remove adherent materials. Some orthopaedic instruments such as burs and saw blades may require more aggressive cleaning with either soft brass or stainless steel wire brushes designed for the purpose. Do not use DIY wire brushes or wire wool, which will damage the instrument surface.

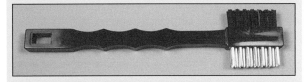

2. Rinse in tap water.
3. Submerge the instruments with joints open, or in a disassembled state, in an enzyme solution for 20 minutes. Pay particular attention to cannulated or tubular instruments to ensure that the cleaning solution enters areas inaccessible to brushes.
4. Rinse in tap water.
5. Submerge the instruments in an ultrasonic cleaning bath filled with a proprietary cleaning agent. Do not use domestic dishwashing agents, which are too alkaline. The ultrasonic action penetrates areas that cannot be accessed by brushes. Run the cleaner for 10 minutes at 50°C. If instruments have a build-up of baked-on debris, this stage may be repeated several times.
6. Rinse thoroughly in distilled water.
7. Immerse jointed instruments in a solution of instrument milk (an emulsion of instrument oil in water). The emulsion penetrates the joints. When the instrument is autoclaved the water is evaporated, leaving a film of oil inside the joints. An alternative to this stage is to dry and lubricate the joints directly, using instrument oil.
8. Wipe off excess instrument oil.
9. Examine for damage, faults and function.
10. Dry for storage, or pack for autoclaving (see Chapter 2).
11. Carefully follow the autoclave manufacturer's instructions to ensure that at the end of the cycle the instrument packs or boxes are dry. If they are not, they must be left in a warm dry place to dry out before storage.

3.12 Standard protocol for care of instruments.

The regime in Figure 3.12 is designed for routine instrument care in a large clinic or hospital. If space or resources are limited, doing nothing is not an option. The principles of keeping instruments clean, lubricated and dry will eliminate 99% of problems.

PRACTICAL TIP

In addition to the standard protocol, certain precautions should be observed:

- Separate instruments of different metals (e.g. remove carbon steel blades before cleaning)
- Place sharp edges so that they do not contact each other
- Protect cutting edges with silicone caps (see Figure 3.13).

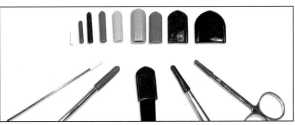

3.13 Protection of sharp and delicate tips using silicone caps.

Marking instruments

Most instruments are marked with the supplier's name and coding. This mark is made using either a laser marker or chemical etcher. Both processes require passivation after marking.

It is sometimes desirable to mark instruments as belonging to a particular clinic or to allocate an instrument to a certain kit within the clinic. Permanent marking of instruments with the clinic name without causing significant damage to the instrument is difficult. Vibro-etching is not recommended, as it scratches the surface through the protective chromium oxide layer and provides a starting point for fatigue cracks. Once stainless steel is damaged, the time to fatigue failure is significantly shortened.

The semi-permanent marking of instruments to show which kit they belong to is much easier and safer. Autoclave-tolerant tape of different colours is available (Figure 3.14a). It should be noted that the tape is designed to stick to stainless steel rather than to itself and so it is necessary to minimize any overlap. An alternative for single-piece instruments, such as scalers and elevators, is the use of coloured elastic silicone rings (Figure 3.14b).

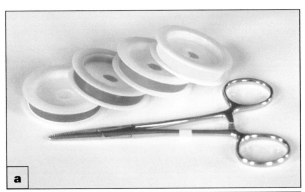

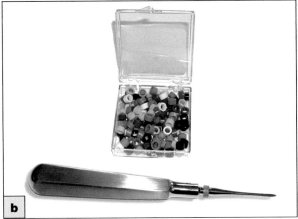

3.14 Instrument marking systems: **(a)** coloured autoclave-resistant tape; **(b)** silicone rings.

Problem identification and management

During surgery the surgeon should draw attention to any instrument that is not performing well, so that it can be put on one side for further examination. Once cleaned, dried and lubricated, all instruments should be periodically checked for wear and faults. Particular attention should be paid to dissecting

instruments (scissors, dissecting forceps and needle-holders) as problems with these items can be particularly frustrating.

- **Scissors** in good condition will 'feel right' (a skill worth acquiring). The action should be smooth and the blades should be in contact along the full cutting length. Scissors with any roughness of action, or bluntness, should be sent for repair. The cut may be tested on a plastic carrier bag: it is not an exact substitute for living tissues but there are similarities. The scissor should cut along the full length of the blade but should be especially efficient at the tip. Sharpening surgical scissors is not straightforward; it requires great skill and should not be attempted without appropriate training.
- **Needle-holders** are required to grasp needles firmly and pick up the finest of suture materials. Even needle-holders with tungsten carbide inserts wear. They can be examined by holding them up to the light: the tips should meet, excluding all light. Where the tips do not meet, through either wear or misuse, the needle-holder must be discarded or repaired.
- **Artery forceps** should be checked for alignment of jaws and interlock of teeth. Misaligned jaws may be gently brought back into position. Mosquito forceps should be capable of holding fine tissue on the first ratchet.
- **Dissecting forceps** usually have teeth, though some are very fine. Where present, the teeth should interlock.

Some of the more common instrument problems are illustrated in Figures 3.15 to 3.19.

Good quality surgical instruments are designed and manufactured to last a lifetime with normal use. Adherence to the principles of keeping instruments clean, lubricated and dry, and avoiding inappropriate use will ensure that they do.

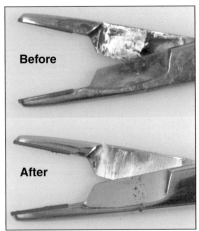

3.15 Before and after removal of biological residues from the joint of a pair of Olsen-Hegars. Most of the visible discoloration here is not rust but baked-on residues. These will contain chloride molecules which, in solution, act as reducing agents, stripping the protective chromium oxide layer and exposing ferric elements to corrosion. In the 'after' photograph the residues have been removed by repeated cycles through an ultrasonic bath. The newly cleaned surface reveals pits of corrosion.

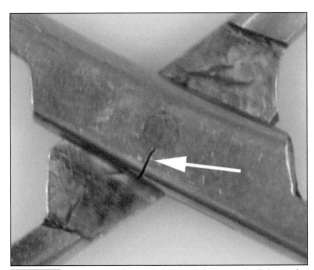

3.16 Cracking of a joint (arrowed) due to build-up of biological residues in a pair of Allis tissue forceps. A build-up of residues with resulting corrosion in the joints of instruments creates increased friction, which makes the instrument difficult to use and leads ultimately to cracking and failure. Once cracked, the instrument is beyond repair.

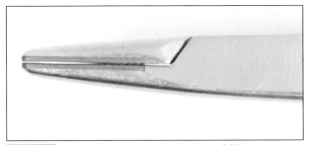

3.17 Areas of wear towards the tips of Olsen-Hegar tungsten carbide needle-holders.

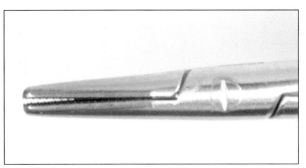

3.18 Castroviejo needle-holders damaged by inappropriate use with a large needle.

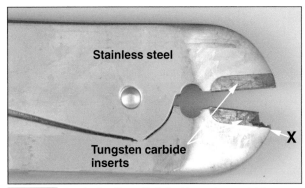

3.19 Implant cutter with failed tungsten carbide inserts (arrowed). Tungsten carbide, while being very hard, is also very brittle and relies on the surrounding stainless steel for support. If the support from the stainless steel is insufficient, the stainless support will deform and the tungsten carbide insert will break. At the tips of implant cutters the stainless steel support tapers down for improved access. This makes the tungsten carbide vulnerable (X). It is important to avoid cutting at the very tip, especially when using on materials outside the specification of the instrument. Stainless steel implants have a high tensile strength and are difficult to cut.

Surgical instruments – types and use

Nicholas J. Bacon

Introduction

In most veterinary practices an extraordinarily broad range of surgical procedures are performed and it may not be immediately obvious which instruments are needed to perform a procedure effectively and with as little trauma as possible. Veterinary surgeons, regardless of skill or experience, are all guilty, at some time or other, of knowingly using the wrong instrument for the wrong purpose. This is because of speed, laziness, indifference or emergency. There should be no strong ergodynamic or tissue-oriented reasons to misuse instruments, as they have often been designed, re-designed and improved, sometimes over generations, to fit comfortably in the hand and address one surgical technique or tissue type. Although many instruments may appear to be multipurpose, they are not as versatile as some believe, or try to make them.

Intentional misuse is likely far outweighed by surgeons *unknowingly* using the wrong instrument for the wrong purpose, such as tissue forceps to hold the skin, artery forceps to secure drapes, needle-holders to twist orthopaedic wire, or Metzenbaum or Mayo scissors to cut suture material. It is this aspect that this chapter hopes to reduce, not only by describing the types of instruments that are widely available, but also by providing many examples of appropriate use.

Manufacture, repair and maintenance of instruments are described in Chapter 3; correct use of instruments is covered in Chapter 21. Further information on orthopaedic instruments is available in the *BSAVA Manual of Small Animal Fracture Repair and Management* and the *BSAVA Manual of Canine and Feline Musculoskeletal Disorders*. Dental instruments are covered in the *BSAVA Manual of Canine and Feline Dentistry*. Instrument catalogues are often well illustrated and informative.

Scalpels

Scalpels consist of a scalpel handle and a scalpel blade.

Handles

Various scalpel handles are available, of which the most commonly used in small animal surgery is the

Bard Parker No. 3 (Figure 4.1). The handle is flat with various grooved patterns etched into the sides to increase handling security. Some have centimetre markers down one side, useful for measuring, for example, skin margins prior to tumour removal. The ends of some handles taper to a point and can be used during surgery as a crude periosteal elevator. It is wise to remove the blade before use in this manner.

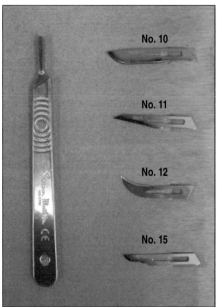

4.1 Bard Parker No. 3 scalpel handle with a selection of blades. (Courtesy of T Hutchinson)

No. 10
No. 11
No. 12
No. 15

Attaching a scalpel blade to a handle is best performed by firmly grasping the blade with the cutting edge away from the operator and pushing the central ridge of the handle into the central blade socket from below until the angled end of the blade snugs firmly into place in the handle. This can be done by holding the blade, carefully, between the finger and thumb of the dominant hand or using a dedicated pair of forceps. Needle-holders and artery forceps should not be used as they are not designed for this purpose and may become damaged.

To remove the blade, the angled end of the blade is gently lifted above the level of the handle ridge. The handle is then pulled backwards off the blade, rather than pushing the blade away from the body.

The Bard Parker No. 7 handle is long and slender, but has the attachment for the same blades as the No. 3 handle. The Swann Morton Beaver type handle has a different form of attachment and a different range of very fine blades, particularly suited to intricate work, especially ophthalmic surgery.

Blades

The scalpel blades most commonly used in small animal surgery (all of which attach to a No. 3 handle) are numbers 10, 11, 12 and 15.

- **No. 10**: These all-purpose scalpel blades for general surgery have a large convex cutting edge and are used for most linear skin incisions, cutting the thick linea alba, taking incisional biopsy samples from masses, and sharp cutting of intestines, vessels and nerves.
- **No. 11**: These sharply pointed blades are used for making stab incisions into a hollow viscus (e.g. stomach, bladder), arthrotomies, or when an accurate delicate incision is required (e.g. urethrotomy).
- **No. 12**: These large concave hooked blades are primarily used for suture removal. This is more easily achieved and safer if the blade is attached to a scalpel handle. Swann Morton also make dedicated disposable suture-removing blades, which are longer and cannot be attached to a handle.
- **No. 15**: A blade with a much smaller convex cutting edge than No. 10, the No. 15 is useful for small skin incisions, or for general surgery in small patients (Figure 4.2). It also has many similar uses to the No.11, in particular stab incisions into hollow viscera.

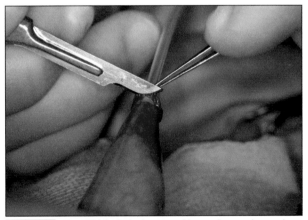

4.2   No. 15 blade being used to excise prolapsed urethral mucosa.

Scissors

Scissors are used for either blunt dissecting or sharp cutting. More expensive pairs of scissors come with tungsten carbide inserts to improve instrument life and cutting consistency. The inserts must be replaced when blunt, as sharpening is not possible.

Scissors are more traumatic than a scalpel, because tissue is cut by the shearing action generated as the blades close rather than the sharp incision of the scalpel. The tips of scissors vary according to use: sharp/sharp, sharp/blunt and blunt/blunt

configurations are all available. There is also a range of scissors with the blade sharpened to a tapered edge, which reduces the crushing action.

Different scissors are required for different functions (Figure 4.3).

- The heavy **Mayo** scissors are ideal for cutting thick connective tissue, fascia, the linea alba, muscle, skin and fibrous tissue.
- The finer, lighter and typically longer **Metzenbaum** scissors are used when accurate precise dissection is needed through loose delicate tissue. Examples include dissection of subcutaneous tissues, and within the abdomen, neck or chest.

Both types come with straight or curved blades. The curved blades improve visibility and control, as the tips are more easily visible in the field of dissection. Straight blades provide a greater mechanical advantage when cutting tough fibrous tissue.

- **Ophthalmic** scissors (e.g. iris or tenotomy scissors) (Figure 4.4) have two sharp tips and are usually straight. Some surgeons also use these for perineal urethrostomy surgery in cats, and other general surgery procedures where fine precise cuts are needed.
- **Suture** scissors should be a dedicated instrument in an operating pack, to prevent tissue scissors being misused and blunted by cutting suture materials. They can be recognized by a blunt-ended top blade, which minimizes the risk of inadvertently cutting tissues deep to the suture material. This risk is further reduced by only using the tips of the scissors to cut suture material, and by never cutting suture material unless the whole blade and tips can be seen by the surgeon.

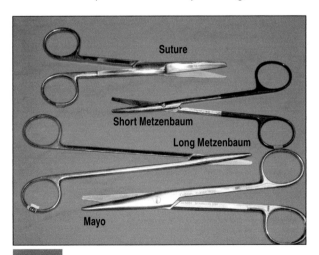

4.3   Scissors.

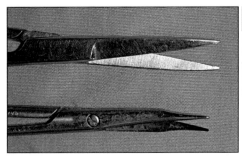

4.4

Iris (top) and tenotomy (bottom) scissors.

Needle-holders

Various sizes and styles of needle-holder are available, depending on the size of needle being used and the body cavity, location or tissue requiring suturing (Figure 4.5). The **Mayo-Hegar** needle-holder is of medium size and is the most commonly used in general surgery, whereas longer needle-holders can be used for suturing in deep body cavities. The tips of needle-holders are blunt-ended and short, as they are never required to grasp anything more than a few millimetres in diameter. Compared with artery forceps, the tips are smoother and cross-hatched rather than grooved.

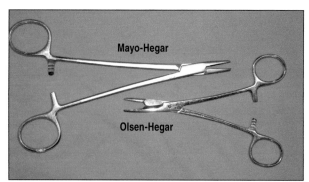

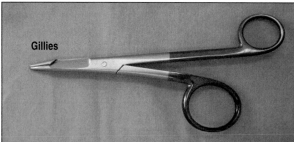

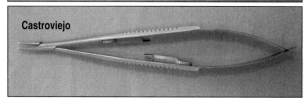

4.5 Needle-holders. (Middle and bottom: courtesy of T Hutchinson)

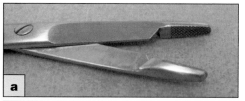

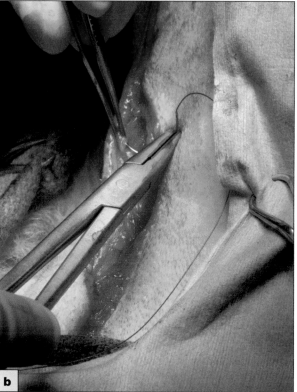

4.6 **(a)** Needle-holder tips, showing scissor section and tungsten carbide inserts. (Courtesy of T Hutchinson) **(b)** The tungsten carbide inserts on the Mayo-Hegar needle-holders improve grip on the needle.

The needle-holder is held in the dominant hand with the thumb and ring-finger. When in use the ratchet is typically engaged to stabilize the needle, especially when passing it through dense tissue.

Needle-holders are designed with robust jaws and specially hardened tips (Figure 4.6a). They often have tungsten carbide inserts to improve the grip on the needle and to prolong the life of the instrument (Figure 4.6b). They should only be used for holding needles and suturing, not (for example) to twist wire during orthopaedic procedures.

Some needle-holders, such as **Olsen-Hegars** (Figure 4.5), combine grasping jaws with a scissor just distal to the joint, which allows sutures to be tied and cut with the same instrument (Figure 4.6a). These take some familiarity to use properly and inadvertent cutting of the suture is a common frustration. For this reason they are not recommended while learning to suture, but can increase efficiency of a skilful surgeon operating without an assistant.

Another combined scissor/needle-holder is the **Gillies** (Figure 4.5), distinctive in appearance with asymmetric handles, having a short upper handle, bending upwards and sideways to fit ergonomically in the palm. They have no ratchet and so the handles need to be gripped tightly whilst suturing, potentially making needle placement less accurate and the operator's hand less comfortable when a large amount of suturing is required. The same problem seen with the Olsen-Hegars of cutting the suture material inadvertently also exists with Gillies.

MacPhail needle-holders have a spring ratchet and so by squeezing the handle, the jaws open and release the needle. Tightening the grip on the handles to open the jaws is not immediately intuitive and so these take some time to master. For that reason they are not widely used in general practice.

Shorter needle-holders such as the **Castroviejo** (Figure 4.5) are specialized for fine ophthalmological procedures, such as suturing the conjunctiva or nictitating membrane, which require delicate pencil-grip suturing. These typically do not have a ratchet but instead have a spring and latch mechanism for locking.

Needle-holders should be used to grasp a curved needle towards its mid-point, perpendicular to the needle-holder, and the curved needle passed through tissue with a twist of the wrist to minimize trauma but maximize ease of tissue penetration.

Thumb forceps

Held in a pencil grip, typically in the non-dominant hand, thumb forceps are tweezer-like instruments that are an extension of the thumb and index finger and are used to help to stabilize tissue that is being sutured, cut or clamped (Figure 4.7). The tips of most thumb forceps have interlocking 'rat teeth' to improve the grip on the tissue.

Treves are cheap general purpose rat-tooth forceps commonly used in practice with a single rat tooth on one tip, interdigitating with a pair on the opposing tip. Much less traumatic are the **Adson** forceps, which have finer tips and so can only grasp a tiny fragment of tissue (Figure 4.8). They can be used for suturing fascial tissue, and because of the delicate grip, can also be used to stabilize skin during wound closure. **Brown–Adson** forceps look similar in many respects, but have multiple intermeshing teeth at the

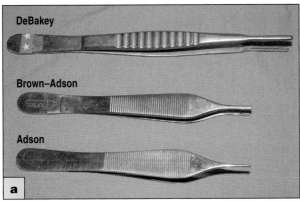

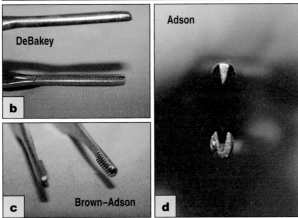

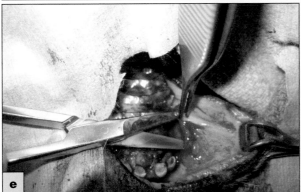

(**a**) Thumb forceps. (**b–d**) Details of tips.
4.7 (**e**) Raising a labial flap to close an oronasal fistula: non-crushing Babcock tissue forceps extend the lip; Adson forceps are used to stabilize the cut edge; and Metzenbaum scissors undermine the mucosa.

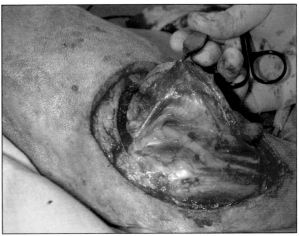

4.8 The single rat-tooth of the Adson tissue forceps maintains a secure grip on the tough fascia beneath a soft tissue sarcoma excision.

tip that provide a broad yet delicate grip without causing major trauma (Figure 4.9). They are often misused to grasp needles during suturing but this will rapidly blunt the teeth, ultimately increasing the amount of tissue damage caused.

The least traumatic thumb forceps are **DeBakeys**. Originally developed for vascular surgery to minimize endothelial damage, they have a role in general, abdominal and thoracic surgery whenever minimally traumatic grasping of tissue is required. They have relatively smooth tips and are ribbed in a longitudinal direction with two rows of tiny transverse striations. They provide very delicate tissue handling and should be used for grasping intestines, bladder, lung, blood vessels, lymph nodes and hepatobiliary structures, when stay sutures (which are even less traumatic) are not employed.

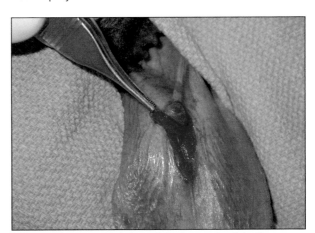

4.9 The multiple interdigitating teeth of the Brown-Adson forceps offer a broad gentle grip during the excision of a sublingual mass.

Haemostatic forceps

Haemostatic forceps tend to be identifiable by the instrument size and the location and direction of serrations on the tips. Common types of forceps with transverse grooves include the **small Halsted mosquito** and the **Spencer Wells, Kelly, Crile** and **Rochester Pean** (Figure 4.10). The transverse groove pattern helps to grasp and secure bleeding vessels through the crushing action of the serrations. For ligation of a

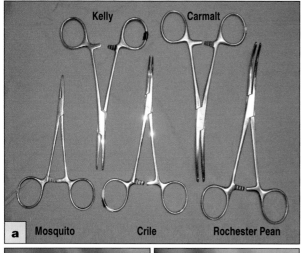

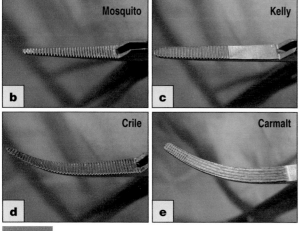

4.10 (a) Haemostatic forceps. (b–e) Details of tips.

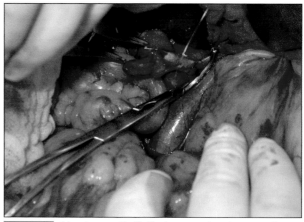

4.11 Non-traumatic Satinsky vascular clamp on the vena cava during removal of an adrenal gland mass with a small phrenicoabdominal vein tumour thrombus.

Tissue forceps

Allis tissue forceps (Figure 4.12) have traumatic grasping jaws that should not be applied to the skin or delicate tissues. Their grip is secure and can be used to grasp fascia or tissue being excised. The number of teeth in the intermeshing jaws varies – three to four is common. They are also commonly used to secure drapes around suction and diathermy lines to keep these in place.

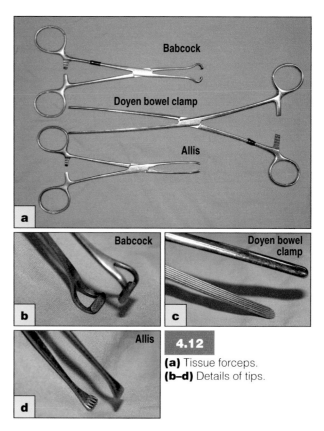

4.12 (a) Tissue forceps. (b–d) Details of tips.

vessel or tissue pedicle, the instrument is placed transversely so that the striations run parallel to the blood flow. The smaller Halsted mosquito forceps are used to clamp isolated bleeding vessels and are most effective when the tips are used. Mosquito, Spencer Wells and Rochester Pean haemostatic forceps offer the surgeon different options to clamp tissues of various thicknesses.

Forceps can either be straight or curved, depending on the desired use. Straight forceps are suitable for dealing with easily visible superficial bleeding vessels. When working with reduced visibility (for example, in a cavity), the use of curved forceps allows the surgeon to see the bleeding vessel more easily and direct the tips of the haemostat to it without the hand obscuring the surgical field.

The larger **Carmalt** forceps have longitudinal grooves over the majority of their tips and are used primarily for ligating stumps and pedicles, for example during ovariohysterectomy. The very end of the tips have transverse grooves for grasping vessels. The longitudinal grooves make for easier removal of the forceps from a pedicle whilst tying a ligature.

Specialized **cardiovascular forceps** (e.g. Satinsky) (Figure 4.11) have large U-shaped tips with minimally traumatic serrations, in a pattern similar to DeBakeys. These can be used to occlude a portion of a vessel if part of the vessel wall needs opening, resecting and/or repairing. A detailed description of cardiovascular instruments can be found in the *BSAVA Manual of Canine and Feline Head, Neck and Thoracic Surgery*.

Babcock tissue forceps (Figures 4.12 and 4.13) have large triangular jaws with fine longitudinal striations on the tips. They are less traumatic than Allis tissue forceps because they lack teeth, but they tend to crush tissue as they have to be applied with more force to prevent slipping. They may be used to grasp and manipulate tissues as an alternative to stay sutures (e.g. stomach, pericardium).

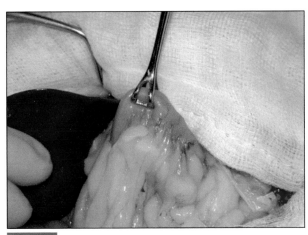

4.13 Babcock tissue forceps on the pylorus of a cat.

Right-angled tissue forceps (e.g. Mixter and Lahey) have blunt or rounded tips and transversely (Mixter) or longitudinally (Lahey) striated jaws. These are used for blunt dissection around the back of tubular structures (e.g. blood vessels and the biliary tract). They are available in a variety of sizes for use in the deeper areas of the abdominal and thoracic cavities.

Non-crushing forceps allow for atraumatic clamping of a hollow viscus (e.g. the intestine). **Doyen** intestinal clamps (Figures 4.12 and 4.14) have thin longitudinal striations along the whole length of the clamp and should be used gently to occlude the open end of the intestine being sutured. Doyens are very useful when performing resection and anastomosis of the bowel, to occlude the bowel lumen and gently manipulate the bowel ends to bring them into apposition before performing a tension-free anastomosis. The two ends of the intestinal section being resected can be clamped with crushing **Carmalt** forceps. Doyens are also useful when operating alone, i.e. when a sterile assistant is not available to occlude the intestines with their fingers to avoid intestinal spillage during simpler enterotomy procedures.

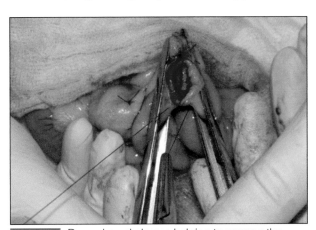

4.14 Doyen bowel clamps helping to appose the jejunum and ascending colon during anastomosis, following an intestinal resection for a large ileocaecocolic mass.

Retractors

Retractors increase visibility, exposure and access to deeper tissues and structures. They increase the accuracy and efficiency of surgery. Better exposure allows for more accurate tissue recognition (reducing

the risk of complications), less traumatic handling of tissues and improved visibility of bleeding points; it places tissue under tension, which makes it easier to cut or dissect and allows more accurate tissue apposition when closing the wound.

Self-retaining retractors

Self-retaining retractors can be divided into those used to hold open body cavities and those that retract soft tissues.

Abdominal

The **Balfour** retractor is the most widely used self-retaining abdominal retractor (Figure 4.15). There are two fenestrated side blades applying lateral distraction on the laparotomy wound and a solid curved spoon to hold open the cranial end of the wound. Removing the falciform fat prior to inserting the spoon is helpful, especially when performing surgery on the stomach or liver. Wound edges can be protected by moistened laparotomy swabs, and any exposed or exteriorized viscera (especially the small intestines) should be covered by gauze and regularly moistened to reduce the risk of tissue desiccation and evaporative heat loss.

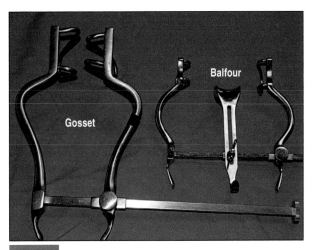

4.15 Abdominal retractors.

The **Gosset** abdominal retractor (Figure 4.15) is similar in appearance and use to the Balfour, but lacks the central spoon and so is prone to twisting, due to the lack of three-point fixation provided by the spoon. Both Gossets and Balfours are available in a variety of sizes that are suitable for cats through to giant-breed dogs.

Thoracic

The **Finochietto** (Figure 4.16) is the most widely used thoracic cavity retractor, used in both intercostal thoracotomies and median sternotomies. It has two sturdy outwardly facing arms, with a heavy toothed ratchet and handle connecting them. Although the ratchet allows for progressive distraction of the surgical site, the increase in tension is less obvious to the surgeon, which may lead to over-distraction that could result in rib fracture in an intercostal approach. The Finochietto or an alternative, the Tuffier retractor, is useful for a midline pubic osteotomy approach to the pelvic canal.

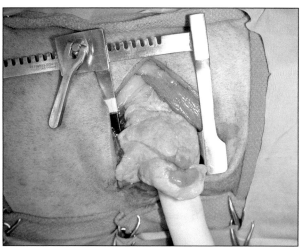

4.16 Finochiettos retracting the ribs during an intercostal thoracotomy in a cat, allowing a solitary lung mass to be fully evaluated.

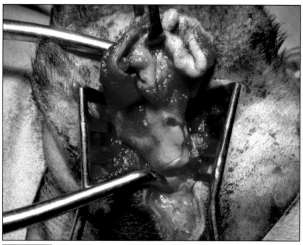

4.18 Weitlaner and Gelpi self-retaining retractors improve exposure during a total ear canal ablation in a cat. The ear canal is being manipulated by Allis tissue forceps.

General purpose

The **Gelpi** retractor (Figures 4.17a and 4.18) is possibly the most widely used self-retaining general purpose retractor, indispensible for head and neck, orthopaedic, perineal and neurosurgery. In cats and small dogs Gelpis can also be used to retract thoracotomy and laparotomy incisions. The retractor is hinged and the tips can be either sharp or round ended; some surgeons file them flat for vertebral distraction in neurosurgical procedures. When using sharp-ended pairs, the surgeon must be cautious to avoid iatrogenic neurovascular damage. Some have ball tops for tips to prevent them from entering the tissues too deeply. Often two pairs of Gelpis are placed in a wound at 90 degrees to each other to achieve maximal exposure. They retain their retraction with either a curved ratchet with a finger-release trigger for rapid adjustment, or a spin-lock version when prolonged periods of retraction without repositioning are required. Mini-Gelpis with a ratchet are also available and have many uses, especially in delicate head and neck surgery in cats.

The tips of the **Weitlaner** or **Wests** self-retaining retractors (Figures 4.17b and 4.18) have three to four outwardly facing curved prongs, which increase contact between the retractor and wound, making them less likely to rotate in the surgical site, and also allow a larger cross-section of tissue to be retracted than a single Gelpi. A retractor of similar size, however, requires a larger wound bed than the Gelpi, which can be inserted into fairly small incisions to aid exposure. Weitlaner and Wests retractors are very similar, but the arms of Wests are angled so that the handles and ratchet part of the instrument sits snugly against the drape, improving access for the surgeon.

Hand-held retractors

Needless to say, hand-held retractors (Figure 4.19) require a scrubbed assistant during surgery. The advantages over self-retaining retractors are that the

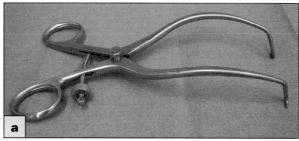

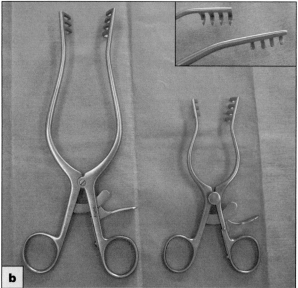

4.17 **(a)** Gelpi self-retaining retractors with spin-lock. **(b)** Weitlaner self-retaining retractors of two different sizes, with sharp and blunt tips (inset). (Courtesy of T Hutchinson)

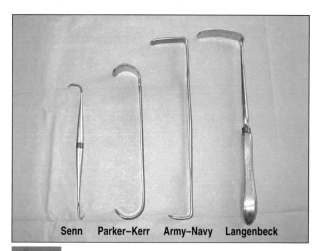

Senn   Parker–Kerr   Army–Navy   Langenbeck

4.19 Hand-held retractors. (Courtesy of V Lipscomb)

tips can be more accurately placed to retract specific tissues; they may be replaced within the wound more readily; and tension applied to different tissues can vary within a single wound.

The **Senn** retractor is double-ended with a smooth blunt right-angled end and a three-pronged 'rake' or 'claw' on the other end. Commonly used for muscle and fascia, the Senn's ends are small and so are useful for retracting small amounts of tissue (e.g. the infrapatellar fat pad, or small muscle bellies during orthopaedic surgery).

The larger **Army–Navy** retractors have longer blunt right-angled ends and can be used to retract large muscle bellies, especially during amputations or large tumour resections.

Malleable retractors are thin flat smooth-edged round-ended blades of metal that can be moulded to any angle to fit their purpose. They are most useful when working deep within the abdomen to gently retract friable tissues such as the liver (Figure 4.20) or gastrointestinal tract, for example during nephrectomy, adrenalectomy or liver lobectomy. It is helpful to protect the organ by placing a moist laparotomy swab between the retractor and the organ.

Hohmann retractors (Figure 4.21) are hourglass shaped with either a blunt or sharp central 'beak' on the end. This tip is used for leverage of the retractor against patient tissues, thus opening the surgical site to increase exposure. One example is inserting a Hohmann over the caudal edge of the proximal tibia

during stifle arthrotomy, to lever the tibia cranially to help inspection of the meniscus. Hohmanns can also be used to lever bone fragments past each other to aid in fracture reduction.

Suction tips

Three types of suction tip are used in general surgery: the Frazier, Yankauer and Poole (Figure 4.22). Suction removes blood and other fluids from the surgical site, increasing visibility, decreasing operative and anaesthesia time, improving haemostasis and decreasing the risk of infection. Suction is provided by wall-mounted or portable suction units.

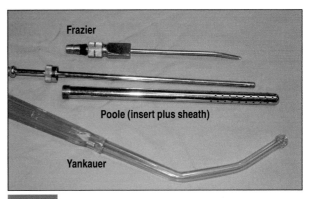

4.22 Suction tips.

The **Frazier** tip is the smallest of the three and has a small hole in the handle that must be occluded by a finger for sufficient suction to be achieved through the tip. Frazier tips are usually an angled tube (metal or plastic) and allow for fine control of suction, but can cause inadvertent trauma if they come into direct contact with tissue. The small diameter of the suction tip means that they are liable to become blocked during surgery. Most come with a stylet that can be inserted into the tip to dislodge any blockage and push it out of the larger handle.

The **Yankauer** suction tip has a wider diameter than the Frazier and so is suitable for dealing with larger fluid volumes, thicker fluid (e.g. salivary mucocele) or when higher rates of suction are needed. It has a rounded tip with multiple holes, meaning that suction can be directed but minimally traumatic and is more suitable for working in the abdomen amongst friable organs. It still only has one hole in the end and so is prone to becoming obstructed by tissue.

The **Poole** suction tip comprises two parts: a narrow diameter cannula with a single hole at the tip; and a longer fenestrated outer sheath into which the cannula slides and is screwed into position. The multiple holes in the outer cover allow large volumes of fluid to be drained from the abdominal cavity with little risk of tissue, such as the omentum, blocking the tip, unless it completely wraps around the outer cover. It is therefore the suction tip of choice when dealing with any type of abdominal effusion, or when performing abdominal lavage. Thoracic lavage can be performed with either a Poole or Yankauer suction tip, but care must be taken not to let the open end of the Yankauer directly touch the lung as this may cause trauma. A swab placed over the distal end of a Yankauer suction tube may allow the tip to behave like a Poole tip.

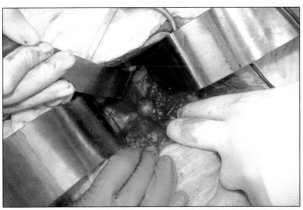

4.20 Three malleable retractors holding back the liver (narrower retractor) and other organs deep within the abdomen during a left-sided adrenalectomy.

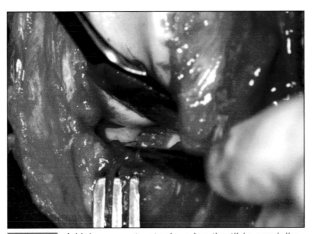

4.21 A Hohmann retractor levering the tibia cranially to allow the medial meniscus to be inspected, as the fat pad is tractioned by a Senn retractor.

Towel clamps

Small pointed towel clamps are used to attach towels and drapes to the patient. The most commonly used types in veterinary medicine are the cross-action towel clamp (Jones) and the Backhaus towel clamp (Figure 4.23). The **cross-action** types have no handle but instead use a sprung design of a single piece of bent metal. The **Backhaus** clamp has a ringed handle with a ratchet, which allows more control over placement and clamp security. The tips penetrate the skin, making a secure sterile boundary immediately surrounding the prepared surgical site. They should not be used to secure electrocautery lines or suction tubing away from the surgical site, as the tips will penetrate the drape and break the sterile field.

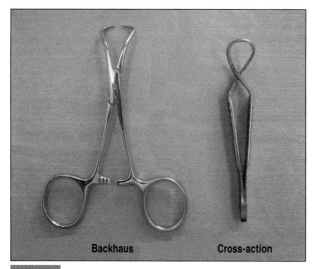

Backhaus   **Cross-action**

4.23   Towel clamps. (Courtesy of T Hutchinson)

Other instruments

Rongeurs

Rongeurs (Figure 4.24) are used for removing bone fragments in a variety of situations and therefore come in a variety of sizes and designs. In soft tissue surgery, they are most frequently used for sinusotomies, rhinotomies, occasionally for mandibular and maxillary tumour resections, and in aural surgery to remove mineralized ear cartilage and for bulla osteotomies. Orthopaedic uses include debriding the ends

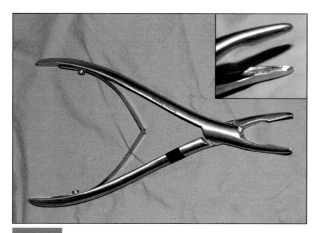

4.24   Rongeurs, with close-up of tip.

of fracture fragments and removing mineralized joint capsules during excision arthroplasties. Rongeurs are used in neurosurgery to assist in removing articular facets, spinous processes and laminae.

They can be single- or double-action instruments, with the double-action giving greater mechanical advantage so that less force is required. The jaws can be in line with the handle, or curved or angled for better visibility. The **Lempert** is commonly used and has tapered jaws with a relatively sharp tip and cutting edge. The **Kerrison** is a different style of rongeur and has two long slender blades. The upper blade has a sharp cutting end and runs along the lower blade to a footplate at the end against which it cuts. The footplate is inserted between the spinal cord and lamina in neurosurgery procedures and the upper blade cuts down on to it to remove small bone fragments.

Curettes

Curettes are typically long straight instruments with a sharply edged oval spoon on one or both ends (Figure 4.25). The spoons are usually of slightly different sizes and are most often used for debridement of soft tissues from within or on bony surfaces. Examples of use in soft tissue surgery include removing the middle ear epithelium from the tympanic bulla during total ear canal ablation and removing turbinates from within the nasal chamber during turbinectomy. Orthopaedic indications include removing cancellous bone from the humerus during a bone graft harvest, removing remnants of the teres ligament during total hip replacement, removing cartilage during arthrodesis surgery, removing periosteum, debriding the lining of bone cysts and removing fibrous tissue from the end of bone fragments when dealing with chronic or non-healing fractures. Neurosurgeons often use curettes to remove the nucleus pulposus during intervertebral disc fenestration. The **Volkmann** is a double-ended curette, and the **Spratt** has a single cup on the end of a stainless steel handle.

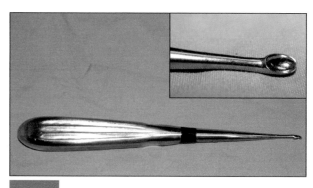

4.25   Spratt curette, with close-up of tip.

Periosteal elevators

Periosteal elevators (Figure 4.26) are designed to reflect muscle from bone by elevating the periosteum (and attached muscle) from the bone. They are used in a pushing fashion against the cortical bone to lift the periosteum, ideally in a single layer (Figure 4.27). They can be wooden handled with a single end, or double-ended such as the **Freer** elevator. Tips may be square or rounded.

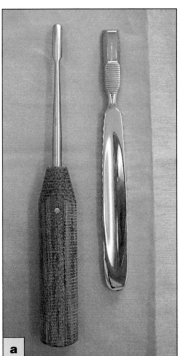

4.26

(a) Periosteal elevators: round-ended and flat-ended. (b) Close-up of tips. (Courtesy of T Hutchinson)

a

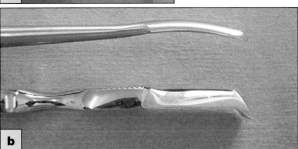

b

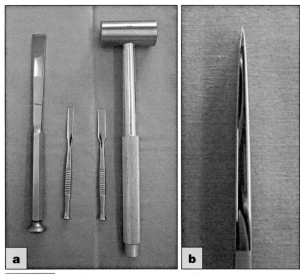

a   b

4.28   (a) Osteotomes of three different sizes and mallet. (b) Close-up of osteotome profile. (Courtesy of T Hutchinson)

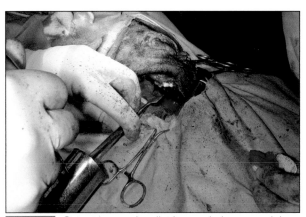

4.29   Osteotome and mallet in use during a caudal maxillectomy/orbitectomy for invasive squamous cell carcinoma in a spaniel.

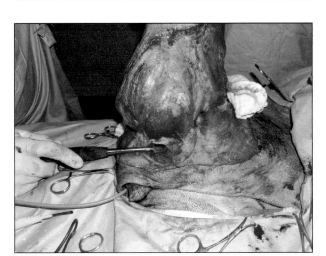

4.27   Broad periosteal elevator removing muscles from the pubic symphysis during a large pelvic resection for neoplasia, prior to pubic symphysiotomy.

Osteotomes and chisels

Osteotomes (Figure 4.28) and chisels are outwardly similar in appearance, except that:

- Osteotomes have a double bevel on the end
- Chisels have a single bevel and are flat on one side.

Both are used for cutting bone and require a mallet (Figure 4.29). The symmetrical cutting end of the osteotome tends to maintain the direction of cut better than the chisel. The double bevel also makes it easier to withdraw from bone. The striking surface on the end of both instruments can be round or rectangular.

Bone-cutting forceps (Figure 4.30) can be single- or compound-action and are used for removing, for example, bony prominences, sharp edges of bone during osteotomies, femoral head and neck excisions in small patients, and vertebral spinous processes during neurosurgery or tumour resections.

Bone can also be cut with **power instruments**, which are invaluable although expensive. Surrounding soft tissues should be carefully protected and any osteotomy should have the soft tissues on the far side

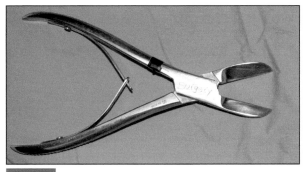

4.30   Bone cutters.

protected by either a swab or metal barrier, such as an Army–Navy, Hohmann, or malleable retractor.

Saws are classified according to the direction of blade movement relative to the drive shaft. **Oscillating** saws use a circular blade which moves in an arc of 5–6 degrees at right angles to the drive shaft. These are most commonly used as cast saws. **Sagittal** saws have the blade working parallel to the drive shaft and have more diverse veterinary surgical uses. The blade only moves by 5–6 degrees but is used to cut bone in most situations, including sternotomies, oral surgery and appendicular osteotomies.

Right- and left-handed instruments

Most instruments, especially scissors, are designed for use with a right-handed grip. The pushing of the thumb and pulling of the fingers creates the shear forces between the blades necessary to generate the cutting force. When used in a left-handed grip, the push of the thumb actually loses shear and torque forces between the blades, making cutting awkward and ineffective. Most instrument companies also manufacture left-handed instruments.

Suggestions for a basic surgical pack

Instruments should be used for their intended purpose only and so there needs to be sufficient diversity in a general pack to minimize misuse. Instruments to include in a basic surgical pack include:

- Backhaus towel clips × 8
- Mosquito artery forceps (straight) × 6
- Mosquito artery forceps (curved) × 6
- Rochester Pean or Kelly forceps (curved) × 6
- Mayo needle-holders × 1
- Adson forceps × 1
- Brown-Adson forceps × 1
- Mayo scissors (straight) × 1
- Metzenbaum scissors (straight) × 1
- Suture scissors × 1
- Allis tissue forceps × 2
- Scalpel handle No. 3 × 1
- Army–Navy retractor × 2
- Mayo bowl × 1
- Bulb syringe × 1 (Figure 4.31)
- 10 × 10 cm surgical swab pack (radiopaque marker) × 1 (10 count)
- Drape × 4 for field draping
- Single patient drape × 1 (for more detail on drapes, see Chapter 16).

Once the pack is opened on the instrument trolley (Figure 4.32), the instruments should be arranged so that the most commonly used can be readily reached by the surgeon or the assistant. Similar instruments should be grouped together (e.g. haemostatic forceps, scissors).

The surgical swabs are counted at the beginning of surgery and each new pack is counted to ensure that the total number on the back table is accurate.

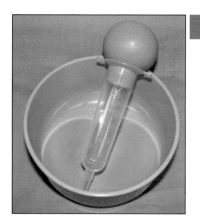

4.31 Mayo bowl and syringe.

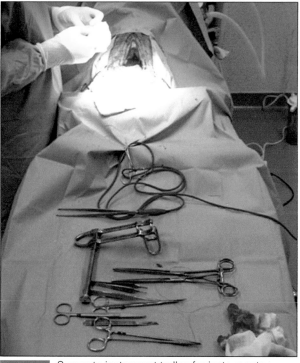

4.32 Separate instrument trolley for instruments contaminated during intestinal resection and anastomosis, to avoid their being placed back amongst sterile instruments.

The swabs are also counted prior to wound closure to ensure that all are accounted for. Radiopaque lines are present in the more expensive swabs and these are typically also 100% woven cotton in an open-mesh gauze. They can be both absorbent and abrasive, though the weave rarely separates and unravels even with aggressive use. Less expensive alternatives include non-woven synthetic fabrics, which can often fragment when wet or abraded and more commonly leave lint particles in the wound, which ultimately might lead to granuloma formation. Cheap synthetic swabs can also be squeezed more tightly, which means that there is an increased risk of leaving them in a wound. Large laparotomy swabs come with firmly attached cotton ties.

In conclusion, putting some thought into selecting an appropriate instrument for a specific task will minimize tissue trauma and maximize efficiency during surgery, which is in keeping with Halstead's principles of surgery.

Suture materials

Stephen J. Baines

Introduction

Suture material is used for a number of purposes during surgery:

- Closure of tissues
- Ligation of blood vessels
- Anchoring of drains and tubes
- Atraumatic tissue manipulation with stay sutures.

There is no ideal suture material for all purposes. If there were, the surgeon would only have to choose the correct size. To make a rational choice of the most appropriate suture material, the surgeon must understand the properties of the material, the intended use of the material and the nature of the wound. The ideal properties of a suture material are given in Figure 5.1.

Interaction with tissue

- Maintenance of adequate tensile strength until purpose served.
- Rapid resorption once it is no longer required (absorbable).
- Encapsulated without postoperative complications (non-absorbable).
- Minimal tissue reaction.
- Should not favour bacterial growth.
- Minimal drag through tissues.
- Suitable for all wounds.

Interaction with surgeon

- Easy to handle.
- Good knot security without fraying.

Material properties

- Easy to sterilize without changing its material properties.
- Non-capillary.
- Non-electrolytic.
- Non-corrosive.
- Non-allergenic.
- Non-carcinogenic.

Practicalities

- Inexpensive.
- Readily available.

5.1 Ideal properties of a suture material.

At the present time, no single material can provide all of the characteristics listed. Under different situations and with differences in tissue composition throughout the body, the requirements for wound closure will require different suture material characteristics. The essential properties are:

- Sterility
- Uniform diameter and size
- Pliability for ease of handling and knot size
- Uniform tensile strength by suture type and size
- Freedom from impurities that might elicit a tissue reaction.

Materials are described individually later in this chapter. Comparative details for the different materials, including classification, composition, manufacture, absorption, loss of strength, tissue interaction, handling, use, advantages and disadvantages, are summarized in the suture material monographs at the end of this chapter.

Suture material production and characteristics

The properties that are generally used to determine the choice of an appropriate suture material under given circumstances are shown in Figure 5.2.

Manufacture
Some natural fibres, such as silk, are harvested, spun into thread and braided to an appropriate size. Other natural fibres, such as catgut, require harvesting, stripping, washing, tanning, twisting and polishing. Synthetic fibres are usually polymerized from liquid resins, which are then extruded into uniform fibres.

Handling
The handling qualities of a suture material are influenced by all the physical characteristics of the material, including pliability, memory, ductility, surface friction and knot security. Silk is considered to be the suture material with the best handling qualities and is often the standard against which the handling qualities of other materials are gauged.

- Persistence: absorbable *versus* non-absorbable.
- Number of filaments: monofilament *versus* multifilament.
- Size of braid: relatively large (e.g. Vicryl) *versus* small (e.g. Polysorb).
- Coating: reduces reactivity and drag but worsens knot security.
- Dyed colour: improves visibility but may affect absorption.

Strength and mechanical properties

- Tensile strength: ability to resist deformation; breaking strength per unit area.
- Straight pull strength: linear breaking strength of material.
- Knot-pull tensile strength: breaking strength of knotted material (10–40% weaker than straight pull strength).
- Knot strength: amount of force required for knot to slip.
- Elasticity: ability to regain original form and length after deforming.
- Plasticity: ability to deform without breaking and keep new shape.
- Rate of loss: percentage of original tensile strength present after implantation.
- Mechanism of loss: hydrolysis, proteolysis or macrophage activation.

Handling characteristics

- Pliability: ease of handling; ability to adjust tension and knots.
- Memory: tendency to revert to the packaged shape on handling.
- Knot security: frictional ability of knot to resist untying.
- Chatter: noise made by non-smooth suture materials on knotting.
- Tissue drag: frictional trauma to tissue when passing suture material.

Suture/tissue interaction

- Inflammation: foreign body reaction.
- Potentiation of infection: reduction in bacterial load required to cause infection.
- Capillarity: ability to wick fluid through tissue planes.
- Suture pull-out value: force required to induce tissue failure around suture loop.
- Wound breaking strength: force required to cause wound edge separation.

5.2   Properties used to determine choice of appropriate suture material under given circumstances.

Pliability

Pliability is the tendency of a suture material to change from its current shape when subjected to an external force. The scale of pliability runs arbitrarily from limp (silk) to stiff (steel), with the more pliable or limp materials having superior handling characteristics. Braided materials are usually more pliable than monofilament materials of the same diameter, although the physical characteristics of the material and its manufacture will play a part. Monofilament polyglactin 910 is very stiff and brittle and would only be useful in very small diameters; however, when braided, a versatile suture material with good handling is produced. Polypropylene may be extruded to give a monofilament suture material of almost any size. Poliglecaprone, despite being a monofilament material, has handling characteristics that are closer to the multifilament materials than the rest of the monofilament materials.

Memory and plasticity

Memory refers to the tendency to return to the shape adopted while the material was packaged. Memory is inversely correlated with plasticity (or ductility for metals), with materials of high plasticity having low memory, i.e. the strand can assume and hold a new shape. Memory is generally a poor trait in suture materials, since it makes them hard to handle and they knot poorly. Plasticity confers improved handling and knot security, but plastic materials may also take on

unwanted shapes during use. This includes coiling (particularly with synthetic monofilament materials) or kinking (particularly with steel) during use and makes handling the material more difficult. The high memory of some materials may be reduced by grasping the ends of the material and applying tension to encourage it to adopt a new, straighter shape.

Surface friction

Surface friction is beneficial for knot security, but it produces tissue drag as the suture material is passed through the tissue. In this respect, monofilament suture material has less tissue drag. To reduce tissue drag some suture materials are lubricated with beeswax, polytetrafluoroethylene, silicone or stearates.

Knotting characteristics and security

The security of knots tied with a particular suture material depends on the pliability, memory, surface friction and diameter. Wetting of the suture may also play a part, but most suture materials are wetted by placement in tissue, so the knot security of the dry material is of little significance. For instance, catgut has excellent knot security when dry, but it absorbs fluid on wetting and begins to untie.

Knot security also depends on the physical characteristics of the material and its process of manufacture. For example, Polysorb and Vicryl have a very similar chemical composition, but the finer braid and filament size of Polysorb means that the knot security is higher and the tissue drag is lower than for Vicryl.

PRACTICAL TIPS

- Smaller diameter materials have improved security because they may be tied more tightly: the increased pliability of small-gauge materials allows them to bend into sharper curves, making knot loosening less likely.
- Surface friction influences knotting by increasing resistance of the surfaces within the knot to sliding against one another.
- Suture materials with high memory tend to have poor security, whereas those with high plasticity have better security.
- Plastic materials such as polypropylene deform when the strands are tensioned, which causes flattening of the strands as they pass over one another and gives excellent knot security.
- Ductile materials such as steel have the best knot security, since once the limbs are twisted around each other there is no tendency to revert to the original shape.

Capillarity or wicking

All braided suture materials possess the property of capillary attraction, known as 'wicking'. This is a problem if the braided material is likely to be contaminated with bacteria, either during the surgical procedure (e.g. use in the gastrointestinal or urogenital tracts) or prior to use (e.g. break in aseptic technique). This may potentiate wound infection and lead to a chronic wound infection that will not resolve until the suture material is absorbed or removed. This is a major disadvantage of multifilament non-absorbable suture materials.

Colour

Following manufacture, most suture materials are white or clear. Dying the suture material generally enhances visualization during surgery, though this depends on there being a contrast between the colour of the suture material and the colour of the tissues within the wound. Darkly coloured materials are visible in most surgical wounds, but they are less easy to see against darkly pigmented skin.

Packaging

Suture materials are generally packaged by coiling in card or plastic trays wrapped in foil packets, sometimes with an outer polyethylene/paper wrapper. Suture materials are usually sterilized by gamma irradiation or ethylene oxide (see Chapter 2). Suture materials may also be provided on a reel in a cassette; such suture materials should be regarded as surgically clean, but not sterile.

Tensile strength and loss of strength

Suture material requires a certain tensile strength to be of use in coapting wound edges and must maintain this for as long as the wound needs supporting. The tensile strength is normally tested with dry suture material, despite the fact that most sutures will be wetted and this will affect their strength.

PRACTICAL TIPS

- A suture material is generally strongest when linear tension is applied along its long axis as soon as it is removed from the packet.
- The suture material is weakened by any manipulation or use, and these factors should be considered and minimized to reduce any loss of initial tensile strength.
- Tensile strength is reduced by:
  - Knotting
  - Wetting
  - Natural absorption in tissues
  - Placement in a hostile environment (e.g. infected wound, contact with gastric acid)
  - Abuse of the material by grasping any part other than the end with instruments
  - Repeated autoclaving of unused portions of suture material.

If a suture material is selected whose diameter is too small or whose tensile strength is too weak, breakage and subsequent wound dehiscence are possible. Simply choosing a large-gauge suture material for all applications is not suitable, however, since this will reduce knot security (as this is inversely proportional to diameter) and increase the risk of infection (as this is proportional to the amount of suture material in the wound).

Classification of suture material

Factors affecting the classification of suture material are shown in Figure 5.3.

Composition

- Natural material.
- Synthetic fibre.

Persistence

- Absorbable (loss of strength in <60 days).
- Non-absorbable (tensile strength persists >60 days).

Structure

- Monofilament.
- Multifilament.
- Pseudomonofilament (i.e. sheathed).

Other factors

- Coating.
- Memory.

5.3 Classification of suture material.

Composition

- Naturally occurring materials are generally associated with inflammatory reactions within the tissues and their absorption may be variable.
- Synthetic materials are usually chemical polymers and their absorption characteristics are generally more predictable.

Persistence

Absorbable suture materials: Ideally, absorbable suture materials provide temporary wound support, while the wound is still healing, and are then absorbed once the wound has sufficient strength to withstand normal stresses. Although suture materials are classified as absorbable or non-absorbable according to their maintenance of breaking strength at 60 days, some 'non-absorbable' suture materials (e.g. silk) will be absorbed after a prolonged period of time. In addition, absorbable suture materials may be categorized into those of:

- Short duration, i.e. appreciable strength persists for <21 days (e.g. poliglecaprone)
- Long duration, i.e. appreciable strength persists for >21 days (e.g. polydioxanone).

Absorption consists of two main phases, which overlap. The first phase is linear, with a predictable loss of strength over days to weeks. The second phase consists of loss of suture material mass and is mediated by phagocytes, which remove cellular debris and suture material. Synthetic materials are absorbed primarily by hydrolysis, which proceeds at a predictable rate. Catgut is absorbed by phagocytosis and proteolysis, and varies according to various patient and wound factors.

For absorbable suture materials, the rate of absorption may vary considerably according to the properties of the material itself, the presence of external coatings or sheaths, treatments applied to the material (e.g. treatment of catgut with chromium salts) and the environment in which they are placed (e.g. increased loss of strength in the acid environment of the stomach). In addition, changes to the manufacturing process may enhance absorption (e.g. Vicryl Rapide *versus* Vicryl).

Non-absorbable suture materials: These elicit a tissue reaction that results in encapsulation of the material by fibrous tissue. If applied percutaneously for skin closure, sutures should be removed before this process has progressed very far to avoid suture sinuses. For implanted non-absorbable suture material, the suture is permanently encapsulated in tissue.

Non-absorbable suture materials are classified according to the United States Pharmacopoeia (USP) into three categories:

- **Class I**: silk, monofilament and sheathed suture materials
- **Class II**: cotton and linen fibres, coated synthetic fibres (e.g. polyester)
- **Class III**: steel (monofilament and multifilament).

All class II suture materials have the disadvantage that they may allow bacteria to become lodged in the interstices of the material, where they are inaccessible by the immune system. This may result in a chronic localized infection, with a draining tract, which persists until the suture material is removed. Silk and braided nylon may be absorbed within 6 months if they become infected. For this reason, the use of these is limited.

General figures for loss of tensile strength are given in this chapter. However, these may be variable depending on the experiment conducted, the characteristics of the wound and, in some cases, the gauge of suture material and whether it is dyed or not. This may account for the fact that different figures may be found in different sources. It is not possible to give a single figure that represents the rate of loss of tensile strength of any individual suture material in all circumstances.

Structure

Monofilament suture materials are made of a single strand. This structure allows the suture material to pass through the tissues with less resistance and is relatively more resistant to harbouring bacteria. Care must be taken in handling and tying this type of suture material, because any crushing or crimping may nick or weaken it, resulting in premature failure.

Multifilament suture material is composed of several filaments, which are twisted (e.g. catgut, polymerized caprolactam) or braided (e.g. polyglactin 910) together. These materials are less stiff to handle, but have a higher coefficient of friction. Multifilament material generally has a higher tensile strength, better pliability and flexibility, and better handling and knot security. However, multifilament materials have increased capillarity, which results in the suture material absorbing fluid and may result in wicking of bacteria through the tissues.

Other factors

Coating of some suture materials improves their handling characteristics and reduces tissue drag. Excessive tissue drag may injure the tissue and slow wound healing.

Types of suture material

Figure 5.4 summarizes the categorization of different suture materials.

Absorbable suture materials

Multifilaments

Surgical gut (catgut and collagen): Catgut is derived from the submucosal layer of sheep intestine or the serosal layer of cattle intestine. It is sterilized by gamma irradiation and cannot be sterilized by autoclaving.

- **Plain catgut** maintains tensile strength for approximately 7–10 days post-implantation and absorption is complete within 70 days. It is used in rapidly healing tissues requiring little support, for ligation of superficial blood vessels and for apposing subcutaneous fatty tissues.
- **Chromic gut**, which has been pre-treated with chromium salts, persists longer in the tissues, because the chromium salts are locally toxic to macrophages. Treatment with chromium salts results in light, medium and heavy chromic gut, which persist for different times. Tensile strength is maintained for 10–14 days and absorption is prolonged (90 days). The tissue reactivity is also lessened by this treatment.

Catgut produces an intense tissue reaction and shows a rapid loss of tensile strength, which varies between individual patients and local wound environments, thus limiting its use in surgery. Absorption is more rapid in infected, vascular and more acidic wounds (e.g. the stomach) and it should be avoided in these wounds. Treatment with chromium salts (chromic gut) improves tensile strength and decreases tissue reactivity.

Catgut is a foreign protein and hence stimulates an intense tissue reaction. Absorption occurs by macrophage phagocytosis and this process continues for a relatively long time after it has lost its effective strength. Hence, it acts as a continued stimulus for tissue inflammation. Poor knot security means that the ends should be longer.

Collagen suture materials are prepared from a homogeneous dispersion of bovine tendon that has been highly purified. Extrusion of this collagen dispersion ensures a strand of uniform diameter, with consistent strength and smoothness. Collagen suture materials tie easily and flatten when knotted, giving extra security. Their purity is such that virtually all non-collagenous material has been removed, thus minimizing tissue reaction and assuring a uniform rate of absorption. Like catgut, collagen is available in plain and chromic forms. Its use is limited to fine sizes in ophthalmic surgery.

Persistence	Group	Type	Examples
Absorbable suture materials	Multifilament	Surgical gut	Catgut; collagen
		Polyglycolic acid	Dexon
		Polyglactin 910	Vicryl
		Lactomer 9-1	Polysorb
		Poly(L-lactide/glycolide)	Panacryl
	Monofilament	Polyglytone 6211	Caprosyn
		Poliglecaprone 25	Monocryl
		Glycomer 631	Biosyn
		Polydioxanone	PDS; PDS II
		Polyglyconate	Maxon
Non-absorbable suture materials		Silk	Mersilk; Permahand
		Cotton	
		Stainless steel	Flexon
		Polyamide: ■ Monofilament nylon ■ Braided multifilament nylon	Ethilon; Monosof; Dermalon Surgilon; Nurolon; Bralon
		Polypropylene	Prolene; Surgipro; Surgilene
		Polyethylene	
		Polymerized caprolactam	Supramid; Vetafil
		Polyester	Surgidac; Mersilene
		Polybutester	

5.4   Categorization of different suture materials.

Polyglycolic acid: Polyglycolic acid (e.g. Dexon) is a synthetic absorbable braided multifilament suture material composed of a polymer of glycolic acid. Absorption is by hydrolysis and this progresses more rapidly in an alkaline environment. Absorption is minimal until approximately 14 days after implantation and is complete by 120 days. Absorption is generally associated with little tissue reaction, although a marked reaction may be seen in the acute stages of infection. Absorption is enhanced in urine *in vitro* and while the clinical significance of this *in vivo* is not clear it is not recommended for use in the bladder.

Polyglycolic acid is relatively strong and loses 33% of its initial strength at 7 days and approximately 80% within 14 days. Polyglycolic acid tends to drag through tissues, will cut friable tissue and has relatively poor knot security. Friction is reduced by wetting the suture material before use.

Although polyglycolic acid provides little tensile strength beyond 3–4 weeks, the material may still be detected in the wound. In the bladder, this has the potential to be calculogenic.

Polyglactin 910: Polyglactin 910 (e.g. Vicryl) is a braided synthetic multifilament material composed of glycolic and lactic acids in a ratio of 9:1. It is more hydrophobic and more resistant to hydrolysis than polyglycolic acid. It is coated with a copolymer of lactide and glycolide (polyglactin 370). The water-repelling qualities of lactide slow the rate of loss of tensile strength, and the bulkiness of lactide leads to rapid absorption of the suture mass once the tensile strength is lost. The suture material is also available coated with calcium stearate, which permits easy tissue passage, precise knot placement and smooth tie-down.

Absorption is by hydrolysis, as for polyglycolic acid, and polyglactin 910 has a similar pattern of loss of tensile strength. Both these have little detectable strength by 21 days. Absorption is minimal for 40 days and complete by 56–90 days. Polyglactin 910 is well tolerated in many different wound environments.

Polyglactin 910 has an excellent size-to-strength ratio, is relatively easy to handle, is stable in contaminated wounds and elicits minimal tissue reaction. It is the most widely used coated braided synthetic suture material.

Vicryl Rapide is polyglactin 910 that has been manufactured so that it loses its tensile strength at a more rapid, but predictable, rate compared with standard polyglactin 910. It was created to provide a suture material that matched the absorption characteristics of collagen or catgut. At implantation, it has approximately two-thirds of the tensile strength of polyglactin 910. Half the initial tensile strength is lost at 5–6 days and all tensile strength is lost at 10–14 days. When implanted beneath the skin, it is completely absorbed in 42 days. It is indicated for approximation of rapidly healing superficial soft tissues such as the skin and mucosa, where only short-term support is needed. These sutures will fall out at 7–10 days post-implantation, making the material useful for paediatric, exotic or fractious patients because suture removal is not required.

Lactomer 9-1: Lactomer 9-1 (e.g. Polysorb) has very similar characteristics to polyglactin 910 but the finer filament diameter provides a softer and more compliant strand, with superior handling characteristics and less memory than Vicryl and the other synthetic absorbable multifilaments. The fine filament diameter also allows a more flexible braid and lactomer 9-1 has a superior knot security to other suture materials of a similar construction.

Lactomer 9-1 is the strongest braided absorbable suture material available, being up to 40% stronger than others with a similar construction. The rate of loss of tensile strength and time to absorption of the material is more favourable than other similar materials. At 21 days, this material retains 30% of its initial tensile strength. However, lactomer 9-1 has a more rapid rate of absorption.

Poly(ʟ-lactide/glycolide): Poly(ʟ-lactide/glycolide (e.g. Panacryl) is the only absorbable braided synthetic material that provides long-term support over a minimum of 6 months. It has a similar appearance and handling characteristics to polyglactin 910. It was initially introduced in a wide variety of sizes, attached to a range of needles, and was intended for closure of fascia and other tissues where prolonged support is required. It is now only available attached to tissue or bone anchors and its main use is in the prosthetic replacement of ligaments for joint stabilization. In this respect it encompasses the advantages of other absorbable materials (ease of handling and knot security) and non-absorbable materials (prolonged tissue support), without using a non-absorbable multifilament material.

Monofilaments

Polyglytone 6211: Polyglytone 6211 (e.g. Caprosyn) is similar in composition to poliglecaprone (see below), but loses tensile strength more rapidly. Although these two materials have essentially lost all their tensile strength at 21 days, polyglytone is absorbed more rapidly than poliglecaprone. Thus, suture material is not left in the wound for a long time after it has lost all its tensile strength. The absorption characteristics of polyglytone are similar to those of light or medium chromic gut and its major application is to replace catgut for closure of subcutaneous tissues and ligation of vessels.

Poliglecaprone 25: Poliglecaprone 25 (e.g. Monocryl) is a copolymer of glycolide and E-caprolactone. It has a high tensile strength and good pliability for a monofilament absorbable suture material. Its smooth surface and low memory, coupled with its pliability, result in very low tissue drag and good handling. It is absorbed at a predictable rate, even in the presence of infection. Tensile strength is reduced to 50% by 7 days; and 100% is lost by 21 days. However, the material stays in the wound for up to 4 months. Tissue reaction is minimal. The high initial tensile strength allows the surgeon to select a smaller diameter than would normally be used with other synthetic absorbable monofilaments, which results in improved knot security. It may be used for soft tissue approximation in place of surgical gut or synthetic absorbable multifilament suture materials.

Glycomer 631: Glycomer 631 (e.g. Biosyn) is the strongest monofilament absorbable suture material available and is second in strength only to steel. This strength is maintained over the critical wound-healing period but is then lost rapidly, absorption being complete by 90–110 days, compared with 180 days for polydioxanone. Glycomer 631 has good handling characteristics with low memory and smooth passage through the tissues with little tissue drag. However, some surgeons find that the material is relatively brittle. The knot security is good, but good surgical technique must be used to ensure that successive throws lock properly.

Polydioxanone: Polydioxanone (e.g. PDS, PDS II) is a polymer of *p*-dioxanone. Compared with synthetic absorbable multifilaments, polydioxanone has a greater flexibility and less tissue drag. Its handling characteristics are slightly poorer, but still acceptable. It has the tendency to coil (pig-tail) when handled, which makes grasping the end of the material more difficult. Knot security is relatively poor and seven throws are recommended at the end of a continuous suture line.

Polydioxanone has a greater tensile strength than nylon or polypropylene when implanted. It is absorbed by hydrolysis, but at a slower rate than polyglactin or polyglycolic acid. Absorption is minimal for the first 90 days and is essentially complete within 6 months. It elicits only a mild tissue reaction and, like other monofilament materials, it has a low affinity for microorganisms.

Polyglyconate: Polyglyconate (e.g. Maxon) is composed of a copolymer of glycolic acid and trimethylene carbonate. It has a high initial tensile strength, with little or no loss of strength during the critical period of wound healing. It then loses strength relatively rapidly. Its tensile strength half-life is 3 weeks compared with 6 weeks for polydioxanone. Polyglyconate is absorbed by the action of macrophages between 6 and 7 months after implantation.

Non-absorbable suture materials

Silk

Silk is a natural fibre that is obtained from the cocoon of the silkworm. It is available as a twisted or braided suture material and may be coated with beeswax or silicone to reduce tissue drag and capillarity. Silk is considered to have the best handling characteristics of any suture material and is cheap. However, compared with other suture materials, it is inferior in terms of tensile strength and knot security. Coating further reduces the knot security.

Although it is classified as a non-absorbable suture material, silk is absorbed by proteolysis and is often undetectable in the wound by 2 years. The tensile strength is decreased by moisture and is lost by 1 year. Silk will initiate a stronger inflammatory reaction than other non-absorbable suture materials and this results in its encapsulation by fibrous tissue. Silk sutures will potentiate infection and should not be used at potentially contaminated sites.

Silk has certain limitations in its application, since it may result in ulceration if it protrudes into the lumen of the gastrointestinal tract and serves as a nidus for calculi formation if used in the urinary bladder or gall-bladder. However, it is often used for ligation of large-diameter blood vessels.

Cotton

Surgical cotton is a natural non-absorbable fibre made of twisted long-staple cotton fibres. It is an inexpensive material that may be autoclaved, although this method of sterilization will decrease its tensile strength. Cotton is unusual in that it gains in tensile strength and knot security when wet. Tensile strength is reduced to 50% at 6 months and 30–40% by 2 years. It is non-absorbable and is encapsulated by the body tissues. The main disadvantages of cotton are its capillarity, tissue reactivity, inferior handling due to electrostatic properties and its ability to potentiate infection. There are few, if any, indications for this material and it is included here only for completeness.

Stainless steel

Surgical steel (e.g. Flexon) is made of stainless steel (iron with chromium, nickel and molybdenum) and is available as a monofilament and twisted multifilament. It is biologically inert and non-capillary as a monofilament, and is easily sterilized by autoclaving. It is flexible and may be made into fine sizes. It has high tensile strength, with little reduction in strength over time, and has excellent knot security. It shows negligible tissue reactivity, but sharp cut ends may cause mechanical irritation.

Surgical steel is difficult to handle because of its stiffness, and kinking makes it more difficult to manipulate and tie knots. Cutting or tearing through the tissues may occur and repeated bending within tissues may cause suture failure. Fragmentation and migration of implanted material, particularly the multifilament form, may occur. The use of surgical steel may be associated with electrolytic reactions in the patient if used with other metallic implants of different composition, which may result in loosening of the implants. Surgical steel may be used effectively in infected wounds because it does not support infection.

Polyamide

Nylon is a polyamide suture material derived from hexamethylenediamine and adipic acid, available in monofilament (e.g. Ethilon, Monosof, Dermalon) and multifilament (e.g. Nurolon, Surgilon, Bralon) forms. Its inherent elasticity makes it useful for retention sutures and skin closure. Nylon is fairly pliable, particularly when moist. The braided forms are coated with silicone. Nylon has reasonable handling characteristics, although its memory tends to return the material to its straight form. It has an intermediate tensile strength, similar to polypropylene. Monosof appears to have greater plasticity, which results in better handling, and improved compliance, leading to greater knot security, compared with other polyamide monofilaments.

Nylon is hydrolysed slowly but is stable for at least 2 years, retaining 72% of its initial strength at this time. As a monofilament it is biologically inert and non-capillary. Nylon is recommended for use as a skin suture, but should not be used within a serous or synovial cavity because the buried sharp ends may cause frictional irritation. The main disadvantages of nylon are its poor handling and knot security. Knots in nylon exhibit

the greatest degree of slippage and at least four or five carefully placed throws are required to overcome this, which results in bulky knots.

Polypropylene

Polypropylene (e.g. Prolene, Surgipro, Surgilene) is a synthetic monofilament suture material, composed of polymerized propylene. It may be sterilized by ethylene oxide. It is ductile and tough, but with a relatively low tensile strength and tendency to break if handled roughly. It does not adhere to tissue, which makes it easy to remove; it elicits very little tissue reaction and has the lowest potentiating effect in promoting wound infection. Its plasticity allows the suture material to flatten when knotted, giving it the best knot security of all the non-metallic synthetic monofilament materials. In the tissues, it is not subject to degradation and maintains tensile strength for up to 2 years. It is the least thrombogenic suture material and is therefore used in vascular surgery. Its high flexibility makes it suitable for use in tissues with a great capacity for elongation, such as skin and cardiac muscle.

Polyethylene

Polyethylene is a synthetic monofilament material composed of a polymer of ethylene. It has excellent tensile strength but poor knot security. It may be autoclaved a number of times without significant loss of tensile strength. Like polypropylene, it shows minimal tissue reactivity and has a low potential for encouraging wound infection.

Polymerized caprolactam

This twisted multifilament polyamide suture material (e.g. Supramid, Vetafil) is enclosed in a smooth sheath of proteinaceous material. It is available on a reel in a cassette, but chemical disinfection does not sterilize it for safe implantation in the tissues. Ethylene oxide or steam sterilization is required if the material is to be implanted, but autoclaving increases the difficulty in handling the material. It is only available in relatively large diameters. It has a superior tensile strength to nylon. It has an intermediate reactivity in tissues: skin wounds closed with this material often show more inflammation and suture tracts.

Polyester

Polyester (e.g. Surgidac, Mersilene) is a synthetic non-absorbable braided suture material composed of a polymer of polyethylene terephthalate. It is available uncoated (e.g. Mersilene, Dacron) or coated with polybutylate (e.g. Ethibond), Teflon (e.g. Ethiflex) or silicone (e.g. Ticron), or impregnated with Teflon (e.g. Tevdek). The coating reduces friction for ease of passage through the tissues and improves pliability and tie-down, but reduces knot security. A minimum of five throws is required for a secure knot.

Polyester suture material elicits the greatest tissue reaction among the synthetics, which is increased if the coating is lost. It has a very high initial tensile strength, which is not lost with time, and offers prolonged support for slowly healing tissues. However, this persistence, coupled with its multifilament nature, may potentiate local wound infection, and persistent local infection with sinuses may be seen following implantation.

Polybutester

Polybutester is a monofilament material made from a copolymer of polyglycol terephthalate and polytriethylene terephthalate. It has many of the advantages of polypropylene and polyester. It is slippery and plastic, and yet has good tensile strength and knotting characteristics. The material has approximately twice the flexibility of polypropylene or nylon and has a low coefficient of friction. These properties are ideal for surface closure, permitting adequate tissue approximation, while allowing for postoperative swelling of tissue and its resolution. There is no absorption or loss of tensile strength.

Rational selection of suture materials

Much of the process of selecting a suture material depends on a surgeon's training and individual preference. For each particular application of suture material, a number of possible choices usually exist. Selection of an appropriate suture material is based on a few principles (Figure 5.5). The factors governing the rational choice of a suture material for a particular wound are given in Figure 5.6 (see also Figure 5.2).

Principle	Considerations
Tensile strength should match strength of tissue	Depends on collagen content: fascia and skin > viscera > muscle/fat
Rate of loss of strength should match gain in wound strength	Rate of healing: viscera > skin > fascia
Consider whether suture will alter healing biologically	Tissue reaction Potentiation of infection Sinus formation Potentiation of calculi, thrombi and ulcers
Mechanical properties of the suture should match the tissue	Physical characteristics: durability, handling, knot security, flexibility Biological characteristics: absorption, reactivity, infection

5.5　Principles of suture material selection.

Suture characteristics

- Initial strength.
- Knot security.
- Handling characteristics.

Suture/tissue interaction

- Tissue reactivity.
- Loss of tensile strength.
- Mechanism of degradation.
- Potentiation of infection.

Tissue characteristics

- Resistance to suture pull-out – collagen content.
- Normal rate of healing.

Wound characteristics

- Elective *versus* traumatic wound.
- Degree of contamination.
- Normal rate of healing.

Patient factors

- Alterations in normal rate of healing:
  - o Drug therapy (e.g. corticosteroids, chemotherapy)
  - o Disease (e.g. hyperadrenocorticism, diabetes mellitus).

Surgeon factors

- Individual preference and training.
- Experience with materials.

5.6　Factors influencing the rational choice of suture material.

A suture is only needed until the wound has healed. The loss of tensile strength of the suture material should match the gain in strength of the healing wound. In addition, once the suture material has lost significant tensile strength, it should not persist in the wound.

PRACTICAL TIPS

- Visceral and cutaneous wounds heal rapidly and are no longer reliant on the suture material for wound strength after 14–21 days.
- Fascia heals at a slower rate and regains only approximately 20% of its original strength at 28 days and only about 70% at 9 months postoperatively. Hence healing of fascia relies on the inherent strength of the suture material to support the wound for a longer period of time.

Multifilament suture materials are a poor choice in contaminated or infected wounds, since the interstices of the braid provide a haven for bacteria, and blood and serum soaked into the suture provide an ideal medium for bacterial growth. Approximately 10^5 to 10^6 bacteria per gram of tissue are required to produce a wound infection, but the addition of a silk suture reduces the number of bacteria required by a factor of 10^3 to 10^4.

PRACTICAL TIPS

To avoid complications associated with incorrect suture material choice:

- Avoid multifilament material in contaminated wounds
- Avoid non-absorbable suture materials in hollow organs
- Avoid burying any suture material from a multi-use cassette
- Avoid using catgut in inflamed, infected or acidic wounds
- Avoid reactive material for stoma creation
- Use slowly absorbable material in fascia/tendons
- Use inert material in the skin.

Some guidelines as to the most appropriate type of suture material for given tissues are detailed in Figure 5.7; these may be modified in animals with impaired healing of those tissues.

Tissue	Persistence	Structure
Skin	Non-absorbable	Monofilament
Subcutis	Absorbable (short duration)	Monofilament/multifilament
Fascia	Absorbable (long duration)/non-absorbable	Monofilament
Muscle	Absorbable (long duration)/non-absorbable	Monofilament
Hernia repair	Absorbable (long duration/non-absorbable	Monofilament

5.7　Suitable suture materials for various tissues. (continues) ▶

Tissue	Persistence	Structure
Viscera	Absorbable (short duration)	Monofilament
Tendon	Non-absorbable	Monofilament
Vessel ligation	Absorbable (short duration). A non-absorbable multifilament such as silk may be used for large vessels (e.g. renal/pulmonary artery/vein)	Multifilament
Vessel repair	Non-absorbable	Monofilament
Nerve	Non-absorbable	Monofilament

5.7 (continued) Suitable suture materials for various tissues.

Size

Two classification systems are in use: United States Pharmacopoeia (USP) or European Pharmacopoeia (PhEur); and the metric system (Figure 5.8). Both sizes are displayed on the packet, with the USP/PhEur size usually being displayed more prominently.

Metric	USP/PhEur
0.2	10/0
0.3	9/0
0.4	8/0
0.5	7/0
0.7	6/0
1	5/0
1.5	4/0
2	3/0
3	2/0
3.5	0
4	1
5	2
6	3

5.8 Conversion table of metric to USP/PhEur.

USP/PhEur system

In the USP/PhEur system, suture materials are assigned a size that is based on a combination of diameter, tensile strength and knot security. The precise criteria vary according to:

- Whether it is a natural or synthetic fibre
- Whether it is absorbable or non-absorbable
- What class of non-absorbable suture material it is.

Larger integers represent suture materials of larger diameter; integers followed by a zero represent smaller sizes.

Metric system

In the metric system, each metric unit represents 0.1 mm. This results in the system having a number of advantages:

- The marks on the scale actually mean something: '3 metric' is 0.3 mm in diameter, whereas '2/0' in the USP system tells us nothing about its size

- The metric system is an ascending scale, with larger numbers representing larger suture material sizes. In the USP system, for suture material sizes smaller than 3.5 metric (0 USP), an increasing number refers to a smaller suture material
- The metric suture material is a linear scale, with no points missed out. The USP scale does not have 1/0
- The metric system has regular increments. In the USP scale, equal increments from 5/0 to 2/0 represent metric increments of 0.05 or 0.1 mm
- The metric scale is the same for all suture materials. The USP scale is different for catgut compared with synthetic suture materials.

One potential drawback of the metric system is that the dramatic differences in tensile strength between various suture materials can make it difficult to compare a standard size of suture material. For example, 2 metric Vicryl has a greater tensile strength than 2 metric silk.

Choice of suture material size

The surgeon should choose the smallest size of suture material that will provide adequate support to the tissues. The advantages of choosing a smaller gauge suture material are:

- Less tissue trauma (tract and strangulation)
- Smaller knots
- Greater knot security with small-diameter suture material
- Adherent bacteria less viable on small-gauge suture material.

PRACTICAL TIPS

Rule-of-thumb guide for selection of suture material size:

- 3 metric for dogs; 2 metric for cats
- Reduce by 1 size for delicate tissue
- Increase by 1 size for tough tissue.

Suture needles

General properties

The characteristics of a suture needle are described in Figure 5.9 and the classification of suture needles is shown in Figure 5.10.

The ideal suture needle should be:

- Of high-quality stainless steel
- Of the smallest diameter possible
- Stable in the grasp of the needle-holder
- Capable of allowing passage of suture material with minimal trauma
- Sharp enough to pass through tissue with minimal resistance
- Sterile
- Resistant to corrosion
- Strong enough to resist deformation during normal working conditions.

Attachment to suture material

Suture needles may be eyed, for threading, or may have suture materials swaged on (Figure 5.11).

Characteristic	Definition
Strength	Resistance to deformation during passage through tissue
Ultimate moment	Measure of maximum strength by bending needle to 90 degrees
Surgical-yield moment	Amount of angular deformation before permanent deformation
Ductility	Resistance to breakage under a given amount of bending
Sharpness	Ability to penetrate tissue
Clamping moment	Stability of needle in needle-holder
Point	Portion of the needle extending from the tip to the area of maximum cross-section
Body	The majority of the length of the needle
Swage	The attachment of the suture material to the needle
Needle length	Distance along the needle from needle tip to swage
Chord length	Distance in a straight line from needle tip to swage
Radius	Distance from body of needle to centre of circle along which the needle curves
Diameter	Gauge or thickness of wire from which the needle is made

5.9   Characteristics of a suture needle.

Attachment to suture	Swaged-on Eyed needle
Number of strands	Single strand Double strand
Number of needles	Single armed Double armed
Size *(note: length is normally <8 × diameter)*	Length Diameter Gauge
Shape	Straight (superficial wounds) Curved (deeper wounds: 1/4, 3/8, 1/2 or 5/8 of a circle) Half-curved (curved point, straight shaft) J-shape (deep wounds with poor access)
Needle point	Non-cutting: ■ Round-bodied ■ Taperpoint Cutting: ■ Tapercut ■ Standard cutting ■ Reverse cutting ■ Side-cutting – spatula

5.10   Classification of suture needles.

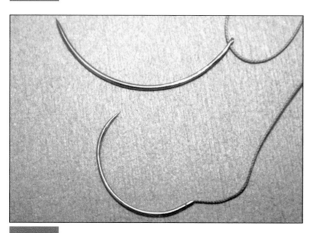

5.11   An eyed needle (top) and a swaged-on needle.

Swaged-on needles

The advantages of swaged-on needles are:

■ Available for use immediately, without the need to attach the suture material
■ Cause less tissue trauma as the needle/suture material junction is passed through tissue
■ Less likely to have the suture material become detached prematurely
■ Less handling of the suture material required, thus maintaining suture integrity
■ Less likely to cause fraying of suture material compared with corners of eyed needle
■ More likely to be sharper than eyed needles
■ Guaranteed to be sterile if used straight from the packet.

Channel-swage needles have a channel into which the suture material is introduced before the channel is crimped over the suture material. The diameter of the channel-swage is greater than that of the suture material. **Drill-swage** needles have metal removed from the end by drilling; the suture material is introduced and the end of the needle is crimped over the suture material. The diameter of the drill-swage is less than the diameter of the suture material.

Swaged-on needles may be constructed as **controlled release**, which allows the suture material to be detached from the needle with a sharp tug. A hand tie may then be performed without the encumbrance of a needle.

Eyed needles

Eyed needles are available with a standard circumferential 'hole' in the end of the needle or with a spring-eye. A spring-eye (French) needle has a slot at the end of the needle where the suture is to be attached. The suture is passed through the slot easily, but ridges prevent the suture from being withdrawn easily.

Eyed needles may be re-used, but suture material must be reloaded on to the needle before each use. The suture material should not be knotted to the eye of the needle, since this will increase tissue trauma.

For large-gauge suture material, passing the suture material through the eye from the convex to the concave side, followed by skewering the suture material on the concave side with the point of the needle, has been reported as a way of preventing the suture material pulling out of the eye, without tying a knot. However, this still increases the bulk of suture material passed through the tissue.

> **PRACTICAL TIP**
>
> Passing the suture material through the eye from the concave to the convex side will reduce the likelihood of the suture material pulling out of the eye.

Multiple strands and needles

Most suture materials are formulated as a single strand of suture material and are attached to a single needle. Single needles armed with a double strand of suture material allow two strands of material to be passed through the tissue for increased strength of closure, and allow the needle to be passed through the loop created by the two strands after the first pass across the wound, so that a continuous suture line may begin without tying a knot.

Single strands of suture material armed with a needle at either end allow a continuous closure to start at a single point and to continue along two aspects of the tissue to close the wound. For instance, during simple continuous closure of the circumference of the intestine following enterectomy, the suture material may be knotted at the mesenteric border and passed towards the anti-mesenteric border, with one needle used at each side. Double-armed suture materials are often used in cardiovascular surgery and polypropylene is often provided this way.

Needle size and needle-holders

Heavy-gauge needles are thicker to prevent bending of the needle during passage through tough tissue. They are usually attached to large-gauge suture material. **Vascular-type** needles are thin and their diameter approximates the diameter of the suture material, to ensure that the hole left in the tissue by the needle is filled with suture material. This is to prevent leaks in vascular structures.

The stability of the needle within the jaws of the needle-holder will affect control and performance. The jaws of the needle-holder must be appropriate for the size of the needle to hold it securely:

- If the needle-holder is too small, the needle is likely to be subject to rocking, turning or twisting
- If the needle-holder is too large, the jaws will bend the needle, thus increasing tissue trauma as the needle is passed through the wound.

An ovoid cross-section of the needle body will maximize both the surface contact of the needle with the jaws of the needle-holder and the bending moment of the needle.

Needle shapes

A range of different needle shapes is available (Figure 5.12).

- **Curved needles** are used in deep wounds with restricted access.
- With progressively more superficial wounds, a less curved needle may be used, with **straight needles** being used in the skin. A straight needle is passed through the tissues with the hands rather than using instruments.
- **Half-curved needles** have a straight shaft, with a curve at the point. These needles are difficult to handle, as the flat portion of the needle does not follow the curved point.
- **Compound curved needles** have a different radius of curvature along the shaft of the needle. They are designed for anterior segment ophthalmic surgery and vessel anastomosis. These needles have a tight 80 degree curvature at the tip, which becomes a 45 degree curvature throughout the remainder of the body.

Needle points

Non-cutting round-bodied needles are used in parenchymatous organs (e.g. liver), fat and muscle. Cutting needles are used in tissues with a higher collagen content (e.g. fascia, skin). Needle points as illustrated on packaging are shown in Figure 5.13.

Round-bodied needles

Round-bodied needles are generally less traumatic to the tissues than are cutting needles. However, it is certainly more traumatic to the tissues to attempt to pass a round-bodied needle through tough tissue, because of the likelihood of damaging the tissue from excessive handling with thumb forceps.

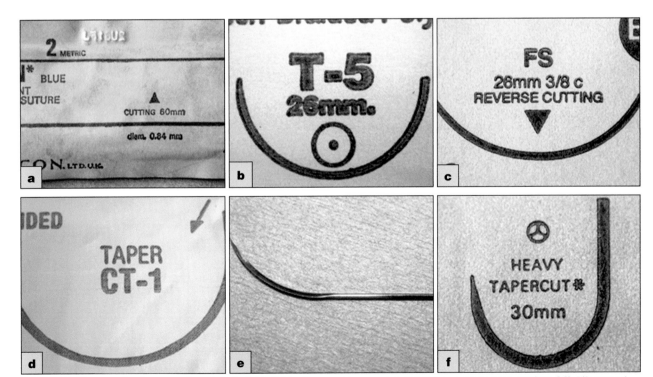

5.12 Shapes of suture needles: **(a)** straight; **(b)** half-curved taperpoint; **(c)** 3/8 curved reverse cutting; **(d)** 5/8 curved taper; **(e)** curved on flat; **(f)** J-shaped tapercut.

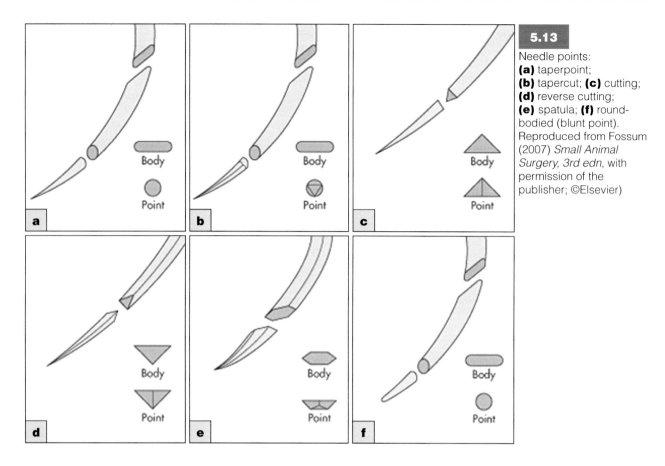

5.13

Needle points:
(a) taperpoint;
(b) tapercut; **(c)** cutting;
(d) reverse cutting;
(e) spatula; **(f)** round-bodied (blunt point).
Reproduced from Fossum (2007) *Small Animal Surgery, 3rd edn*, with permission of the publisher; ©Elsevier)

Cutting needles

- The **tapercut** needle represents a compromise between a round-bodied needle and a standard cutting needle.
- A **conventional cutting** needle has the cutting edge along the concave aspect of a curved needle.
- A **reverse cutting** needle has the cutting edge along the convex side. The reverse cutting needle has a stronger construction and minimizes suture cut through, since the suture material abuts the flat side of the triangular hole in the tissue rather than the pointed apex (Figure 5.14).

- **Spatula cutting** needles are used for very small-gauge suture material for ophthalmic surgery. They have a flat top and bottom and allow maximum ease of tissue penetration and control as they pass through tissue.

Needle selection

Factors governing the rational choice of a suture needle include:

- Wound characteristics: depth; accessibility
- Tissue characteristics: tissue strength
- Surgeon's preference: use of hands or instruments to pass the needle.

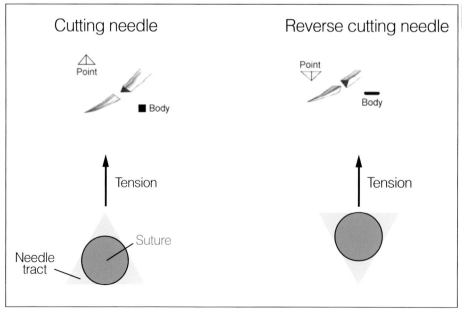

5.14 Cutting *versus* reverse cutting needles. Reproduced from Fossum (2007) *Small Animal Surgery, 3rd edn*, with permission of the publisher; ©Elsevier)

Handling and use of suture material and needles

Information given about the suture material and needle type inside a packet is illustrated in Figure 5.15.

PRACTICAL TIPS

Guidelines for correct suture material handling:

- Protect suture materials from heat and moisture
- Do not autoclave absorbable suture materials
- Do not soak absorbable suture materials in fluid
- Use suture material directly from the packet – do not handle before use
- Do not kink or crush suture material with instruments
- Straighten suture material with memory, using a gentle tug
- Check suture material for fraying or defects during use.

PRACTICAL TIPS

Principles for correct use of suture needles:

- Swaged-on needles are less traumatic
- Use straighter needles for more superficial wounds
- Grasp the needle at the correct point:
  - Standard use: one-third to halfway from the suture material end
  - Delicate tissue: closer to the suture material
  - Tough tissue: closer to the point
- Hold the needle at the tips of the needle-holder
- Use taper needles if possible (change if difficult to pass)
- Length should allow a bite through both sides of the wound.

The surgical knot

Types of knots and how to tie them are described and illustrated in detail in Chapter 22 along with suture patterns. A surgical suture consists of three components:

- The **loop** (the loop of suture material within the tissue or around a pedicle)
- The **knot** (composed of a number of throws)
- The **ears** (the cut ends that prevent the knot from untying due to slippage).

The basic surgical knot is a **square knot** (reef knot), which is formed by two single throws (left strand over right, then right strand over left). The ear and loop of each end of the suture material are on the same side of the knot. The **granny knot** (left strand over right, then left strand over right again) is weaker and may untie.

The so-called **surgeon's knot** is formed by passing the two strands around each other twice on the first throw (a double throw). The advantage of this knot is that the first double throw will resist tension in the wound and reduce the likelihood of the throw unwrapping before the second throw is secured. However, it produces a bulky and uneven knot; it may damage monofilament suture materials; and it is not recommended. Tension in the wound should be managed using a different technique, such as use of a sliding knot, apposing the wound edges with pre-placed sutures or use of Galiban forceps.

The knot is the weakest part of the suture and failure of the knot may result in disastrous complications, e.g. dehiscence or exsanguination. To reduce the risk of suture breakdown, sutures of slightly greater strength than the holding power of the tissue are placed. Care is taken during the placement of throws while knot-tying, such that each throw lies flat and is apposed to the previous throws to reduce the likelihood of untying. Monofilament material has poorer knot security because of more memory and less friction and so greater care should be taken.

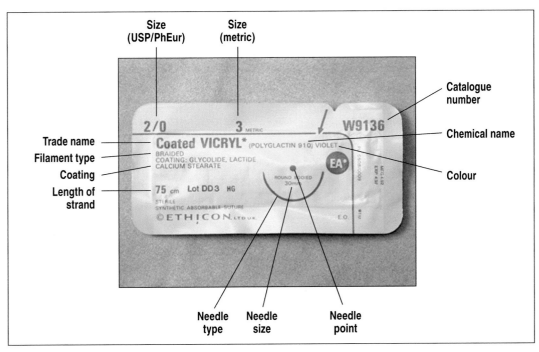

5.15

Example of a suture material packet, explaining the label information.

Knot security is inversely proportional to the diameter of the suture. Hence choosing the smallest diameter suture material consistent with matching the tensile strength of the wound allows a more secure knot. In this respect, choosing a suture material with a high initial tensile strength (e.g. poliglecaprone) allows the surgeon to select a smaller size with improved knot security.

The minimum number of throws to achieve a stable and secure knot should be used. Increasing the number of throws beyond this does not increase knot security, but will increase the amount of suture material in the wound with a resulting increase in foreign body reaction and potentiation of infection. For instance, for a given suture material, using five throws rather than three will increase the bulk of the knot by 50%. The minimum number of throws to achieve a stable knot for various suture materials are shown in Figure 5.16.

Suture material	Interrupted suture	Continuous suture	
		Start knot	End knot
Catgut	3	4	5
Polyglactin 910	3	3	6
Polyglycolic acid	3	3	5
Polydioxanone	4	5	7
Polyamide	4	5	6
Polypropylene	3	3	5

5.16   Minimum number of throws for a stable knot.

PRACTICAL TIPS

Rule-of-thumb:

- For interrupted patterns, a minimum of three throws is required for multifilament material and four throws for monofilament material
- For continuous patterns, one throw should be added to the start knot and one or two throws added to the end knot.

Tissue adhesives for wound closure

Cyanoacrylate tissue adhesives have been available for many years. The very early products had a number of problems and did not gain wide acceptance. These problems related primarily to poor strength and cracking or peeling of the glue and the poor results from their inappropriate use. The newer generations of tissue glue have improved characteristics and are more widely used, with more rational guidelines, though hand-sutured or stapled wound closure remains the standard technique.

The cyanoacrylates are most widely used. Cyanoacrylate monomers are converted to strong insoluble polymers on contact with water on tissue surfaces. The setting time ranges from 2 to 60 seconds, depending on the thickness of the glue film, the amount of moisture present and the length of the alkyl chain molecule in the glue.

A variety of monomers have been used:

- Methyl and ethyl
- Butyl
- Octyl.

Figure 5.17 summarizes some of the veterinary tissue adhesives.

Methyl and ethyl cyanoacrylate-based polymers

Methyl-based and ethyl-based polymers are present in commercially available adhesives, such as Superglue. These polymers are toxic to normal tissue and were prone to cracking and peeling. They are not recommended for use on living tissue, though they have been evaluated for this function. Before a human product (Dermabond) was licensed for use, a comparison was made between (butyl-based) Vetbond and commercially available Superglue. No material difference was found between the two products in the toxicological profile or in the impact on wound healing. Superglue was found to be considerably cheaper (more than 25 times) and had a superior delivery system from the tube.

Butyl cyanoacrylate-based polymers

Butyl-based polymers were the first-generation medicinal cyanoacrylate adhesives. They were approved primarily for use in veterinary medicine and were not licensed for human use by the US Food &

Product	Distributor	Group	Notes
Nexaband S/C	Abbott Laboratories	2-Octyl	Clear, flexible, viscous. Includes plasticizers and stabilizers for greater stability and strength. Setting time 4–5 seconds Shelf life 18–24 months (at room temperature) Glass vial/stock bottle with disposable pipettes
Nexaband Liquid	Abbott Laboratories	n-Butyl-2	Clear, lower viscosity. Includes thickeners and stabilizers. Dropper bottle with disposable tip
Vetbond	3M	n-Butyl	Setting time: 1 second. Shelf life: 12 months at room temperature (longer if refrigerated) Squeezable bottle with narrow tip
Vet-Seal	Braun	n-Butyl-2	Must be refrigerated (shelf life 22 months). Squeezable bottle with narrow tip

5.17   Some veterinary tissue adhesives.

Drug Administration (FDA). Their bond strength is greater than that of methyl or ethyl polymers. The addition of an indicator dye allows good visualization of these products.

Octyl cyanoacrylate-based polymers

Octyl-based polymers are the next generation of medicinal cyanoacrylates and are licensed for both human and veterinary medicine. Compared with the other cyanoacrylates, the octyl-based products have a greater bond strength (2–4 times that of butyl-based cyanoacrylates) and are less toxic to tissue. Their bond strength is approximately equivalent to a sutured closure. Their higher viscosity improves the ability to limit the application of the adhesive to the target areas.

Nexaband is intended for use in closure of skin wounds. Its formulation as a stock bottle with a number of fine disposable pipettes allows accurate delivery of the adhesive and eliminates blockage at the tip of the bottle.

Action

The polymer provides a colourless, waterproof barrier and acts as a tissue bridge to hold the wound edges together. Thus the wound is protected from external contamination, there is no oozing from the wound and postoperative comfort is good. These products also promote haemostasis and will reduce bleeding from vascular tissue (e.g. in the oral cavity), although they will not stop bleeding from large vessels.

Epithelialization of the wound proceeds below the adhesive, which is sloughed from the wound when the repair is complete. The tissue glue may have some antibacterial effect *in situ* in the wound.

Uses of tissue glue

Tissue adhesives have been used effectively in oral surgery, intestinal anastomosis, management of corneal ulceration, control of haemorrhage from the cut surface of parenchymatous organs, microvascular incisions, skin incisions and skin grafts.

Wounds

Use in cutaneous wounds and incisions is most widespread. Skin wounds should not be under tension and should not be contaminated or infected. Thus the most likely application is for elective surgical wounds rather than traumatic wounds. Tissue glue may be used to ensure apposition of edges in wounds that are under tension, but only if the tension is managed using an alternative technique, e.g. tension sutures. Examples of use include:

- Small stab incisions made for percutaneous biopsy needles
- Surgical incisions in intractable patients
- Surgical incisions in patients likely to chew at sutures or who will not tolerate a collar restraint.

In some human studies, glued wounds had a reduced incidence of inflammation of the wound edges and a superior long-term cosmetic appearance compared with sutured wounds.

Corneal ulcers

In human and equine medicine, tissue glue has been used to protect both superficial and deep corneal ulcers. It has been used to attach contact lenses for emergency treatment of deep corneal ulcers that are near to perforation; the glue and contact lens are sloughed by desquamation of the corneal epithelium over an extended period. Tissue glue may also be used to attach conjunctival pedicle flaps to the cornea to avoid the need for sutures.

Other uses

Other reported uses in human and veterinary medicine include:

- Attachment of feeding tubes with a tape butterfly to the skin
- Sealing of the percutaneous wound following placement of a long-stay catheter
- Closure of oral wounds (e.g. following dental work)
- Augmentation of intestinal anastomoses
- Augmentation of sutured tendon repair
- Enteroplication
- Fixing punch-free skin grafts to the recipient bed
- Topical haemostasis for parenchymatous organs (e.g. following liver laceration).

Application technique

1. Lavage the wound with sterile isotonic crystalloid fluid or bicarbonate solution (to enhance polymerization in an alkaline environment) and gently blot dry with a swab.
2. Gently appose the edges with fingers or forceps.
3. Run the tissue glue along the top of the apposed wound edges. The glue may be applied using the applicator supplied, or may be dispensed with a small-gauge syringe, with or without an intravenous catheter.
4. Polymerization and adhesion occur rapidly, but ideally apposition should be maintained for 1–2 minutes until full strength is achieved.

It is important to glue only the skin surface and not the deeper tissues. Incorporation of tissue glue into the deeper layers of the wound will impede normal wound healing. The fresh adhesive will cause any blood in the wound to coagulate. Polymerization is an exothermic reaction and better results are achieved with a thin coating of glue.

WARNING

Do not use tissue glue in:

- Infected wounds
- Deep puncture wounds
- Wounds subject to tension or movement.

PRACTICAL TIPS

- Do not apply tissue adhesive in excessive quantities.
- Do not bury tissue adhesive in deeper tissue layers.
- Do not apply tissue adhesives over a pool of blood or fluid.

Advantages and disadvantages of tissue glue

Advantages and disadvantages of using tissue glue for wound closure are summarized in Figure 5.18.

Advantages
■ Rapid closure of wounds (approximately 3–4 times quicker than a sutured closure).
■ Easy to apply.
■ No pain on wound closure in conscious patients.
■ Reduced cost of wound closure (approximately 25% of cost of a sutured closure).
■ No sutures to remove from the patient.
■ Reduced self-trauma to the wound.
■ Effective haemostasis when applied.
■ Antimicrobial effect.

Disadvantages
■ Introduction of foreign material into wound.
■ Impairment of healing if glue separates wound edges.
■ Cracking or peeling of glue results in poor closure.
■ More difficult to achieve good apposition in irregular wounds.
■ More likely to result in dehiscence if under tension.
■ Necessity to place sutures in longer wounds.
■ Adhesion of glue to swabs, gloves or instruments.
■ Necessity to learn a new technique.

5.18 Proven advantages and disadvantages of tissue glue for wound closure.

As well as the disadvantages described in Figure 5.18, potential problems associated with the use of tissue adhesives include:

■ Tissue toxicity (particularly with earlier cyanoacrylates)
■ Granuloma formation
■ Potentiation of wound infection
■ Delayed wound healing if the edges are separated by the presence of tissue glue
■ Poor adherence to moist surfaces
■ Interference with cortical bone healing if used near bone.

If the glue adheres to skin other than the wound or inanimate objects (e.g. instruments), it can be removed once polymerized by soaking in acetone.

Despite potential concerns over the use of tissue glue for the closure of elective or traumatic wounds, a number of reports have demonstrated that closure with tissue glue has a similar outcome to suture closure, in terms of cosmetic appearance and wound infection rates. However, improper use of tissue adhesive has the potential to delay healing, reduce cosmesis and potentiate infection.

Suture material monographs

Surgical gut – catgut and collagen	
Classification	Natural, absorbable, twisted multifilament (polished)
Composition	SI submucosa (sheep) and serosa (cattle)
Manufacture	Plain gut: formaldehyde-treated collagen Chromic gut: light, medium or heavy chromium salt solutions Polishing reduces drag but weakens suture Chromium reduces rate of phagocytosis because of toxicity to macrophages
Absorption	Macrophages: initial hydrolysis > late proteolysis Variable: rapid in stomach, infected and vascular tissue
Loss of strength	33% loss at 7 days (chromic gut) 67% loss at 28 days (chromic gut) All lost at 7 days (plain), 14 days (light), 21 days (medium), 28 days (heavy) More rapid in infected, vascular and gastric wounds
Tissue interaction	Marked foreign body reaction
Handling	Dry: good Wet: swells, weakens (50%), poor knot security
Use	Vascular ligature, ophthalmic surgery (collagen)
Advantages	Cheap Excellent handling
Disadvantages	Intense tissue reaction and some tissue drag Variability in loss of tensile strength Variability in strength along strand Occasional sensitivity reaction (cats) Fraying during tying

Polyglycolic acid (e.g. Dexon)	
Classification	Synthetic, absorbable, multifilament
Composition	Polymer of glycolic acid ± coating
Manufacture	Available coated or uncoated Coating is polycaprolate
Absorption	Hydrolysis, especially in alkaline environment and urine Minimal for 14 days, complete at 120 days Degradation products have antibacterial activity
Time to absorption	60–90 days
Loss of strength	35% loss at 14 days 65% loss at 21 days
Tissue interaction	Marked reaction in acute infection
Handling	Tissue drag, cut-through and relatively poor knot security Improved by coating (Dexon-II)
Use	Tolerated in infected wounds
Advantages	Strong
Disadvantages	Not recommended in bladder

Polyglactin 910 (e.g. Vicryl)	
Classification	Synthetic, absorbable, multifilament
Composition	Polymer of glycolic and lactic acids (9:1) ± coating
Manufacture	Available dyed or undyed and coated or uncoated Coating is copolymer of lactide and glactide and calcium stearate
Absorption	Hydrolysis at predictable rate, may be increased in urine More hydrophobic and resistant than polyglycolic acid ▶

Time to absorption	56–70 days
Loss of strength	Similar to polyglycolic acid, but stronger 25% loss at 14 days 50% loss at 21 days 75% loss at 28 days Good size:strength ratio
Tissue interaction	Well tolerated, minimal reaction
Handling	Good knot security, some tissue drag Coating improves handling (similar to silk)
Use	General soft tissue approximation Vessel ligation
Advantages	Stronger than polyglycolic acid to 21 days, more rapid absorption
Disadvantages	Very few – more tissue drag than monofilament materials

Lactomer 9-1 (e.g. Polysorb)

Classification	Synthetic, absorbable, multifilament
Composition	Lactomer 9-1: copolymer of glycolide (90%) and lactide (10%)
Manufacture	Available coated or uncoated and dyed or undyed Coated with caprolactone/glycolide copolymer and calcium stearoyl lactylate
Absorption	Hydrolysis
Time to absorption	56–70 days
Loss of strength	20% loss at 14 days 70% loss at 21 days
Tissue interaction	Well tolerated
Handling	Smooth passage through tissue – little drag Smooth knot rundown
Use	Approximation of most soft tissues Not for use in cardiovascular or neurological surgery
Advantages	Smaller braid than polyglactin 910, better handling and knot security
Disadvantages	Potentially calculogenic in urinary bladder and gallbladder

Poly(L-lactide/glycolide) (e.g. Panacryl)

Classification	Synthetic, absorbable, multifilament
Composition	Polymer of L-lactide (95%) and glycolide (5%)
Manufacture	Only available undyed (white) Coated with 90% caprolactone and 10% glycolide
Absorption	Slow absorption by hydrolysis
Time to absorption	1.5–2.5 years
Loss of strength	10% loss at 6 weeks 20% loss at 3 months 40% loss at 6 months 80% loss at 12 months
Tissue interaction	Minimal tissue reaction, similar to polyglactin 910
Handling	Excellent handling characteristics Knot tying similar to monofilament suture material
Use	Soft tissue closure where long-term support needed Prosthetic replacement of ligaments

Advantages	Long-term support Knot less bulky than monofilament non-absorbable material
Disadvantages	Slightly more expensive than other materials (e.g. Vicryl) Absorption delayed in tissue of poor vascularity

Polyglytone 6211 (e.g. Caprosyn)

Classification	Synthetic, absorbable, monofilament
Composition	Glycolide/lactide/caprolactone/trimethylene carbonated
Manufacture	Undyed
Absorption	Hydrolysis
Time to absorption	<56 days
Loss of strength	40–50% loss at 5 days 70–80% loss at 10 days 100% loss at 21 days
Tissue interaction	Minimal tissue reaction
Handling	Satisfactory for a monofilament material
Use	Soft tissue closure where prolonged support is not needed
Advantages	Rapid loss of tensile strength and absorption
Disadvantages	Rapid loss of strength prevents its use in many tissues

Poliglecaprone 25 (e.g. Monocryl)

Classification	Synthetic, absorbable, monofilament
Composition	Copolymer of glycolide and epsilon-caprolactone
Manufacture	Dyed or undyed forms available
Absorption	Hydrolysis
Time to absorption	Complete by 91–119 days
Loss of strength	Quicker than PDS or Maxon 30–50% loss at 7 days 60-80% loss at 14 days 100% loss at 21 days (dyed) or 28 days (undyed)
Tissue interaction	Minimal tissue reaction
Handling	One of the strongest and most pliable synthetic monofilaments Initial tensile strength high, so can use smaller gauge Knot security fair to poor
Use	Instead of gut and synthetic multifilament General soft tissue approximation, vessel ligation
Advantages	High tensile strength, maintained for critical period and then rapidly lost Low memory Easy to handle
Disadvantages	Knot security not as good as multifilament Rapid absorption unsuitable for sites where healing is prolonged

Glycomer 631 (e.g. Biosyn)

Classification	Synthetic, absorbable, monofilament
Composition	Glycomer 631: copolymer of glycolide (60%), dioxanone (14%) and trimethylene carbonate (26%)
Manufacture	Available dyed (violet) or undyed
Absorption	Hydrolysis
Time to absorption	90–110 days

Loss of strength	25% loss at 14 days 60% loss at 21 days
Tissue interaction	Minimal tissue reaction
Handling	Excellent handling characteristics, smooth passage through tissue Knot security similar to braided material
Use	Soft tissue approximation where extended support is required
Advantages	Strongest absorbable monofilament material
Disadvantages	Unfamiliar material Secure knotting requires good technique

Polydioxanone (e.g. PDS, PDS II)

Classification	Synthetic, absorbable, monofilament
Composition	Polymer of p-dioxanone
Manufacture	Available dyed (violet) or undyed
Absorption	Hydrolysis
Time to absorption	182 days, slow and predictable
Loss of strength	14–20% loss at 14 days 30–42% loss at 28 days 40–75% loss at 42 days 86% loss at 56 days
Tissue interaction	Minimal as for polyglactin/polyglycolic acid Less wicking than multifilament
Handling	Flexibility and strength > polyglactin/polyglycolic acid Less drag than multifilament High memory and plasticity (PDS II more pliable than PDS) Coiling during use Knot security requires seven throws
Use	Soft tissue approximation where extended support is required Closure of abdominal and thoracic wall
Advantages	Stronger than polyamide and polypropylene at implantation
Disadvantages	Memory greater than multifilament Associated with calcinosis circumscripta in a few young dogs

Polyglyconate (e.g. Maxon)

Classification	Synthetic, absorbable, monofilament
Composition	Polymer of glycolic acid and trimethylene carbonate
Manufacture	Available dyed (green) or undyed
Absorption	Macrophages, minimal until day 60
Time to absorption	180 days
Loss of strength	As polydioxanone; tensile strength half-life 3 weeks versus PDS 6 weeks 19–30% loss at 14 days 35–45% loss at 21 days 41–50% loss at 28 days 70% loss at 42 days
Tissue interaction	Similar to polydioxanone
Handling	Strength and performance similar to polydioxanone Knot security excellent, less memory
Use	Soft tissue approximation where extended support is required ▶

Advantages	Better handling than polydioxanone High initial tensile strength No increase in absorption at sites of infection/inflammation
Disadvantages	Sharp ends if cut short

Silk

Classification	Natural, non-absorbable, multifilament
Composition	Silkworm cocoon
Manufacture	Treatment with oil, wax or silicone to reduce capillarity
Absorption	Absorbed within 2 years (within 6 months in infected site)
Loss of strength	Relatively low, slow loss
Tissue interaction	Moderate tissue reaction
Handling	Excellent, but poor knot security (especially if treated)
Use	Vascular ligature (PDA) Soft skin sutures
Advantages	Excellent handling Cheap
Disadvantages	Ulceration in gastrointestinal tract Calculogenic nidus in bladder Potentiates wound infection $\times 10^3$–10^4 Relatively weak

Cotton

Classification	Natural, non-absorbable, multifilament
Composition	Natural fibre
Manufacture	Usually available undyed
Absorption	Not absorbed
Loss of strength	50% at 6 months 70% at 2 years
Tissue interaction	Moderate tissue reaction
Handling	Poor – electrostatic properties Gains tensile strength and knot security when wet
Use	Not in current use
Advantages	None
Disadvantages	Potentiates infection

Stainless steel (e.g. Flexon)

Classification	Synthetic, non-absorbable, mono/multifilament
Composition	316L steel wire
Manufacture	Not coated or dyed
Absorption	Not absorbed
Loss of strength	No loss
Tissue interaction	Inert, no reaction
Handling	Poor handling and knot tying Greatest tensile strength and knot security ▶

Use	Few indications – tissues with slow healing (e.g. body wall and sternal closure) Infected tissue – no potentiation of infection
Advantages	Inert and strong Visible radiographically
Disadvantages	Tissue irritation from rigid ends May fragment or break Tissue cut-through Fatigue breaking with movement Poor handling Visible radiographically May interfere with magnetic resonance imaging Requires special scissors to cut

Polyamide (e.g. Ethilon, Monosof, Dermalon, Bralon)

Classification	Synthetic, non-absorbable, mono/multifilament
Composition	Polymer of hexamethylenediamine and adipic acid
Manufacture	Available dyed (black or blue) or undyed
Absorption	Little – chemical degradation
Loss of strength	19% loss at 1 year 28% loss at 2 years 34% loss at 11 years Or approximately 15–20% per year Multifilament: 100% at 6 months
Tissue interaction	Minimal reaction
Handling	Poor handling and knot security (slippage – four to five throws) Strong memory, although elastic rather than plastic Intermediate tensile strength, as for polypropylene
Use	Wide application, particularly skin
Advantages	Inert and non-capillary
Disadvantages	Frictional irritation in serous/synovial cavity Sharp ends if cut short

Polypropylene (e.g. Prolene, Surgipro, Surgilene)

Classification	Synthetic, non-absorbable, monofilament
Composition	Polymer of propylene
Manufacture	Dyed blue
Absorption	Resistant to enzymes
Loss of strength	No loss of strength for years
Tissue interaction	Inert, least thrombogenic material, no potentiation of infection
Handling	Poor handling – slippery, high memory Plastic suture material: excellent knot security (flattening) and flexible Low tensile strength Good knot strength

Use	Vascular surgery Flexible tissue (cardiac muscle, skin) Hernia and tendon repair
Advantages	Best knot security of monofilament materials Least reactive suture material
Disadvantages	Poor handling Poor knot security if tension not applied

Polymerized caprolactam (e.g. Supramid, Vetafil)

Classification	Synthetic, non-absorbable, multifilament
Composition	Polyamide polymer
Manufacture	Smooth sheath of polyethylene/proteinaceous material
Absorption	Not absorbed
Loss of strength	0.5% loss after 10–20 cycles in autoclave
Tissue interaction	Intermediate tissue reaction
Handling	Poorer after autoclaving Stronger than monofilament nylon Knot security better than monofilament (Sheath cracks on knotting)
Use	Few indications (skin closure) – better products are available
Advantages	Cheap Elasticity allows use in areas subject to movement or tension
Disadvantages	Not sterile – subcutaneous swelling and sinuses Not available in small diameters

Polyester (e.g. Surgidac, Mersilene)

Classification	Synthetic, non-absorbable, mono/multifilament
Composition	Polymer of polyethylene terephthalate
Manufacture	Coatings: polybutylate, Teflon, silicone
Absorption	Encapsulated by fibrous tissue
Loss of strength	Little or no loss
Tissue interaction	Most reactive of synthetic materials, especially if coat lost
Handling	Poor handling and knot security (five throws) required The strongest suture material Coating reduces drag but also knot security
Use	Slowly healing tissues Prosthetic ligaments Vessel anastomosis Alternative is usually available for all possible indications
Advantages	Very strong
Disadvantages	Potentiates infection which will persist Tissue reaction

▶

Surgical staplers

Vicky Lipscomb

Introduction

Surgical staplers may be used in a wide variety of cutaneous, abdominal, thoracic and other veterinary surgical procedures. Possible advantages of surgical staplers over manual suturing include:

- Reduction of surgical time (operative and anaesthetic)
- Reduced tissue trauma/manipulation
- Reduction or elimination of surgical contamination by intestinal contents
- Easy and secure closure of large vessels, vascular pedicles and gastrointestinal, lung, liver and splenic tissue (which is especially useful in areas that are difficult to reach and dissect manually).

Therefore, the use of stapling equipment may decrease the morbidity associated with a procedure in certain circumstances. Reduction in surgical time is most beneficial for critically ill patients. Using a surgical stapler does not compensate for inadequate surgical technique and may introduce additional complications. The basic principles of soft tissue surgery (see Chapter 21) and the principles of application of surgical staplers (Figure 6.1) must be followed.

- Do not staple tissue that is inflamed, oedematous or not viable.
- Every staple must penetrate all the layers of the tissue.
- Choose the correct staple size. In particular, the tissue must not be too thick or too thin for the closed staple to hold it securely.
- Do not place excessive amounts of tissue in the stapler.
- Inspect the tissue before firing to ensure that it is correctly aligned within the stapler and that no other tissue is caught up in the stapler.
- Carefully remove the stapler after firing, so as not to disrupt the staple or the staple line.
- Inspect the staple or staple line for haemorrhage, leakage or loose staples, especially at both ends of a staple line.

6.1 Principles of application of surgical staplers.

Linear staplers

Linear staplers (Figure 6.2) are also known as **thoracoabdominal** (TA) staplers.

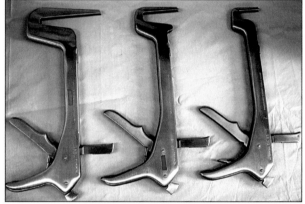

6.2 Selection of reusable linear staplers for use with different cartridge lengths.

Method of action

Linear staplers have a long handle with a pistol-type grip that facilitates stapling within the abdominal or thoracic cavity and a U-shaped end into which the tissue to be stapled is inserted. The staple cartridges (Figure 6.3) consist of the staples and an opposing anvil against which the staples are fired. The cartridge has a retaining pin which helps to ensure that the correct amount of tissue is placed, aligned correctly and kept within the jaws of the stapler during firing.

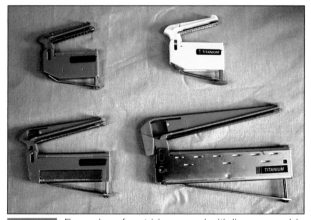

6.3 Examples of cartridges used with linear reusable staplers, including three lengths of a standard cartridge staple size (blue) and a 30 mm long vascular staple cartridge (white).

Tissue in the stapler is compressed by closing the approximating lever (see Figure 6.6d). If placement is unsatisfactory, the approximating lever can be opened and re-closed as required. If the approximating lever cannot be closed easily, the tissue is too thick to be stapled (many disposable staplers have markers on the approximating lever which, when lined up, confirm full compression of tissue). A safety lever keeps the handle of the stapler locked 'open', preventing inadvertent firing. The handle of the stapler cannot be moved until after this lever has been released.

The stapler is fired by squeezing the handle firmly and fully to ensure that the staples form properly into an inverted 'B' shape (Figure 6.4). It fires two or three staggered rows of titanium staples. The staggered rows and the staple configuration are designed to secure the tissues and achieve haemostasis whilst still allowing bloodflow through the microcirculation so that the tissue beyond the staple line does not become necrotic.

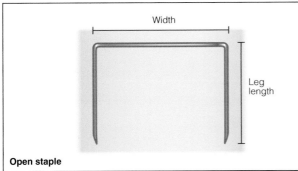

Open staple

Width

Leg length

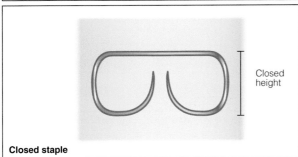

Closed staple

Closed height

6.4 B-shaped staple showing open and closed staple width, leg length and closed height.

Before releasing and removing the stapler, the cartridge unit is used as a guide for resection of the tissue beyond the stapler using a scalpel.

Types, sizes and cartridges

Linear staplers are available either as reusable stainless steel instruments that can be steam-sterilized, or as disposable instruments that may be sterilized in ethylene oxide and used a limited number of times. The stainless steel instruments are likely to be more cost-effective in the long term if stapling equipment is being used regularly, but the cost differential is not substantial. Both types accept single-use disposable cartridge units.

Linear staplers and corresponding cartridge units are available in various lengths ranging from 30 to 90 mm. The 'closed height' of the staple is the most important staple dimension for the surgeon because this determines the thickness of tissue to which the stapler may safely be applied.

- The '**standard**' size of staple cartridge usually contains staples that close tissue to a height of 1.5 mm, which means that they can only be used on tissues that can easily be compressed to 1.5 mm and must not be used on tissues that compress to less than 1.5 mm, as this might prevent an adequate seal at the stapled site.
- For thicker tissues (e.g. stomach), a larger ('**thick**') cartridge is available that can only be used on tissues that can easily be compressed to 2 mm and must not be used on tissues that compress to less than 2 mm.
- A '**vascular**' cartridge is available that closes tissues to a height of 1 mm and provides the increased security of three rows of staggered staples. This type of cartridge is only available in a 30 mm length.

Stapler cartridges are typically colour coded for convenience, e.g. blue for 'standard' cartridges, green for 'thick' cartridges and white for 'vascular' cartridges. Linear staplers that allow for variable adjustable final closed-staple height, or that have rotating or articulating heads to maximize access in deep cavities, are available but used less commonly.

Applications

Linear staplers are extremely versatile (Figure 6.5).

- Closure of the intestinal ends in the final stage of a functional end-to-end anastomosis procedure.
- Partial gastrectomy.
- Gastropexy.
- Partial or complete lung lobectomy.
- Partial or complete liver lobectomy.
- Partial splenectomy.
- Rectal tumour excision following a rectal eversion approach.
- Typhlectomy.
- Partial pancreatectomy.
- Partial prostatectomy.
- Excision of prostatic cysts.
- Closure of the vascular pedicle (e.g. during nephrectomy).
- Resection of right atrial appendage tumours.
- Closure of the vaginal or uterine pedicle during vaginectomy or hysterectomy.

6.5 Common applications of linear staples.

Linear staplers and linear cutter staplers may be used interchangeably in many situations. For example, a partial gastrectomy can be completed using a linear cutter stapler and/or a linear stapler (Figure 6.6). Vascular pedicles and stumps are often closed with 30 mm cartridge lengths.

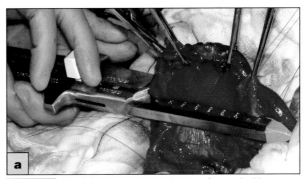

a

6.6 Partial gastrectomy being performed with a combination of **(a,b)** linear cutter staplers and **(c,d)** linear staplers. (continues) ▶

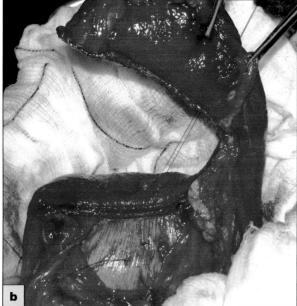

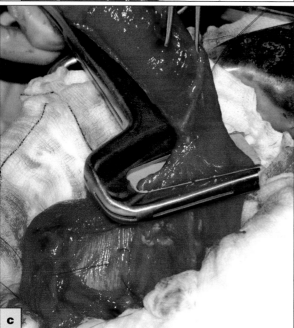

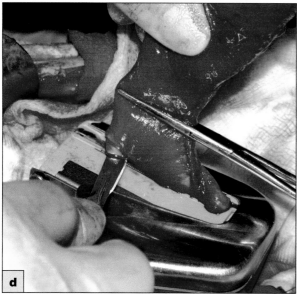

6.6 (continued) Partial gastrectomy being performed with a combination of **(a,b)** linear cutter staplers and **(c,d)** linear staplers.

Liver and spleen

When used on liver (Figure 6.7) or splenic tissue, the staple line must be very carefully inspected. Haemorrhage is unlikely if a vascular cartridge has been used, but if a larger staple cartridge has been used due to the thickness of the tissue (>1 mm) or the length required (>30 mm) additional sutures, vascular clips, application of a topical haemostatic agent and/or omentalization may be needed. The hilar vessels of the spleen should not be incorporated in a stapled partial splenectomy (Waldron and Robertson, 1995).

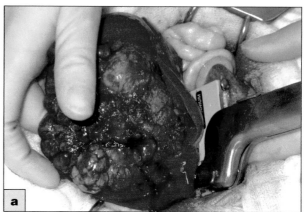

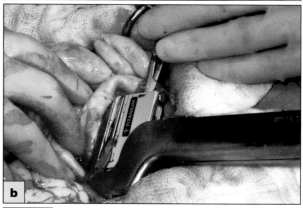

6.7 Complete liver lobectomy **(a)** before and **(b)** after placement of a linear stapler.

When linear staplers are used for hepatic lobectomy there is less haemorrhage, necrosis and inflammation compared with manual techniques (Lewis *et al.*, 1990). The liver lobe still needs to be dissected free of its attachments, which is more challenging on the right side due to the presence of the vena cava, but the surgery is still simpler than manual techniques because individual lobar vessels and hepatic ducts do not have to be isolated.

Lung lobectomy

For stapled complete and partial lung lobectomies, the closure is tested for leaks by filling the thoracic cavity with sterile saline as for manual closure. Any air leaks should be addressed by additional vascular clips or sutures (the bronchus is not routinely oversewn).

En bloc stapling of the bronchus and hilar vessels is regarded as safe, but in approximately 5% of animals the hilar vessels need additional sutures or vascular clips (LaRue *et al.*, 1987). Vascular cartridges that compress tissue to 1 mm are ideal for complete or partial lung lobectomy (Figure 6.8) but cartridges that compress tissue to 1.5 mm may also provide adequate haemostasis for thicker hilar stumps.

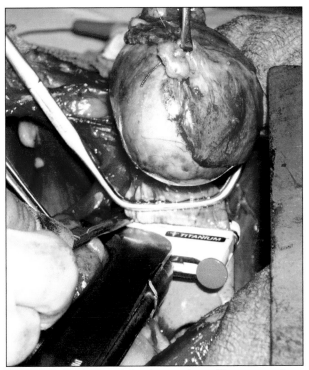

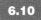 Partial lung lobectomy using a 30 mm vascular
staple cartridge.

Use of a stapling device for complete lung lobectomy in dogs with pneumonia does not affect the complication or perioperative mortality rates compared to conventional suturing (Murphy *et al.*, 1997).

Linear cutter staplers

Linear cutter staplers (Figure 6.9) are also known as **gastrointestinal anastomosis (GIA)** or **intestinal linear anastomosis (ILA)** staplers, though they also have applications outside the gastrointestinal tract.

Method of action

Linear cutter staplers consist of two straight interlocking arms, one of which accepts the staple cartridge containing the staples and a bisecting blade. Each arm is placed on either side of the tissue to be divided and the two arms are locked together. The lock lever must be fully closed and there is usually an audible click that confirms this. The lock lever can be released

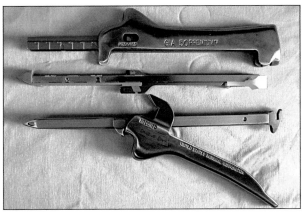

6.9 Reusable linear cutter with the two arms disassembled and a single-use cartridge in the middle.

to allow repositioning. There is no retaining pin and the surgeon must ensure that the tissue in the stapler does not extend beyond the length of the staple cartridge. If excessive force is required to lock the two arms around the tissue, the tissue is too thick or too oedematous to be stapled.

The push-bar handle slides forward to fire four rows of staggered B-shaped titanium staples and the blade divides between rows 2 and 3 (see Figure 6.6). The incision made by the blade stops 8 mm before the end of the staple line. The push-bar handle slides all the way back to its original position before the two arms of the stapler can be uncoupled and removed.

Types, sizes and cartridges

Linear cutter staplers are available as reusable stainless steel or disposable instruments. The surgeon must choose the correct cartridge length and staple size for the tissue being stapled.

- Reusable stainless steel GIA instruments are available in 50 or 90 mm lengths and only accept staple cartridges that close tissue to 1.5 mm.
- An ILA reusable instrument is available for use with a cartridge 100 mm long that closes tissue to a height of 2 mm.
- Disposable GIA staplers are available that accept 55, 60, 75, 80 and 100 mm cartridge lengths (depending on the manufacturer) and staples that close tissue to 1.5 mm or 2 mm.
- A 60 mm disposable GIA stapler is also available that accepts a vascular staple cartridge that closes tissue to a height of 1 mm.

Applications

Uses of linear cutter staplers are listed in Figure 6.10.

- Partial gastrectomy.
- Functional end-to-end anastomosis of intestine.
- Partial lung lobectomy.
- Partial liver lobectomy.
- Resection of oesophageal or rectal diverticula.
- Prostatic cyst resection.
- Typhlectomy.
- Side-to-side anastomosis of small intestine to stomach (e.g. Bilroth II surgery).

6.10 Uses of linear cutter staplers in clinical veterinary practice.

Partial gastrectomy

One of the most useful applications of a linear cutter stapler is for rapid partial gastrectomy during gastric dilatation–volvulus surgery (see Figure 6.6). In this situation 20–50% of the stomach is often resected, necessitating the use of multiple staple cartridges, which should be overlapped. A staple size that compresses tissue to 2 mm is usually used and it is recommended that staple lines are oversewn with a manual continuous inverting suture pattern, because there is a risk of gastric mucosal necrosis even if the serosa appears viable in dogs with gastric dilatation–volvulus (Pavletic, 1990).

End-to-end anastomosis

A very useful application of a linear cutter stapler is to perform a functional end-to-end anastomosis (Technique 6.1).

TECHNIQUE 6.1
Performing a stapled functional end-to-end intestinal anastomosis

1 Place two stay sutures through opposing edges of both intestinal lumens to assist manipulation of the tissues and placement of the staplers.

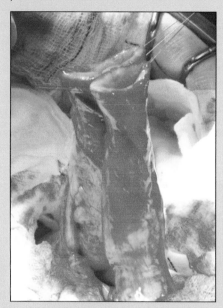

2 Appose the anti-mesenteric surfaces of the intestinal ends (this will produce an anti-peristaltic side-to-side anastomosis) and fully insert each arm of the linear cutter stapler (55–75 mm cartridge length, depending on the manufacturer) into the ends of the intestinal lumen. Couple and lock stapler in place and fire to produce a linear intestinal anastomosis with two rows of staggered staples either side of the stoma.

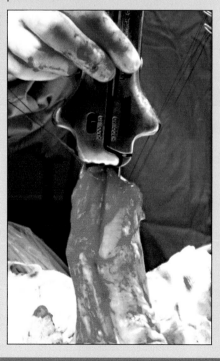

3 Carefully withdraw the stapler and use the stay sutures to inspect the staple line internally and externally. Use the stay sutures to offset the staple lines by approximately 0.5–1.0 cm so that they are not directly in contact with each other when the intestinal lumen is closed.

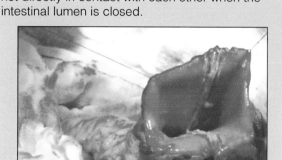

4 Place a linear stapler or linear cutter stapler across the now common opening of all the intestinal edges to close them. It is important to ensure that the staple lines stay offset and that all layers of the intestine are fully included and do not slip out as the stapler is closed.

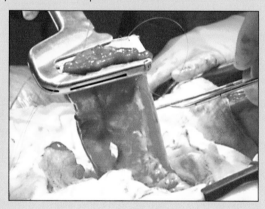

5 Place a partial-thickness anchoring suture at the base of the first staple line ('crotch of the trousers'). This is where there is greatest tension and suture placement minimizes the risk of staples being pulled out.

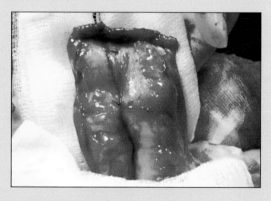

6 Close the mesenteric defect using sutures. There is no need to oversew the staple line but it should be omentalized as for any other intestinal anastomosis.

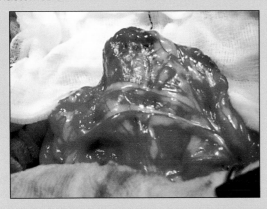

An obvious advantage of a stapled functional end-to-end anastomosis is that luminal disparity is easily accommodated. Complication rates for animals undergoing a stapled functional end-to-end anastomosis compare favourably with manually sutured anastomoses: in one case series no complications relating to the surgical anastomosis procedure were reported (White, 2008); and in another case series 2 of 24 animals had minor leakage (requiring one or two simple interrupted sutures) that was discovered incidentally on re-exploration for abdominal closure following postoperative open peritoneal drainage for pre-existing peritonitis (Ullman et al., 1991). Additionally, there are no consistent differences in dehiscence rates between stapled and manually sutured anastomoses in randomized human trials. Strictures are not encountered following the use of the linear cutter stapler, because it creates a stoma that is larger than the original intestinal lumen.

Partial liver and lung lobectomies

Partial liver and lung lobectomies can be performed with linear cutter staplers (Figure 6.11) or linear staplers (see Figures 6.7 and 6.8). The benefit of using a linear cutter compared with a linear stapler is that both ends are sealed, which is extremely convenient, but linear cutter staplers do need more room for placement.

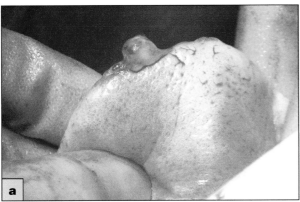

6.11 Partial lung lobectomy performed with a linear cutter for excision of **(a)** a pulmonary bleb. (continues) ▶

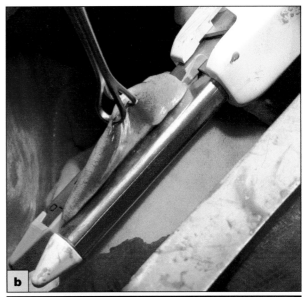

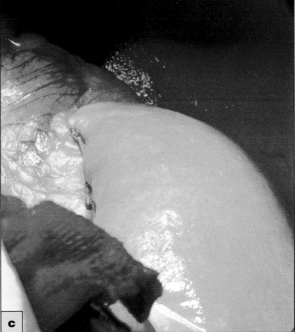

6.11 (continued) Partial lung lobectomy performed with a linear cutter for excision of a pulmonary bleb. **(b)** Application of stapler and **(c)** appearance of the staple line.

Bilroth II procedures

Clinical reports of Bilroth II procedures, either stapled or manually performed, are scarce in the veterinary literature. A stapled Bilroth II procedure that was fast and reliable in experimental dogs has been described (Ahmadu-Suka et al., 1988). In this study, there was no leakage or mechanical problems but additional sutures were occasionally required at the tissue margin, and some or all of the complications (vomiting, anorexia, diarrhoea, weight loss) that have been reported in humans undergoing Bilroth II surgery were seen in all dogs.

Circular staplers

Circular staplers are used to perform end-to-end anastomoses (EEA) in the gastrointestinal tract (Figure 6.12).

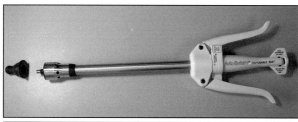

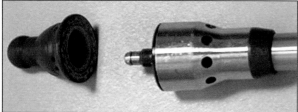

6.12 Circular stapler for performing end-to-end anastomosis. Reproduced from *BSAVA Manual of Canine and Feline Abdominal Surgery.*

Method of action

Circular staplers place two staggered circumferential rows of B-shaped titanium staples full thickness through each inverted gastrointestinal wall and cut two circular segments of redundant gastrointestinal tract tissue from each end to produce a two-layer inverting anastomosis.

The stapler has a long handle with a central rod at the end on to which a circular staple cartridge with a circular blade is inserted. A dome-shaped anvil screws on to the central rod after it has passed through the staple cartridge.

Types, sizes and cartridges

Circular staplers are available as reusable stainless steel or disposable instruments with outer diameters ranging from 21 mm to 34 mm. Newer disposable circular staplers have the widest range of available outer diameters and a curved shaft with a tilting mechanism to aid placement in areas that are difficult to access.

- Staple cartridges that close tissue to a height of approximately 2 mm are available for most circular staplers.
- Staple cartridges that close tissue to approximately 1.5 mm are also available for use with some of the smaller circular staplers.

Reusable or disposable ovoid sizers are available in sizes that match the outer diameters of the various staplers. They are lubricated and used to dilate the bowel gently prior to insertion of the stapler and enable the surgeon to select the correct cartridge size.

The inner diameter of the staple cartridge corresponds to the diameter of the stoma that will be created in the anastomosis. A stapler should not be used if the intestine is stretched by introducing the cartridge. Intestinal lumen size should be slightly larger in diameter than the stapler, but as big a stapler as possible should be used to ensure an adequate stomal size.

Applications

Circular staplers are much more limited in their application than other types of staplers in small animal practice. They are technically more demanding to apply and they can only be used if the size of the

bowel lumen is big enough to accept the currently available sizes of circular stapler. A further consideration in cats and small dogs is that the bowel lumen diameter may be compromised by the inverting nature of the anastomosis.

Colorectal anastomosis

The circular stapler can be introduced through the anus for a colorectal anastomosis or through an access incision in the adjacent gastrointestinal tract. Access to the colon and rectum within the pelvic canal may be difficult, particularly in cats and male dogs with small or narrow pelvic canals. Each end of gastrointestinal tract to be anastomosed is tied down using a purse-string suture over the anvil and cartridge end of the stapler, respectively. There must be sufficient tissue present to allow proper inversion of the intestinal edges.

A disposable automatic purse-string device can be used or a purse-string suture can be placed manually, which is recommended if the tissue is likely to compress to <1 mm. Disposable automatic purse-string devices have two jaws and ring handles that are squeezed together to clamp the device perpendicularly around the bowel. They place a circumferential suture secured by stainless steel staples (the suture type and length vary depending on the manufacturer). Another alternative is a reusable Furniss clamp purse-string device, which is secured around the bowel perpendicular to the long axis and allows quick passage of a straight needle with swaged-on suture material through the clamp to create a circumferential suture. The stapling procedure is described below.

1. Any redundant tissue beyond the purse-string is excised and the suture ends are cut short.
2. The wing nut of the circular stapler is turned to compress the two segments of gastrointestinal tract together until the indicators on the stapler are aligned (the tissues are also visualized during this process to check that sufficient inverted gastrointestinal tract wall from both ends is fully incorporated within the stapler).
3. The stapler is fired by squeezing the handle and the wing nut is loosened to allow careful removal of the stapler.
4. The stapler removes with it the two purse-string sutures and two doughnut-shaped segments of gastrointestinal tract excised from the inverted gastrointestinal tissue.
5. The excised tissues are inspected to ensure that both full-thickness walls of gastrointestinal tract have been included around the full circumference of the anastomosis, i.e. two complete rings of tissue are present. The excised tissue can also be submitted for histopathology if evaluation of margins in relation to tumour excision is required.
6. The staple line is checked and the access site, if present, can be closed manually or using a linear stapler.
7. The stapled anastomosis is omentalized as for a manually sutured anastomosis.

Colorectal masses

Circular staplers have been used in dogs and cats for distal colonic or proximal rectal anastomoses using a combined transrectal and laparotomy approach. They are most useful for excision of colorectal masses that cannot be manually anastomosed via a single laparotomy, rectal pull-through or dorsal approach because there is insufficient room due to the mass being too large and/or located too far within the pelvic canal (Banz *et al.*, 2008). Circular staplers may also be used to avoid the potential increased morbidity associated with these other approaches or a pubic symphysiotomy approach (Banz *et al.*, 2008).

Subtotal colectomy in cats

Circular staplers have been used in cats for performing subtotal colectomy to treat acquired megacolon (Kudisch and Pavletic, 1993). In these cats the circular stapler was introduced into the colon via the caecum (instead of transanally), which simplifies the surgery because everything is performed via one approach. Successful use of circular staplers in combination with a dorsal approach to the rectum has been reported in experimental cats (Fucci *et al.*, 1992). Long-term clinical problems associated with defecation were not reported by owners of these cats following subtotal colectomy, for which prognosis appears to be excellent, although two cats in this study did require a blood transfusion to treat haemorrhage in the immediate postoperative period.

Other applications

Other reported uses include gastro-oesophageal anastomosis (e.g. following subtotal gastro-oesophageal resection to treat extensive gastric necrosis resulting from gastric dilatation–volvulus), oesophageal anastomoses, end-to-end gastrointestinal anastomosis as part of a Bilroth I procedure and end-to-side gastrointestinal anastomosis as part of a Bilroth II procedure (Pavletic, 1990). However, a Bilroth II is probably easier to perform using a combination of linear cutter and linear staplers (see above).

Experimentally, early strength of circular stapled gastrointestinal anastomoses has been reported as being similar (Stoloff *et al.*, 1984) or less than (Dziki *et al.*, 1991) manually sutured end-to-end anastomoses. Clinically, anastomoses using circular staplers are reported to save time (Dziki *et al.*, 1991) without increasing the risk of postoperative dehiscence (Kudisch and Pavletic, 1993; Banz *et al.*, 2008).

Strictures are a frequently reported complication following the use of circular staplers (Dziki *et al.*, 1991; Banz *et al.*, 2008) and so the surgeon must try to use the largest size that can be accommodated by the intestinal lumen.

Ligate and divide stapler (LDS)

The LDS stapler (Figure 6.13) places two U-shaped staples around a vessel and divides the tissue between them.

Method of action

The LDS stapler has a handle in the shape of a pistol. The vessel or vessels to be ligated are placed within the C-shaped jaws of the stapler and the stapler is fired by squeezing the handle. Care must be taken to keep the instrument steady when firing, because movement during application can tear the vessel. Vessels up to 7 mm wide that can be compressed to less than 0.75 mm can be safely secured using this technique. There is a safety mechanism that prevents firing of the stapler when the cartridge is empty.

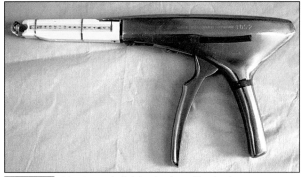

6.13 Ligate and divide stapler with single-use cartridge inserted.

Types, sizes and cartridges

A reusable stainless steel LDS stapler is available that accepts a disposable cartridge containing stainless steel staples. Single-use gas-powered LDS staplers accept disposable cartridges containing titanium staples but cannot be reloaded and so are relatively expensive.

The tissue should be thick enough for the staple not to slip on the pedicle, but excessive tissue should not be forced into the jaws of the stapler: as an approximate guide, the vessel/tissue pedicle should measure between one-third and two-thirds of the staple width. Vessels that require double ligation (e.g. major arteries and veins such as the splenic artery and vein) must have an additional single staple or manual ligature applied before the stapler is used.

Applications

LDS staplers save the surgeon considerable time during procedures that require multiple vessel ligations, e.g. splenectomy (Figure 6.14) or resection of omental adhesions, and their use is associated with minimal complications.

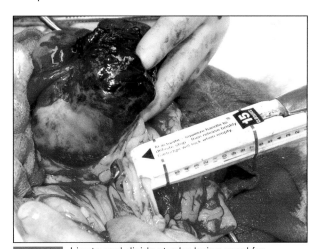

6.14 Ligate and divide stapler being used for splenectomy.

Vascular clip applicators

Vascular clip applicators (Figure 6.15) place a metallic V-shaped clip around a vessel. Their small fine jaws make these applicators useful for ligation of small vessels, compared with the relatively bulky LDS staplers, which are suited to larger vessels and vascular pedicles.

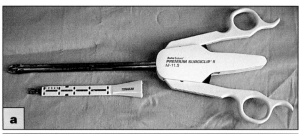

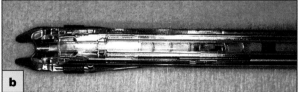

6.15 **(a)** Vascular clip applicator, where **(b)** the staple is automatically reloaded at the tip after firing.

Method of action

Vascular clip applicators have a long handle with a scissor-type grip, which is squeezed firmly to secure the staple in place and then released carefully so as not to disturb the staple during removal. The vessel must still be adequately dissected and exposed so that application of the clip can be performed accurately and leave enough tissue (e.g. 2–3 mm) beyond the clip to prevent its slippage. As a general guide the vessel width should not exceed half to three-quarters of the vascular clip width.

Types and sizes

There is a wide selection of clip applicators available that have different features, including:

- The number of clips they hold
- The size of clips available
- Whether or not the device holds multiple clips which automatically replace at the tip on firing (see Figure 6.15), compared with those where single clips are manually loaded into the device after every use
- Whether or not the clips have a locking mechanism for increased security
- Whether or not the devices are single-use or may be reloaded with additional cartridges
- Whether or not they can be re-sterilized and by what method
- What the staple is made of (e.g. metal *versus* absorbable material).

Variations in these features will affect whether a particular vascular clip applicator is suitable for a particular surgical use and/or cost-effective for individual veterinary practices. The most useful and economic choice for veterinary surgery is usually a device that holds multiple clips (e.g. 10–20), allowing rapid and easy application during surgery, but which can be re-sterilized until all the remaining clips have been used.

Applications

Vascular clips can be used in almost any surgical procedure in place of suture ligatures but are particularly useful where surgical access is limited, where traditional ligatures may be difficult to apply and during surgeries requiring application of many vessel ligatures (e.g. tumour excision).

An added advantage in oncological surgery is that postoperative imaging of the clips can be performed to help with any radiation treatment planning. Stainless steel clips can be used as radiopaque surgical markers; titanium clips have the added advantage of not interfering with computed tomography or magnetic resonance imaging studies.

Vascular clips have been used for attenuation of patent ductus arteriosus (PDA) in dogs via a conventional thoracotomy (Corti *et al.*, 2000) or a thoracoscopic approach (Borenstein *et al.*, 2004) but complete elimination of ductal flow is not a consistent finding and some PDAs are too big for total occlusion using vascular clips.

Vascular clips have few drawbacks but great care must be taken where they have been used, because they are more easily dislodged than traditional ligatures.

Skin staplers

Skin staplers are the most commonly used stapler in veterinary surgery and their proposed advantages and disadvantages are outlined in Figure 6.16. As for skin sutures, all the wound tension should be borne by the underlying tissues and not the skin staples. Placement of a subcuticular or intradermal suture layer prior to stapling achieves this and places the skin edges in close apposition, producing an ideal wound for skin stapling. This is a crucial step and skin wounds closed with staples but without appropriate suturing of the underlying tissues are less secure and will be at increased risk of wound breakdown and/or infection. If the skin edges are not perfectly aligned they may be held together with thumb forceps to facilitate accurate placement of the skin staple.

Advantages
- Increased speed of wound closure.
- Do not increase risk of delayed healing, infection or poor wound cosmesis (provided they are applied correctly).
- Cost-effective.

Disadvantages
- Correcting malapposed skin is more difficult.
- Skin staplers slightly evert skin edges of wound.
- Less secure wound closure.
- Tend to rotate (becoming ineffective or stuck in tissues) in very mobile areas (e.g. groin, axilla) or thin skin (e.g. cats).
- If there is increased wound tension, manual sutures are still preferred.

6.16 Advantages and disadvantages of skin staplers.

Method of action

Skin staples form a rectangle when fired into the closed position. The skin stapler should be placed directly perpendicular to the skin incision to optimize apposition of the skin edges. As with skin sutures, a gap should be left between the wound and the skin staple to allow for postoperative swelling and they should be placed approximately 0.5–1.0 cm apart. A dedicated staple remover is required to remove skin staples.

Types and sizes

There are many different designs of skin stapler but those typically used in veterinary surgery have a palm grip, fixed head and stainless steel staples, because these are easy to use and cost-effective. The ideal properties of palm-grip fixed-head skin staplers include:

- An audible click to confirm that staple formation is complete
- A staple counter
- Easy staple alignment (low-profile head; open clear nose piece with distinct arrows; pre-cock mechanism)
- Secure staple placement (firm attachment to skin, no rotation)
- Good staple depth control
- Easy staple removal.

These properties have been compared for various brands of skin stapler in an experimental dog cadaver study (Smeak and Crocker, 1997). Most skin staplers are manufactured to be for single use but in practice they may be re-sterilized using ethylene oxide or hydrogen peroxide gas plasma without any significant decrease in function, so that all the preloaded staples in the unit can be utilized (Smeak and Crocker, 1997).

Skin staples are usually between 5 mm and 7 mm wide, depending on the manufacturer and whether a regular or wide staple width has been selected.

Applications

In addition to skin wound closure, skin staplers have been used clinically to attach skin grafts, close gastrotomy and enterotomy wounds and perform intestinal anastomoses (Coolman et al., 2000ab). They may also be used in a wide variety of situations to secure drains, dressings and tubes to animals.

Current and future developments

Endoscopic versions of some of the staplers described, including linear and linear cutters, have been used successfully in minimally invasive surgery, which is a rapidly expanding field of veterinary surgery. The small size of endoscopic staplers may also be useful during conventional open surgery, e.g. to perform a cholecystoduodenostomy (Morrison et al., 2008).

Absorbable staples have not yet found common uses in the veterinary field but are particularly useful for gynaecological surgery in women and applications in veterinary surgery may yet be discovered. Sutureless biofragmentable anastomosis rings (BARs) are used widely in the human field for intestinal anastomosis and have been used to perform subtotal colectomy in cats with idiopathic megacolon (Ryan et al., 2006).

Conclusion

Surgical staplers save time during surgery without increasing the risks, which is most beneficial for critically ill animals. There are some procedures where the use of staplers is now the preferred method. Complications following the use of stapling devices are low provided that they are applied correctly by a surgeon trained in their use, using good surgical judgement.

The two main manufacturers of stapling products worldwide are Autosuture (Covidien) and Ethicon (Johnson & Johnson). It has not been the intention here to promote or omit discussion of any specific stapling product and readers are advised to contact the individual distributors of these products in the UK for current recommendations on all available products, details of specific product dimensions, their indications and limitations.

References and further reading

Ahmadu-Suka F, Withrow SJ, Nelson AW et al. (1988) Bilroth II gastrojejunostomy in dogs. Stapling technique and postoperative complications. Veterinary Surgery **17**, 211–219

Banz WJ, Jackson J, Richter K et al. (2008) Transrectal stapling for colonic resection and anastomosis (10 cases). Journal of the American Animal Hospital Association **44**, 198–204

Borenstein N, Behr L, Chetboul V et al. (2004) Minimally invasive patent ductus arteriosus occlusion in 5 dogs. Veterinary Surgery **33**, 309–313

Clark GN and Pavletic MM (1991) Partial gastrectomy with an automatic stapling instrument for treatment of gastric necrosis secondary to gastric dilatation–volvulus. Veterinary Surgery **20**, 61–68

Coolman BR, Ehrhart N and Marretta SM (2000a) Use of skin staples for rapid closure of gastrointestinal incisions in the treatment of canine linear foreign bodies. Journal of the American Animal Hospital Association **36**, 542–547

Coolman BR, Ehrhart N, Pijanowski G et al. (2000b) Comparison of skin staples with sutures for anastomosis of the small intestine in dogs. Veterinary Surgery **29**, 293–302

Corti LB, Merkley D, Nelson OL et al. (2000) Retrospective evaluation of occlusion of patent ductus arteriosus with haemoclips in 20 dogs. Journal of the American Animal Hospital Association **36**, 548–555

Dziki AJ, Duncan MD, Harmon JW et al. (1991) Advantages of handsewn over stapled bowel anastomosis. Diseases of the Colon and Rectum **34**, 442–448

Fucci V, Newton JC, Hedlund CS et al. (1992) Rectal surgery in the cat: a comparison of suture versus staple technique through a dorsal approach. Journal of the American Animal Hospital Association **28**, 519–526

Kudisch M and Pavletic MM (1993) Subtotal colectomy with surgical stapling instruments via a trans-cecal approach for treatment of acquired megacolon in cats. Veterinary Surgery **22**, 457–463

LaRue SM, Withrow SJ and Wykes PM (1987) Lung resection using surgical staples in dogs and cats. Veterinary Surgery **16**, 238–240

Lewis DD, Bellenger CR, Lewis DT et al. (1990) Hepatic lobectomy in the dog: a comparison of stapling and ligation techniques. Veterinary Surgery **19**, 221–225

Morrison S, Prostredny J and Roa D (2008) Retrospective study of 28 cases of cholecystoduodenostomy performed using endoscopic gastrointestinal anastomosis stapling equipment. Journal of the American Animal Hospital Association **44**, 10–18

Murphy ST, Ellison GW, McKiernan BC et al. (1997) Pulmonary lobectomy in the management of pneumonia in dogs: 59 cases (1972–1994). Journal of the American Veterinary Medical Association **210**, 235–239

Pavletic MM (1990) Surgical stapling devices in small animal surgery. Compendium on Continuing Education for the Practicing Veterinarian **12**, 1724–1740

Pavletic MM (1994) Stapling in esophageal surgery. Veterinary Clinics of North America: Small Animal Practice **24** (2), 395–412

Ryan S, Seim H III, Macphail C et al. (2006) Comparison of biofragmentable anastomosis ring and sutured anastomoses for subtotal colectomy in cats with idiopathic megacolon. Veterinary Surgery **35**, 740–748

Smeak DD and Crocker C (1997) Fixed-head skin staplers: features and performance. Compendium on Continuing Education **19**, 1358–1368

Stoloff D, Snider TG III, Crawford MP et al. (1984) End-to-end colonic anastomosis: a comparison of techniques in normal dogs. Veterinary Surgery **13**, 76–82

Swiderski J and Withrow S (2009) A novel surgical stapling technique for rectal mass removal: a retrospective analysis. Journal of the American Animal Hospital Association **45**, 67–71

Tobias KM (2007) Surgical stapling devices in veterinary medicine: a review. Veterinary Surgery **36**, 341–349

Ullman SL, Pavletic MM and Clark GN (1991) Open intestinal anastomosis with surgical stapling equipment in 24 dogs and cats. Veterinary Surgery **20**, 385–391

Waldron DR and Robertson J (1995) Partial splenectomy in the dog: a comparison of stapling and ligation techniques. Journal of the American Animal Hospital Association **431**, 343–348

White RN (2008) Modified functional end-to-end stapled intestinal anastomosis: technique and clinical results in 15 dogs. Journal of Small Animal Practice **49**, 274–281

Surgical lasers

Noel Berger and Peter H. Eeg

Introduction

LASER is the acronym for Light Amplification by Stimulated Emission of Radiation. Increasing knowledge and availability has made it more practical for veterinary surgeons to own and operate surgical lasers. With a full understanding of laser physics and safety and following the basic preparations discussed below, veterinary surgeons can quickly master surgical lasers and make use of them in a variety of procedures.

At present, the most commonly used form of laser for small animal soft tissue surgery applications is carbon dioxide gas (CO_2). Yttrium–aluminium–garnet (**YAG**) lasers such as erbium-doped YAG (**Er:YAG**), holmium-doped YAG (**Ho:YAG**) or neodymium-doped YAG (**Nd:YAG**) are less commonly used.

Possible advantages of surgical lasers include:

- Decreased postoperative pain
- Decreased haemorrhage
- Reduced tissue swelling.

Physics of laser light

Laser light is distinctly different from other light in how its photons are generated, organized, confined and transmitted. This can be illustrated by comparing white light produced from an incandescent light bulb with light from a laser (Figure 7.1). White light is composed of wavelengths radiating in all directions at varying amplitudes and frequencies. In the laser beam,

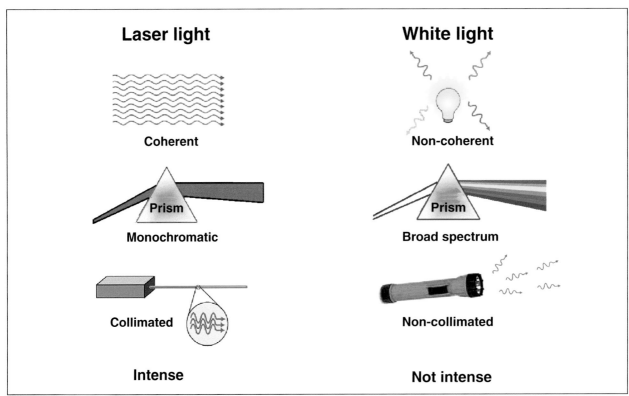

Laser light	White light
Coherent	Non-coherent
Monochromatic	Broad spectrum
Collimated	Non-collimated
Intense	Not intense

7.1 Laser light is coherent, monochromatic, collimated and intense. Note the differences between laser light and the white light produced by an incandescent light bulb.

photons are emitted in parallel and in phase with each other and are collimated. Photons emitted from a single compound or atom producing consistent energy released at the same wavelength, amplitude, frequency, direction and time are considered a laser beam. A laser therefore produces a beam of one type of photon (monochromatic) and is a very intense form of energy. Measurements of laser output are shown in Figure 7.2.

- Laser light output is described in terms of:
  o **Energy**, measured in **joules** (J)
  o **Power**, measured in **watts** (W).
- Laser energy dose delivered to an area is described in terms of **fluence**, or **energy density**, and is expressed in joules/cm² (J/cm²).
- The very important concept of **power density** refers to the amount of energy delivered to a given area per unit of time and is expressed in watts/cm² (W/cm², where W = J/second).

7.2   Measurements of laser output.

The power that a laser delivers can be controlled by changing either the diameter of the beam or the amount of time that the energy is delivered. When a laser beam contacts a target tissue, the diameter of the circular pattern produced is called the **spot size** and can be altered by using either focusing tips or a lensed focusing handpiece. For a given power, a small spot size has a higher power density than a large spot size, and increasing the spot size will decrease the power density.

PRACTICAL TIPS

- If the distance between a focusing tip and the target is altered, it will change the intensity delivered.
- If a non-focused beam is used, the intensity can only be altered by changing the power.

Successful surgical laser use requires an understanding of the relationship between:

- Power output
- Spot size of the beam
- Distance to the target tissue
- Angle of targeting
- Length of delivery time.

Modes

A laser can be operated in three modes, which alter the way in which energy is delivered to the target tissue:

- **Continuous wave mode** (**CW**), in which laser energy is continually released through an open shutter during activation
- **Pulsed wave mode** (**PW**), which allows laser energy to be released in repeated bursts (milliseconds in duration)
- **Superpulse mode** (**SP**), which provides bursts of laser energy at high peaks, accompanied by rests in a shorter pulse duration (microsecond range). This higher peak energy release, coupled with increased rate of pulse repetition, effectively eliminates heat accumulation in the peripheral tissue. Superpulse waveforms minimize thermal damage to normal tissue adjacent to surgical sites. The added benefit is cooling of the peripheral tissue between pulses, which maximizes vaporization effects and minimizes thermal accumulation, together reducing heat trauma over time.

Absorption and scatter

Changes to the wavelength of the emitted beam will alter the degree to which it is absorbed or scattered by the target tissue. There is no single wavelength produced by a laser that will optimally assist every surgical procedure.

- Lasers whose wavelengths are predominantly *absorbed* by tissue but experience little or no scatter make exceptional incisive *tissue vaporizers* but poor coagulators. Examples of these 'what you see is what you get' lasers are the CO_2 at 10,600 nm and the Er:YAG at 2940 nm.
- Lasers whose wavelengths are *scattered* significantly more than they are absorbed by tissue, or are absorbed by multiple tissue components, produce more coagulating effects. Typically, lasers with wavelengths between 600 nm and 1400 nm are good *tissue coagulators* because of the increased tissue that becomes thermally excited. Diode lasers (635–1064 nm) and the Nd:YAG laser at 1064 nm are examples of a coagulative tool.

Laser types

A variety of lasers are commercially available (Figure 7.3). Each wavelength of laser energy has unique properties that can be utilized for specific techniques and procedures. The major wavelengths are:

- CO_2 laser: 10,600 nm
- Semiconductor diode lasers: 635–1064 nm
- Nd:YAG laser: 1064 nm
- Holmium laser: 2100 nm
- Excimer lasers: 193 nm.

Biostimulation laser wavelengths vary (see section on Laser therapy).

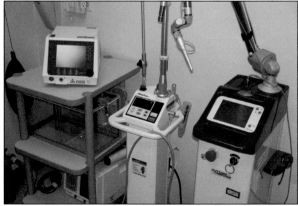

7.3   Three common commercially available surgical lasers: (left to right) Accuvet 25D-980 Diode Surgical Laser; Novapulse 20 watt CO_2 laser; Cutting Edge ML030 30 watt CO_2 laser.

Carbon dioxide lasers

The CO_2 laser wavelength (10,600 nm) is ideal for cutting and vaporization because it is highly absorbed by water at the peak of the 10.6 µm absorption band. It can cut tissue cleanly when the beam is focused and can debulk tissue, providing adequate haemostasis when the beam is defocused. At the tissue interface, blood vessels <0.6 mm in diameter can be coagulated and sealed, improving visibility of the surgical field. Lymphatics are also sealed, so postoperative oedema may be reduced and the number of secondary chemotactic factors initiating inflammatory responses decreased. In the authors experience, using a visual analogue scale, there seems to be less pain associated with a laser incision compared with the apparently more painful effect of a scalpel incision (Mison *et al.*, 2002).

Light from the CO_2 laser generator can be delivered to the target tissue by either an articulated arm or a hollow reflective wave guide. An articulated arm usually has a series of straight sections and allows light transmission by a series of highly reflective mirrors perfectly aligned within the mechanical system. The mirrors may be fixed in position, or they may be mounted within jointed elbows. The collimated beam arising from such an articulated arm is the same as at the source generator; it can therefore be used unaltered, or passed through a focusing tip. An alternative for wavelengths not suited to fibreoptic transmission is to use a hollow wave guide (essentially a highly reflective flexible cylindrical tube), but the resulting beam will have reduced energy and will no longer be collimated, so must be used through a focusing tip.

Focusing tips produce a range of beam diameters, from 0.25 mm to 1.4 mm. The tips may be straight or curved and come in a variety of lengths. The spot size will be the same as the diameter of the focusing tip if held at the focal distance (usually 1–3 mm from the target tissue).

PRACTICAL TIPS

- The focused beam diverges distal to the focal area, so the power density of the spot can be reduced by moving the handpiece away from the tissue. Since the area of this circular spot is related to the square of the diameter, the power density of the beam will diminish exponentially by increasing the spot size using the same power setting.
- For example, the power density of 8 W focused by the 0.8 mm tip is the same as the power density of 2 W focused by the 0.4 mm tip.

Scanner attachments can be used to ablate large areas of tissue, by generating a scanned laser pattern of up to 3–5 mm in diameter *versus* the standard spot size of 0.25–1.4 mm, making quicker work of ablating larger surface areas with less peripheral tissue damage.

Semiconductor diode lasers

Recent engineering and commercial applications have allowed development of diode lasers producing wavelengths from approximately 635 nm to 980 nm. Diode lasers used in veterinary medicine typically are in the range of 808–980 nm, delivering power up to 25 W, but higher power is also available commercially. It must be noted that increased peripheral tissue heating is a side effect of their use.

The lasers can be used with a variety of delivery fibre tips through an endoscope, otoscope or bronchoscope. They can be used in non-contact mode for non-focused deep tissue coagulation and vascular effects. Carbonization of the cleaved tip allows precise cutting

or vaporization in tissue contact mode. Diode wavelengths also make up the majority of therapy lasers currently being utilized. The diode laser can significantly complement CO_2 laser use in veterinary practice.

Nd:YAG lasers

The neodymium-doped YAG laser differs greatly from the CO_2 laser because light of this wavelength (1064 nm) is transmitted though tissue, in addition to the observed surface tissue effect. Nd:YAG lasers can deliver high powers of up to 100 W through silicon-based optical transmitting fibres, which can easily be inserted into working channels of standard gastrointestinal endoscopes, otoscopes and bronchoscopes. Fairly rapid tissue vaporization is possible with a bare fibre, but collateral thermal injury may be substantial and produce unrewarding postoperative effects. In the authors' opinion this laser wavelength should only be used by very knowledgeable and experienced laser practitioners.

Holmium lasers

Clinical holmium lasers are used sparingly in veterinary medicine for arthroscopic surgery, lithotripsy and very limited general surgery. While this wavelength of laser (2100 nm) interacts with water much like the CO_2 laser, it has a very shallow depth of penetration (0.3 mm). Small thermal necrosis zones provide better surgical precision and adequate haemostasis in very sensitive anatomical regions. This wavelength of laser energy is provided in slow pulse rates and is therefore inappropriate for general incisional uses. The acoustic energy of the holmium laser can provide energy for lithotripsy of gallstones or urological calculi disruption via a photo-disruptive effect. However, this is a slow process and up to 3 hours may be required to complete photo-disruption of stones.

Excimer lasers

The 193 nm excimer laser has the ability to incise tissue and leave a peripheral thermal event of less than 1 µm. The incision heals rapidly and there is minimal inflammation. The excimer laser is superior for corneal refractive sculpting. This wavelength is currently in high demand for use in radial keratotomy, but it is ineffective in a blood-filled field. Currently cost, size and safety considerations provide too many disadvantages for inclusion in the average veterinary practice.

Safety considerations

It is imperative that all veterinary surgeons and technicians who work in a facility where lasers are used are trained in laser hazards and safety.

Lasers are divided into four classes according to the degree of hazard they present, particularly with respect to ocular damage through inadvertent exposure (Figure 7.4). Class III and IV lasers pose serious hazards to nearby personnel as well as to the laser surgeon. Warning signs, optical shielding and built-in safety components to shut off the laser in an emergency may be required. A laser safety officer must be named and a log must be kept when these lasers are being used clinically. Although no mandatory training is required to use a surgical laser, the clinician should check with appropriate agencies that regulate healthcare lasers.

Laser class	Degree of hazard	Output and labelling
I: Exempt	No more harmful than electric light bulb or barcode scanner. Do not emit levels of optical radiation above exposure limits for the eye under any circumstances. No known damage potential, even after long-term intentional viewing of direct beam	Very low-power lasers: output a few microwatts or less in continuous wave mode. No warning label required
II: Low-power	Laser pointer is best example. Can be hazardous to eyes if intentionally viewed for several seconds or longer; but natural pain aversion reflex normally prevents accidental eye damage even with direct eye exposure	Less than 5 mW in continuous wave mode. Warning label required
III: Medium-power	Used at laser light shows. May be hazardous for direct viewing as has potential to damage eye tissue faster than natural aversion reaction (<0.25 seconds) Class IIIa: only hazardous to eye when focused by optical device, e.g. binoculars Class IIIb: hazardous even when not artificially focused	Output 5–500 mW. Warning label required
IV: High-power	Includes most surgical lasers. Can cause serious eye and skin injuries. Can set fire to many materials. Direct and reflected beams both hazardous to the eye. Potential serious hazards to eye and skin from accidental exposure to either direct or diffusely reflected laser light	Includes all lasers that exceed 0.5 W average power over 0.25 seconds, or exceed 10 J/cm^2. Warning label required

7.4   Laser classes and degree of hazard.

- A standard 'Laser in use' warning sign (Figure 7.5) should be highly conspicuous near the operating room as a warning to passers-by.
- A smoke evacuation system must be used to remove the plume created by laser interaction with tissue.
- A laser surgery mask should be worn over the nose and mouth during any procedure (Figure 7.6). These masks have very fine pores (<1 µm) that filter out any suspended airborne particles missed by the smoke evacuator and also protect the patient from the contaminated gases exhaled by the surgeon.
- Veterinary technicians should monitor the time that the smoke evacuating systems have been used, and ensure that this vital safety equipment is functioning properly.
- Direct or indirect laser light can be permanently harmful to the eye.
  - Everyone within the surgical suite should wear goggles or other eyewear that will attenuate harmful laser wavelengths and intensities. These protective goggles (Figure 7.7) are specific for the wavelength of laser light that they can filter, and are also rated by the diminished ten-fold factor of attenuated light intensity they provide to the user.
  - The eyes of the patient should also be shielded from potential stray laser beams.

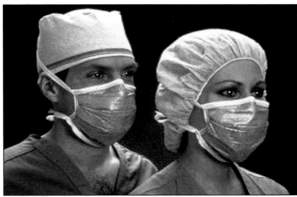

7.6   High-filtration particulate surgical masks have a pore size of <1 µm. This small diameter protects the surgeon and assistant from inhaling heavy plume material.

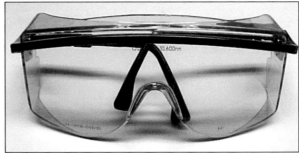

7.7   Protective goggles for CO_2 laser surgery use. The pair shown are rated OD6 because they reduce the intensity of 10.6 µm laser light by a factor of 10^6.

Potential laser safety hazards

The use of lasers in a clinical setting can present hazards to the laser operator and nearby personnel, including the following.

Fire hazards

High-power lasers, particularly infrared devices (e.g. CO_2, diode and Nd:YAG lasers), can induce combustion of tissue, surgical gowns, anaesthetic gases and tongue depressors. Smoke arising from laser-induced combustion can obscure vision, and may dangerously scatter the laser beam.

- Preparation with wetted gauze and sterile water or saline is important to reduce the potential for injury.

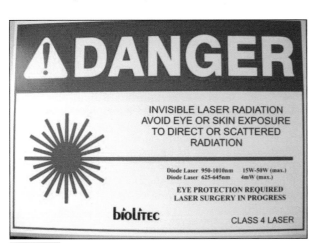

⚠ DANGER

INVISIBLE LASER RADIATION
AVOID EYE OR SKIN EXPOSURE
TO DIRECT OR SCATTERED
RADIATION

Diode Laser 950-1010nm   15W-50W (max.)
Diode Laser 625-645nm   4mW (max.)

EYE PROTECTION REQUIRED
LASER SURGERY IN PROGRESS

bioLiTEC   CLASS 4 LASER

7.5   Standard laser safety warning sign.

- Attention to where the laser beam targets the surgical site will reduce or eliminate the potential for adverse outcomes due to errant laser beam contact.
- Use of high-proof alcohol on the surgical or therapeutic site could cause combustion so should be avoided.
- A fire extinguisher should be readily available.

Potential damage to the eyes
Accidental or intentional irradiation of the exposed eye via direct, reflected or scattered laser light can result in damage to the ocular tissues and may lead to temporary or even permanent damage, including loss of vision.

- Direct and reflected laser beam exposure to wavelengths between 400 nm and 1400 nm may cause ocular transmission hazards.
- Focusing through the cornea and lens may increase the power density at the level of the retina by five orders of magnitude.
- Chronic exposure may result in cataract formation or degradation of the corneal surface, iris, lens or retina.

Potential damage to exposed skin
Laser energy can be produced from the ultraviolet to infrared regions of the light spectrum, and each has its own potential for skin damage.

- Laser irradiation of exposed skin can result in severe burns when high-power lasers are used.
- Long-term exposure to medium- and low-power lasers can lead to sunburn-like symptoms.
- Actively aiming the laser beam away from exposed skin surfaces not being targeted for treatment minimizes this potential.

Electrical hazards
As with any high-voltage electrical device, routine safety precautions should be taken. The laser housing should never be opened and only certified technicians should be allowed to carry out repairs.

Chemical hazards

- Toxic chemical hazards may exist from organic solvents that interact with or are altered by the laser energy.
- Coolant gases or liquids in radiator-cooled units also present potential dangers.
- Laser cavity byproducts (i.e. excimer lasers) are sometimes produced and can be toxic if inhaled.
- Photochemical reactions may occur within laser-irradiated material that escapes in the plume and is not contained in the plume evacuation unit.
- Several chemicals may be emitted as vapours, e.g. alcohols and iodophors used in skin preparation; the former is a combustion risk and the latter is toxic. This risk can be minimized by flushing the surgical site with sterile 0.9% saline prior to using a surgical laser beam.

Biological hazards

- The laser plume can have components that are irritating or injurious to the mucous membranes.
- The respiratory tract may also be at risk of infection, irritation, allergic reaction or long-term debilitating effects of small-particulate inhalation.

- Some bacterial, viral, or fungal organisms can survive in the plume.
- Components of the chemicals in and on the patient can be altered to become carcinogenic and potentially damaging. These components can also be drawn up into the plume.

Patient protection
A key consideration of patient protection is that anaesthetized animals do not have pain reflexes. They cannot respond to or move away from noxious odours or painful stimuli.

The laser-producing devices and the laser energy itself use heat to work on the target tissue and produce heat as a byproduct. It is also important to remember that varying wavelengths of laser energy interact differently with tissues, depending on the pigments present. Actions that might be taken to avoid damage to patients are given in Figure 7.8.

- The patient's eyes should be protected by using backstop titanium rods, quartz rods, saline-soaked tongue depressors, or saline-soaked gauze sponges. Ophthalmic lube protection can also be considered if the wavelength that is being used is highly absorbed by water and as an additional protectant for the cornea.
- Tooth enamel can also be protected in this way. Periosteal elevators can serve as backstops for procedures performed in the oral cavity. However, only instruments with matt surfaces should be used to reduce light reflection.
- It is critical to observe safe lasing procedures when working near the endotracheal tube because of the increased combustion risk in the potentially oxygen-rich local environment. Moist packing such as sterile fluid-soaked gauze or laparotomy sponges surrounding tissue structures can reduce or eliminate peripheral tissue injury and decrease thermal relaxation time.
- It is important to protect against ignition of intestinal gases, anaesthetic gases within endotracheal tubes and vapours from surgical preparation solutions by paying attention to anatomical orientation and the direction of the laser beam.
- Plume evacuation must always be considered for the patient, especially when working in the oral cavity.
- Standard operating procedures detailing the response to an emergency should be posted prominently for the attention of all staff.
- Only trained personnel should use the laser.
- Safety monitoring should occur at all times, with the staff permitted to make recommendations and comment on any issues of safety that might occur.

7.8 Precautions to maximize patient safety.

Applications of the CO_2 laser

The CO_2 laser's more predictable and controllable soft tissue effect, coagulation properties, broader range of applications and inherently shorter learning curve make it the ideal laser for the general veterinary practitioner. Optimum vaporization of the target tissue is achieved through a minimum power density of 5000 W/cm^2.

The CO_2 laser wavelength has a high absorption coefficient in water, which makes it ideal for soft tissue incisions and ablations because it results in the least amount of collateral tissue damage and postoperative tissue necrosis due to heat. Because this particular wavelength does not pass through cellular water but is strongly absorbed by it, tissue is vaporized layer by layer, minimizing energy transmission to underlying cellular structures.

Skin incisions
Skin incisions should, whenever possible, be made with a spot diameter of <0.8 mm with the skin held

under slight tension. Adequate power density of at least 5000 W/cm^2 will allow a smooth single-pass full-thickness dermal penetration with minimal char (Figure 7.9). The non-contact aspect of CO_2 laser energy also reduces tissue distortion, especially in delicate regions on the body surface. The authors prefer a 0.25 to 0.4 mm spot size with superpulse continuous wave parameters to incise the skin.

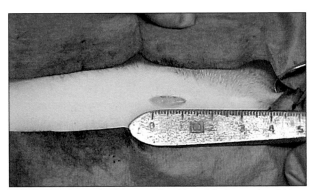

7.9 A skin incision made with a CO_2 laser should be clean, dry and less painful than a scalpel incision. The superpulse temporal pattern is an ideal setting for skin incisions and, if available, can be pulsed for a greater reduction in char formation.

Excision of cutaneous lesions

For the excision of cutaneous lesions, after incising the skin the laser is used to undermine subcutaneous fat and connective tissue using a 0.25–0.8 mm spot size at power density of 4500–5000 W/cm^2 to continue vaporization. Power densities in the 1500–2000 W/cm^2 range, without superpulse function, allow for coagulation of vessels <0.6 mm in diameter after skin incision is completed.

The CO_2 laser can provide excellent vaporization of connective tissue deep to the dermis. A spot size of 0.25–0.8 mm is optimal for this technique. The laser beam should be perpendicular to the dermis and at the level of the connective tissue interface. As the tissue is cut, the skin should be lifted to allow adequate visualization and access for vaporization. Care should be taken to avoid moving the laser beam too close to the dermis, because peripheral thermal energy release may damage dermal blood supply.

When submitting specimens for histopathology, larger tissue margins should be submitted since some shrinkage due to desiccation may occur. The use of laser energy to resect the mass should also be noted in the pathology request.

Other techniques

Below are examples of other techniques that can be performed using a 20–30 W CO_2 laser with superpulse capability. In general, the techniques vary little from the standard protocol, with the exception that a handpiece delivering focused laser energy replaces the traditional steel scalpel.

Canine and feline ovariohysterectomy

The laser is used for the skin and linea alba incisions. It is not recommended to use the laser to cut the ovarian pedicle or cervix without additional ligation, due to the larger diameter vessels, but it can be very useful in reducing seepage if used to cut the broad ligament.

Canine and feline orchiectomy

The laser is used for the scrotal and subcutaneous incisions. In young kittens the laser can be used to transect the cord, but this is not recommended in mature cats or dogs, due to the larger diameter of the vessels.

Elongated soft palate correction

This procedure requires a backstop on the laser delivery handpiece, or wet gauze placed behind the soft palate to prevent inadvertent lasing of tissues at the back of the oropharynx. The laser incision is begun at one lateral margin and continued to the contralateral side. It is extremely important to keep the laser beam perpendicular to the target tissue, because tangential beams are less efficient at vaporization and cause thermal necrosis, postoperative discomfort and potentially disastrous bleeding into vital supporting tissues (e.g. the palatine artery). After the desired tissue is excised, visual inspection confirms that the soft palate rests just above the epiglottis (Figure 7.10). Many dogs and cats that have elongated soft palates corrected also benefit from correction of stenotic nares. These procedures may be performed with a CO_2 laser.

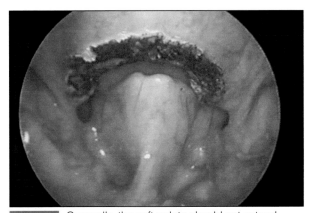

7.10 Generally, the soft palate should not extend beyond the level of the caudal pole of the tonsil. The goal for laser-assisted staphylectomy is for the new soft palate to conform to the shape of the epiglottis and just barely make contact with it.

Anal sacculectomy

An open technique is used, with the laser being applied to incise the skin and dissect the anal sac tissue from the attached muscle (Figure 7.11).

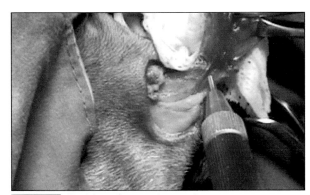

7.11 Excision of an anal sac using an open technique. The laser is used to vaporize tissue surrounding the glandular serosa. The spherical gland is removed from its bed using gentle traction.

Laser therapy

Laser devices may also be used for therapeutic rather than surgical applications. Techniques include:

- Photomodulation, also known as cold or low-level laser therapy (**LLLT**) or laser biostimulation
- High-power laser therapy (**HPLT**), which is claimed to achieve deeper penetration than LLLT.

LLLT devices are generally class IV laser devices, though earlier LLLT models were class IIIb. They use an infrared (808–910 nm) wavelength of light that is non-destructive to living tissues at the power level it delivers. Generally, LLLT delivers power of <500 mW; whereas HPLT delivers power >500 mW and in some cases up to 15 W. In either case the spot size is focused from 10–25 mm up to 5 cm in diameter.

Clinical evaluation of HPLT is providing increasingly compelling evidence that the effect of these wavelengths of laser energy on tissue may provide pain relief, stimulate wound healing, reduce oedema and inflammation, or produce alteration in other damaged biological processes (Tunér and Hode, 1999). The release of chemotactic factors or increased blood flow via vasodilation or tissue modifiers may be the result of local cytokine amplification as a result of this low-level energy stimulation. There is no heat-altering effect on tissue structures as exists for the higher power lasers noted earlier. The entire concept is still being explored but has gained a significant following in both human and animal physical therapy.

Conclusion

Laser equipment is now more affordable and easier to use. The application of a surgical laser does not guarantee success, but its judicious use may provide perioperative advantages such as reduced pain, bleeding and swelling. An appropriate level of veterinary surgical training and experience for the procedure being performed is still essential and may even be required at a higher level than performing the same procedure using a conventional surgical technique. The CO_2 laser is currently the most useful and flexible choice of surgical laser for small animal practice.

References and further reading

Bartels K and Peavy G (2002) *Veterinary Clinics of North America. Small Animal Practice.* **32**(3) 495–746

Berger NA and Eeg PH (2006) *Veterinary Laser Surgery: A Practical Guide.* Blackwell, Ames, Iowa

Brdecka D, Rawlings C, Howerth E *et al.* (2007) A histopathological comparison of two techniques for soft palate resection in normal dogs. *Journal of the American Animal Hospital Association* **43**, 39–44

Bussieres M, Krohne SG, Stiles J and Townsend WM (2005) The use of carbon dioxide laser for the ablation of meibomian gland adenomas in dogs. *Journal of the American Animal Hospital Association* **41**, 227–234

Davidson EB, Davis MS, Campbell GA *et al.* (2001) Evaluation of carbon dioxide laser and conventional incision techniques for resection of soft palates in brachycephalic dogs. *Journal of the American Veterinary Medical Association* **219**, 776–781

Dye T, Teague HD, Ostwald DFA and Ferreira SD (2002) Evaluation of a technique using the carbon dioxide laser for the treatment of aural hematomas. *Journal of the American Animal Hospital Association* **38**, 385–390

Holt T and Mann F (2003) Carbon dioxide laser resection of a distal carpal pilomatricoma and wound closure using swine intestinal submucosa in a dog. *Journal of the American Animal Hospital Association* **39**, 499–505

Lopez N (2002) The basics of soft tissue laser surgery. *Veterinary Medicine* **97**, 294–300

Lopez N (2002) Using CO_2 lasers to perform elective surgical procedures. *Veterinary Medicine* **97**, 302–312

Lucroy M (2004) Histologic comparison of skin biopsy specimens collected by use of carbon dioxide or 810nm diode lasers from dogs. *Journal of the American Veterinary Medical Association* **225**, 1562–1566

Mison M (2003) Comparison of the effects of the CO_2 surgical laser and conventional surgical techniques on healing and wound tensile strength of skin flaps in the dog. *Veterinary Surgery* **32**, 153–160

Mison M, Bohart G, Walshaw R *et al.* (2002) Use of carbon dioxide laser for onychectomy in cats. *Journal of the American Veterinary Medical Association* **221**(5), 651–653

Tunér J and Hode L (1999) *Low Level Laser Therapy, Clinical Practice and Scientific Background.* Prima-Books, Grängesberg, Sweden

Upton M, Tangner CH, Payton ME *et al.* (2006) Evaluation of carbon dioxide laser ablation combined with mitoxantrone and piroxicam treatment in dogs with transitional cell carcinoma. *Journal of the American Veterinary Medical Association* **228**, 549–552

Xiaogu W (2005) Healing process of skin after CO_2 laser ablation at low irradiance: a comparison of continuous-wave and pulsed mode. *Photomedical Laser Surgery* **23**, 20–26

Preoperative assessment

Kathryn M. Pratschke

Introduction

The success or otherwise of a surgical procedure can depend largely on good planning, awareness of potential risk factors and selection of the appropriate procedure. It is therefore critical that thorough preoperative patient evaluation is performed in every case, to ensure that surgical risk is minimized and that the chance of a successful outcome is maximized.

Selecting the right patient for the right procedure, and *vice versa*, is where the gap between knowing the theory and having sound clinical judgement based on experience and an ability to evaluate information critically is most likely to come to the fore. The best place to start, regardless of level of experience, is by collecting as much information as possible about the patient. In this way, any decisions that are reached, or discussions that may be had with colleagues or the client about the patient, are based on an accurate and complete picture rather than one that lacks essential information because shortcuts were taken. An example of this might be taking an animal to surgery to remove a large tumour without having identified the presence of metastatic disease that means a likely survival time of only a month or two, or taking a vomiting dog to exploratory abdominal surgery without running the blood tests that would identify it as Addisonian or having renal failure.

A number of the procedures referred to in this chapter can be found in the *BSAVA Guide to Procedures in Small Animal Practice*.

Taking a clinical history

A complete history (Figure 8.1) and thorough physical examination form the mainstay of patient assessment. The consultation prior to surgery may be the first point of contact with the owners, and as such it will influence their perception of the veterinary surgeon and the level of confidence that they have in the surgeon's judgement and abilities. It is an opportunity to determine the owners' expectations and wishes, explore what financial restrictions there may be and any other issues that may influence their decisions and what the veterinary surgeon recommends. For example, where an animal

- How long the client has had the animal, and where it came from (e.g. breeder *versus* rescue centre with an unknown history).
- Vaccination and worming status.
- Patterns of urination and defecation.
- Food and water intake, including the type of food and how often the animal is fed.
- Weight gain or loss – it is worth recording a body condition score (see Figure 8.2) as well as the weight, as they are not the same.
- Any recent changes to the animal's environment.
- Is it an indoor or outdoor pet?
- How many other animals does the owner have?
- Has the animal been abroad at any stage, and if so where and when?
- Any concurrent or previous problems (the temptation to focus solely on the current problem should be avoided), including information regarding recent illnesses or traumatic episodes, as well as chronic conditions and any medications or treatment.
- Previous anaesthetic episodes and problems or complications resulting from them.
- Previous surgical procedures and problems or complications resulting from them.
- Any known adverse drug reactions in the animal's history, or any known allergies or food intolerances.
- Any alteration in energy levels, exercise tolerance, enthusiasm for normal activities.
- How long the current condition has been present and how it has progressed since the owner noticed the first signs, bearing in mind that the owner's first awareness of the problem may not be the same thing as the first clinical indication (for example, the overt respiratory noise and dyspnoea associated with laryngeal paralysis will usually have been preceded by a history of coughing, gagging, voice change and reduced exercise tolerance, while marked unilateral muscle atrophy of a limb may suggest an acute-on-chronic pattern to lameness rather than merely acute).
- Any investigations or treatments that have been carried out so far, including any remedies that the owner may have given (including homeopathic or naturopathic remedies, over-the-counter or prescription medications that the owners may have at home).
- Any history of bleeding tendencies (e.g. in at-risk breeds such as the Dobermann) and whether the patient has ever required a blood transfusion; if so, whether they were cross-matched and blood typed.
- For certain conditions, any similar problems in the siblings, dam or sire.
- More detailed questioning on a specific body system for certain breeds (for example, brachycephalic breeds have a higher incidence of airway problems; regardless of whether they form the main presenting problem or not, they should be taken into account).

8.1 Factors to consider when taking a history of the patient.

requires tumour removal that should ideally be followed by chemotherapy, but the owner of that animal is pregnant, the ideal plan may not be feasible for health and safety reasons. If the available finances are limited, it is important to prioritize where money should be spent.

It is also wise to find out early on whether the animal is intended for working or performance use, for breeding, or as a family pet. A dog intended as a family pet may cope very well with a mild to moderate reduction in performance from carpal or tarsal arthrodesis or a total ear canal ablation–lateral bulla osteotomy, but reduction in athletic or other function could be a crucial factor for a working dog expected to earn its keep or one that is specifically required for competition performance.

When taking a history it is important to enquire not only about the current condition, but also about the general health status. This includes (but is not necessarily limited to) the factors listed in Figure 8.1.

Clinical examination

It is often tempting to focus on the most obvious problem (e.g. a visible tumour, a fractured limb) but the preoperative examination should always evaluate the entire animal; anaesthetic and surgical complications may be reduced in this way. A 'whole body' approach is important in every case, but particularly so in older patients, trauma cases and young or neonatal patients.

The physical examination does not have to be a prolonged or time-consuming process, just one that is efficient, practised and thorough.

Despite the unfortunately widespread perception amongst both owners and veterinary surgeons that old age is a reason to withhold treatment, older age in itself is not a negative prognostic factor, nor does it necessarily influence outcome. It does increase the risk of concurrent organ dysfunction or other disease (e.g. renal insufficiency or cardiac disease), hence the importance of the full examination to allow both the veterinary surgeon and the owner to decide how serious the risk is, what can be done to alleviate it and what this means for treatment. Young patients and neonates are more prone to anaesthetic risk factors such as a relative inability to regulate body temperature and blood glucose, and the potential for prolonged action of drugs should be borne in mind.

Before the in-depth examination is commenced, the animal's demeanour, mentation and gait, hydration and nutritional status (Figure 8.2) should be observed. A thorough systematic examination should then be performed, ensuring that core elements are examined in every case, every time. These include, but are not necessarily limited to, the following areas.

Cardiovascular function
Colour of the mucous membranes should be recorded along with capillary refill time, but it should be remembered that these provide only a crude estimate of

Category	Description
BCS 1	▪ Ribs, vertebrae, pelvic bones and all bony protuberances evident from visual examination ▪ No discernible body fat ▪ Obvious loss of muscle mass
BCS 2	▪ Ribs, vertebrae and pelvic bones easily identified by visual examination ▪ Other bony protuberances may be evident ▪ No palpable fat ▪ Minimal loss of muscle mass
BCS 3	▪ Ribs easily felt and may be visible as there is little fat over rib cage ▪ Dorsal vertebral processes of the lumbar vertebrae visible ▪ Obvious 'waist' with prominent pelvic bones
BCS 4	▪ Ribs easily palpable, with minimal fat covering ▪ Waist can be seen from above when looking down at the dog ▪ An abdominal tuck can be seen
BCS 5	▪ Ribs easily palpable, with only mild to moderate fatty covering ▪ Waist can be seen from above when looking down at the dog ▪ Abdominal tuck can be appreciated when viewed specifically
BCS 6	▪ Some excess fat over ribs but they are palpable ▪ Waist can be seen when viewed from above but not prominent ▪ Abdominal tuck present but again not prominent
BCS 7	▪ Ribs can only be palpated with difficulty due to fat cover ▪ Fat deposits over lumbar spine and base of tail may be visible ▪ Little or no evidence of waist or abdominal tuck
BCS 8	▪ Ribs cannot be palpated beneath fat cover without applying significant pressure ▪ Large fat deposits present over lumbar spine and base of tail ▪ No identifiable waist or abdominal tuck ▪ Abdomen may be visibly distended
BCS 9	▪ Extensive fat deposits over thorax, lumbar spine and base of tail as well as neck (sometimes colloquially referred to as 'coffee table appearance') ▪ Fat deposits may also be present over limbs ▪ Obvious abdominal distension

8.2 Assessment of body condition score (BCS) based on a system developed by Purina (www.purina.co.uk). Categories 1–3 are considered too thin, 4–5 are good and 6–9 are too fat. See *BSAVA Manual of Canine and Feline Rehabilitation, Supportive and Palliative Care* for more information.

cardiovascular function, peripheral perfusion and the presence of anaemia. The heart should be carefully auscultated and the peripheral pulses checked both for correlation with the heart rate (to identify pulse deficits) and for the pulse quality.

Dehydration

There should be an assessment of the degree of dehydration, if present. It is important to be aware that physical examination findings generally underestimate the degree of dehydration. During the acute phase of volume depletion, however, these classical physical examination findings may be the only assessment option available.

- Where an animal is <5% dehydrated there may be a history of fluid loss but there are no findings on physical examination.
- At 5% dehydration the patient will have dry oral mucous membranes but no panting or pathological tachycardia.
- At 7% dehydration there will be mild to moderate decreased skin turgor, dry oral mucous membranes, mild tachycardia and decreased pulse pressure.
- At 10% dehydration there will be moderate to marked decreased skin turgor, dry oral mucous membranes, tachycardia and decreased pulse pressure.
- At 12% dehydration there will be marked loss of skin turgor, dry oral mucous membranes and significant signs of shock.

Respiratory function

Respiratory function should be assessed carefully. The lung fields should be auscultated and percussed, the respiratory rate and pattern checked and ventilation assessed.

Ventilation is the ability of the chest wall and diaphragm to move an adequate volume of air into the chest. This requires normal brainstem control, spinal cord function to the level of C3/4, spinal and phrenic nerve function, muscle and chest wall integrity, absence of pleural disease and a patent airway. Abnormality of any one of these will result in inadequate ventilation. If presented with a patient with a history of chronic respiratory pathology, or one currently showing very marked respiratory signs, a check should be made for signs of respiratory muscle fatigue and the posture the animal favours should be noted.

- In the normal animal, chest wall movements are almost undetectable.
- During normal inspiration, the ribs are pulled cranially and laterally by the external intercostal muscles, contraction of the diaphragm creates negative pressure within the thorax and the abdominal wall moves outwards.
- Expiration is usually a passive event during quiet breathing.

Signs of respiratory difficulty are as follows:

- Diaphragmatic excursions become more marked and secondary muscles of respiration are recruited, including the scalenus muscles (to elevate the first two ribs), the sternomastoideus muscles (to pull the sternum cranially) and the alae nasi muscles (to flare the nostrils)

- Expiration may become an active event, with contraction of the abdominal wall muscles and the internal intercostal muscles
- In more severe respiratory compromise, open-mouth breathing and dilatation of the nares can be seen
- If an animal has suffered chronic respiratory difficulty, respiratory movements may become paradoxical and oppose normal expansion of the chest wall, thereby exacerbating an already bad situation.

Animals in severe respiratory distress adopt a posture that minimizes the work of breathing. They often stand or sit, and if exhausted tend to lie in sternal rather than lateral recumbency. They may lift and extend the head and neck, in order to reduce nasal and pharyngeal airway resistance, and favour abduction of the elbows to allow for maximal movement of the chest wall with each breath.

> **WARNING**
>
> Animals showing signs of severe respiratory compromise or possible respiratory muscle fatigue should be treated as emergencies.

A dyspnoeic/tachypnoeic animal may exhibit either a rapid and shallow pattern of breathing, or slow and deep, depending on the underlying lesion.

> **PRACTICAL TIPS**
>
> - Restrictive lesions such as pleural effusion, pneumothorax or parenchymal disease (e.g. pneumonia) tend to cause a rapid shallow pattern.
> - Obstructive disease such as laryngeal paralysis tends to cause slower deeper breaths.

Ocular and nasal abnormalities

Any ocular or nasal discharge should be recorded and characterized. Checks should be made for abnormalities such as strabismus, nystagmus (positional or otherwise), protrusion of the third eyelid, or facial swelling.

Lymph nodes

Lymph nodes that are palpable superficially should be checked for changes in size, shape, attachment to surrounding tissues and pain.

Abdominal palpation

Gentle abdominal palpation may assist in identifying organomegaly, or localizing pain. For example, pancreatic disease is typically associated with cranial abdominal pain; prostatitis or prostatic abscessation will manifest with caudal abdominal pain.

Abdominal pain may be associated with a variety of disorders in companion animals and may be classified as visceral, parietal or referred.

- **Visceral pain** is usually dull and poorly localized; it occurs secondary to rupture, ischaemia, inflammation or distension of abdominal organs.
- **Parietal pain** is usually sharp, severe and localized.

■ **Referred pain** is due to pathological changes at another site of the body, e.g. intervertebral disc disease.

An animal will manifest pain by guarding the abdomen when it is touched or palpated, but the extent to which abdominal palpation is useful depends on many factors, including anxiety, species or obesity as well as pathological processes. Other clinical signs that may be noted concurrently include adopting the 'praying' posture, restlessness and inability to settle.

Musculoskeletal system

Musculoskeletal integrity, initially assessed via gait and mobility, may need to be analysed further through palpation for pain, assessment of range of motion for all joints, evaluation of muscle mass and comparison between opposite sides, or the use of specific tests for joint stability such as the cranial drawer, or the cranial tibial thrust tests for stifle stability. If there is a history of trauma associated with lameness and a fracture or luxation is suspected, it is very important to check for neurovascular compromise. This relates to how the treatment plan is formulated as well as to prognosis; for example, identifying a humeral fracture that is associated with radial nerve transection, a pelvic fracture with severe sciatic trauma, or distal antebrachial fractures associated with significant soft tissue damage (such as a degloving injury with severe vascular injury).

Neurological examination

In appropriate cases a neurological examination may be indicated. Depending on the presenting history, a screening neurological examination may include assessment of gait and posture, tests for conscious proprioception, assessment of eye position and movements, pupil size, pupillary light reflexes, menace response, palpebral reflex, jaw tone, gag reflex, tail function, anal reflex and mental status. Detailed information regarding full neurological evaluation and interpretation can be found in the *BSAVA Manual of Canine and Feline Neurology*. Neurological problems that need to be identified promptly for further evaluation and treatment include stupor, hepatic encephalopathy, seizures and loss of consciousness.

Rectal examination

Where appropriate, a rectal examination can provide valuable information regarding abnormalities such as strictures, colorectal masses, perineal hernia with rectal dilatation or deviation, anal sac problems, enlarged sublumbar lymph nodes and prostatic size/symmetry/pain/mobility/shape.

Vaginal examination

In bitches with a history of dysuria, haematuria, incontinence, vaginal haemorrhage or swelling, a digital and if possible visual vaginal examination should be performed, though in some cases sedation will be required for a useful examination. This may allow identification of such abnormalities as vaginal tumours, vestibulovaginal stenosis, hermaphroditism, imperforate hymen, or neoplasia affecting the urethra.

Breed-related problems

Certain breeds may come with additional inherent problems, such as brachycephalic animals that present for ophthalmic problems, gastrointestinal signs or with severe ear disease. Even in the absence of overt recorded respiratory problems, a full respiratory assessment should be carried out or at the very least advised prior to anaesthesia and surgery. An animal that was apparently coping under normal circumstances may actually have an elongated soft palate with everted laryngeal saccules, so that the additional stress of anaesthesia and surgery results in a respiratory crisis, pulmonary oedema and possibly death. If severe complications result from a failure to recognize breed-related problems, it will be that much worse for everyone concerned if the animal was anaesthetized for a routine procedure when the whole disaster could have been avoided with proper patient assessment.

The critical patient

There are some cases where the history taking and clinical examination outlined above may need to take second place to a rapid survey examination and emergency treatment. In these situations, only the essential data required for triage are collected until such time as the animal is stable enough to undergo further examination and tests. An example of such a case might be the cat that presents with urinary tract obstruction and severe acid–base imbalance (metabolic acidosis), post-renal renal failure, hyperkalaemia and cardiac dysfunction as a consequence. In these cases it is crucial to be thorough and systematic in the approach to the case, and to remember that instituting life-preserving measures is of paramount importance.

In critical patients the **ABC** of airway, breathing and circulation must be assessed first. Once this is done a general system examination can be completed.

1. Start at the head, assessing the colour of the mucous membranes and capillary refill time.
2. Check for pupillary dilatation or constriction, failure of the pupils to respond to light, or asymmetry (anisocoria).
3. Auscultate the heart and palpate the peripheral pulses simultaneously, checking for pulse deficits or arrhythmias. As a rough rule-of-thumb, if a femoral pulse cannot readily be palpated, blood pressure is dangerously low (though it is important to be aware that pulse pressure is the *difference* between systolic and diastolic pressures and that reduction of the difference between the two is not necessarily the same as a reduction in either one or the other, or in both). It is always a good idea, in a critical patient, to palpate the peripheral pulse in more than one location.
4. Auscultate the lung fields and abdomen, percuss both the thorax and abdomen, and assess the respiratory rate and pattern.

It should always be remembered that trauma cases may have a dramatically obvious musculoskeletal problem, such as pelvic fractures that are painful and cause marked disability, and are immediately visible on even a single radiograph. However, if there are concurrent problems, such as urethral rupture, diaphragmatic rupture, renal haemorrhage, pulmonary contusions or myocardial contusions, it is crucial that these are recognized and prioritized for treatment (Figures 8.3 and 8.4). A pelvic fracture is unlikely to be life threatening, but a diaphragmatic rupture or urethral rupture may be.

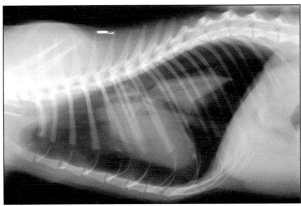

8.3 Lateral thoracic radiograph of a cat showing some typical findings associated with pneumothorax: a 'floating' cardiac silhouette, atelectasis of caudal lung lobes and straightening of diaphragmatic outline. In this case the cause of the pneumothorax was a tracheal lesion cranial to the carina, resulting in a one-way valve effect and ultimately rupture of the pulmonary parenchyma.

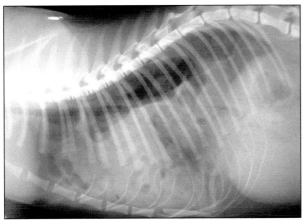

8.4 Lateral thoracic and cranial abdominal radiograph of a cat showing loss of diaphragmatic outline and cardiac silhouette, dorsal displacement of lung fields and numerous tubular radiolucent structures within thorax. These findings are consistent with diaphragmatic rupture and the presence of abdominal viscera within the thorax.

Clinical pathology

Laboratory tests should complement the clinical evaluation, not be used as a substitute for it. They should be interpreted in light of the patient's condition.

PRACTICAL TIP

The tests required preoperatively depend on the patient and presenting complaint, as well as the proposed procedure: e.g. a young animal in good health undergoing an elective surgery will require less testing (if any) than one due to undergo a more complex procedure, or with a more complicated disease condition.

As a general rule the tests should be the minimum required for thorough evaluation of the presenting problem, its systemic manifestations and the significance of any concurrent disease conditions. Preoperative tests may also be important in establishing a baseline against which to assess postoperative progress.

Economic factors will often determine which laboratory tests to use, but should not prevent necessary tests; rather these factors increase reliance on the clinician's judgement in deciding which tests to prioritize. Treating the patient appropriately the first time round is cheaper in the long run than treating unexpected but avoidable complications, not to mention avoiding an unpleasant discussion with an unhappy client.

Haematology and biochemistry

A minimum database (PCV, total solids, urea, creatinine, electrolytes and urinalysis) may be sufficient for many cases, but a geriatric patient, a seriously ill patient, or one that has suffered extensive trauma may warrant more extensive testing, such as a full haematology and a serum biochemistry screen. A thorough history and clinical examination should be used to guide the decision regarding which tests to perform. A platelet count should be included in all routine haematology tests, as this can give an indication of the risk of bleeding due to thrombocytopenia. Although amylase and lipase are often included in the initial work up for dogs, their accuracy in evaluating pancreatitis is poor and analysis of canine pancreatic lipase, or feline trypsin-like immunoreactivity in cats, is likely to be more useful.

The buccal mucosal bleeding time (BMBT; Figure 8.5) is a very useful test for preoperative assessment of platelet function and number. Most animals will stop bleeding within 2–3 minutes, but up to 5 minutes is considered normal. This test is described in detail in Chapter 20.

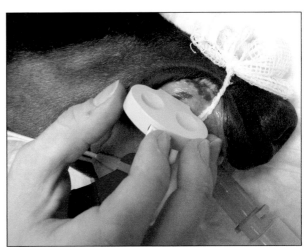

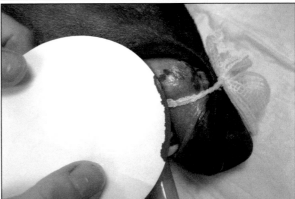

8.5 BMBT is a useful and simple preoperative test that many dogs will tolerate either conscious or with light sedation. It is important not to wipe off a forming clot inadvertently when blotting the site, as this will artificially prolong the BMBT. (See also Chapter 20.)

Any animal with neoplastic disease requires complete staging as an integral part of their assessment. A coagulation screen should be performed for those with a history of bleeding, liver disease or neoplasia affecting the spleen or liver. This typically includes activated partial thromboplastin time (aPTT) and prothrombin time (PT).

Opinions vary as to the usefulness of PIVKAs (proteins induced by vitamin K antagonism or absence) in suspected warfarin toxicities or hepatopathies (Giger, 2003; Mount *et al.*, 2003) and currently their use is not commonplace.

If it is available, blood gas analysis can be invaluable for assessment of patients with respiratory compromise, being considerably more sensitive than pulse oximetry for such analysis (see Chapter 10).

- Normal P_aO_2 in patients breathing room air should lie between 80 and 100 mmHg. Cyanosis is not usually seen until 50–55 mmHg, though patients require oxygen therapy below 60 mmHg.
- Normal P_aCO_2 acts as a marker of effective ventilation and should lie between 35 and 45 mmHg.
- P_aCO_2 is usually low in conditions that cause hyperventilation, such as pulmonary contusions, but is usually high in conditions that cause hypoventilation, such as pneumothorax, pain, pneumonia, raised intracranial pressure or trauma.

Pleural fluid

If a sample of pleural fluid is obtained, the following tests should be considered:

- Preparation of direct smears for cytology
- Submission for both aerobic and anaerobic culture
- Determination of specific gravity, protein content, clotting characteristics, presence of chylomicrons and triglycerides (along with concurrent evaluation of serum triglycerides)
- Total cell count and centrifuged cell concentrate smears.

Although pleural effusions are typically categorized (Figure 8.6) as transudate, modified transudate or exudate and as chylous, haemorrhagic or neoplastic, it is worth remembering that there may be considerable overlap between these 'categories', and therefore clinical data should always be taken into account when interpreting test results.

	Transudate	Modified transudate	Exudates
Total nucleated cell count (TNCC)	<1500/µl	1000–7000/µl	>7000/µl
Total protein (TP)	<25 g/l	25–75 g/l	>30 g/l

8.6 Assessment and classification of effusions.

Peritoneal fluid

If peritoneal fluid is obtained, tests should include cytological examination and pertinent laboratory tests. If only a tiny amount of fluid is obtained from a patient with an acute abdominal crisis, cytology is the most useful test and should ideally be performed on both a direct smear and a spun sediment sample.

> **PRACTICAL TIP**
>
> A combination of degenerate neutrophils and bacteria indicates that septic peritonitis is present, which requires emergency exploratory surgery.

If the fluid is bloody, it should be collected and monitored for clotting. If it is free blood in the abdomen, it should not clot (since mechanical defibrination and activation of the fibrinolytic system occurs). If blood has been obtained by unintentional organ puncture, the fluid will clot within 5–15 minutes when placed in a glass tube unless the animal has a coagulopathy. Use of plastic tubes may significantly delay or otherwise alter the onset of coagulation and thus give a misleading result.

Measurement of potassium and creatinine in abdominal fluid should be performed concurrently with measurement of the same parameters in peripheral blood. Higher levels of potassium and creatinine in abdominal fluid than in the peripheral circulation are highly suggestive of uroperitoneum. Equilibration will develop over time and so the sample analysis should not be delayed.

Amylase/lipase evaluation where pancreatitis is suspected may be useful but does not provide a definitive diagnosis.

Where bile leakage is suspected, measurement of bilirubin (with concurrent determination of serum levels) may be useful but is not definitive. Slow leakage from a small defect can result in focal bile peritonitis within a fibrous walled-off pocket, which may be missed on routine abdominocentesis without ultrasound guidance. As the presence of bilirubin within peritoneal fluid due to necrotizing cholecystitis without any overt clinical signs of peritonitis has been documented (Babin *et al.*, 2006), it is also important to be aware that this test must be interpreted correctly in order to make the right decision as to which cases warrant surgical intervention. Ascites with pre-hepatic or hepatic icterus will also contain bilirubin, due to diffusion from the blood into the ascitic fluid. To determine whether the source of the bilirubin is the blood or the biliary tract, concurrently collected samples should be compared; bilirubin levels will typically be significantly higher where the biliary tract is ruptured.

Anaesthetic risk assessment

The use of routine pre-anaesthetic blood sampling, testing for clinically silent disease as a means of risk assessment, remains a controversial subject in both medical and veterinary anaesthesia. For example, in humans it is recognized that electrocardiograms (ECGs) in patients without cardiovascular risk factors do not predict cardiovascular complications, and running routine blood tests on patients with no evidence of disease is not predictive of anaesthetic complications.

A study that reviewed findings from 1537 client-owned dogs undergoing surgery at the University of Leipzig (Alef *et al.*, 2008) concluded: 'In dogs, pre-anaesthetic laboratory examination is unlikely to yield additional important information if no potential problems are identified in the history and on physical examination.' A summary of recommendations from an Expert Round Table Discussion (Senior *et al.*, 2009) stated this position even more strongly, saying: 'The routine use of pre-anaesthetic blood tests is unnecessary and unjustified unless indicated by the findings of the medical history and a full physical examination.'

Diagnostic imaging

There are numerous situations where diagnostic imaging is crucial to preoperative planning for surgical cases, such as identification of an articular fracture, pulmonary metastatic disease on thoracic radiographs from patients with neoplastic disease, or contrast studies or ultrasonography to investigate urinary tract disease or lesions. The type of diagnostic imaging that is selected will be dictated by the facilities and expertise available, the suspected pathological changes, the animal's condition, and the finances available.

- Ultrasound examination can often be performed with manual restraint without either sedation or anaesthesia.
- For radiography or computed tomography (CT), health and safety radiation concerns mandate chemical restraint.
- For magnetic resonance imaging (MRI), anaesthesia is required for diagnostic films in veterinary patients.
- Where diagnostic imaging requires general anaesthesia it may be feasible to consider combining diagnosis and treatment in one anaesthetic episode, e.g. CT scan of the tympanic bullae (Figure 8.7) followed immediately by surgery based on the scan combined with the physical findings and clinical history, or radiography of a fracture followed immediately by surgical repair.

> **WARNING**
>
> In an unstable patient, diagnostic imaging should never be performed at the expense of the patient's welfare. These cases require appropriate assessment and prioritization of procedures.

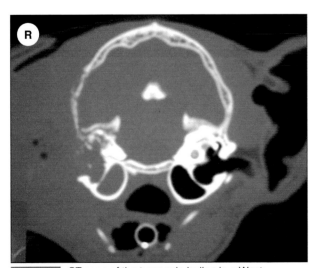

8.7 CT scan of the tympanic bullae in a West Highland White Terrier with severe right-sided chronic otitis externa and media with para-aural abscessation. This is an example of an imaging procedure that can be followed immediately by surgery under the same anaesthetic.

Radiography

With radiographic examination, two views of a region are generally required, but if conventional views are not obtainable standing, sitting or sternal views with a horizontal beam may provide another option, provided they can be performed without compromising radiation safety. Patients with abdominal pain may be unwilling to tolerate ventrodorsal positioning, as it will tend to exacerbate their discomfort.

> **WARNING**
>
> In cases with marked respiratory compromise the ventrodorsal view should be avoided, as turning an animal on its back may lethally reduce its ability to compensate.

Ultrasonography

If free fluid is suspected within the thorax or abdomen, plain film radiography may be unrewarding (Figure 8.8), whereas ultrasound examination can take advantage of a fluid window (Figure 8.9). Ultrasonography is also very useful for evaluating parenchymal organs within the abdomen and for identifying lymphadenopathy associated with neoplastic processes, although lymph node enlargement in itself is not necessarily diagnostic for neoplasia without either cytology or histology to confirm the suspicion.

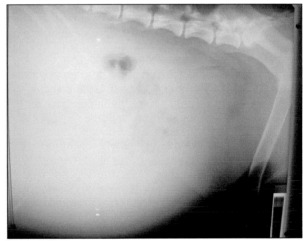

8.8 The presence of free abdominal fluid severely impairs radiographic interpretation. Ultrasonography could be considered as an alternative.

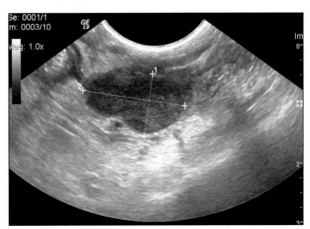

8.9 Ultrasound scan showing lymph node enlargement in the mesenteric region of a patient with an intestinal carcinoma.

CT and MRI

Investigation of nasal disease in dogs, and especially in cats, by means of radiography does not always yield a diagnosis, whereas a CT scan is very useful. In contrast, evaluation of a fracture or luxation is probably best done from well positioned radiographs.

MRI is ideal for certain body systems, such as the brain, if a CNS lesion is suspected (such as a brain tumour), or to evaluate disc extrusion. MRI is not appropriate if the neurological signs are caused by either an insulinoma-induced hypoglycaemic crisis or an episode of hepatic encephalopathy, and this illustrates the usefulness of a good history and clinical pathology testing prior to diagnostic imaging. The cost of MRI must also be considered: there is little benefit in superior quality diagnostic images if euthanasia is to be performed because the client cannot afford any further treatment.

Fluoroscopy

Fluoroscopy is very helpful for assessment of conditions where dynamic images are required, such as assessment of swallowing function and investigation of regurgitation or tracheal collapse. As with conventional radiography and CT, there are radiation safety issues that must be given attention.

Critical and emergency presentations

Thoracic trauma

Pneumothorax: Typical radiographic findings with pneumothorax include elevation of the cardiac silhouette off the sternum, collapse of lung lobes (especially caudal lobes), absence of bronchovascular markings in the periphery and the presence of pneumomediastinum. 'Barrelling' of the rib cage and flattening of the diaphragm may indicate tension pneumothorax, which requires immediate intervention.

Pulmonary contusions: Pulmonary contusions can be detected radiographically, but it is important to remember that they will not become visible immediately; they may take 6 hours or more to develop and therefore early radiographs may miss the presence of clinically significant contusions. Contusions appear as patchy asymmetrical areas of alveolar and interstitial patterns that do not follow an anatomical pattern. There will often be evidence of other traumatic injuries, such as fractured ribs, pleural effusion, or diaphragmatic rupture.

Diaphragmatic rupture: Typical radiographic findings include loss of diaphragmatic outline, loss of the cardiac silhouette, presence of gas-filled structures within the thorax and the presence of soft tissue structures within the ventral thorax. Atelectasis may be present, as well as displacement of abdominal organs or alterations in topographical anatomy (altered gastric axis). Ultrasonography is particularly useful in animals with pleural effusion secondary to diaphragmatic rupture (with liver entrapment and transudation), as fluid is an excellent medium for signal transmission of signal, whereas with radiography fluid obscures detail. Contrast radiography is indicated in suspected diaphragmatic ruptures only when conventional radiographs are non-diagnostic and ultrasonography is unavailable, i.e. it should not be required very often.

Acute abdominal crisis

Plain radiography: Plain radiographs should be obtained initially where conditions such as gastric dilatation–volvulus (GDV), peritonitis, prostatic abscessation, gastrointestinal foreign body obstruction, urinary tract rupture or pyometra are suspected, bearing in mind that taking two orthogonal views is essential and a single radiograph will often be inadequate and may be misleading. These two views can be a lateral and either a dorsoventral or ventrodorsal (dorsoventral may be tolerated better by an animal with acute abdominal pain, but will be more difficult to interpret).

- An alteration in size or shape of an abdominal organ is potentially suspicious.
- Loss of normal detail or a 'ground glass' appearance suggests ascites or peritonitis.
- Free gas indicates a ruptured gastrointestinal tract, urogenital tract, a penetrating wound or recent surgery (within the last 10–14 days).
- GDV is likely if the pylorus is gas-filled and located dorsally, and the fundus gas-filled and located caudoventrally on a right lateral view (Figure 8.10). A line of compartmentalization may be seen.
- A caudal abdominal mass of soft tissue/fluid opacity with or without calcification suggests prostatic disease, such as abscessation, cyst, or tumour (which may be accompanied by abscessation).
- Distension of intestinal loops may suggest ileus, intussusception, incarceration, volvulus or foreign body obstruction (not all foreign bodies will be radiopaque).

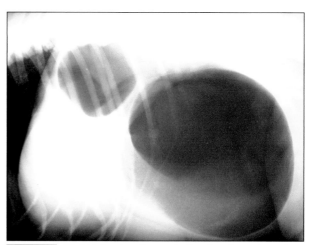

8.10 Right lateral radiograph showing the pylorus in a dorsal position and gas-filled, while the fundus is also gas-filled and located caudoventrally. With these findings, gastric dilatation–volvulus is likely. A compartmentalization line is also seen, suggesting the presence of volvulus.

Contrast radiography: Contrast radiographs are most commonly indicated where a ruptured urinary tract is suspected, e.g. intravenous urogram (IVU) for suspected ureteral rupture, or urethrocystogram for bladder (Figure 8.11) or urethral ruptures. These are not commonly used where rupture of the gastrointestinal tract is suspected but may be used, for example, if ultrasonography is not available. Water-soluble iodine-based contrast medium should be used in these situations,

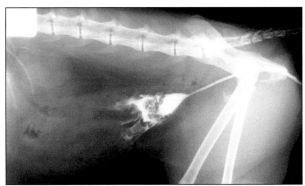

8.11 This patient suffered prolonged urinary tract obstruction due to a urethral calculus. A ruptured bladder was confirmed with a positive-contrast retrograde urethrocystogram. At surgery the apical third of the bladder was necrotic, necessitating partial cystectomy to excise the devitalized tissue.

though the study may be difficult to interpret due to dilution of the medium. Use of barium is contraindicated as it may induce chemical peritonitis if spilled into the peritoneal cavity and will exacerbate any other coexisting abnormalities such as gastrointestinal spillage, bile leakage or uroabdomen.

Ultrasonography: Ultrasonography is a very useful diagnostic tool for acute abdominal crises. It is capable of detecting very small quantities of abdominal fluid (4 ml/kg bodyweight – far less than abdominal radiography). Areas that should be particularly evaluated for fluid accumulation are:

- Between and around liver lobes
- Between the body wall and the spleen
- At the apex of the bladder.

The location of fluid accumulation may sometimes suggest an aetiology: for example, pocketing of fluid in the right cranial quadrant around the stomach, duodenum and right kidney suggests pancreatic disease; retroperitoneal fluid accumulation suggests haemorrhage or ureteral leakage.

Prostatic abscessation and/or cysts are readily identifiable on ultrasonography as loculated areas of varying echogenicity. Dilated or enlarged uterine loops may suggest pyometra, hydrometra, or torsion. Intussusceptions can be visualized directly with ultrasonography with a bullseye appearance on cross-section, and intestinal lesions and motility may also be assessed, though gas within the intestinal tract secondary to obstruction or stasis may interfere with the ultrasound examination.

An additional benefit to ultrasonography is that changes within parenchymal organs such as the spleen, liver or kidneys can also be assessed, as opposed to only their outline and position as seen on radiography. Lesions most likely to be missed on abdominal ultrasonography prior to surgery are gastrointestinal ulceration or perforation (Pastore *et al.*, 2007).

Other investigations

Other investigations may include, but are not limited to, needle thoracocentesis/abdominocentesis, diagnostic peritoneal lavage, endoscopy, ultrasound-guided aspiration or biopsy, and cytology.

Needle thoracocentesis

This may be diagnostic or therapeutic, as well as contributing to patient stabilization in certain conditions.

TECHNIQUE 8.1
Needle thoracocentesis

1 Pre-oxygenate if possible and have all equipment collected in one place. Gentle restraint is often all that is necessary, though chemical restraint may be preferable in some cases. If possible, place the animal in sternal recumbency.

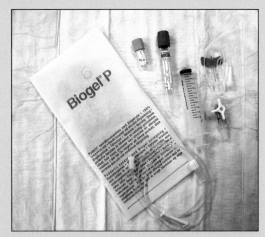

2 Clip and aseptically prepare the sites, as time permits.

3 Whether to infiltrate local anaesthetic prior to thoracocentesis is a matter of personal preference. The usual site for thoracocentesis is at the seventh or eighth intercostal space. If pneumothorax is present the needle should be inserted in the dorsal third of the intercostal space, while fluid may be better accessed in the ventral third of the chest with the patient in sternal recumbency.

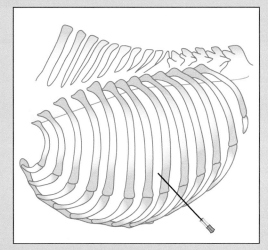

Reproduced from the *BSAVA Guide to Procedures in Small Animal Practice.*

4 Connect the needle/catheter to extension tubing and a three-way tap, and introduce cranial to the rib, since the intercostal arteries and veins run along the caudal margins of the ribs. A needle of sufficient length to penetrate the intercostal muscles and into the pleural cavity is needed; this will vary in length from half-inch in cats to 2 inches in larger or obese dogs. The bore required depends on size of animal but is usually between 14 and 22 gauge.

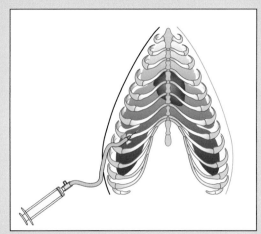

Reproduced from the *BSAVA Guide to Procedures in Small Animal Practice*.

5 Initially the needle/catheter should be introduced perpendicular to the skin, but once through the intercostal muscles it should be redirected more parallel with the skin to reduce the risk of iatrogenic trauma to thoracic structures.

6 With a moderate to severe pneumothorax the pressure within the pleural cavity may be quite high, sometimes even greater than atmospheric, in which case gas/fluid will egress under the positive pressure as soon as the needle tip enters the pleural space. Suction should be applied *gently* when aspirating gas/fluid from the pleural space. What is removed from each site tapped should be measured and recorded.

7 Any fluid aspirated should be kept for laboratory evaluation as described in the section on laboratory tests.

Abdominocentesis

This is indicated where abdominal effusion is suspected or confirmed. Abdominocentesis may facilitate diagnosis of a range of conditions including peritonitis, uroabdomen and haemoabdomen, and may also provide an assessment of severity. It is a very easy and quick technique, but it requires that large volumes of fluid (5–25 ml/kg) are present. Abdominocentesis can be performed with the patient standing or in lateral or dorsal recumbency. Any fluid obtained should be kept for laboratory evaluation.

TECHNIQUE 8.2
Abdominocentesis

1 Clip abdomen and aseptically prepare as for surgery.

2 Palpate the spleen and urinary bladder if possible, as this facilitates avoiding them.

3 Use a 20–22 gauge needle, depending on patient size, and insert it 2–3 cm caudal to the umbilicus and 1 cm to the right of midline. Do not attach a syringe straight away – if only small amounts of fluid are present capillary action is relied on to draw fluid into the hub of the needle, so fluid should be allowed to drip from the needle first.

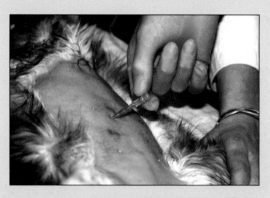

4 If no fluid is obtained from this site, proceed to a four-quadrant tap.

5 If no fluid is obtained from a four-quadrant tap, proceed to diagnostic peritoneal lavage.

Diagnostic peritoneal lavage

Diagnostic peritoneal lavage (DPL) is a far more sensitive technique than abdominocentesis: it can detect as little as 1.1–4.0 ml fluid/kg. Relative contraindications for DPL include severely dyspnoeic patients, suspected diaphragmatic rupture, or suspected or severe organomegaly. DPL can be carried out with the patient in lateral or dorsal recumbency. The use of local analgesia and/or sedation is a matter of personal preference. Sufficient fluid samples should be collected for cytology, laboratory tests and both aerobic and anaerobic culture and sensitivity.

TECHNIQUE 8.3
Diagnostic peritoneal lavage

1 Clip the abdomen and aseptically prepare as for surgery.

2 Empty the bladder if possible.

3 Use a multi-lumen dialysis catheter, an angio-catheter with additional holes cut in it or a large intravenous catheter. Introduce the catheter in the same location as described for abdomino-centesis, angled caudally towards the pelvis.

4 Infuse 20–22 ml of sterile warmed normal saline/kg body weight and then rock the animal gently to disperse fluid throughout the abdomen.

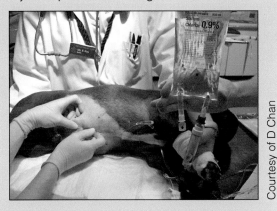

Courtesy of D Chan

5 Aspirate a sample for examination, or alternatively attach a closed system and allow drainage by gravity. It will not be possible to remove all the instilled fluid.

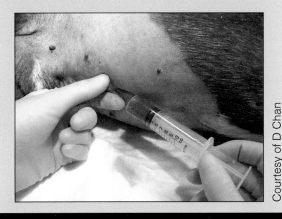

Courtesy of D Chan

Endoscopy

Endoscopy is very useful for assessment of patients with nasal disease, lower airway disease, lower urinary tract disease and upper and lower gastrointestinal disease. It complements the information gained from diagnostic imaging studies by providing a magnified view of intraluminal and mural lesions and allows lesion biopsy under direct visualization. In nasal disease it may allow confirmation of suspected fungal disease, or in a patient that presents with a history of coughing it can allow accurate grading of tracheal collapse. A more detailed discussion of endoscopy in veterinary patients can be found in the *BSAVA Manual of Canine and Feline Endoscopy and Endosurgery.*

In addition to visual examination, biopsy should be routinely considered for the gastrointestinal tract, as the mucosa can appear normal even in the presence of inflammatory or neoplastic disease (Figure 8.12). Biopsy samples taken endoscopically are mucosal only; therefore they do not provide information about

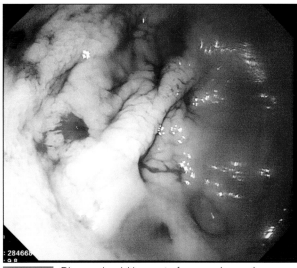

8.12 Biopsy should be part of any endoscopic examination of the gastrointestinal tract, as gross visual inspection is not accurate in identifying abnormal from normal. When taking biopsy samples from the gastrointestinal tract, caution needs to be exercised when sampling areas that appear diseased or abnormal or if taking multiple samples from a single site.

pathological changes within the deeper layers of the wall and can on occasion be non-diagnostic. As they are typically very small tissue fragments, they are also prone to crush artefact. The possibility of a non-diagnostic yield can be a particular problem when taking samples from mass lesions. Repeat biopsy from the same site may provide deeper samples, but in the gastrointestinal tract this should be done with caution to avoid a rupture. As endoscopy requires general anaesthesia, patient stability should be considered first.

Ultrasound-guided fine-needle aspiration or biopsy

Potential risks of ultrasound-guided aspiration or biopsy include haemorrhage, leakage of abscess contents, seeding of neoplastic cells along the needle tract and a non-diagnostic or inaccurate result. If samples are collected for cytology rather than histology, the potential limitations of the information acquired need to be appreciated: no information will be gained about the architecture or cellular structure of the lesion, and tumour grade cannot be assigned for neoplastic masses. It is wise to check coagulation panels prior to aspirating organs with a good vascular supply such as the liver, spleen or kidneys. More detailed information regarding aspiration and biopsy techniques, which can be very useful for patient assessment, may be found in the *BSAVA Manual of Canine and Feline Clinical Pathology.*

Cytology: slide preparation following sample collection

A good quality microscope is necessary with magnification up to x1000, otherwise interpretation will be compromised. For in-house analysis smears should be prepared as soon as possible after sample collection in EDTA tubes. Options for smear preparation include:

- Standard smear technique
- Concentration technique
- Squash preparation.

The choice of technique depends on the cellularity, volume and viscosity of the sample. Artefacts and incidental findings, including ruptured and damaged cells, may result from poor sample preservation or excessive force in smear preparation.

The most commonly used and generally useful stains are the Romanowsky type (e.g. Diff-Quik). These stains are generally good for cytoplasmic staining (Figure 8.13) and for organism detection. Nuclear detail is usually adequate.

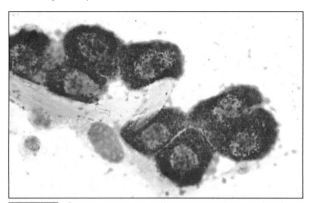

8.13   Cutaneous mast cell tumour aspirate stained with Diff-Quik (original magnification x1000).

Basic cytological analysis can be carried out in-house as long as the limitations of the technique are understood. It is also important to be aware of certain well recognized areas of confusion or diagnostic dilemma that may arise. Some of the more common potential diagnostic dilemmas with cytology include the following:

- Is it a chylous or lymphosarcoma-associated pleural effusion?
- Reactive mesothelial cells masquerading as neoplastic cells: which is it?
- Interpretation of the significance of abnormal appearing cells in regional lymph nodes: is it metastatic disease or not?
- If no neoplastic disease is identified from a single site aspirate, is that conclusive?

These can all be crucial factors in patient assessment. If there is any doubt, cytology should be backed up by additional tests such as tissue biopsy or an expert opinion.

Establishing surgical risk

The benefits of treatment must be weighed against the risks and potential adverse effects of anaesthesia and surgery. A physical status can be assigned on the basis of the American Society of Anesthesiologists (ASA) classification table (Figure 8.14) following the physical examination alone in many cases.

Surgical risk is influenced by the animal's primary condition, but also by any secondary conditions, current overall health status, age, the surgeon's experience, facilities and personnel available. Surgical risk also takes into account the long-term prognosis, the likely quality of life following surgery and the potential for complications.

First and foremost, the veterinary surgeon should always remember the recommendation contained in Hippocrates' book *Of the Epidemics*, written in 400 BC, 'to do good or to do no harm'; or the more popular version (which is of unknown origin): 'First do no harm.' This means that whatever decisions or recommendations are made regarding patients must be guided by what offers the best outcome and quality of life with minimum risks or adverse effects.

If surgery is unlikely to benefit the patient significantly, the question of whether it should be done at all should be addressed. Just because something *can* be done does not always mean that it *should* be done.

Communication with the client

Once the preoperative assessment is complete, surgical risk has been assessed, an ASA grade assigned and a treatment plan decided, all of this information must be communicated to the client in such a way that they can understand it and make an informed decision about what to do. This is a crucial stage in proceedings, and it is important that the veterinary surgeon should not only have a full, frank and informed discussion with the client, but should also record this fact and a summary of what was discussed. This is important from the point of view of avoiding a 'he said, she said' situation if complications arise, but it also facilitates a review of how the case has progressed, and case management if another clinician happens to see the patient at a later stage.

Physical status	Definition	Examples	Likely prognosis
I	Healthy patient, no organic disease	Elective surgery, not for therapeutic purposes (e.g. neutering)	Excellent
II	Local disease but no systemic signs	Non-elective surgery, but patient is healthy (e.g. suturing a skin laceration, repair of simple fracture)	Good
III	Disease that causes moderate systemic dysfunction	Patient exhibits problems such as heart murmur, anaemia, pneumonia, moderate dehydration	Fair
IV	Disease that causes severe systemic dysfunction, possibly life threatening	Conditions such as traumatic diaphragmatic rupture, GDV, severe thoracic trauma, diaphragmatic rupture	Guarded
V	Patient moribund, not expected to live longer than 24 hours either with or without surgery	Endotoxic shock, DIC, septic peritonitis, severe multi-system trauma	Very poor
E	Emergency	(This used to be a qualifier of categories listed above)	Variable

8.14   American Society of Anesthesiologists (ASA) Classification System for Physical Status.

What the client wants may not always be the same as what the veterinary surgeon would want but it is important that *all* the options are presented rather than just the surgeon's preference, to avoid doing both the client and patient a disservice. It is also necessary to be able to recognize whether the patient assessment indicates a condition, surgical intervention or level of aftercare that the surgeon is uncomfortable with or not equipped to provide, and the option of referral should be offered where appropriate.

Another vital part of client communication is the likely cost of treatment, or of alternatives where this applies, such as the cost of a tibial plateau levelling osteotomy (TPLO) compared with extracapsular repair for a ruptured cruciate ligament. Any discussion about likely costs or estimates should be recorded and updated as and when necessary in the patient's file.

References and further reading

Alef M, von Praun F and Oechtering G (2008) Is routine pre-anaesthetic haematological and biochemical screening justified in dogs? *Veterinary Anaesthesia and Analgesia* **35**, 132–140

Aronson LR, Brockman DJ and Cimino Brown D (2000) Gastrointestinal emergencies. *Veterinary Clinics of North America: Small Animal Practice* **30**, 555–579

Babin J, Langlois S, Friede J, Guay G and Agharazii M (2006) Green dialysate: asymptomatic perforated cholecystitis without peritonitis. *Nephrology Dialysis Transplantation* **21**, 1121–1122

Boag A and Hughes D (2004) Emergency management of the acute abdomen in dogs and cats. 1. Investigation and initial stabilisation *In Practice* **26**, 476–483

Fossum T (2002) Preoperative assessment of the surgical patient. In: *Small Animal Surgery, 2nd edn*, ed. TW Fossum, pp. 18–22. Mosby, St Louis

Giger U (2003) Differing opinions on value of PIVKA test. *Journal of the American Veterinary Medical Association* **222**, 1070–1071

House A and Brockman DJ (2004) Emergency management of the acute abdomen in dogs and cats. 2. Surgical treatment. *In Practice* **26**, 530–537

Mount ME, Kim BU and Kass PH (2003) Use of a test for proteins induced by vitamin K absence or antagonism in diagnosis of anticoagulant poisoning in dogs: 325 cases (1987–1997). *Journal of the American Veterinary Medical Association* **222**, 194–198

Pastore GE, Lamb CR and Lipscomb VJ (2007) Comparison of the results of abdominal ultrasonography and exploratory laparotomy. *Journal of the American Animal Hospital Association* **43**, 264–269

Schmon C (2003) Assessment and preparation of the surgical patient and the operating team. In: *Textbook of Small Animal Surgery, 2nd edn*, ed. D Slatter, pp 162–178. WB Saunders, Philadelphia

Senior M, Hird JF, Taylor PM *et al.* (2009) *Pre-medication and Anaesthesia in Dogs and Cats: summary of recommendations from 2009 Expert Round Table Discussion.* Vetoquinol Academia, Vetoquinol UK, Buckingham

Preoperative stabilization

9

David Holt and Jeffrey Wilson

Introduction

The best results from surgery come from following an appropriate plan, based on an accurate preoperative diagnosis. This plan includes a thorough evaluation and investigation of the presenting complaint and any other concurrent disease an animal may have.

Many animals requiring surgery in general practice are young and healthy and are presented for routine ovariohysterectomy or castration. After a thorough history, complete physical examination, evaluation for possible congenital abnormalities and, if indicated, a minimum database (including packed cell volume (PVC), total protein, evaluation of urea and blood glucose level), the majority of these animals require little if any stabilization prior to anaesthesia and routine surgery. Intravenous access, careful endotracheal intubation, strict attention to asepsis and meticulous surgical technique all ensure a successful surgical outcome.

Other animals, with a variety of diseases, require a more involved preoperative evaluation (see Chapter 8) and more intensive preoperative stabilization before anaesthesia and surgery can be considered. The aim of preoperative stabilization is to restore physiological functions to as close to normal as possible before anaesthesia and surgery. In some situations this is not always possible. The clinician must monitor the re-sponse to treatment carefully and assess when best to proceed with anaesthesia and surgery. This chapter describes the considerations and strategies for preoperative stabilization of animals with diseases affecting different body systems.

Gastrointestinal diseases

Oesophageal foreign bodies

Animals with oesophageal foreign bodies may be significantly dehydrated if the oesophageal obstruction and discomfort have prevented the swallowing of liquids for several days. The animal's hydration status is assessed from physical and laboratory parameters, including skin turgor, capillary refill time, PVC and total protein levels.

The choice of fluid for intravenous rehydration is based on preoperative serum electrolyte levels.

Ideally fluid deficits are replaced within 4 hours and prior to the induction of anaesthesia.

At the same time the animal is evaluated for evidence of possible oesophageal perforation, aspiration pneumonia and gastrointestinal disease associated with linear foreign bodies attached to needles or fishhooks lodged in the oesophagus.

- Perforation of the thoracic oesophagus causes mediastinitis, pleural effusion and, rarely, pneumothorax.
- Perforation of the cervical oesophagus causes pneumomediastinum and subcutaneous emphysema, and ultimately leads to cellulitis of the cervical tissues and mediastinitis.
- Exudation associated with mediastinitis and pleural effusion results in loss of fluid and protein from the vascular space that must be replaced before anaesthesia and surgery.
- Bacterial contamination often results in systemic inflammation and sepsis (the treatment of sepsis is described in the Peritonitis section of this chapter, and an in-depth discussion of shock, sepsis and systemic inflammatory response (SIRS) is presented in Chapter 11).
- Any animal regurgitating or vomiting frequently is at risk of aspiration (treatment of aspiration pneumonia is described in the Respiratory system section of this chapter).

Gastric dilatation–volvulus

Dogs with gastric dilatation–volvulus (GDV) have severe perfusion deficits. Compression of the portal vein and caudal vena cava cause decreased venous return to the heart, resulting in decreased cardiac output and poor tissue perfusion. Preoperative stabilization involves:

- Increasing the intravascular blood volume
- Decompressing the stomach.

Intravascular blood volume

Two large-bore catheters are placed in the cephalic veins (Figure 9.1), or, if these are not accessible, the jugular vein. Vessels in the caudal half of the body should not be used for fluid administration until full

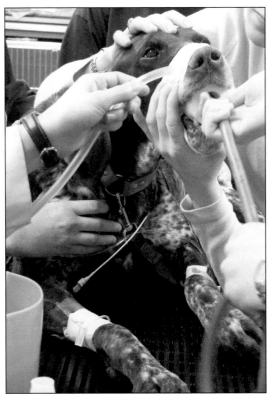

9.1 Dog with gastric dilatation–volvulus. Two cephalic catheters have been placed to administer intravenous fluids. Orogastric intubation is being attempted. (© David Holt)

decompression of the stomach at surgery has been accomplished. Samples are obtained for a minimum database and, ideally, for levels of serum electrolytes and lactate along with venous blood gas analysis.

Rapid volume resuscitation: Rapid volume resuscitation is often necessary, using crystalloids at 60–90 ml/kg in the first hour. A goal-directed approach to therapy has demonstrated benefits over delivering set volumes of fluid (see also Chapters 10 and 11). A rational approach is to administer rapid boluses of intravenous crystalloid at 20–30 ml/kg while assessing the response in perfusion parameters (heart rate, blood pressure, capillary refill time, etc.).

In large or giant dogs, or in dogs with profound hypoperfusion:

- A combination of hypertonic saline (7–7.5%) and a colloid (4–7 ml/kg i.v. given slowly over 10–15 minutes) can be used for rapid intravascular volume expansion
- This must then be followed by a crystalloid infusion to sustain the effect on volume expansion and offset the effects of the large shifts in fluid between body compartments which result from hypertonic saline administration
- Synthetic colloids or blood products may be required, depending on the severity of concurrent hypoproteinaemia or intra-abdominal haemorrhage.

Monitoring: The dog's mucous membrane colour, capillary refill time, heart rate, pulse quality and, ideally, blood pressure, electrolyte and serum lactate levels are monitored to assess the response to treatment.

Cardiac arrhythmias: An electrocardiogram (ECG) is monitored for arrhythmias such as ventricular premature contractions (VPCs) and ventricular tachycardia. The main cause of cardiac arrhythmias in dogs with GDV is thought to be associated with poor perfusion, so increasing intravascular volume is the first treatment for this condition. Anti-arrhythmic drugs (lidocaine 2 mg/kg bolus with a 30–80 µg/kg/min infusion) should be considered in dwogs with persistent high-rate ventricular tachycardia (>160 beats/min), or with multifocal VPCs or evidence of an R-on-T arrhythmia, or any time the arrhythmia is deemed to affect perfusion and cardiac output negatively, as assessed by pulse quality and/or blood pressure measurements.

Stomach decompression

Once resuscitation has commenced, the distended stomach is decompressed.

- This is initially attempted by passing a lubricated large-bore tube through the mouth and down the oesophagus (see Figure 9.1). The tube is measured and marked before passage so that the approximate length necessary to reach the stomach is known.
- In some animals the stomach tube can be passed through the lumen of a roll of tape held in the mouth with the dog conscious.
- Less tractable animals are sedated using an opioid/benzodiazepine combination, or the stomach may be trocharized.
- If airway protective reflexes are obtunded or lost with sedation, tracheal intubation should be secured to allow safe passage of the stomach tube.
- Gastric contents are removed and the stomach is lavaged several times with warm water.

In many dogs with gastric volvulus the tube does not pass easily at the level of the caudal oesophageal sphincter. The tube should not be forced, as this can tear the abdominal oesophagus or cardia of the stomach. Passage of a smaller diameter tube is attempted, but if this is unsuccessful the stomach is trocharized (Figure 9.2).

Stomach trocharization is a very useful and quick technique that often allows enough stomach decompression by removal of air to aid initial patient stabilization prior to removal of all stomach contents by tube decompression later (either following initial stabilization or intraoperatively once the stomach has been repositioned).

To trocharize the stomach:

1. The abdomen is carefully palpated and a tympanic area selected. The spleen, although often displaced in a dog with GDV, is engorged and palpable and should be avoided.

2. The area is clipped and scrubbed.

3. A 14 or 16 gauge catheter is placed through the skin and abdominal wall and into the stomach.

4. As soon as the stomach is entered the catheter is advanced off the stylette.

5. As much gas as possible is removed using a large syringe. Fluid or food material may obstruct the catheter and impede decompression.

9.2 Stomach trocharization.

Anaesthesia

Anaesthesia should be induced only when the clinical parameters, blood pressure and ECG confirm that perfusion has been improved as much as possible.

- Pre-oxygenation is essential as these dogs commonly have severe changes in ventilation and reduced functional residual capacity as a result of compression by the enlarged stomach.
- Many combinations of drugs can be used but protocols should centre around use of opioids and benzodiazepines, along with careful titration of all these agents to effect.
- Maintenance of anaesthesia can be achieved with inhalant anaesthetics, but it is useful to combine this with infusions or serial injections of other drugs (lidocaine, opioids, ketamine) to achieve minimum alveolar concentration (MAC) reduction and analgesia.

Crystalloid infusions should be continued through the induction and surgical period and any decreases in perfusion should be aggressively treated with fluids, positive inotropes and vasopressors, as indicated.

Gastric foreign bodies

Gastrointestinal foreign bodies are one of the most common conditions requiring exploratory laparotomy. The amount and type of stabilization required for an animal with an intestinal foreign body depends on the location, duration and severity of the intestinal obstruction.

Fluid loss

Dogs ingest 40–60 ml water/kg bodyweight each day. Salivary, gastric, pancreatic and biliary secretions add to the fluid presented to the intestines. The vast majority of this fluid load is reabsorbed by the small intestine and, to a far lesser degree, by the colon. Large quantities of many electrolytes (including sodium, chloride, potassium, hydrogen and bicarbonate) are also secreted into and reabsorbed from the intestines.

- In animals with intestinal obstruction, secretions into the intestines are increased and fluid resorption is decreased.
- Vomiting results in loss of both fluids and electrolytes.
- Additional fluid is sequestered in distended intestinal loops.
- The severity and nature of the fluid and electrolyte loss depends on the level (high *versus* low) and degree (partial *versus* complete) of the obstruction.

Hypochloraemia and metabolic alkalosis

Dogs with gastric foreign bodies or masses that obstruct gastric outflow lose large amounts of acidic stomach contents from vomiting and often have a substantial hypochloraemic metabolic alkalosis with a compensatory increase in the arterial carbon dioxide level.

- The metabolic abnormality should be recognized and corrected using intravenous 0.9% sodium chloride supplemented with potassium chloride.

Sodium chloride solution has a higher chloride concentration and is more acidic than other commercially available crystalloids.

- Electrolytes should be monitored closely and a balanced solution (Nomosol R) instituted as the primary problem is corrected.

> **PRACTICAL TIP**
>
> It is important to recognize that the increased carbon dioxide level due to hypoventilation is a normal compensatory response to the metabolic alkalosis and the veterinary surgeon should refrain from hyperventilating the dog once it is anaesthetized. This would only worsen the alkalosis.

Small intestinal surgery

Dogs vomiting because of small intestinal obstruction lose fluid and sodium, potassium, hydrogen and chloride ions, plus variable amounts of pancreatic bicarbonate. Experimentally, mechanical intestinal obstruction predisposes dogs to hypokalaemia, hyponatraemia and hypochloraemia. Animals may have a metabolic acidosis due to excessive bicarbonate loss worsened by acidosis secondary to poor tissue perfusion. It is not possible to give general recommendations on restoring perfusion, acid–base and electrolyte levels in animals with intestinal obstruction: each case must be evaluated and treated individually.

The animal's degree of dehydration and perfusion status are assessed from the physical examination. Electrolyte levels and acid–base status are measured and blood lactate levels provide objective information on tissue perfusion.

Rehydration

Stable animals should be rehydrated with a balanced electrolyte solution for 2–4 hours. The fluid rate is determined based on the degree of dehydration, an estimation of ongoing losses from vomiting and diarrhoea, and an allowance for maintenance fluid requirements (see also Chapter 10).

For example, a 20 kg dog that is judged to be 5% dehydrated, losing 200 ml/h through vomiting and with a maintenance requirement of 50 ml/h, would require 2 litres over 4 hours (1000 ml dehydration + 800 ml for ongoing losses + 200 ml for maintenance over 4 hours), i.e. a fluid rate of 500 ml/hour (or 25 ml/kg/h).

Antibiotics

The use of perioperative antibiotics in dogs with small intestinal obstruction has become routine, based largely on theoretical considerations rather than controlled clinical trials. The benefits of antibiotics are well documented in dogs with strangulating intestinal obstructions, but those with non-strangulating obstructions receive antibiotics based on the increased number of bacteria in the stagnant intestine and the concern for intraoperative contamination.

When used, antibiotics should be administered intravenously immediately before surgery so that they are at bactericidal levels in the serum and tissues during the procedure. The normal intestinal flora includes coliforms, enterococci and anaerobes. A combination of either ampicillin and a fluoroquinolone or an aminoglycoside, or a second-generation cephalosporin (e.g. cefuroxime), is a reasonable choice for antimicrobial prophylaxis.

Mesenteric volvulus

Dogs with mesenteric volvulus are often in severe shock when presented and are difficult to stabilize. Large amounts of fluid and protein are rapidly lost into the lumen of the entrapped intestines. Poor intestinal perfusion quickly compromises the mucosal barrier and increases the likelihood of translocation and systemic absorption of bacteria and endotoxins. Resuscitation will not completely stabilize these animals, as any increase in intravascular volume from resuscitation will rapidly be lost into the entrapped intestines.

■ Two large-bore intravenous catheters are placed in affected dogs and goal-directed infusions of intravenous crystalloid (20–30 ml/kg boluses, repeated as required) and colloid (Hetastarch 5–10 ml/kg) are administered over 30–45 minutes. Colloids may benefit compromised intestine by maintaining mucosal oxygen tension and preventing intestinal oedema formation.

■ The animal is carefully anaesthetized and an immediate abdominal exploration performed.

Large intestinal surgery

Dogs most frequently require surgery on the large intestine for neoplastic masses affecting the caecum (leiomyoma, leiomyosarcoma, gastrointestinal stromal cell tumour) or for colonic perforations secondary to trauma, ulcers and, rarely, endoscopic biopsy.

■ Dogs with caecal tumours may have few clinical signs and be diagnosed as part of the investigation for another abdominal condition.

■ Conversely, if the tumour ruptures and caecal contents begin to leak, the animal requires prompt stabilization and surgery for peritonitis (stabilization of dogs with colonic perforations is discussed in the section on Peritonitis, below).

Cats frequently undergo subtotal colectomy to treat megacolon. A thorough evaluation and clinical investigation are necessary, as many affected cats are older and have concurrent diseases (hyperthyroidism, hypertrophic cardiomyopathy and renal disease). Stabilization of hyperthyroid cats is discussed in the Endocrine disease section of this chapter.

■ Preoperative enemas are avoided in both species. Enemas administered in the immediate preoperative period turn any faecal material into a loose liquid that is difficult to manipulate and likely to contaminate the surgical field.

■ Similarly, oral cathartics are contraindicated immediately prior to surgery.

■ Perioperative antibiotics are administered parenterally and should be effective against anaerobes and Gram-negative bacteria.

Peritonitis

Dogs and cats develop aseptic peritonitis caused by pancreatitis and leakage of gastric contents with minimal bacterial contamination. Peritonitis secondary to urine or bile leakage can be septic or aseptic. Leakage of small or large intestinal contents or rupture of a pyometra or prostatic abscess rapidly causes septic peritonitis.

■ In all cases, capillaries in the parietal and visceral peritoneum dilate and capillary permeability increases.

■ The peritoneal surface area is extensive and massive amounts of fluid and protein are quickly lost from the vascular space.

■ Cytokines and endotoxins released as part of the inflammatory response and secondary to systemic bacterial infection affect vascular tone, resulting in substantial vasodilatation.

■ The net result is decreased intravascular volume in the face of increasing intravascular space and decreased cardiac output resulting from a substantial drop in preload. This leads to maldistribution of blood flow and poor tissue perfusion.

■ Poor perfusion and thrombosis associated with disseminated intravascular coagulation and vascular endothelial dysfunction cause organ failure if aggressive treatment is not instituted quickly (see Chapter 11 for an in-depth discussion of shock, sepsis and SIRS).

Fluid therapy

Stabilization of an animal with peritonitis requires intravenous access with large-bore catheters in two peripheral veins, or a peripheral and a central vein. The choice of fluids and rate of resuscitation are determined by assessment of tissue perfusion, concurrent diseases (cardiac, pulmonary) and the initial laboratory data.

■ In most instances a combination of crystalloids and colloids is necessary, with colloids being preferred if endothelial dysfunction and increased vascular permeability are suspected.

■ Fresh frozen plasma provides albumin and clotting factors, but is often not immediately available to the general practitioner. In addition, a relatively large volume of plasma is required to increase serum albumin levels.

Synthetic colloids (Hetastarch, Dextran 70) are administered with crystalloid fluids as an initial bolus. In severe septic peritonitis 30–40 ml crystalloid/kg and 10 ml colloid/kg may be administered initially. The rate of ongoing fluid administration is determined by the response to therapy, which is monitored by clinical parameters, direct and indirect blood pressure measurements, and changes in acid–base status and blood lactate levels.

In advanced care settings, monitoring central mixed venous oxygen saturation and cardiac output provides useful objective information to guide resuscitation therapy.

Vasopressors

In some cases blood pressure and perfusion do not improve in spite of appropriate volume expansion, because of cytokine-mediated disruption of normal vascular tone. In these cases vasopressor therapy may be necessary. Vasopressors are most effective at improving perfusion when combined with appropriate fluid therapy and positive inotropes. The goal is to re-establish vascular smooth muscle tone so that delivery of oxygen is achieved without the occurrence of vasoconstriction and organ hypoxia. This is often a delicate balance to achieve and it should be remembered that improving blood pressure alone with vasopressors is not the most important determinant of improved tissue perfusion.

PRACTICAL TIP

Once volume resuscitation has been achieved, the addition of a positive inotrope (dopamine 5–10 µg/kg/min, or dobutamine 2–15 µg/kg/min) may be effective in improving perfusion.

As indicated previously, however, peritonitis is often accompanied by systemic inflammatory disease and circulating endotoxins, which result in inappropriate vascular tone. In this situation careful titration of a vasopressor (phenylephrine 1–3 µg/kg/min, noradrenaline 0.05–1 µg/kg/min) is often effective at re-establishing vascular tone and improving organ perfusion.

The combination of a vasopressor and positive inotrope is more effective at maintaining organ perfusion than a vasopressor alone. Vasopressors are titrated to achieve a mean arterial pressure of at least 70 mmHg without creating hypertension. Additional variables such as lactate, jugular venous oxygen saturation and central venous pressure may aid in evaluating the success of treatment if available.

Antibiotics

In septic peritonitis, intravenous antibiotics are administered immediately, based on knowledge of both the normal bacterial flora in the suspected source organ and antimicrobial pharmacokinetics. Bacteria commonly found in the intestine include enterococci, coliforms and anaerobes. Appropriate antibiotics to treat these infections include a combination of a penicillin or first-generation cephalosporin with an aminoglycoside or fluoroquinolone, or a second-generation cephalosporin. An antibiotic specifically targeting anaerobes, such as metronidazole, is often added to this regimen.

PRACTICAL TIPS

- Penicillins and cephalosporins are time-dependent antibiotics: their effectiveness depends on maintaining serum and tissue concentrations above the minimum inhibitory concentration (MIC) by frequent dosing, generally every 6 hours.
- Aminoglycosides and fluoroquinolones are concentration-dependent antibiotics: their maximum effect is dependent on obtaining the highest possible concentration using a single daily dose.

The location and nature of the source infection is also considered when deciding on appropriate antibiotic therapy. Fluoroquinolones are concentrated in phagocytes and penetrate abscesses far better than aminoglycocides; they are a more appropriate choice for peritonitis secondary to prostatic abscessation.

Haemoperitoneum

The two most common causes of haemoperitoneum in dogs are rupture of splenic masses and blunt abdominal trauma associated with a road traffic accident or a fall. Canine splenic masses associated with haemoperitoneum can be malignant (haemangiosarcoma) or benign (haematoma). Loss of blood into the peritoneal space frequently results in hypovolaemia.

Tissue oxygen delivery is dependent on both cardiac output and arterial oxygen content.

- Cardiac output is the product of heart rate and stroke volume.
- Arterial oxygen content is largely determined by the haemoglobin concentration.

Maintaining tissue oxygen delivery in haemoperitoneum is therefore largely dependent on restoring and maintaining an appropriate intravascular volume and an adequate haemoglobin concentration.

Crystalloids *versus* blood products

The choice of crystalloid or blood products for resuscitation depends on a thorough assessment of the animal's perfusion, blood pressure and PCV. Some animals that are relatively stable with non-life-threatening abdominal haemorrhage may respond to conservative (20 ml/kg) intravenous boluses of crystalloid fluids. Animals with more severe perfusion deficits require more aggressive intravenous resuscitation.

WARNINGS

- Aggressive volume resuscitation may increase blood pressure but this may, in turn, promote re-bleeding.
- The use of crystalloids or synthetic colloids for intravascular volume expansion in animals with haemoperitoneum may cause haemodilution and may lower the haemoglobin concentration enough to adversely affect tissue oxygen delivery.

Re-bleeding

Temporary application of a tight abdominal bandage ('abdominal counterpressure') (Figure 9.3) can slow or arrest parenchymal or venous bleeding by raising intra-abdominal pressure. However, increasing intra-abdominal pressure for prolonged periods can adversely affect renal and hepatic blood flow. There are many experimental studies in animal models investigating intravenous resuscitation, blood pressure and re-bleeding. Depending on the model, some studies show that re-bleeding occurs at a systolic blood pressure of 90 mmHg, yet limited volume resuscitation may not improve the outcome unless rapid access to surgical control of bleeding is available. In veterinary medicine it is usually effective to titrate resuscitative therapy with a goal of achieving a mean arterial pressure not higher than 60–70 mmHg until surgical haemostasis can be achieved.

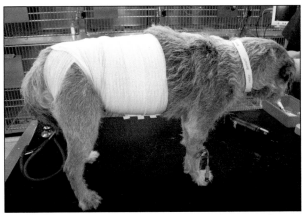

9.3 Dog with progressive haemoabdomen and tachycardia following a Tru-cut liver biopsy. An abdominal counterpressure bandage has been firmly placed using elasticated adhesive bandage material. (Courtesy of V Lipscomb)

Haemodilution

In general, oxygen delivery is well preserved at lower haemoglobin values (>6–7 g/dl) as long as cardiovascular parameters are maintained. Decreased blood viscosity occurs with haemodilution and may result in improved microcirculatory blood flow. Animals that have clinical or laboratory evidence of poor perfusion and a low PCV at presentation should be resuscitated with both crystalloid/colloid fluids and stored packed red blood cells (PRBCs) or fresh whole blood. The PCV should ideally be maintained above 25%.

Blood transfusion

Blood typing

Dogs should be blood typed before donating blood or receiving a transfusion. They can be tested for the dog erythrocyte antigen (DEA) 1.1 either by a reference laboratory, or in-house using a card test kit.

PRACTICAL TIPS

- Dogs that are DEA 1.1-negative should not receive DEA 1.1-positive blood as they will become sensitized and produce antibodies that will induce an acute haemolytic transfusion reaction if a second DEA 1.1-positive transfusion is administered.
- Dogs that are DEA 1.1-positive may receive either DEA 1.1-positive or DEA 1.1-negative blood.

Blood typing of donor and recipient cats prior to transfusion is imperative. Cats have three blood types: A, B and, rarely, AB. Type A cats have alloantibodies in their plasma against the type B antigen and *vice versa*. There is thus a high risk of a serious reaction if a cat receives an incompatible blood transfusion. A detailed discussion of blood collection, typing, cross-matching, storage and administration is presented in Chapter 20.

Whole blood and packed red blood cells

In a dog without ongoing haemorrhage:

- Transfused whole blood (with a PCV in the normal range) at 2 ml/kg will raise the PCV by 1%

- PRBCs at 1 ml/kg will raise the PCV by 1%.

It would be reasonable to expect most animals with haemoperitoneum, anaemia and poor perfusion requiring surgery to receive an initial bolus of whole blood at 10 ml/kg, or an equivalent quantity of PRBCs. The volume of blood administered and rate of administration will, however, depend upon the initial severity of the anaemia, the response to the transfusion and the amount of ongoing haemorrhage. In cases with severe ongoing haemorrhage, large volumes of blood may be required in a short time to maintain PCV and blood pressure.

Citrate as an anticoagulant

Citrate is used as an anticoagulant in blood collection systems. It will bind calcium in the patient's peripheral blood and may result in hypocalcaemia and hypotension in animals receiving massive transfusions. Intravenous calcium may be required to maintain blood pressure and normal cardiac rhythm (10% calcium glutamate, 0.5–1.5 ml/kg i.v. very slowly).

Oxyglobin

Haemoglobin-based oxygen-carrying solutions and autotransfusions are two possible alternatives when fresh or stored blood products are not available in emergency situations. Oxyglobin, a solution containing sterile purified polymerized bovine haemoglobin, has been approved for use in dogs (see Chapter 10 for a detailed description). In addition to increasing blood oxygen-carrying capacity, it is an effective colloid and increases intravascular volume. The recommended dose of Oxyglobin in anaemic normovolaemic dogs is 10–30 ml/kg administered at a rate of <10 ml/kg/h. With Oxyglobin administration the PCV becomes an inaccurate measure of oxygen-carrying capacity, but haemoglobin concentration can reliably be used to direct further therapy. A goal of 7–8 g/dl is sufficient to establish adequate delivery of oxygen if cardiovascular parameters are maintained. It is possible, however, that Oxyglobin will no longer be available to the veterinary market in the future.

Autotransfusion

Autotransfusion can be life-saving in the appropriate patient when other alternatives are not available. It is contraindicated in any cases with haemorrhage secondary to neoplasia (i.e. canine splenic haemangiosarcoma) or those associated with potential contamination (i.e. traumatic haemoperitoneum with a concurrent intestinal rupture).

- In cases of traumatic haemoperitoneum, blood is withdrawn from the abdomen through a large-bore intravenous catheter or peritoneal dialysis catheter into syringes and quickly transferred to a blood collection bag.
- A blood smear is made and evaluated microscopically to rule out bacterial contamination.
- The blood is then re-infused intravenously through an in-line blood filter (170–260 μm) provided with standard blood infusion sets.
- For smaller animals, blood may be collected into syringes containing 1 ml of 3.8% citrate for every 9 ml of blood withdrawn and re-infused directly from the syringe through a micro-aggregate filter (18–40 μm).

Hepatic disease

Animals with liver disease may require surgery for biopsy, correction of congenital portal vascular anomalies, relief of biliary obstructions, removal of gallbladder mucoceles or ruptured gallbladders, and removal of neoplasms. The liver performs several vital functions directly relevant to anaesthesia. In all animals with liver disease a serum biochemical panel, including albumin and full coagulation screen, are mandatory, as are a blood type and the availability of compatible fresh frozen plasma.

Albumin

In addition to biotransformation and metabolism of drugs, the liver produces albumin, the most abundant plasma protein that binds many drugs, including anaesthetic agents. Decreased production of albumin by a diseased liver results in decreased drug–protein binding and an increased amount of the free or active form of the drug. This is one of several reasons why lower doses of anaesthetic drugs are often required in animals with liver disease and why anaesthesia in these animals in particular should be carefully titrated to effect.

Albumin is also the primary determinant of plasma colloid oncotic pressure (the difference between the osmotic pressure of blood and that of the lymph or tissue fluid). Severe decreases (<2 g/dl) lead to tissue oedema, especially with delivery of large volumes of crystalloids as may be required in stabilization and anaesthesia. Hetastarch (5 ml/kg + 1–2 ml/kg/h) is effective at restoring and maintaining the plasma oncotic pressure and should be used in place of large volumes of crystalloid.

Vitamin K

Liver disease may also affect production of the coagulation factors vital for surgical haemostasis. Several of the coagulation factors (II, VII, IX and X) require vitamin K for post-translational modification and normal function. As vitamin K is fat-soluble, biliary obstruction or biliary leakage can decrease its absorption. In animals with suspected biliary leakage or obstruction, vitamin K is administered subcutaneously at a rate of 1 mg/kg bodyweight.

Serum ammonia levels

Some dogs with portosystemic shunts and other dogs with severe liver disease present with clinical signs of hepatic encephalopathy, a complex metabolic condition associated with increased serum ammonia levels. Serum ammonia levels should be reduced and clinical signs of hepatic encephalopathy ameliorated before anaesthesia and surgery are considered.

Diet

Animals are placed on a restricted protein diet (14–17% protein on a dry matter basis in dogs; 30–35% protein in cats) that is high in carbohydrates. The protein should be of high quality and have a high level of branched chain amino acids. The diet should be a low-residue easily digestible food to minimize the amount of material reaching the colon. It must contain adequate amounts of arginine for cats, as this is an essential amino acid necessary for the urea cycle.

Lactulose

Lactulose is an osmotic cathartic that decreases gastrointestinal transit time and reduces the pH of the intestinal contents, trapping ammonia within the gastrointestinal tract as ammonium ions and decreasing the number of urease-producing colonic bacteria. It is administered orally at a dose of 1–3 ml/10 kg q6–8h and the dose rate and interval are titrated to produce two to four moderately soft stools daily. Lactulose may be administered as an enema to animals in status epilepticus or animals with such severe neurological depression that oral administration is not possible.

Antibiotics

Antibiotics are administered to decrease the number of urease-producing bacteria in the intestines.

- Neomycin sulphate (20 mg/kg orally q6–8h) is generally considered non-absorbable, but should be avoided in animals with concurrent renal disease.
- Metronidazole (10–20 mg/kg orally or i.v. q12h) is a reasonable alternative, but neurotoxicity may occur more commonly in animals with hepatic disease.
- Amoxicillin (12 mg/kg orally q12h) has also been used.

The effect of long-term therapy with antibiotics on the intestinal flora of dogs and cats is not clear. Since the therapeutic effect of lactulose depends on its metabolism by colonic bacteria, the benefit of combined lactulose and antibiotic therapy is open to question in small animals.

Antacids

Some animals with severe liver disease have concurrent gastrointestinal haemorrhage, which serves as a high protein source for gastrointestinal ammonia production. Antacids or gastrointestinal protectants such as famotidine (0.25–1 mg/kg orally or i.v. q12–24h), omeprazole (0.5–1.5 mg/kg i.v. or orally, q24h), misoprostol (2–3 µg/kg orally q8h) and sucralfate (0.25–1 g/25 kg orally q6–8h) may be used to minimize gastrointestinal haemorrhage.

Seizures

Animals with seizures prior to surgery may need emergency stabilization with propofol (0.5 mg/kg i.v., then 0.05–0.1 mg/kg/min) to stop seizure activity. Phenobarbital has also been used for this purpose, but liver metabolism is variably affected by the shunt, making dose recommendation difficult for an individual animal.

Respiratory system

Upper airway diseases

Dogs often present with conditions causing upper airway obstruction (laryngeal paralysis, brachycephalic obstructive airway disease (BOAS), tracheal collapse) that require stabilization prior to definitive treatment. Other less common conditions affecting the upper airways include granulomatous laryngitis in cats, laryngeal or tracheal crushing injury, foreign bodies, neoplasia and tracheal tearing or avulsion.

The stabilization required before anaesthesia and surgery is determined by the severity of the animal's respiratory compromise. One study of arterial blood gas values in dogs with laryngeal paralysis showed that the severity of clinical signs approximated the degree of hypoxia but hypoventilation (increased P_aCO_2) did not occur, even in severely affected dogs (Love *et al.*, 1987).

Many animals with upper airway obstruction respond to oxygen supplementation, mild sedation and systemic medication (dexamethasone 0.01–0.02 mg/kg i.v.) to decrease airway swelling. Intravenous access is mandatory, in case respiratory signs worsen.

Oxygen supplementation

Options for oxygen supplementation include an oxygen cage (Figure 9.4a), oxygen piped into a modified human incubator, 'flow-by' oxygen (Figure 9.4b), or mask supplementation. Nasal catheter placement for oxygen supplementation is not appropriate, as this requires restraint and often causes the animal to struggle, increasing oxygen consumption.

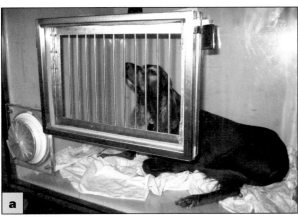

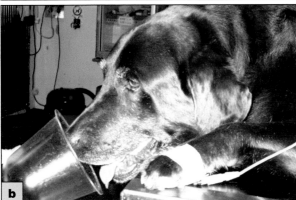

9.4 Oxygen supplementation. **(a)** Dog with dyspnoea due to laryngeal paralysis in an oxygen cage. **(b)** Dog with laryngeal paralysis receiving 'flow-by' oxygen whilst awaiting placement of an intravenous catheter. (a, © David Holt; b, courtesy of V Lipscomb)

Sedation

Sedation with acepromazine (0.005–0.02 mg/kg i.v.) ± an opioid (butorphanol 0.2–0.4 mg/kg) in animals with normal blood pressure often substantially improves signs of respiratory distress. It is important to note that acepromazine decreases laryngeal abduction in normal dogs, making definitive diagnosis of laryngeal paralysis during laryngoscopy more difficult in affected animals.

Hyperthermia

The increased muscular activity required by animals to ventilate effectively with an upper airway obstruction often generates substantial heat and marked hyperthermia. Cool intravenous fluids are the most effective method of decreasing core body temperature in a controlled manner.

> **PRACTICAL TIP**
>
> To avoid 'overshoot' hypothermia, aggressive cooling should stop when the temperature drops to <39.5°C.

Arrhythmias

An ECG should be closely monitored in cases of upper airway disease. High vagal tone is often present in animals with chronic upper airway malformations or disease, and severe bradyarrythmias or arrest may occur with laryngeal stimulation. It is not uncommon to see ventricular arrhythmias in animals with laryngeal paralysis.

Intubation

In some animals with severe upper respiratory obstruction, rapid intubation is necessary to prevent respiratory and subsequently cardiac arrest. Intravenous access is mandatory. An ECG and a well organized emergency trolley (Figure 9.5) or box containing a range of endotracheal tubes, stylettes, polypropylene catheters, laryngoscopes and emergency drugs greatly facilitates this process.

- The minimum doses of drugs necessary to allow intubation are administered and the trachea is intubated with direct laryngeal visualization.
- In cases of suspected tracheal tearing, a small tube is used and passed with great care to avoid worsening of the tear or complete separation of the torn ends (in cats with tracheal rupture due to an endotracheal intubation injury or a road traffic

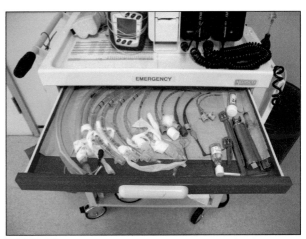

9.5 Crash trolley stocked with an organized system of endotracheal tubes, stylettes, polypropylene catheters, laryngoscopes, and emergency drugs. (Courtesy of V Lipscomb)

injury, the tracheal tear is likely to be around the level of the thoracic inlet).

- In animals with laryngeal paralysis or BOAS where there is going to be a delay in instituting definitive treatment (e.g. further stabilization or investigation is required, treatment of aspiration pneumonia, transfer to a referral institution), a temporary tracheostomy tube may be placed before recovering the animal from anaesthesia.

Lower airway and pleural space diseases

Diseases affecting the lower airways and pleural space in animals requiring surgery include pneumothorax, pleural effusions, diaphragmatic rupture, pneumonia, pulmonary contusions, pulmonary oedema and asthma.

Pneumothorax

Pneumothorax is most commonly secondary to thoracic trauma or associated with rupture of pulmonary bullae (so-called primary spontaneous pneumothorax). In many instances the pneumothorax is mild enough that the animal is able to compensate for the decrease in lung volume; and ventilation and gas exchange are not affected substantially. In such animals requiring surgery there is some debate as to when it is safe to perform general anaesthesia and surgery, centred on the concern that positive pressure ventilation may cause damaged lung to start leaking again. There is no general answer for this question, but ideally anaesthetic protocols should be designed to allow the animal to breathe spontaneously as much as possible and positive pressure ventilation should be limited, with peak inspiratory pressures (PIP) kept below 10 cmH$_2$O.

Thoracocentesis: In more severely affected animals an initial chest tap is performed using a butterfly catheter and extension set for smaller dogs and cats and an intravenous catheter in larger dogs (see Chapter 8 for technique).

- Air is carefully removed by an assistant using a syringe and three-way stopcock.
- When negative pressure is obtained, the needle/catheter is removed and the animal's clinical signs are reassessed. Some air will invariably remain in the pleural space radiographically.
- If negative pressure cannot be reached, the

connections between the catheter, three-way stopcock and syringe are checked.

Chest drains: Persistent or worsening respiratory distress associated with continued leakage of air into the pleural space is an indication for placement of a chest drain. Although this can be performed using only sedation and local anaesthesia, careful general anaesthesia and intubation are preferred as this gives the veterinary surgeon more time, the ability to ventilate the patient with 100% oxygen and complete control of the airway in case of an emergency. The exception to this is if a small-bore wire-guided chest drain is placed: this technique has recently been described in veterinary patients (Valtolina and Adamantos, 2009) and is typically performed under sedation.

- Whichever method of chest drain placement is used, the patient is usually placed in lateral recumbency and the lateral thorax is clipped.
- To obtain an anaesthetic block of skin, muscle and parietal pleura, 2% lidocaine (0.2 ml/kg) is infused at the site of incision.
- Manual ventilation is stopped during insertion of the chest drain and a syringe should be immediately attached to the tube following placement to remove residual fluid or air and prevent iatrogenic pneumothorax.
- After placement, the chest drain is secured with a purse-string suture and a Chinese finger-trap suture.
- A clamp is placed over the tube and a three-way stopcock is placed on the end of the tube to provide two points of secure tube closure.
- It is often useful to radiograph the thorax following chest drain placement in order to document its position and reassess for any thoracic disease that was not apparent before complete removal of pleural fluid and/or air.
- If intermittent aspiration of the chest drain is not sufficient to deal with the pneumothorax (uncommon), the chest drain is connected to a continuous suction drainage device (e.g. Pleurovac) with the initial drainage pressure set between 10 and 15 cmH$_2$O.

The placement, advantages and disadvantages of three non-surgical chest drain techniques used by the authors or the editors are summarized in Figure 9.6.

Type	Advantages	Disadvantages
Trochar chest drain (Figure 9.7a): PVC tube with two to four distal fenestrations, 16–30 Fr (Technique 9.1)	Procedure is quick to perform Larger bore tubes support removal of thick fluid	General anaesthesia is recommended PVC tube is quite rigid and therefore likely to be more uncomfortable for the patient than softer silicone tubes (the diameter of the chest tube will also affect patient comfort) Risk of iatrogenic damage to intrathoracic structures if introduction into chest is not carefully controlled, especially in cats and small dogs
Chest drain placement using haemostat forceps: PVC trochar or silicone non-trochar chest drain (with two to four additional distal fenestrations cut in by surgeon; Figure 9.7a), 16–30 Fr (Technique 9.2)	Silicone tube is softer and less irritant than PVC tube Larger bore tubes support removal of thick fluid Negligible risk of iatrogenic damage to intrathoracic structures	General anaesthesia is recommended May require 'mini thoracotomy' to enter pleural cavity

9.6 Comparison of three non-surgical techniques for chest drain placement. (continues) ▶

Type	Advantages	Disadvantages
Small-bore wire-guided chest drain (modified Seldinger technique) (Technique 9.3): polyurethane multi-fenestrated catheter, 14 gauge, 20 cm long (Figure 9.7c)	Polyurethane small diameter tube is likely to be more comfortable for patients (especially cats and small dogs) Procedure is quick to perform Negligible risk of iatrogenic damage to intrathoracic structures Typically placed under sedation only	Once in the pleural space, the operator has little control over the guidewire trajectory; therefore catheter placement may not always be optimal The tube is 14 gauge so is likely to be more prone to dislodgement, blockage or incomplete removal of thick exudate (e.g. in pyothorax cases) compared with large-bore tubes

9.6 (continued) Comparison of three non-surgical techniques for chest drain placement.

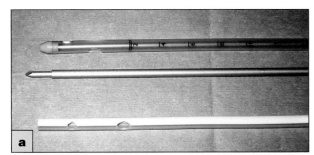
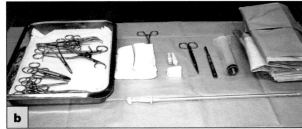
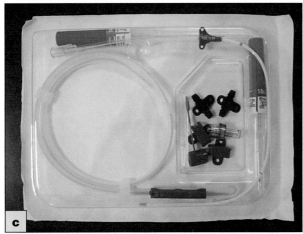

9.7 **(a)** PVC chest drain (top) with its trochar (middle), and (bottom) a silicone non-trochar chest drain with extra side holes cut in by the clinician (holes should be approximately one-third of the tube diameter). **(b)** Equipment for trochar chest drain placement. **(c)** Multi-fenestrated chest drain catheter (Chest Tube – Guideware Inserted; MILA International). (a, © David Holt; b,c, courtesy of R Goggs)

TECHNIQUE 9.1
Placement of a trochar chest drain

1 A stab skin incision is made in the dorsal region of the thorax around the 9th or 10th intercostal space, through which the chest drain is introduced and tunnelled subcutaneously in a cranial direction for approximately three rib spaces.

2 The chest drain is then positioned perpendicular to the chest and held firmly distally and proximally whilst slowly increasing pressure and gently twisting the tip of the drain until it enters the 6th or 7th intercostal space. It is important to control the rate of pressure increase and keep a firm grasp of the distal end of the chest drain to prevent uncontrolled or sudden chest penetration. (NB: There is no need to 'hit' or aggressively punch the trochar.)

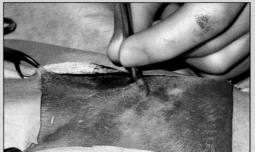
(Courtesy of V Lipscomb)

3 The chest tube is clamped to prevent iatrogenic pneumothorax whilst the correct connectors and a syringe are attached.

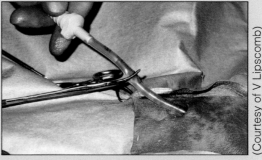
(Courtesy of V Lipscomb)

4 A security clamp, connector and three way-tap are attached to the chest drain. The chest can be drained by attaching a syringe to the end of the three-way tap.

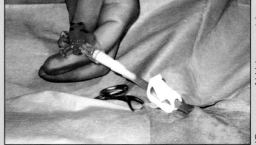
(Courtesy of V Lipscomb)

TECHNIQUE 9.2
Chest drain placement using haemostat forceps

1 A small incision is made directly over the 6th or 7th intercostal space.

2 A pair of haemostats are used to make a small opening into the pleural space.

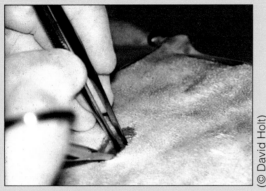
(© David Holt)

3 The chest tube is placed directly into the pleural space with haemostats or a trochar and passed cranially.

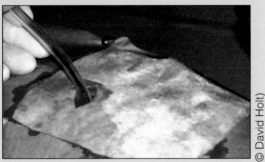
(© David Holt)

4 A second incision is made 6–8 cm caudally. A pair of haemostats are passed through the second incision into the first; the distal end of the tube is grasped and pulled back out of the second incision, creating a subcutaneous tunnel for the chest drain.

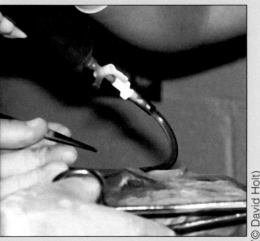
(© David Holt)

5 Both incisions are closed and the tube is secured with a purse-string and Chinese finger-trap suture.

TECHNIQUE 9.3
Placement of a small-bore wire-guided chest drain

1 A stab skin incision is made around the 9th or 10th intercostal space (one-third or halfway down from top of thorax for pneumothorax or pleural effusion, respectively).

2 The 14 gauge introducer catheter is tunnelled subcutaneously in a cranial direction for one or two rib spaces and then inserted into the pleural cavity at the 7th or 8th intercostal space. Aim to enter the pleural space off the cranial edge of the rib to minimize risk of injury to the caudally situated neurovascular bundle.

3 Advance the introducer catheter fully into the thorax over the stylette.

4 Remove the stylette and rapidly thread a J-wire through the catheter in a cranioventral direction for 12–20 cm or until resistance is met.

5 Remove the introducer catheter but leave the guidewire in place.

6 Advance the 14 gauge chest tube into the pleural cavity over the guidewire.

7 Drain any air that may have been introduced during placement.

8 Secure the chest drain to the skin using the suture holes on the catheter.

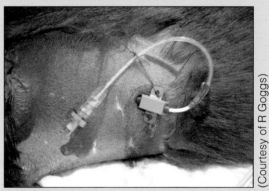
(Courtesy of R Goggs)

9 If the drain cannot be fully inserted (small patients) the tube can be secured using a Chinese finger-trap suture or by using the additional suture wing adapters provided in the kit.

10 It is recommended that the drain is flushed with sterile saline several times a day to decrease the risk of tube blockage.

Pleural effusions

Pleural effusions are drained in a manner similar to a pneumothorax (see Chapter 8). Owners should be carefully questioned about possible exposure of their pet to anticoagulants if the nature of the effusion is not known. Samples of the effusion are saved for evaluation. With some large-volume chronic effusions, life-threatening re-expansion pulmonary oedema may occur if all the pleural fluid is drained at once. Depending on the underlying cause of the effusion, pleural drainage may result in rapid re-effusion and depletion of fluid from the intravascular space that may need to be replaced.

Aspiration pneumonia

Any animal presenting for regurgitation or vomiting is at risk for aspiration pneumonia. Although non-acidic fluid (pH >2.4) is less damaging to the lung than acidic fluid, the aspiration of particulate matter increases the severity of pulmonary damage. Bacterial infection of the damaged lung is a potential complication.

The treatment required to stabilize an animal with aspiration pneumonia secondary to an oesophageal foreign body is determined by the severity of the respiratory compromise.

- Humidified oxygen is delivered by mask, nasal catheter or oxygen cage to offset hypoxaemia.
- Bronchodilators such as beta agonists (albuterol, terbutaline) or methyl xanthines (aminophylline) are administered to prevent or treat bronchoconstriction.
- Intubation and ventilation are indicated in animals with severe respiratory compromise that are not responsive to oxygen supplementation.

Affected animals can lose a significant volume of fluid as exudate into the pulmonary interstitium and alveoli. Pulmonary oedema in cases of aspiration often has a high protein content. Careful intravenous fluid administration with crystalloids and high-molecular-weight colloids (Hetastarch) is indicated to replace these losses.

- Ideally the minimum amount of crystalloid and colloid necessary to improve and then maintain tissue perfusion is administered. Excess fluid resuscitation will increase pulmonary capillary hydrostatic pressure and subsequently worsen fluid leakage into the alveoli through the damaged pulmonary capillary endothelium.
- Broad-spectrum bacteriocidal antibiotics effective against Gram-positive, Gram-negative and anaerobic bacterial species are administered intravenously to symptomatic dogs.
- An endotracheal wash through a sterile endotracheal tube is performed immediately after the induction of anaesthesia to obtain specimens for bacterial culture and sensitivity testing.

Diaphragmatic rupture

Animals with diaphragmatic rupture have varying degrees of respiratory compromise and can benefit from oxygen supplementation.

Patients with the stomach trapped in the thorax can rapidly become emergencies. Compression of the pulmonary parenchyma by the stomach causes dyspnoea and swallowing of air, expanding the stomach and worsening the respiratory compromise. This vicious cycle quickly becomes life-threatening.

- It may be possible to pass a naso-oesophageal tube in amenable patients to relieve the trapped air.

- Percutaneous gastrocentesis may also be possible in the conscious patient, but the air in the stomach will quickly reform.
- Anxiety worsens the animal's ability to breathe and struggling increases oxygen consumption. General anaesthesia may therefore be required.
- Spontaneous ventilation is often ineffective until the stomach is decompressed, but gentle positive pressure breaths can be delivered (PIP <10 cmH$_2$O) to maintain oxygenation.
- Based on the radiographic location of the stomach in the thorax (generally on the left side), a large-bore catheter is passed through the 7th–9th intercostal space and into the stomach to remove the trapped air.
- Once the air is removed a stomach tube can be passed to keep the stomach decompressed until the diaphragm is repaired.

Cardiovascular system

The most common conditions affecting the cardiovascular system of dogs and cats that require surgery are valvular heart disease and cardiomyopathy, respectively.

Canine valvular heart disease

In dogs with valvular heart disease, the mitral valve is most often affected. Decreased stroke volume and arterial blood pressure associated with mitral regurgitation results in activation of the renin–angiotensin–aldosterone pathway, sympathetic nervous system, sodium and water retention, and increased blood pressure. Eventually volume retention, dilatation of the left atrium and increased pulmonary capillary hydrostatic pressure result in pulmonary oedema.

When a murmur is detected during a preoperative physical examination, owners should be thoroughly questioned about the dog's exercise tolerance and the presence of a cough or difficulty in breathing. Thoracic radiographs are taken and carefully evaluated for heart size and pulmonary oedema. The caudal cardiac waist, dorsoventral heart size and pulmonary vasculature are evaluated carefully for evidence of heart failure.

In animals with heart failure, elective procedures are postponed until the condition is stabilized. Emergency treatment of heart failure is beyond the scope of this chapter (see *BSAVA Manual of Canine and Feline Emergency and Critical Care*).

The majority of dogs with stable or slowly progressive chronic valvular disease are managed with diuretics (furosemide 1–2 ml/kg orally q12h) and often an angiotensin-converting enzyme inhibitor. Pimobendan, an oral calcium-sensitizing inodilator, may be administered in more advanced cases.

- Prior to anaesthesia and surgery, a careful evaluation of hydration status is performed.
- Thoracic radiographs are repeated and renal function, serum electrolyte levels and acid–base status are assessed from preoperative blood work.
- Several preoperative indirect blood pressure measurements are obtained.
- If possible, these patients benefit tremendously from spending the night prior to the procedure in

the hospital, being slowly fluid-loaded. This helps to ensure that fluid and electrolyte balances are optimized, helps to preserve blood pressure in the face of anaesthetic drugs and decreases the amount of fluids that need to be given during the procedure, therefore lessening the chances of cardiac overload and pulmonary oedema.

■ Oxygen supplementation is provided prior to the induction of anaesthesia.

Many anaesthetic combinations are possible in these patients and the choice of drugs will depend on the level of cardiac compromise, invasiveness and length of the procedure, and the presence of concurrent disease. Avoidance of stress and substantial restraint is desirable and can be achieved by use of opioids and benzodiazepines. Induction agents should be titrated slowly to effect and commonly include propofol or etomidate, depending on the severity of the disease.

Feline cardiomyopathy

In cats, cardiomyopathy is most often associated with ventricular hypertrophy and can occur secondary to hyperthyroidism or be idiopathic.

Hyperthyroidism

In cats with hyperthyroidism, a trial of medical management with methimazole is often instituted prior to definitive surgical or radioactive iodine (I-131) therapy. In some cats, hyperthyroidism increases renal perfusion and masks underlying renal disease.

■ Serum urea, creatinine, electrolyte levels and urine specific gravity are checked before and after normalization of thyroid levels with methimazole (10–15 mg/kg orally divided twice daily).
■ Normalization of serum thyroid hormone levels often reverses the associated secondary hypertrophic cardiomyopathy.
■ Stabilization of cats with idiopathic cardiomyopathy is guided by radiography, echocardiographic findings and blood pressure measurement.

Atrial dilatation

Cats with a murmur but no atrial dilatation are generally not treated preoperatively, but the clinician should be very careful with intraoperative fluid administration.

Cats with atrial dilatation, tachycardia and echocardiographic evidence of diastolic dysfunction are often treated with a beta-adrenergic antagonist (propranolol 0.5–1 mg/kg orally q8–12h). The use of low-dose alpha-2 receptor agonists (dexmedetomidine 2–5 µg/kg) as part of a premedication protocol with opioids helps to decrease stress, prevent tachycardia and may alleviate aortic outflow obstruction in these cases.

Urogenital system

Urinary obstruction or leakage often results in severe dehydration, azotaemia, hyperkalaemia and acidosis.

Hyperkalaemia

Severe hyperkalaemia is truly life-threatening and requires immediate treatment. Animals are often recumbent and semi-comatose.

Hyperkalaemia increases resting membrane potential towards the threshold potential, leading to muscle weakness and cardiac arrythmias. Depression and severely altered mentation in conjunction with changes in the ECG indicate life-threatening hyperkalaemia in situations where rapid measurement of the serum potassium level is not available.

■ Cardiac arrhythmias are first apparent at serum potassium levels >6.5 mEq/l when the P–R interval becomes prolonged and peaked T waves may be seen.
■ As the hyperkalaemia becomes more severe, P waves are absent (atrial standstill) and QRS complexes become progressively wider.

Ten percent calcium gluconate (a functional antagonist of potassium) can be administered *slowly* intravenously (0.5–1 ml/kg) while the ECG is closely monitored. Although calcium does not lower serum potassium, it increases the threshold potential and returns membrane excitability to normal for approximately 20–30 minutes. Soluble insulin (0.5–1 unit/kg) and glucose (1–2 g/unit of insulin) can also be administered to encourage potassium uptake by cells and so decrease extracellular fluid potassium.

Animals with urinary obstruction are often also severely acidotic. Sodium bicarbonate can be administered slowly (1–2 mEq/kg i.v.) to correct the acidosis; however, this can paradoxically lower ionized calcium and so worsen the effects of hyperkalaemia.

Rehydration

Intravenous access is mandatory. Rehydration should begin *immediately*, using warm intravenous fluids. If possible, anaesthesia and surgery should be delayed until rehydration is accomplished and electrolyte abnormalities have been controlled.

The rate of fluid administration is based on the severity of dehydration. Fluid needs should take into account the level of assessed dehydration and plan to correct the deficit over 4–6 hours. The initial rate should also take into account maintenance fluid needs and potential losses from the urinary tract, vomiting and diarrhoea.

The type of fluid used for initial rehydration is controversial. Some clinicians use 0.9% NaCl to avoid administering potassium. Others believe that 0.9% NaCl might worsen the strong ion difference and feel that a balanced electrolyte solution (Normasol R) gives better clinical results. 2.5% Dextrose in 0.45% NaCl has also been recommended. In general, balanced electrolyte solutions are acceptable unless severe hyperkalaemia (>8.5 mEq/l) is present.

Urine drainage

The urinary tract obstruction or leakage should be addressed as resuscitation is commenced, but anaesthesia should not be induced until potassium levels have decreased below 6.5 mEq/l with aggressive therapy. Re-establishing urine drainage and kidney function will allow normalization of serum potassium levels and acid–base status.

Catherization: In cases of urethral obstruction, a urinary catheter should be passed into the bladder if possible. Stones or 'plugs' can often be retropulsed by flushing saline through the catheter.

In some cases, a catheter cannot be passed. The bladder is decompressed by careful cystocentesis and catheterization is attempted again. In some blocked cats a soft flexible wire ('weasel wire' 0.018 inch) can be advanced into the bladder when a regular tomcat catheter will not pass. A 3 Fr red rubber catheter can then be advanced over the 'weasel wire' to allow urine drainage. Alternatively, if fluoroscopy is available, a needle can be placed into the bladder percutaneously. The 'weasel wire' is advanced through the needle into the bladder then normograde out the urethra under fluoroscopic visualization. A catheter is then advanced retrograde into the bladder.

Tube cystostomy: Occasionally, tube cystostomy is required to drain the bladder whilst the animal is stabilized.

1. The ventral abdomen is clipped and prepared for aseptic surgery.
2. Using local anaesthesia with minimal sedation (alpha-2 receptor agonists are contraindicated prior to relief of obstruction), a mini-laparotomy is performed on the caudal ventral midline (or in the peripreputial area in male dogs).
3. A Foley catheter is inserted into the abdominal cavity via a second small stab incision in the body wall, and into the bladder through a purse-string suture.
4. The balloon of the Foley catheter is inflated, the purse-string suture is tightened and the incisions are closed.
5. The catheter is connected to a sterile closed urine collection system.

Emergency drainage: In an emergency, urine can be drained from the peritoneal cavity using a large-gauge fenestrated intravenous catheter or a peritoneal dialysis catheter (Figure 9.8).

1. The caudal abdomen is prepared for aseptic surgery and local anaesthetic is infused.
2. A small stab incision is made caudal to the umbilicus with a scalpel and the catheter is introduced in a caudal direction.

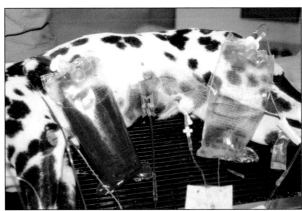

9.8 Dalmatian with a ruptured bladder secondary to prolonged urethral obstruction. The obstruction has been relieved and an indwelling urethral urinary catheter, as well as a peritoneal dialysis catheter draining urine from the peritoneal cavity, have been placed. (© David Holt)

3. The peritoneal cavity is entered cautiously to minimize damage to abdominal viscera.
4. The catheter is advanced off the stylette, sutured in place, and connected to a sterile closed urine collection system.

Pyometra

Older female intact dogs are often presented to veterinary surgeons for treatment of pyometra. Animals with severe infections or a ruptured pyometra may present in septic shock. The degree of dehydration, electrolyte and acid–base abnormalities will depend on the amount of fluid lost through vomiting, into the distended uterus, and in urine. Endotoxin-associated renal dysfunction is common in dogs with pyometra.

- Intravenous access is obtained and blood is sampled for PVC, total protein, urea, creatinine, electrolytes and, if available, blood gas analysis.
- Intravenous fluid therapy is commenced with the goal of rehydrating the stable animal in 2–4 hours.
- Calculations for the rate of fluid administration are similar to those described for small intestinal surgery and are based on an assessment of the degree of dehydration, volume of ongoing losses and an estimation of maintenance fluid requirements.
- In many cases serum creatinine and urea values will not normalize in spite of appropriate fluid resuscitation until the pyometra is surgically removed.

The most common bacterium cultured from pyometra is *Escherichia coli*, but *Staphylococcus* and *Streptococcus* species are also isolated. Antibiotics effective against *E. coli* that can be administered intravenously include the fluoroquinolones, cephalosporins, potentiated penicillins and trimethoprim/sulphonamide.

Treatment for animals in septic shock is similar to the description in the Peritonitis section of this chapter.

Orthopaedic surgical conditions

Many patients presenting with orthopaedic disease are otherwise healthy and require little formal stabilization prior to surgery.

Fracture cases are often associated with significant trauma from road traffic accidents or falls. Stabilization begins immediately after a rapid evaluation of the central nervous, respiratory and cardiovascular systems.

- Stupor or coma indicates the likelihood of cranial trauma.
- Intubation may be required to provide adequate ventilation and blood oxygenation.
- The upper and lower airways and chest wall are carefully evaluated for injury.
- Pulmonary contusions, pneumothorax and diaphragmatic rupture are common in fractures associated with road traffic accidents. These animals also often have poor perfusion secondary to haemorrhage. Goal-directed limited volume resuscitation with intravenous crystalloid fluids (10–20 ml/kg) combined with colloids, hypertonic saline, and blood products as indicated is now advocated in animals with suspected pulmonary contusions to minimize the likelihood of worsening pulmonary oedema.

Once this initial survey has been completed, life-threatening injuries addressed and resuscitation commenced, a more thorough examination is performed.

- The bladder is carefully palpated. An intact bladder does not, unfortunately, rule out urethral laceration or transection that can occur in association with pelvic fractures.
- Limb perfusion and nerve function are evaluated once resuscitation has improved systemic perfusion.
- General anaesthesia is required to treat fractures, luxations and wounds. Until the animal is stable enough for general anaesthesia, any open fracture or wound is covered with a sterile, water-soluble gel and a thick padded bandage comprising sterile gauze, cotton wool or cast padding, a gauze wrap and an elasticated outer layer (Figure 9.9). For fractures proximal to the elbow and stifle the bandage is brought over the shoulder or hip, respectively, and around the body to provide proper immobilization.
- Early administration of appropriate antibiotics decreases infection rates in open fractures. A first-generation cephalosporin antibiotic (e.g. cefalotin) is effective against the many bacteria isolated from open fractures.

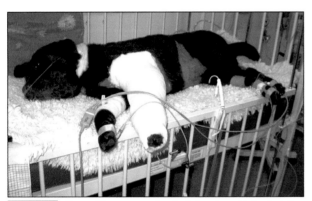

9.9 Dog with an open forelimb fracture and wound that has been dressed with a Robert Jones bandage whilst the dog is stabilized with intravenous fluids for hypovolaemic shock and nasal oxygen for pulmonary contusions. An indwelling urinary catheter has also been placed, due to the dog's recumbency and for monitoring of urine output, and ECG pads have been attached to the dog's paws to monitor ventricular tachycardia. (Courtesy of V Lipscomb)

Pain management

Preoperative pain management is an essential part of stabilizing trauma cases and preparing for orthopaedic surgery. Appropriately treating pain in a multimodal fashion early in the process reduces the overall need for anaesthetic drugs, minimizes central sensitization and wind-up, and allows a more rapid return to function and physical therapy in the postoperative period (see Chapter 14).

Opioids

Opioids are the mainstay of therapy for orthopaedic pain in the acute and perioperative setting. Pure mu receptor agonists are preferred because of the severity of pain associated with orthopaedic surgery and the inhalant anaesthetic reduction that they provide.

Morphine (dogs: 0.1–1 mg/kg; cats: 0.1–0.4 mg/kg), hydromorphone (0.1–0.2 mg/kg), and fentanyl (1–5 µg/kg + 3–10 µg/kg/h) are all effective first line drugs used for acute pain control and anaesthetic premedication.

Non-opioids

Opioid adjunct medications have begun to play a major role in treating aspects of pain that are resistant to opioid therapy.

- Gabapentin (5–10 mg/kg orally) and ketamine (0.5 mg/kg i.v. + 1–3 µg/kg/min) play a key role in treating and preventing wind-up and in treating pain of neuropathic origin in the perioperative period. Ketamine can additionally be used as a component of the anaesthetic induction and maintenance protocol.
- Injectable non-steroidal anti-inflammatory drugs (carprofen 2.2–4.4 mg/kg s.c. or i.v.; meloxicam 0.1 mg/kg i.v. or s.c.) exert a synergistic effect on analgesia when combined with opioids, but should only be administered to stable well hydrated patients.

Local anaesthetics

Local anaesthetics can be used in multiple capacities for regional, neuroaxial and local pain management in both conscious and anaesthetized patients. Significant reductions in the dose of systemic pain and anaesthetic medications can be achieved, with a concurrent reduction in side effects, when local anaesthetics are utilized.

Endocrine diseases

Diabetes

Diabetic animals present the surgeon with several perioperative challenges:

- Unregulated diabetic patients are often significantly dehydrated and have serious electrolyte and acid–base imbalances
- Poorly controlled diabetes increases the risk of postoperative infections and poor wound healing
- The stress associated with hospitalization and surgery may increase insulin requirements.

Elective surgeries should be postponed in diabetic animals until blood glucose levels are well controlled with regular meals and subcutaneous insulin doses. A thorough physical examination, blood count, serum biochemical analysis and urinalysis and culture are performed. Pre-existing infections, especially urinary tract infections, are treated and resolved prior to surgery.

- The animal is fed early on the night before surgery and receives its normal evening dose of insulin.
- On the morning of surgery, food is withheld and half the normal dose of insulin is administered subcutaneously, unless the measured blood glucose level is <8.3 mmol/l in which case no insulin is given.
- An intravenous catheter that allows for intraoperative and postoperative blood glucose sampling is placed.
- Solutions of 2.5% and 5% dextrose are prepared and regular insulin is available to treat perioperative hyperglycaemia.

- Ideally blood glucose levels are maintained between 5.5 and 13.9 mmol/l.
- Perioperative antibiotics are administered based on the surgical procedure and sensitivity of the likely contaminating bacterial flora.

Hyperadrenocorticism

Surgery to treat hyperadrenocorticism secondary to functional adrenal gland neoplasia is performed at referral centres. However, general practitioners may perform surgery on hyperadrenocorticoid dogs for concurrent conditions.

These dogs are generally stabilized with either mitotane, using an induction dose of 50 mg/kg/day divided, then 50 mg/kg/week (i.e. 25 mg/kg twice weekly), or trilostane (3–6 mg/kg daily). The results of treatment are monitored carefully based on clinical signs and ACTH stimulation testing.

Hyperadrenocorticoid dogs are at risk for infection and poor wound healing.

- Prophylactic antibiotics are administered intravenously to minimize the risk of wound infection.
- Vitamin A has been shown to reverse the adverse affects of corticosteroids on wound healing in experimental skin and bowel models in rodents. The exact dose required for dogs is not known, but 10,000 to 20,000 IU given orally q24h has been used by one of the authors in clinical cases. Administration of vitamin A begins several days before surgery and continues for 10–14 days postoperatively.

Conclusion

In summary, good surgical outcomes rely on careful consideration and implementation of preoperative stabilization measures for a particular patient's presenting complaint and any concurrent conditions, based on a thorough patient evaluation and investigation. By monitoring the patient's response to preoperative stabilization measures, the clinician can make an informed judgement as to the least risky time to proceed with anaesthesia and surgery, ideally when the patient's physiology has been restored to as close to normal as possible.

References and further reading

Bentley A and Holt DE (2007) Drainage techniques for the septic abdomen. In: *Kirk's Current Veterinary Therapy IX*, pp. 174–191. WB Saunders, Philadelphia
Boag AK and Hughes D (2004) Emergency management of the acute abdomen in dogs and cats. 1. Investigation and initial stabilisation. *In Practice* **26**, 476–483
Boag AK and Hughes D (2005) Assessment and treatment of perfusion abnormalities in the emergency patient. *Veterinary Clinics of North America: Small Animal Practice* **35**, 319–342
Dugdale A (2000) Chest drains and drainage techniques. *In Practice* **22**, 2–15
Fischer JR (2009) Hemodialysis and peritoneal dialysis. In: *Small Animal Critical Care Medicine*, ed. DC Silverstein and K Hopper, pp. 599–602. Saunders Elsevier, St Louis
King L and Boag A (2007) *BSAVA Manual of Canine and Feline Emergency and Critical Care, 2nd edn*. BSAVA Publications, Gloucester
Love E, Waterman AE and Lane JG (1987) The assessment of corrective surgery for canine laryngeal paralysis by blood gas analysis: a review of thirty-five cases. *Journal of Small Animal Practice* **28**, 597–604
Manning AM (2002) Oxygen therapy and toxicity. *Veterinary Clinics of North America: Small Animal Practice* **32**, 1005–1020
Valtolina C and Adamantos S (2009) Evaluation of small-bore wire-guided chest drains for management of pleural space disease. *Journal of Small Animal Practice* **50**, 290–297

Fluid therapy, and electrolyte and acid–base abnormalities

10

Karen Humm and Sophie Adamantos

Introduction

Abnormalities in electrolytes and in fluid and acid–base balance are commonly seen in surgical patients. Abnormalities may be due to the primary surgical disease process, concurrent illness or surgical intervention. This chapter focuses on identification of fluid, electrolyte and acid–base disturbances, their pathophysiology and treatment.

Fluid therapy

Intravenous fluid therapy is one of the most commonly performed treatments in small animal practice. Although other methods are possible (intraosseous or subcutaneous techniques), intravenous administration combines simplicity and familiarity with efficacy. For other methods of administration see the *BSAVA Manual of Canine and Feline Emergency and Critical Care*.

Fluid therapy is used in:

- Dehydrated animals
- Hypoperfused animals
- Animals undergoing general anaesthesia
- Animals with acid–base and electrolyte abnormalities (covered later in the chapter).

It is very important to appreciate the difference between dehydration and hypoperfusion, in terms of both recognition (related to physical examination findings) and consequences.

- **Dehydration** occurs when loss of water from the body leads to a decreased volume of all body fluid compartments (Figure 10.1) in approximately equal proportions. As most of the water in the body is contained in the extravascular compartment, signs of dehydration are related to loss of interstitial and intracellular fluid, i.e. loss of skin turgor, dry mucous membranes.
- **Hypoperfusion** is defined as circulatory failure leading to inadequate perfusion and oxygenation of the tissues. It occurs most frequently as a result of hypovolaemia, which is loss of fluid from the intravascular compartment (Figure 10.1). It can

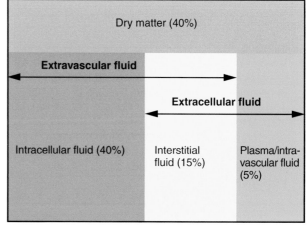

10.1 Contributions of different body fluid compartments and dry matter to total body weight. Note that approximately 60% of the mass of a healthy adult dog or cat is fluid; approximately 65% of that fluid is within the cells and 35% is extracellular. The extracellular fluid is mostly (75%) interstitial (fluid which surrounds the cells), with 25% being within the vessels.

occur independently from dehydration (e.g. due to acute blood loss) or in association with dehydration in the case of severe gastrointestinal losses (vomiting and diarrhoea). Clinical signs of hypoperfusion include tachycardia, abnormal pulse quality, abnormal mucous membrane colour and mentation changes.

Physical examination in conjunction with a thorough history can aid in the identification of both hypoperfusion and dehydration.

Dehydration

Any animal with a history of vomiting or diarrhoea is likely to be at least mildly dehydrated. Physical examination findings such as loss of skin turgor, sunken eyes and dry mucous membranes are often cited as identifying features of dehydration, but they are subjective and inaccurate (Figure 10.2). They can also be disguised or exaggerated; for example, skin turgor changes with age, and dry mucous membranes can be masked by hypersalivation secondary to nausea.

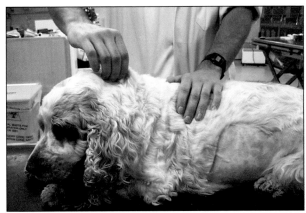

10.2 Physical examination findings such as loss of skin turgor, sunken eyes and dry mucous membranes are often cited as identifying features of dehydration, but they are subjective and often inaccurate.

Measuring an animal's packed cell volume (PCV) and total solids simply using a capillary tube, centrifuge, microhaematocrit reader and refractometer can be a useful way of assessing hydration status, with the caveat that other disease processes such as anaemia or protein-losing disease may affect these measurements (Figure 10.3).

A recent weight (within the previous few days) when the patient was healthy allows accurate assessment of dehydration, as any acute weight loss is typically due to loss of fluid (i.e. water). For example, if a 10 kg patient loses 1 kg of bodyweight over 2 days, this equates to a water deficit of 1 litre (10% dehydration). It is safe to assume that an animal with a history that suggests excessive fluid losses is approximately 5% dehydrated and would benefit from rehydrating fluids. The presence of physical examination findings compatible with dehydration suggests that the animal is >5% dehydrated. Most affected patients will be between 5 and 10% dehydrated.

Packed cell volume	Total solids	Interpretation
↑	↑	Dehydration
↑	N or ↓	Haemorrhagic gastroenteritis Polycythaemia
↓	N	Anaemia – haemolysis or chronic anaemia
N	↑	Hyperglobulinaemia (e.g. FIP) Anaemia and dehydration
N	↓	Hypoproteinaemia (e.g. PLN, PLE) Peracute haemorrhage
↓	↓	Haemorrhage Anaemia and hypoproteinaemia

10.3 Packed cell volume and total solid changes seen with different disease processes. FIP = feline infectious peritonitis; N = normal; PLE = protein-losing enteropathy; PLN = protein-losing nephropathy.

Rehydration

Rehydration with intravenous fluids is ideally performed over 24–48 hours and preferably prior to any surgery, though this is not always possible. Attempting to rehydrate a patient more quickly is generally not effective, as the administered fluid will not redistribute out of the intravascular space effectively and will be excreted via the kidneys. If hypoperfusion is present (see below) this should be corrected prior to the initiation of rehydration therapy. Obviously in many instances waiting 48 hours prior to surgery is not an option and in these cases rehydration will occur both peri- and intraoperatively. Figure 10.4 gives details of how to calculate the fluid requirements of a dehydrated patient.

To calculate total fluid requirement and rate of administration

1. **Calculate the volume of fluid required to rehydrate the patient:**
   Rehydration fluid volume required (litres) = % dehydration × bodyweight (kg).
2. **Calculate the maintenance requirement of the patient** (generally estimated at *2 ml/kg/h*).
3. **Calculate the anticipated abnormal losses** (e.g. fluid loss through vomiting or diarrhoea). This is often difficult to estimate. Attempts can be made to measure the volume of vomitus and diarrhoea, but this is often unsuccessful and very messy; therefore, it is acceptable to estimate a further loss of 0.5–2 ml/kg/h, depending on the level of estimated fluid loss. Regular assessment of hydration status and urine output over the period of fluid therapy can aid in understanding whether ongoing abnormal losses are being compensated for appropriately.
4. **Calculate the total fluid therapy requirement** by adding the results of calculations (1), (2) and (3).

Example

For a dog of 25 kg bodyweight with approximately 7% dehydration due to vomiting

1. Rehydration fluid volume required (litres) = % dehydration × bodyweight (kg)
   = 0.07 × 25 kg
   = **1.75 litres**

2. Maintenance fluid volume required (at 2 ml/kg/h)
   = 2 ml × 25 kg × 24 hours
   = 1200 ml = **1.2 litres**

3. Abnormal fluid losses volume required
   On the expectation that this patient will vomit, say, four times in 24 hours with estimated losses at 1 ml/kg/h:
   = 1 ml × 25 kg × 24 hours
   = 600 ml = **0.6 litres**

4. Total fluid requirement for 24 hours
   = 1.75 + 1.2 + 0.6
   = 3.55 litres/24 hours = 3550 ml/24 hours
   = **148 ml/h** (or just under 6 ml/kg/h)

If the rehydration is performed more slowly over 48 hours (in which case the maintenance and abnormal loss volumes are twice as much as for 24 hours):
Total fluid requirement for 48 hours
= 1.75 + 2.4 + 1.2
= 5.35 litres/48 hours = 5350 ml/48 hours
= **111 ml/h** (or just under 4.5 ml/kg/h)

10.4 Calculations for the fluid requirements of a dehydrated patient.

Hypoperfusion

Hypoperfusion, or shock, occurs when there is inadequate perfusion relative to tissue demands, resulting in decreased oxygen and nutrient delivery and decreased waste removal.

Classification and diagnosis

Hypoperfusion can be categorized into one of four types, according to the underlying pathophysiology (in some instances more than one type of hypoperfusion is present):

- **Hypovolaemia** – decreased blood volume. This can be caused by blood loss, but also by rapid loss of fluid from the intravascular space into another fluid compartment (usually third-space losses such as into the gastrointestinal tract as a result of vomiting and diarrhoea)
- **Distributive abnormalities** – decreased vascular tone due to marked inflammation or infection. Sepsis is a common underlying cause of distributive shock. Septic peritonitis and pyometra can both result in distributive shock
- **Obstruction of venous return** – due to obstruction of the great vessels or of cardiac filling. Gastric dilatation–volvulus (GDV) can cause obstruction of the vena cava and decrease venous return and therefore cardiac output
- **Cardiogenic** – inadequate cardiac output (forward heart failure) due to intrinsic disease such as dilated cardiomyopathy or severe arrhythmias such as ventricular tachycardia. Severe arrhythmias may be seen in association with certain surgical diseases such as a ruptured splenic mass or GDV. Unlike with other types, *patients with signs of cardiogenic hypoperfusion may not require fluid therapy*. Patients with intrinsic myocardial failure require improvement of cardiac output through the use of positive inotropes. Patients with arrhythmias should be managed as appropriate for the rhythm disturbance as diagnosed on an electrocardiogram.

In surgical patients the most common causes of hypoperfusion are hypovolaemia and distributive abnormalities. Cardiogenic and obstructive shock are seen less frequently, but clinicians should be familiar with their clinical signs and management.

Physical examination allows recognition of the hypoperfused patient through:

- Tachycardia
- Abnormal pulse quality
- Abnormal mucous membrane colour
- Mentation changes.

Pulse quality is best described using terms such as normal, tall and narrow ('hyperdynamic') or short and narrow ('weak') (Figure 10.5).

Classifying the form of hypoperfusion can help to tailor therapy and create a diagnostic plan.

- Figure 10.6 outlines the classic physical examination findings in dogs in varying stages of **hypovolaemic** shock.

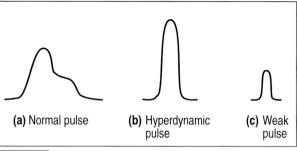

(a) Normal pulse   **(b)** Hyperdynamic pulse   **(c)** Weak pulse

10.5   Pulse profiles from direct arterial pressure measurements.

- Patients with **distributive** shock have abnormal vascular tone, which leads to peripheral vasodilatation and as a result mucous membranes appear congested or injected rather than pale, as would be seen in a patient with hypovolaemia.
- Patients with **obstructive** shock will have a variety of signs depending on the underlying disease process. For example, patients with pericardial effusion may have pulsus paradoxus and jugular distension; patients with GDV may have a distended abdomen; and patients with tension pneumothorax will have dull lung sounds.
- Patients with **cardiogenic** shock may have an audible murmur or arrhythmia.

Feline hypoperfusion
Hypoperfused cats can present with tachycardia and hyperdynamic pulses. However, they can also develop bradycardia and hypothermia and become mentally depressed. Bradycardia is an important presenting sign in cats and should lead to further investigation, including measurement of body temperature and blood pressure and a search for an underlying cause.

Treatment
Treatment of hypoperfusion is a priority.

- Intravascular fluid deficits should be replaced prior to surgery, as this will decrease morbidity and mortality under general anaesthesia. The volume of fluid administered will be dependent on the severity of the patient's clinical signs; patients with mild signs require less fluid than those with more severe signs.
- Hypoperfused patients are treated to effect and therefore a standard dose of fluids cannot be applied to all animals, nor is there an ideal fluid for resuscitation and the argument over which fluid is best is ongoing.

Clinical sign	Mild (compensatory)	Moderate	Severe (decompensatory)
Heart rate	130–150 bpm	150–170 bpm	170–220 bpm
Mucous membrane colour	Normal to pinker than normal	Pale pink	White, grey or muddy
Capillary refill time	Vigorous, <1 second	Reduced vigour, 2 seconds	>2 seconds or absent
Pulse amplitude	Increase	Moderate decrease	Severe decrease
Pulse duration	Mild decrease	Moderate decrease	Severe decrease
Metatarsal pulse	Easily palpable	Just palpable	Absent

10.6   Guidelines for clinical assessement of uncomplicated hypovolaemia in the dog.

Isotonic crystalloids: Isotonic crystalloids are the first choice in the majority of situations as they are familiar, cheap and associated with few side effects. The 'shock dose' of isotonic crystalloid fluids is 60–90 ml/kg for dogs and 40–60 ml/kg for cats. Patients presenting with hypoperfusion should be treated with a proportion of the 'shock dose' administered over a short period, depending on the severity of their signs. The derivation of this dose is based upon a single blood volume and has been shown experimentally to be very safe when administered rapidly.

Fluid resuscitation should target an end point, which should be as close to normal cardiovascular parameters for that animal as possible. After the patient has received their initial dose they should be reassessed. If their cardiovascular parameters are still abnormal, a further dose should be administered (see Figure 10.7 for a case example). Chapter 11 also discusses the recognition and treatment of hypoperfusion/shock in detail.

Generally in dogs, doses of isotonic crystalloid at 10–40 ml/kg are administered as a bolus over 10–30 minutes, with the volume of fluid and the length of time of the infusion varying with the severity of the clinical signs. Hypertonic saline is a useful fluid for very large dogs, where rapid administration of large volumes of isotonic crystalloids can be challenging. A dose of 2–4 ml/kg given over 5–20 minutes will give similar results to those for a full shock dose of isotonic crystalloids.

Artificial colloids: Artificial colloids have also been recommended as resuscitation fluids. They have more potent and longer lasting effects than crystalloids, due to their persistence in the intravascular space. There is no evidence to suggest that they are more effective or associated with a better outcome than isotonic crystalloid fluids. The maximum shock dose of most artificial colloids is 20 ml/kg in 24 hours and for resuscitation an initial dose of 5 ml/kg given over 10–20 minutes is generally used.

Cats: Cats can be more difficult to manage due to their small size and the frequency of undiagnosed cardiac disease. They should be monitored closely and both crystalloid and colloid fluid doses should be titrated carefully. As cats have a lower blood volume on a per kilogram basis and are at higher risk of volume overload, lower volumes are used for resuscitation compared with dogs. Initial volumes of isotonic crystalloid at 10–30 ml/kg over 10–30 minutes, colloid at 5 ml/kg over 20 minutes and hypertonic saline at 2 ml/kg over 5–20 minutes are recommended. Blood pressure is a good indicator of perfusion in cats and fluid therapy can be titrated to a systolic pressure of 80–100 mmHg.

Disease differential diagnosis: Once hypoperfusion has been recognized and measures to stabilize the patient have been initiated, attempts should be made to identify the disease process that has led to hypoperfusion. Frequently historical or physical examination findings lead to refinement of the differential diagnoses, so further investigation can be targeted. For example, a 6-year-old entire bitch with a 2-week history of polyuria and polydipsia and physical examination findings compatible with distributive shock would have pyometra as the most likely diagnosis.

Hypotensive and low-volume resuscitation

Hypotensive resuscitation has been extensively discussed in the human medical literature. It has been shown to be better than rapid high-volume resuscitation in some experimental studies of uncontrolled bleeding (Jackson and Nolan, 2009). It is used in human patients with severe ongoing blood loss, typically secondary to penetrating trauma, prior to emergency surgery. The patient is resuscitated with fluid therapy to a systolic blood pressure of between 70 and 100 mmHg, with further fluid resuscitation limited to prevent increased blood loss. The patient is then rapidly anaesthetized and surgically explored to control the bleeding. Once the bleeding is controlled, the patient is resuscitated.

There have been no studies of hypotensive resuscitation in small animal patients. It is not recommended in veterinary patients, as penetrating trauma (the major indication in humans) is very uncommon. Patients that are to be managed with hypotensive resuscitation require rapid surgical management of their bleeding. Great care needs to be taken with anaesthetizing these hypotensive patients and once control of the bleeding has been achieved aggressive resuscitation can ensue.

Low-volume resuscitation involves the use of hypertonic or colloid products to decrease the volume of fluid administered to a hypoperfused patient. Again, there is much interest in this area in human medical research. However, there is limited clinical evidence to suggest that using lower volumes of fluid leads to decreased patient morbidity or mortality, except where there is concurrent pulmonary parenchymal disease.

Case example

A 10-month-old entire male Staffordshire Bull Terrier presents with:
- 24-hour history of severe vomiting
- Tachycardia (184 bpm) with bounding pulses, pale mucous membranes, capillary refill time (CRT) = 2 seconds
- Appears mentally depressed but is ambulatory
- Has a palpable abdominal mass, suspected to be a foreign body.

Initial management
- Bolus of isotonic crystalloid at 40 ml/kg over 20 minutes.

After the bolus
- Heart rate is 140 bpm.
- Improved pulse quality.
- Mucous membranes are pale pink.
- CRT = 1.5 seconds.

Further management
- Bolus of isotonic crystalloid at 20 ml/kg over 30 minutes.
- Abdominal radiography performed, suggestive of intestinal obstruction.

After the second bolus
- Heart rate is 120 bpm.
- Pulse quality is further improved.
- Mucous membranes are more pink than normal.
- CRT = 0.5 seconds.

The patient can now be prepared for surgery. Fluid should be administered at 10 ml/kg/h with close monitoring of heart rate, pulse quality and mucous membrane colour.

10.7 Treatment of hypoperfusion with isotonic crystalloids.

Fluid therapy during anaesthesia

Fluid therapy is commonly utilized during general anaesthesia. It both counteracts the hypotensive effect of most anaesthetic agents (due to vasodilatation and/or myocardial depression) and compensates for the fluid losses that occur during the anaesthetic period. These include normal losses through urine and faeces and additional losses including blood loss, the fluid lost from the respiratory tract by the use of non-humidified inhalant gases and evaporative losses from open body cavities.

- In the absence of contraindications, such as heart failure, isotonic crystalloid fluid at a rate of 10 ml/kg/h is recommended for patients undergoing general anaesthesia for surgical procedures.
- In patients undergoing general anaesthesia for non-surgical procedures, such as diagnostic imaging, a rate of 5 ml/kg/h may be preferred.
- It is important to remember that isotonic 'replacement' crystalloids should be used for patients undergoing general anaesthesia and low-sodium 'maintenance' fluids are almost never indicated (see Fluid therapy options below for more details).

Whilst this plan is useful for the majority of stable and healthy patients, it should be tailored to the individual where there is underlying or concurrent disease. For example:

- Patients with cardiovascular disease such as mitral valve disease or hypertrophic cardiomyopathy may develop congestive heart failure with this rate of fluid administration and should therefore be monitored carefully and administered lower rates of fluid
- Markedly hypoproteinaemic patients can develop oedema if they are given high rates of isotonic crystalloid fluids. In these patients a much lower dose of crystalloid is recommended to match insensible water losses at 1–2 ml/kg/h and artificial colloid can be used to maintain blood pressure and perfusion.

Once general anaesthesia is underway the patient needs to be monitored closely to assess the adequacy of the fluid therapy plan. The major requirement for a change in the rate of fluid administration would be identification of hypoperfusion, typically associated with excessive blood loss as determined by tachycardia (unrelated to pain or inadequate plane of anaesthesia) or hypotension (not explicable by overdose of anaesthetic agents).

- In this situation, rapid infusion of boluses of fluid, as described above for preoperative stabilization of a patient with hypoperfusion, is appropriate.
- Colloid therapy is often used rather than isotonic crystalloid, as it may improve blood pressure to a greater extent and have a longer lasting effect.

Fluid therapy options

Fluid therapy should be considered a pharmacological intervention; therefore consideration should be given to the correct product for the situation and the dose to be used. Careful monitoring of the effect following administration is also required.

Tonicity and osmolality

The tonicity of a fluid (crystalloid or otherwise) is calculated by adding up the number of osmotically active particles. This value is compared with the osmolality of a healthy animal's plasma to determine whether the fluid is hyper-, iso- or hypotonic. Normal plasma osmolality in dogs is 290–310 mOsm/kg and in cats is 290–330 mOsm/kg.

> ### PRACTICAL TIPS
>
> - **Hypotonic** crystalloids are often referred to as maintenance fluids.
> - **Isotonic** crystalloids are often referred to as replacement fluids.

Crystalloid fluids

Whilst there are many different options, the majority of patients can be treated with one of a small number of products. Isotonic crystalloids such as Hartmann's solution and 0.9% saline are the most commonly used fluid products. They are solutions of electrolytes and small non-electrolyte substances.

Hypotonic fluids

These fluids are all low in sodium and are hypotonic to the plasma, which leads to distribution of the water present in the fluid throughout the intravascular, interstitial and intracellular spaces (see Figure 10.1). Some of these fluids are initially isotonic, as they contain glucose to prevent erythrocyte lysis (which can occur when extremely hypotonic fluids are administered). However, *in vivo* the glucose is rapidly metabolized, leading to the effective administration of a hypotonic fluid.

Hypotonic fluids are rarely indicated, as they contain very low levels of sodium and chloride and are deficient in potassium. Administration to sick patients commonly results in hyponatraemia, hypochloraemia and hypokalaemia. In patients where maintenance fluids are required, isotonic fluids with the addition of potassium can be used. Although this will provide excessive sodium and chloride, this is not a problem in the majority of patients. Specific hypotonic fluids available in the UK are discussed below.

0.18% NaCl with 4% dextrose: This fluid can be used in patients with *no abnormal fluid losses* if fluid is not being taken orally. It should be used with caution, as the sodium concentration is 20% of that in a healthy dog's plasma. It commonly leads to a number of severe electrolyte, metabolic and acid–base abnormalities, including hyponatraemia, hypochloraemia and hypokalaemia as well as hyperglycaemia and metabolic alkalosis. Hyponatraemia can result in severe neurological effects that can be difficult to correct.

- It is important to realize that this fluid cannot be used as a method of administering nutrition, as the calories provided by a safe administration rate are not sufficient to provide the resting energy requirements of an animal.

- It also should not be used for treating hypoglycaemia, as side effects related to electrolyte abnormalities are common. A more appropriate fluid would be an isotonic crystalloid with added glucose, or a commercially available preparation such as 0.9% NaCl with 5% dextrose.
- If 0.18% NaCl with 4% dextrose is to be used as a maintenance fluid, it should be supplemented with potassium chloride at 40–50 mmol/l to prevent hypokalaemia. The resultant high potassium concentration means that the fluid should not be administered at high rates.

5% Dextrose/glucose: Once the glucose in the fluid is metabolized (as described above) this solution is solely water. It has been recommended for replacement of maintenance losses, but generally these losses include potassium, sodium, chloride and bicarbonate as well as water and so the use of 5% dextrose is not recommended.

- As with 0.18% NaCl and 4% dextrose, this fluid *cannot* be used as a source of energy or for the management of hypoglycaemia.
- It is suggested in some texts for the management of hypernatraemia, but this is not recommended by the authors (see Hypernatraemia section).
- Its sole use should be as a dilution agent for certain drugs, such as sodium nitroprusside.

0.45% NaCl (half-strength saline): This fluid is not as markedly hypotonic as 0.18% NaCl with 4% dextrose or 5% dextrose, but it is still half the tonicity of a healthy cat's or dog's plasma and so its use can be associated with marked hyponatraemia.

- Its major indication is for the management of hypernatraemic patients. Great care should be exercised in these patients, as rapid reduction of sodium concentrations can cause marked neurological signs. Therefore, the judicious use of an isotonic fluid such as Hartmann's is often more appropriate.
- The low sodium content of 0.45% NaCl means that it is also recommended for the replacement of fluid losses secondary to dehydration in heart failure patients. Fluid therapy in patients with heart failure is a tightrope and extreme care should be taken, as the risk of overload and congestive heart failure is high. Intravenous administration should only be performed when all other routes, including oral administration, have been excluded.

Isotonic fluids

Hartmann's solution (compound sodium lactate): Hartmann's solution is the most 'physiological' of all the fluid therapy options available in the UK and is therefore a good first choice in most situations. It contains sodium, chloride, calcium and potassium as well as lactate.

- Lactate acts as a bicarbonate precursor so the fluid may be beneficial in patients with metabolic acidosis (the most common acid–base disturbance in dogs and cats).

- It can be used as a replacement fluid to replace gastrointestinal or third-space losses and can also be used to support the cardiovascular system during blood loss.
- Concern about using Hartmann's solution in patients with hyperkalaemia is commonplace (as it is a potassium-containing fluid) but unfounded. A study of cats with urethral obstruction showed the use of a potassium-containing balanced electrolyte solution did not appear to affect the rate of normalization of blood potassium adversely (Drobatz and Cole, 2008).
- Hartmann's should not be used as an infusion in the same intravenous port as blood products, as it contains calcium. Calcium can combine with the citrate anticoagulant used in blood products, leading to the formation of microemboli.

Lactated Ringer's solution: This fluid is very similar in its electrolyte balance to Hartmann's, with minor changes in the electrolyte composition. The two fluids can be considered as equivalent.

Normal saline (0.9% NaCl): Sodium chloride is an appropriate isotonic crystalloid for most situations, but its high chloride content has an acidifying effect that can lead to a worsening of metabolic acidosis.

- It is used in preference to Hartmann's solution in patients with hypercalcaemia, as its high sodium concentration aids calciuresis.
- It is also the fluid of choice in hypochloraemic patients, particularly if there is an associated metabolic alkalosis. These patients require chloride to restore their acid–base equilibrium and therefore the high chloride content of normal saline is beneficial (see 'Acid–base' section).
- Normal saline has been recommended as the fluid of choice for Addisonian (hypoadrenocorticoid) patients as they are hyponatraemic and hyperkalaemic. However, rapid correction of hyponatraemia can be detrimental to the central nervous system and therefore an isotonic crystalloid with a lower sodium concentration such as Hartmann's may be preferable.

Ringer's solution: Ringer's solution was developed from normal saline to be a more physiological fluid. However, as it lacks lactate or any other bicarbonate precursor and has a high chloride concentration, it is still an acidifying solution. It can be used as an isotonic replacement or maintenance fluid but has no specific advantage over normal saline and Hartmann's solution.

Hypertonic fluids

Hypertonic saline (7.2% NaCl): The percentage of NaCl in hypertonic saline can vary, but commercially available veterinary preparations in the UK contain 7.2%. Hypertonic saline is a crystalloid with excellent resuscitative powers via a number of effects. Its high tonicity results in a large osmotic 'pull' of water into the intravascular space. However, the sodium and chloride quickly equilibrate with the interstitial space and therefore its intravascular space expansion is not long lasting. It has direct cardiac effects resulting in increased myocardial contractility.

- The large expansion of the intravascular space per millilitre of fluid administered means that it is very useful for large patients, as a shock dose can be administered rapidly in a manageable volume. For example, to achieve comparable effects a 60 kg Great Dane with a GDV could be given a 40 ml/kg bolus of Hartmann's over 20 minutes (2.4 litres) or a 4 ml/kg bolus of hypertonic saline (240 ml) over 15–20 minutes.
- As hypertonic saline 'pulls' water from the intracellular and interstitial spaces it needs to be followed by a balanced electrolyte solution to allow rehydration.
- Hypertonic saline should be given over at least 5 minutes, as faster administration can lead to bronchoconstriction, bradycardia and other adverse effects.
- It should be avoided in patients with hypernatraemia or dehydration as this may be worsened.
- Repeat administration should be avoided as this will result in hypernatraemia and hyperchloraemia.

Colloid fluids

Colloids are fluids containing large molecules that are retained within the intravascular compartment, maintaining a pull for fluid in the vascular space. Both artificial and natural colloids are available for veterinary use. Artificial colloids are more commonly used and indications for their use include:

- Hypoperfusion
- Modulation of low colloid osmotic pressure (COP)
- Peripheral oedema related to vascular leak.

Artificial colloids are useful for the management of hypoperfusion as a result of hypovolaemia or distributive abnormalities, as they result in a larger expansion of intravascular volume on a per millilitre administered basis than that produced by crystalloids, and therefore can be used at lower doses. As they do not redistribute into the interstitial compartment quickly, their effect is also longer lasting than crystalloids. They are, however, more expensive and can have more serious adverse effects.

Colloid osmotic pressure

In hypoproteinaemic patients, colloids may be used to increase COP. This is the 'pull' provided by colloids (including natural colloids such as albumin) in the intravascular compartment. This 'pull' retains water within the intravascular space and prevents interstitial fluid overload. If the innate COP is decreased (e.g. due to a protein-losing enteropathy), oedema can result (Figure 10.8), particularly if the hydrostatic pressure (which 'pushes' fluid out of the vessel) is increased by crystalloid fluid therapy.

Many patients with chronic protein loss can cope with a very low COP, as the COP gradient between the vasculature and the extravascular space is maintained at normal levels. However, if crystalloid fluid therapy is administered the gradient may not be maintained and tissue oedema can result. It is important to realize that the lungs are well protected from oedema as a result of the low COP and so peripheral oedema will occur in advance of pulmonary oedema.

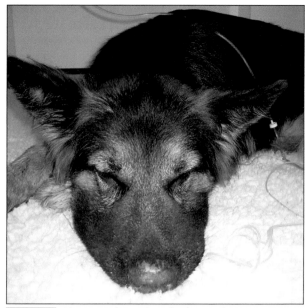

10.8 Hypoproteinaemic animals may become oedematous. Administering colloid instead of crystalloid fluids in these patients is useful to increase the colloid osmotic pressure, thereby retaining water within the intravascular space and reducing interstitial fluid overload.

As it is not common to measure COP in practice, it is often inferred from a low total solids or protein level. Low total protein in itself is not an indication for colloid administration, but if the patient requires fluid therapy the possibility of interstitial fluid overload should be considered and monitored. If marked hypoproteinaemia is present (e.g. albumin <15 g/l, total protein <30 g/l), intraoperative crystalloid fluid rates should be reduced and a colloid added.

A low COP may increase the likelihood of tissue oedema, which may have implications for wound healing; therefore, colloid administration may be beneficial.

Artificial colloids

Gelatines: Gelofusine and Haemaccel are both authorized for veterinary use in the UK. They are produced by hydrolysis of bovine collagen. They contain small colloidal particles (average molecular weight 30 kDa) when compared with the other available artificial colloid solutions. This leads to rapid degradation and excretion, and so their colloidal effects are short acting.

- They are often used to give a rapid but fairly brief 'boost' to intravascular volume and are useful in patients that are acutely hypoperfused under anaesthesia.
- They are less useful when longevity of a colloid is important, such as in patients with hypoproteinaemia.
- Rare adverse effects, including anaphylactic reactions, have been reported. If anaphylaxis occurs, symptomatic treatment with antihistamines should be administered and the gelatine infusion should be stopped. Oxygen, corticosteroid and vasopressor (usually adrenaline) therapy may be required in severe cases.

PRACTICAL TIPS

- Haemaccel contains calcium and so should not be administered in the same line as blood products.
- Gelofusine contains negligible calcium and therefore can be administered in conjunction with blood products.

Hydroxyethyl starches: Hydroxyethyl starches (HES) are produced by partial hydrolysis of amylopectin (a plant starch). Although they are *not* authorized for veterinary use in the UK, they have advantages over gelatine products as they contain larger colloidal molecules and are therefore longer lasting.

Various products are available in the UK. There are differences between them (Figure 10.9) but they are all used in a similar way. They are useful for both volume resuscitation and for patients with low COP.

- Bolus therapy (5–20 ml/kg over 10–30 minutes) can be used in patients with hypoperfusion.
- For patients with a low COP an infusion rate of 1 ml/kg/h is often used.
- Pentafraction (a medium molecular weight starch) has benefits in patients with increased capillary leakage, which can be seen in animals with marked systemic inflammation. However, this specific starch is not available as a commercial product for infusion.
- All colloids can adversely affect coagulation to varying degrees by interfering with factor VIII and von Willebrand factor function. For this reason hetastarch and pentastarch should not be administered at doses above 20–30 ml/kg/24h.
- Tetrastarches (such as Voluven) have a human dose limit of 30–50 ml/kg/24h, as their smaller average molecular size and lower substitution level (Figure 10.9) seem to result in fewer adverse effects on coagulation (Langeron *et al.*, 2001).

HES colloids generally have their **name** followed by **two numbers** written on the bag, e.g. 'Pentastarch 200/0.5'.

- The **first number** (e.g. '200') is the **average molecular weight** of the starch in kilodaltons (kDa). The higher the molecular weight, the longer the lifespan of the HES, as excretion requires hydrolysis to a size that can be excreted via the kidneys (generally <60 kDA).
- The **second number** (e.g. '0.5') is the **substitution ratio**, which is the average number of hydroxyethyl groups per glucose unit in the polymer. Higher levels of substitution result in greater resistance to hydrolysis; therefore, the higher the number, the longer the colloid will last in the body.
- The substitution ratio gives the HES its **name**, with a ratio of 0.5 seen in a pentastarch, 0.4 in a tetrastarch and 0.6 or 0.7 seen in hetastarches.
- There is a final number that is important in the longevity of a colloid but which is not present in the standard description of an HES. This is the **C2:C6 ratio**, which describes the level of hydroxyethyl substitution at the C2 carbon in the glucose molecule compared with the level of substitution at the C6 carbon. A high ratio (i.e. higher level of C2 substitution) leads to greater resistance to degradation and therefore greater longevity. This is clinically important, as a commercially available tetrastarch (Voluven 130/0.4) would be expected to have a short half-life due to its relatively low molecular weight and substitution but, due to its high C2:C6 substitution level, it actually has fair longevity.

10.9 Nomenclature of hydroxyethyl starches (HES).

- Other adverse effects that can occur with HES colloids include anaphylaxis and renal dysfunction, but both are very rare.

Dextran 70: Dextran-based colloids are not commonly used in the UK but are more popular in the USA. They are macromolecular polysaccharides produced by bacterial fermentation of sucrose. They are large colloids (70 kDa) and can be used in a similar fashion to HES. Their use has been associated with rare anaphylactic reactions and interference with coagulation.

Haemoglobin-based oxygen-carrying fluids: Oxyglobin is a stroma-free polymerized bovine haemoglobin solution. It is a potent colloid that also has oxygen-carrying capacity. It is currently only authorized for administration to dogs in the UK, but has been used successfully in cats (Weingart and Kohn, 2008).

- It is useful for patients with acute blood loss to provide oxygen-carrying capacity and colloidal effects.
- It can also be used in euvolaemic anaemic patients, such as those with bone marrow disease or immune-mediated haemolytic anaemia. If Oxyglobin is administered to a euvolaemic patient, care should be taken to prevent volume overload (Adamantos *et al.*, 2005). The authors usually use a rate of 1 ml/kg/h for administration to euvolaemic patients.
- Signs of fluid overload include the development of pleural effusion or pulmonary oedema.
- Other adverse effects are very rare.
- Oxyglobin does cause discoloration of the mucous membranes, urine and serum, particularly at higher dose rates. This is due to the free haemoglobin in the product, which can also interfere with colorimetric biochemical analysers.
- The product should be used within 24 hours of opening the foil overwrap in which it is provided, as it is susceptible to oxidation once the bag is exposed to oxygen.
- Oxyglobin has a dose-related duration of action, but this can be affected by the patient's underlying disease process (i.e. ongoing blood loss).

Biopure USA, the manufacturers of Oxyglobin, have ceased production and stocks are running low. There is the potential for another manufacturer to recommence production, but it is also possible that this fluid will no longer be available to the veterinary market.

Natural colloids

Legislation changes in 2005 now permit canine blood banking in the UK. Using natural colloids is appealing, as they replace exactly what is missing and are therefore a more 'appropriate' fluid. However, natural products are inherently variable and reactions are not uncommon.

Individual products and their applications are discussed below (see also Chapter 20), but it should be noted that natural colloids are rarely the first choice for a patient in shock. Anticoagulated blood products should never be administered with fluids that contain calcium, as this can result in the formation of calcium salts and microthrombi.

Selection of blood donors, collecting and processing blood products and their storage is beyond the scope of this chapter (see Chapter 20). Further information is available in the *BSAVA Manual of Canine and Feline Haematology and Transfusion Medicine* and the *BSAVA Manual of Canine and Feline Emergency and Critical Care*.

Whole blood and packed red blood cells: Whole blood is most appropriate for patients with acute blood loss. As it is very rarely available immediately in practice, patients should be resuscitated with crystalloid or colloid therapy prior to blood product therapy.

- As there is no commercial closed system available for storing and handling feline blood, whole blood (rather than blood products) is most frequently used in cats.
- Canine packed red blood cells (PRBCs) are produced by centrifugation of whole blood and are available from canine blood banks. They can be useful in the management of patients with blood loss or euvolaemic anaemia. In animals with blood loss they can be administered with other fluids for resuscitation.
- Stored PRBCs may not be fully effective immediately following transfusion, which means they are rarely required in an emergency. If the blood is not required as an emergency, it should be given at a rate of 1 ml/kg/h for 30 minutes to monitor for transfusion reactions. The remainder of the unit should be administered over a maximum of 4–6 hours.
- In an emergency, a fast rate of administration may be required but rates above 22 ml/kg/h are not recommended: if a faster rate is used the patient should be carefully monitored for volume overload, hypocalcaemia and coagulopathy.
- Whenever PRBCs are administered, care must be taken to prevent damage to the cells and only fluid pumps suitable for blood administration should be used.

Autotransfusion

Autotransfusion has been described in veterinary species and can be life-saving. However, it is a salvage technique and should only be used when there are no other alternatives. The technique is used to recover blood that has been lost into the pleural or abdominal cavity. Blood is collected using a sterile percutaneous technique with a syringe and catheter, or intraoperatively using sterile suction. The blood will not clot, as it should be defibrinated, but it is recommended that blood is collected into an anticoagulant (1 ml 3.8% sodium citrate per 9 ml blood or 1 ml CPDA per 7 ml blood). The use of heparin as an anticoagulant is not recommended, as it has a long half-life in the recipient and causes platelet activation. The blood should be administered through a blood filter as microthrombi may be present. Autotransfusion is not recommended if there is any risk of septic contamination of the blood (e.g. penetrating trauma) or a neoplastic cause of blood loss (e.g. ruptured spleen).

- Whole blood (donated or autotransfused) and PRBCs should be filtered during administration to the patient, using a blood-giving set or an in-line filter, in order to prevent the administration of microthrombi.
- As cats have preformed alloantibodies to non-self blood types, both donor and recipient cats must be blood typed prior to transfusion as ***administration of the incorrect blood type to a cat can be fatal***.
- As dogs do not have preformed alloantibodies, they can receive blood from any other dog for their first transfusion. However, it is recommended that blood should be obtained prior to transfusion to allow blood typing (even if the procedure is performed later).
- Although it is likely that antibodies to non-self blood types take 10–14 days to develop, it is recommended that any canine or feline red blood cell transfusions carried out more than 4 days after the first transfusion are cross-matched prior to administration.

Fresh, fresh frozen and stored plasma: Plasma is produced by separation of whole blood by centrifugation. It can then be stored in a variety of different ways. In dogs it is not necessary to administer blood type-matched plasma, although this is vital in cats.

- **Fresh plasma** can be stored at 1–6°C for up to 24 hours after collection and maintains adequate levels of all clotting factors.
- **Fresh frozen plasma** is frozen at –30°C and stored for up to 12 months.
- After this time the levels of all clotting factors are decreased, particularly the labile clotting factors (V and VIII and von Willebrand factor), and the plasma is termed **stored frozen plasma**.
- If plasma is stored in a household freezer rather than a –30°C freezer, the labile factors will begin to degrade straight away and so it should also be classed as **stored plasma**.

The only indication for plasma is provision of clotting factors in coagulopathic animals (as measured by prothrombin (PT) and partial thromboplastin (PTT) times) that are at risk of bleeding or have bleeding diatheses. It can also be used preoperatively in patients with inherited coagulopathies such as haemophilia A or von Willebrand's disease (vWD). Doses of 10–20 ml/kg are required for correction of a coagulopathy.

- Stored plasma has adequate levels of factors II, VII, IX and X (vitamin K-dependent factors) and can therefore be used in patients suffering from rodenticide toxicity as an alternative to fresh frozen plasma.
- Fresh frozen plasma should be used in animals suffering from other coagulopathies.
- Plasma has not been shown to be useful in human patients with pancreatitis and is unlikely to be of benefit to dogs with this disease (Leese *et al.*, 1991).
- It is a common misconception that plasma is useful in the treatment of hypoproteinaemia to increase plasma protein concentrations and COP.

The volume of plasma required to increase albumin serum levels by 10 g/l is 45 ml/kg (Wardop, 1997). At these doses, plasma proves prohibitively expensive and could potentially cause volume overload. Other products such as starch colloids or human serum albumin are more effective at increasing COP at smaller volumes and with less financial cost.

Cryoprecipitate: Cryoprecipitate is a concentrated fraction of plasma containing von Willebrand factor, factors VIII, XI and XII and fibrinogen. In this concentrated form, low volumes can be given prior to surgery in dogs with von Willebrand's disease at a dose of 1 unit/10 kg, decreasing the likelihood of volume overload.

Human serum albumin: This product has been used extensively in humans and is produced from donated blood. In the UK it is available as a 20% solution, which is markedly hypertonic, leading to the movement of extravascular fluid into the intravascular space. Human serum albumin is used as a resuscitative fluid in humans but has repeatedly shown no benefit over crystalloid fluids for this purpose (*Cochrane Review*, 2008). It is not generally used for resuscitation in dogs and cats; it is more commonly used in patients with hypoalbuminaemia and decreased COP.

To determine the amount of albumin required in a patient the following equation can be used:

Albumin deficit =
$$(\ [\text{albumin}]_{\text{desired}} \text{(g/l)} \ - \ [\text{albumin}]_{\text{patient}} \text{(g/l)} \ ) \ \times \ (\ \text{bodyweight} \text{(kg)} \ \times \ 0.3 \ )$$

In the authors' hospital the volume required is given as a slow infusion over at least 6 hours and the patient is monitored closely for reactions to the foreign protein. An initial infusion rate of 0.25 ml/kg/h for 30 minutes is used.

There is increasing literature about the use of human serum albumin in dogs but little in cats (Matthews and Barry, 2005; Trow *et al.*, 2008). There have been reports of both acute and delayed hypersensitivity reactions, some of which were fatal, in healthy dogs administered human serum albumin (Cohn *et al.*, 2007; Francis *et al.*, 2007). A small number of healthy dogs have anti-human albumin antibodies without known prior exposure and therefore all infusions should be carefully monitored (Martin *et al.*, 2008). Both critically ill and healthy animals administered human serum albumin form anti-human serum albumin antibodies and therefore repeated administration of the product is not recommended (Martin *et al.*, 2008).

Given this recent literature, human serum albumin, although not contraindicated in dogs and cats, should only be used after careful consideration and discussion with clients and **should never be used in healthy dogs**. To increase COP, artificial colloids with a greater history of use and less immunogenicity may be more appropriate.

Electrolyte abnormalities

Electrolyte abnormalities are common in patients presenting with surgical diseases. They also commonly develop in hospitalized patients. In many situations these abnormalities are mild and have only minor effects upon the patient; however, some electrolyte abnormalities can significantly impact upon a patient's status.

The introduction of hand-held and bedside biochemical and blood gas analysers allows electrolytes to be measured quickly and accurately, and monitored in patients at risk of abnormalities. As electrolyte concentrations can change quickly, influence patient status and can be managed readily, they are arguably one of the most useful parameters to measure on a regular basis in the hospitalized patient.

Individual electrolytes are discussed below, with the possible causes of and appropriate treatment for imbalances. The deviations seen in surgical conditions are discussed in more detail.

Sodium

Sodium is the primary extracellular cation, making it vitally important in the maintenance of water balance (both intra- and extracellular) and therefore cell volume.

Sodium and water regulation is complex but the osmoreceptors in the hypothalamus play an important role.

- Increased sodium concentration results in hypertonicity, which is detected by the osmoreceptors, leading to thirst and the release of antidiuretic hormone (ADH, also known as vasopressin).
- Decreased sodium concentration (e.g. as a result of excessive water intake) will also be sensed by the hypothalamus and leads to the suppression of thirst and ADH release.

Figure 10.10 lists the potential pathological causes of hyper- and hyponatraemia. Severe sodium abnormalities are fortunately uncommon as their management is extremely challenging.

Hypernatraemia
Pure water deficit:
- Primary hypodipsia
- Diabetes insipidus:
o Central
o Renal.
- Inadequate access to water
- Fever
- High environmental temperature.
Hypotonic fluid loss:
- Vomiting
- Diarrhoea
- Peritoneal fluid
- Pleural fluid
- Burns
- Diuretic administration
- Renal failure
- Diabetes mellitus.
Impermeant solute gain:
- Salt poisoning
- High sodium fluid administration:
o Hypertonic saline
o Sodium bicarbonate
o Parenteral nutrition
o Sodium phosphate enema.
- Hyperaldosteronism
- Hyperadrenocorticism.

10.10   Causes of hypernatraemia and hyponatraemia. (continues) ▶

Hyponatraemia

- Gastrointestinal losses:
  - o Vomiting
  - o Diarrhoea.
- Third-space losses:
  - o Pleural fluid
  - o Peritoneal fluid.
- Burns.
- Hypoadrenocorticism.
- Hypotonic fluid administration.
- Severe liver disease.
- Heart failure.
- Nephrotic syndrome.
- Advanced renal failure.
- Diuretic administration.
- Psychogenic polydipsia.
- Syndrome of inappropriate antidiuresis.
- Antidiuretic drugs.
- High concentrations of other solutes:
  - o Hyperglycaemia
  - o Mannitol.
- Laboratory error (using flame photometry):
  - o Hyperlipidaemia
  - o Hyperproteinaemia.

10.10 (continued) Causes of hypernatraemia and hyponatraemia.

Changes in extracellular sodium concentration result in water movement from or into the intracellular space, causing changes in cellular volume. When plasma sodium levels increase acutely, this leads to the movement of water out of the cells and into the extracellular fluid, with the opposite occurring when plasma sodium levels decrease. In most areas of the body these changes in cell volume can be easily accommodated. In the brain, however, sudden changes in cellular volume can directly lead to central nervous system effects.

- Rapid increases in cellular size lead to cerebral oedema and increased intracranial pressure.
- Decreases cause loss of cellular integrity and myelinolysis.

Where changes in the sodium concentration are chronic, adaptations occur to maintain cell size in the presence of the abnormal sodium concentration. Rapid changes in sodium concentration will therefore lead to either cellular oedema or dehydration.

In most patients it is not possible to discern the chronicity of sodium abnormalities and so treatment should always be performed with care.

- In cases of chronic (more than 48 hours) sodium abnormalities or those of unknown duration, sodium levels should not be changed more rapidly than 0.5 mmol/l/h, i.e. about 12 mmol/l/day. This allows time for the cells to adapt to the new sodium level.
- If an acute onset of sodium abnormality is known (or suspected) due to concurrent appropriate neurological signs, the sodium abnormality can be corrected more aggressively.

Hyponatraemia

Treatment for hyponatraemia depends on the underlying cause of the electrolyte abnormality. Common causes of chronic hyponatraemia include cardiac disease, hepatic disease and hypoadrenocorticism.

Hypoadrenocorticoid (Addisonian) patients require a cautious approach to alteration of their sodium concentration, as there are reports of myelinolysis related to rapid correction of sodium levels. If they are presented with hypoperfusion, the fluid deficits should be replaced with boluses of isotonic crystalloid; and once an ACTH stimulation test has been performed they can be started on mineralocorticoid and glucocorticoid therapy. This will lead to a slow and safe return to normal physiological sodium levels.

Acute hyponatraemia is not uncommon in the pre- and postoperative patient and this is discussed along with treatment below.

Hypernatraemia

Mild hypernatraemia (<170 mmol/l) does not require specific treatment other than isotonic crystalloid fluid therapy at a rate judged necessary to replace any perfusion abnormalities, hydration deficits and ongoing losses (see Fluid therapy section above). The sodium concentration of Hartmann's fluid would make it ideal for this purpose. The patient should also be given free access to water unless contraindicated.

Treatment for moderate to severe hypernatraemia is more challenging. Hypernatraemia indicates a free water deficit, which can be calculated using the following formula:

$$\text{Free water deficit } (l) = \left([Na^+]_{current} (mmol/l) / [Na^+]_{normal} (mmol/l) - 1 \right) \times (\text{bodyweight } (kg) \times 0.6)$$

The normal sodium concentration for a patient can be estimated as the mid reference-range point for the species on the analyser being used.

- In stable patients the total volume of free water required can be administered as 5% dextrose or 0.45% NaCl. The time required to replace the volume required safely (i.e. how long it would take at a rate of 0.5 mmol/h) can be calculated and the fluid replaced over this time period.
  - One difficulty with this approach is that any ongoing losses of free water also need to be replaced and this can be difficult to assess.
  - Also, although simple in theory, in the practical situation changes do not usually happen as calculated and rapid falls in sodium concentration can occur.
- A safer approach is to use a fluid with a higher sodium concentration (e.g. Hartmann's) to replace losses related to dehydration over 24–48 hours, with frequent monitoring of sodium levels to assess efficacy of the therapy and allow alteration as necessary. Unless neurological signs are present or the patient has profuse vomiting, allowing free access to water is important, because if the patient has a normal thirst mechanism this will aid sodium normalization.

Common surgical causes of sodium abnormalities

Gastrointestinal fluid losses: Vomiting, diarrhoea and fluid pooling within the intestinal tract are often seen secondary to intestinal obstruction due to a foreign body, neoplastic mass or intussusception. These fluid losses can lead to both hyper- and hyponatraemia.

- Hyponatraemia can occur if hypovolaemia occurs due to marked gastrointestinal fluid losses. Hypovolaemia leads to the release of ADH, which decreases renal water excretion (to preserve intravascular volume) and therefore leads to the dilution of sodium.
- Hypernatraemia may result as the fluid lost into the gastrointestinal tract is usually hypotonic compared with plasma, leading to an increase in sodium concentration.

The patient's volume and hydration deficits should be assessed as discussed in the Fluid therapy section of this chapter, and isotonic crystalloid therapy should be administered.

Patients with hyponatraemia tend to require more aggressive fluid therapy, due to the concurrent hypovolaemia. It is worth noting that patients with a history of vomiting and diarrhoea may have fluid deficits that require replacement even if abnormalities are not noted on physical examination.

Third-space losses and burns: Loss of fluid into the peritoneum or pleural space or cutaneously via burns can result in either hyper- or hyponatraemia due to similar mechanisms as those described above. Generally these sodium abnormalities should be treated with isotonic crystalloid therapy. Patients with burns lose large volumes of fluid and protein and are prone to oedema formation. Colloid fluids are typically required, often in conjunction with isotonic crystalloid therapy (Figure 10.11).

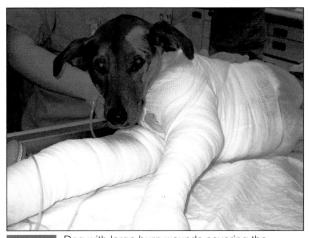

10.11 Dog with large burn wounds covering the forelimbs, hindlimbs, chest and pectoral region. A jugular catheter was placed to administer intravenous crystalloid and colloid fluids to treat the dog for the large volumes of fluid and protein being lost through the burn wounds. (Courtesy of V Lipscomb)

Postoperative hyponatraemia: Mild hyponatraemia is relatively common in postoperative critically ill patients. The pathogenesis is probably multifactorial and may include surgical blood loss, hypoalbuminaemia, postoperative third-space fluid loss and previous fluid therapy. Rarely, a syndrome of inappropriate antidiuresis (SIAD, also known as a syndrome of inappropriate antidiuretic hormone secretion, or SIADH) can be seen postoperatively due to pain, fear, nausea or opioid and other drug administration. It can also be associated with head trauma.

These patients have a higher urine concentration than expected for their low plasma sodium level; they drink an excessive volume of water and can develop peripheral oedema. Diagnosis of SIADH is difficult in veterinary patients.

Renal failure: Chronic renal failure is common in older, particularly feline, patients. Hypernatraemia can develop due to loss of hypotonic fluid through polyuria and the patient not maintaining a sufficient oral intake of water. It is uncommon for hypernatraemia in this situation to be marked and therefore fluid losses (volume and hydration deficits) can be replaced with simple isotonic crystalloid fluid therapy. Hyponatraemia can develop in severe end-stage renal failure when the kidneys are unable to excrete enough water.

Heart failure: If cardiac disease causes a sufficient decrease in cardiac output and blood pressure, ADH release will result in hyponatraemia. Treatment with diuretics can exacerbate the hyponatraemia by decreasing the circulating volume. If these patients require surgery, care should be taken when utilizing fluid therapy as they can easily develop congestive heart failure. In general the hyponatraemia seen in these patients does not require treatment and is more an indication that the patient is suffering from severe disease.

Potassium

Potassium is the major intracellular cation but its concentration is much lower in the extracellular environment. This transcellular concentration difference is important for maintenance of the normal cell membrane resting potential and therefore both hypo- and hyperkalaemia can cause marked skeletal muscle and cardiac signs. Abnormalities in potassium concentration frequently occur; the more common causes of hypo- and hyperkalaemia are listed in Figure 10.12 and the most important are discussed below.

Hypokalaemia

Hypokalaemia is the most common electrolyte abnormality and is often seen in surgical patients due to anorexia, gastrointestinal losses and fluid therapy with inadequate potassium supplementation.

- Mild to moderate hypokalaemia generally does not result in clinical signs.
- Progression to marked hypokalaemia (<2 mmol/l) can result in rhabdomyolysis and severe muscle weakness to the point of hypoventilation and respiratory arrest.

All isotonic fluid therapy being administered for rehydration and ongoing losses should be supplemented with potassium chloride based on the serum potassium concentration of the patient (Figure 10.13).

- The rate of potassium administration should never exceed 0.5 mmol/kg/h.
- If a patient's potassium level is unknown and there is no evidence of acute renal failure or urinary tract injury, it is safe to assume they require at least 20 mmol KCl per litre of isotonic crystalloid.
- Once potassium chloride has been added to a bag of fluid it should be clearly labelled and should never be used to provide bolus fluid therapy.

Hypokalaemia

- Administration of potassium-free or deficient fluid.
- Chronic renal failure.
- Post-obstruction diuresis.
- Gastrointestinal loss:
  - o Vomiting
  - o Diarrhoea.
- Hyperaldosteronism.
- Hyperadrenocorticism.
- Insulin or glucose therapy.
- Alkalosis.
- Drug therapy:
  - o Loop diuretics
  - o Thiazide diuretics
  - o Penicillins
  - o Beta$_2$ adrenergic agonists.

Hyperkalaemia

- Acute renal failure:
  - o Anuric/oliguric renal failure
  - o Urinary tract obstruction
  - o Uroabdomen.
- Repeated pleural fluid drainage.
- Gastrointestinal disease:
  - o Trichuriasis
  - o Salmonellosis
  - o Ruptured duodenal ulcer.
- Hypoadrenocorticism.
- Marked tissue damage:
  - o Tumour lysis syndrome
  - o Reperfusion injury
  - o Rhabdomyolysis.
- Acute mineral acidosis.
- Iatrogenic/drug therapy:
  - o High potassium fluid administration
  - o Concurrent potassium-sparing diuretic and ACE inhibitor administration
  - o Digoxin
  - o Non-specific beta adrenoceptor antagonists.

10.12 Causes of hypokalaemia and hyperkalaemia.

Serum potassium concentration (mmol/l)	Total mmol KCl to be present in 500 ml isotonic crystalloid	Maximal fluid rate (ml/kg/h)
<2.0	40	6
2.1–2.5	30	8
2.6–3.0	20	12
3.1–3.5	14	18
3.6–5.0	10	25

10.13 Potassium supplementation.

Post-obstructive diuresis: Patients with urinary tract obstruction often develop hyperkalaemia (see below). However, once the obstruction has been relieved, patients can develop a post-obstructive diuresis. Urine output should be monitored closely and the volume of intravenous isotonic crystalloid administered matched to urine output to prevent dehydration. This extreme diuresis results in hypokalaemia, which should be treated with potassium chloride supplementation of the isotonic crystalloid fluids.

Hyperkalaemia

Hyperkalaemia is a life-threatening electrolyte abnormality due to its marked cardiovascular effects. Elevated extracellular potassium changes the cardiac resting membrane potential, leading to decreased excitability. Bradycardia and bradyarrythmias result, which can be fatal.

The serum potassium concentration at which a patient develops cardiac abnormalities varies between individuals, but a concentration >7 mmol/l is concerning and should be treated with fluid therapy and monitored closely, even if drug therapy is not yet indicated (i.e. the patient is not bradycardic).

Although it cannot be used to estimate serum potassium concentration, electrocardiography can support a presumptive diagnosis of hyperkalaemia. Commonly seen electrocardiogram (ECG) abnormalities (Figure 10.14) include:

- Tall T waves
- First- and second-degree atrioventricular block
- Absent P waves
- Wide QRS complexes.

If potassium levels cannot be measured and a patient has significant bradycardia and a disease process that could cause hyperkalaemia (e.g. urethral obstruction), treatment should be administered.

Isotonic crystalloid therapy is indicated in nearly all hyperkalaemic patients as part of emergency treatment. It directly reduces the serum potassium concentration through dilution, as well as correcting any fluid deficits.

Emergency treatment of patients *symptomatic* for hyperkalaemia (i.e. those with bradycardia and associated hypoperfusion) can be provided via a number of interventions.

- The most rapidly effective therapy is administration of 10% calcium gluconate at a dose of 0.5–1 ml/kg over 5–10 minutes. The ECG (or heart rate if ECG is unavailable) should be monitored, as too rapid administration can be associated with bradycardia.
- Calcium borogluconate (0.2–0.4 ml/kg of a 23% solution over 5–10 minutes) or calcium chloride (0.5 ml/kg of a 10% solution over 5–10 minutes) can be used if calcium gluconate is not available.
- Calcium administration does not resolve hyperkalaemia but balances the effect of the hyperkalaemia on the resting membrane potential. The effect is not long lasting (approximately 20 minutes) but in most cases will allow enough time for recognition and initiation of treatment of the underlying cause of the hyperkalaemia.

Further therapy may be required in some cases (Figure 10.15).

- Insulin therapy is a rapid method of normalizing potassium concentrations. If it is utilized, patients should be closely monitored for hypoglycaemia, which can develop up to 12 hours after insulin administration.
- The use of a 2.5–5% glucose infusion is necessary in all cases to maintain euglycaemia.
- Sodium bicarbonate is relatively ineffective as therapy for hyperkalaemia and is associated with a significant risk of complications. It should therefore be kept as a last resort. It may be of more use in patients with concurrent metabolic acidosis.

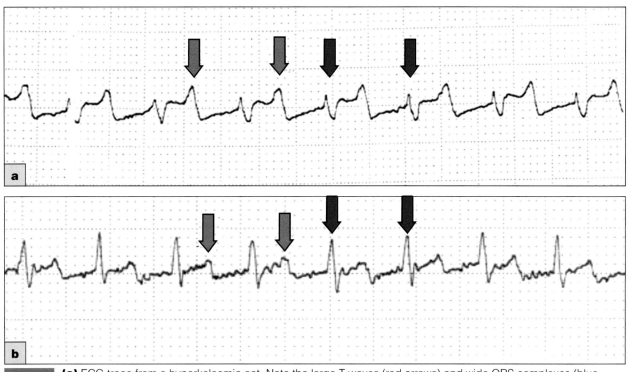

10.14 **(a)** ECG trace from a hyperkalaemic cat. Note the large T waves (red arrows) and wide QRS complexes (blue arrows). **(b)** ECG from the same cat after calcium gluconate therapy. T waves are now smaller and QRS complexes narrower.

---

1. Obtain vascular access with a peripheral intravenous catheter.
2. Administer isotonic crystalloid fluid therapy as required to treat hydration and volume deficits. If fluid therapy is only required to 'dilute' potassium levels, a rate of 4 ml/kg/h is appropriate.
3. If the patient is bradycardic (heart rate <70 bpm in dogs, <160 bpm in cats, or deemed inappropriate), administer 10% calcium gluconate at 0.5–1 ml/kg over 5–10 minutes while monitoring heart rate and/or ECG.
4. Search for an underlying cause of the hyperkalaemia and treat.
5. If hyperkalaemia persists, a repeat dose of calcium gluconate can be administered to counteract the bradycardia.
6. Regular insulin (also known as soluble or crystalline insulin) at 0.2–0.5 IU/kg can be administered in conjuction with dextrose at 1–2 g/kg. Monitor closely for hypoglycaemia over the following 6–12 hours; a dextrose infusion (2.5–5% dextrose in an isotonic crystalloid fluid) is often required. This is rarely required for urethral obstruction, but is useful if anaesthesia is needed for a long surgery and should only be used if there is no alternative.
7. Sodium bicarbonate at 1 mEq/kg can be administered.
8. If all other measures fail, peritoneal dialysis can be attempted.

10.15 Treatment of hyperkalaemia.

Urethral obstruction: This is the most common cause of symptomatic hyperkalaemia seen in practice. Hyperkalaemia is rare in dogs with urethral obstruction, but is commonly seen in cats.

- Treatment should be instigated immediately, with isotonic crystalloid fluid therapy and calcium gluconate administered if there are pronounced cardiac effects related to the hyperkalaemia.
- Patients often require aggressive fluid therapy, as they are hypovolaemic; there is no need to wait until the urethral obstruction has been relieved.
- Passage of a urinary catheter can be attempted if the patient is conscious but collapsed; however, most patients require sedation.

- It is rare for these patients to require further therapy for their hyperkalaemia.
- In cases where a catheter cannot be passed promptly, decompressive cystocentesis may relieve back pressure on the urethra enough to allow a catheter to be passed.
- In patients where a catheter cannot be passed at all, further treatment as described above may be necessary.

Uroabdomen: Mild to severe azotaemia and increased serum potassium in a patient that has recently suffered from trauma should prompt investigation for uroabdomen or urinary tract injury.

- If free abdominal fluid is present, the creatinine and potassium concentrations in the fluid and serum should be compared.
- If the abdominal fluid concentrations are higher than the serum concentrations, uroabdomen should be suspected.
- A urinary catheter should be placed and is often effective at draining urine. Percutaneous drainage of peritoneal fluid may be required in some patients to aid management of electrolyte abnormalities. This drainage, in conjunction with fluid therapy, may be sufficient to decrease potassium to a suitable level for induction of anaesthesia to allow contrast studies and surgical repair to be performed.
- If stabilization is not possible through these methods alone, administration of insulin and glucose provides rapid control of serum potassium concentrations to a level where anaesthesia can be safely performed.
- Care should be taken whenever this therapy is utilized to prevent the occurrence of hypoglycaemia.

Acute oliguric or anuric renal failure: These patients can be difficult to manage, as the kidney is the main route of potassium excretion. The kidney is extremely efficient at excreting excess potassium, so much so that hyperkalaemia is not seen until there is severe oliguria or anuria. As other mechanisms of potassium excretion cannot compensate in the acute situation, these patients will require longer term management strategies.

- In the short term, management with insulin and glucose can be attempted, and if there is severe metabolic acidosis the administration of sodium bicarbonate may be helpful.
- Further treatment will be required if anuria or oliguria is persistent. In the UK, peritoneal dialysis is the only option for these patients, but in other countries haemodialysis or continuous renal replacement therapy are performed.

Metabolic acidosis: Metabolic acidosis is frequently cited as a potential cause of hyperkalaemia due to hydrogen and potassium ion exchange across the cell membrane. However, the situation in the clinical patient is not so clear cut. Although acute mineral acidosis (caused by the administration of ammonium chloride or hydrogen chloride) can cause hyperkalaemia, this type of acidosis is not common clinically and the effect of a mineral acidosis on the potassium concentration is highly variable between patients. The majority of metabolic acidoses seen in veterinary patients are due to organic acids such as lactic or keto acids (see Acid–base abnormalities section) and are not associated with hyperkalaemia.

Calcium

Calcium is required for adequate cardiovascular, neurological, muscular and skeletal function. It is present in three forms in plasma:

- Ionized – free calcium
- Protein-bound – mostly to albumin
- Complexed – with phosphate, bicarbonate and lactate.

Total calcium (the sum of all three fractions above) is measured by most biochemical analysers but it is the ionized fraction that is the biologically active component. Although formulae exist to predict ionized calcium using total calcium, these are inaccurate (Schenck and Chew, 2005). Ionized calcium can be measured on some point-of-care systems but careful sample handling is important.

Causes of hypo- and hypercalcaemia are listed in Figure 10.16. The most important surgical disease processes are discussed below.

Investigation of the underlying causes and appropriate treatment is the most effective way of managing calcium disorders. However, symptomatic treatment for hypo- or hypercalcaemia is often necessary in the interim, or if the underlying cause is not easily controlled.

Hypocalcaemia

Mild total hypocalcaemia is common in critically ill patients and occurs via a number of mechanisms. Calcium supplementation is rarely required.

Hypocalcaemia

- Hypoalbuminaemia (only when measuring total calcium).
- Acute renal failure.
- Chronic renal failure.
- Eclampsia.
- Pancreatitis.
- Ethylene glycol toxicity.
- Hypoparathyroidism:
  - o Primary
  - o Post-surgical removal
  - o Secondary to hypomagnesaemia.
- Hypovitaminosis D.
- Soft tissue trauma/rhabdomyolysis.
- Severe intestinal disease.
- Sepsis.
- Iatrogenic:
  - o Large-volume blood product administration (citrate chelation)
  - o Excessive bisphosphonate administration
  - o Phosphate enema.

Hypercalcaemia

- Neoplasia:
  - o Lymphoma
  - o Thymoma
  - o Anal gland adenocarcinoma
  - o Multiple myeloma
  - o Carcinoma
  - o Bone tumours.
- Hypoadrenocorticism.
- Granulomatous disease:
  - o *Angiostrongylus vasorum*
  - o Fungal disease.
- Idiopathic (cats).
- Hyperparathyroidism.
- Vitamin D overdose:
  - o Iatrogenic
  - o Rodenticide (cholecalciferol)
  - o Plants (calcitriol glycosides) e.g. Day Jessamine (*Cestrum diurnum*) and Yellow Oat Grass (*Trisetum flavescens*)
  - o Psoriasis cream (calcipotriene or calcipotriol).
- Hypervitaminosis A.
- Acute renal failure.
- Chronic renal failure.
- Juvenile patient (mild).

10.16 Causes of hypocalcaemia and hypercalcaemia.

As total calcium is a poor indicator of ionized calcium it is better, where possible, to measure ionized calcium in these patients prior to initiating therapy, except where clinical signs are present. Common clinical signs associated with hypocalcaemia include:

- Muscle tremors
- Facial rubbing
- Stiff gait
- Behavioural changes
- Seizures.

Treatment should be instituted if the hypocalcaemia is severe (ionized calcium of ≤0.7 mmol/l), or if clinical signs are present.

Emergency treatment consists of 0.5–1.5 ml of 10% calcium gluconate/kg given as an intravenous infusion over 10–20 minutes.

- An ECG should be monitored closely (or the patient's heart or pulse rate manually if this is not possible).
- If bradycardia develops, the infusion should be slowed or stopped.

- If calcium gluconate is not available, 10% calcium chloride can be used at a dose rate of 0.5 ml/kg over 10–20 minutes, but it causes a marked tissue reaction if injected perivascularly and so great care should be taken.
- Calcium salts should not be administered by any route other than intravenously or orally, as they can cause marked tissue reactions.
- Further supplementation of calcium will probably be necessary if a patient is displaying clinical signs, and this should take the form of an intravenous infusion of calcium gluconate at a dose rate of 5–15 mg/kg/h.
- In patients requiring longer term supplementation of calcium (e.g. hypocalcaemic post-thyroidectomy patients), oral therapy with calcium salts and vitamin D should be initiated (Figure 10.17). Calcium salt administration can be stopped in the majority of cases once vitamin D therapy has taken effect.

Common causes of hypocalcaemia include thyroid-ectomy, removal of a parathyroid tumour, and eclampsia/puerperal tetany.

Thyroidectomy: Thyroidectomy can result in hypocalcaemia due to damage to or removal of the parathyroid glands. The risk of hypocalcaemia is much greater if a bilateral extracapsular technique has been performed. Hypocalcaemia is generally seen 1–3 days post-surgery, though it can develop as late as 1–2 weeks post-surgery. Cats will frequently exhibit facial pruritis as the first clinical sign and this should prompt measurement of the serum calcium concentration.

- **Emergency treatment** with calcium gluconate should be administered in symptomatic patients (Figure 10.18).
- Oral calcium supplementation should then be instigated with the aim of maintaining mildly subnormal calcium levels to decrease the risk of hypercalcaemia and to provide a continued stimulus for hypertrophy of any remaining parathyroid tissue.

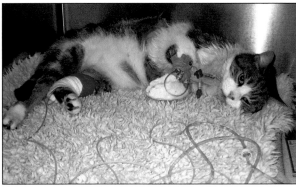

10.18 Cat with hypocalcaemia receiving a calcium gluconate infusion 3 days after bilateral thyroidectomy. The cat had become depressed and displayed twitching and facial rubbing clinical signs.

- In some cats hypocalcaemia persists and vitamin D supplementation is also required.
- Permanent hypoparathyroidism is rare but it may take up to 3 months for residual parathyroid tissue to hypertrophy sufficiently for the maintenance of adequate calcium levels.

Parathyroid tumour removal: The chronic hypercalcaemia seen in patients with parathyroid adenomas results in atrophy of the other parathyroid glands; therefore, hypocalcaemia can develop once the mass is removed. This usually occurs within 24–48 hours of surgery, with clinical signs apparent 3–6 days post-surgery in 50% of dogs.

- The risk of hypocalcaemia is greatest in patients with higher presurgical calcium concentrations. In these patients consideration should be given to preoperative administration of vitamin D metabolites (Figure 10.17) as there is a time lag until they are fully efficacious.
- Otherwise management is as for post-thyroidectomy patients, as described above.

Most affected dogs regain parathyroid function within 2–3 months.

Drug	Trade name	Dose	Comments
Calcium gluconate		25–50 mg elemental calcium/kg orally q8h	
Calcium carbonate		25–50 mg elemental calcium/kg orally q24h	Commonly available as human antacid preparations Contains a high level of elemental calcium and so fewer tablets required compared with calcium gluconate
Dihydrotachysterol	AT-10	0.02–0.3 mg/kg orally q24h initially then 0.01–0.02 mg/kg orally q24–48h	A synthetic vitamin D analogue Onset of action within 24 hours with an increase in serum calcium seen within 1–7 days
Calcitriol	Calcitriol Rocaltrol	10–15 ng/kg orally q12h for 3–4 days, decreasing to 2.5–7.5 ng/kg orally q12–24h	Rapid onset of action (1–2 days) with a short half-life The vitamin D drug of choice but capsule size may make dosing difficult
Alfacalcidiol	One-alpha	10–15 ng/kg orally q12h for 3–4 days, decreasing to 2.5–7.5 ng/kg orally q12–24h	Rapid onset of action (1–2 days) with a short half-life
Ergocalciferol		4000–6000 IU/kg/day orally initially, followed by 1000–2000 IU/kg orally q1–7days	The long onset of action of this drug and its poor action at the vitamin D receptor means that it is not recommended

10.17 Calcium salts and vitamin D analogues available for subacute and chronic hypocalcaemia therapy.

Eclampsia/puerperal tetany: Eclampsia typically occurs in bitches of small to medium breed with large litters at 1–3 weeks postpartum. The disease is rare in cats. Calcium loss in the milk potentially combined with decreased oral intake (poor appetite or inappropriate food) is thought to be the underlying cause of the hypocalcaemia. Hypophosphataemia often coexists.

- Patients usually present with muscular tremors and should be treated with intravenous calcium administration as described above, followed by oral calcium salt administration until lactation has ceased.
- Ideally the puppies should be weaned early but initially calcium supplementation can be attempted.
- If a second episode of hypocalcaemia occurs, early weaning is essential and the puppies need to be hand reared.

Hypercalcaemia

Hypercalcaemia can have marked cardiovascular, renal, gastrointestinal and neurological effects. The following signs are common:

- Polyuria and polydipsia
- Anorexia
- Vomiting
- Lethargy and weakness.

Rarely, cardiac arrhythmias, seizures and twitching may be seen. Hypercalcaemia also disrupts the mechanism for urine concentration and in the longer term causes nephrocalcinosis, commonly resulting in azotaemia.

Neoplastic causes of hypercalcaemia: Neoplasia is the most common cause of hypercalcaemia in dogs and the third most common cause in cats. The most common underlying neoplasm is lymphoma. Other frequently seen tumours associated with hypercalcaemia include thymoma and anal sac adenocarcinoma. Attempts should be made to control hypercalcaemia before surgery, to allow normalization of renal and cardiovascular function prior to anaesthesia. However, full calcium control is often not possible without surgical removal of the neoplasm.

Treatment: Initial treatment aims to cause calciuresis through natriuresis. Fluid therapy with 0.9% NaCl at 4–6 ml/kg/h may be sufficient if hypercalcaemia is not marked. However, more aggressive therapy is indicated if the patient's ionized calcium is 20% higher than the upper end of the reference interval, or if total calcium is >4 mmol/l, or if the patient is displaying clinical signs. This is particularly true if the patient has hyperphosphataemia, as soft tissue calcification is more likely. The calcium phosphate product can be calculated using the following formula:

Calcium phosphate product $= [Ca^{2+}]_{total}$ (mmol/l) x $[HPO_3^-]$ (mmol/l)

If the calcium phosphate product is >5 then the risk of soft tissue mineralization is increased and the hypercalcaemia should be treated aggressively, as it is difficult to address phosphate abnormalities. In conjunction with fluid therapy, drug therapies are available for management of hypercalcaemia (Figure 10.19).

1. **Furosemide** 1–2 mg/kg i.v. q6–12h (promotes natriuresis). This should only be used once dehydration has been corrected. Fluid therapy should be continued at a high rate to allow for the extra fluid losses caused by the diuresis.

2. **Salmon calcitonin** 4–7 IU/kg s.c q6–8h (inhibits bone resorbtion).

3. **Bisphosphonates** (decrease osteoclastic activity):
   a. Pamidronate
      i. Dogs 0.9–1.3 mg/kg i.v. over 2–24 hours, one dose
      ii. Cats 1.5–2 mg/kg i.v. over 2–24 hours, one dose
   OR:
   b. Clodronate
      i. Dogs 5–14 mg/kg i.v. q24h
      ii. Dogs 10–30 mg/kg orally q8–12h
   OR:
   c. Etidronate
      i. Dogs 5–15 mg/kg orally q24h
      ii. Cats 5–20 mg/kg orally q24h

4. **Glucocorticoid** therapy reduces calcium absorption from the gut and increases calciuresis as well as directly treating some of the causes of hypercalcaemia. Glucocorticoids are efficacious for the treatment of many causes of hypercalcaemia but can be detrimental in some conditions, such as renal disease, and can hamper investigation of other causes such as lymphoma. They should only be used once investigation has been completed.

10.19 Drug therapies for the management of hypercalcaemia. These are listed in terms of increasing aggressiveness and should be used in this order.

Phosphate

Phosphate is the main intracellular anion and plays a vital role in cell signalling, energy metabolism, cell membrane structure and enzyme activity. Although many conditions can cause hypo- or hyperphosphataemia (Figure 10.20), very few are surgical conditions other than uroabdomen and urethral obstruction, where other electrolyte abnormalities such as hyperkalaemia are of much greater importance (see above).

Hypophosphataemia

The major effect of hypophosphataemia is haemolysis, but weakness, pain and gastrointestinal signs may also be seen. Treatment of hypophosphataemia is only necessary if patients are symptomatic, the phosphate

Hypophosphataemia

- Post-insulin therapy in diabetic ketoacidosis.
- Feeding post-starvation.
- Hypothermia.
- Primary hyperparathyroidism.
- Renal tubular disorders.
- Eclampsia.
- Vitamin D deficiency.
- Phosphate binders.

Hyperphosphataemia

- Renal failure:
  o Acute
  o Chronic.
- Urethral obstruction.
- Uroabdomen.
- Vitamin D toxicosis (rodenticides, psoriasis cream).
- Tumour lysis syndrome.
- Massive tissue trauma/rhabdomyolysis.
- Juvenile animal.

10.20 Causes of hypophosphataemia and hyperphosphataemia.

concentration is expected to decrease further (e.g. diabetic ketoacidotic animal) or a serum concentration <0.6 mmol/l is present.

- Phosphate can be administered as sodium phosphate, potassium phosphate or a mixture of sodium and potassium phosphate.
- An infusion of phosphate at a rate of 0.05–0.1 mmol/kg/h should be used.
- The patient's serum phosphate concentration should be checked every 6 hours to assess response.

Hyperphosphataemia

The most common cause of hyperphosphataemia is renal failure, including post-renal problems such as uroabdomen and urethral obstruction. Prolonged high phosphate levels, as occurs with chronic renal failure, can result in soft tissue mineralization.

- Intravenous fluid therapy in conjunction with treatment of the underlying cause, if possible, is the optimum method of dealing with hyperphosphataemia.
- In the acute situation, unlike the other electrolytes, there are no alternative methods for controlling phosphate concentrations.
- With chronic hyperphosphataemia, oral phosphate-binding agents can be used to reduce phosphate absorption. These only work to bind ingested phosphate and in combination with a low phosphate diet.

Chloride

Chloride is the major extracellular anion but clinically relevant abnormalities in chloride balance are not as common as with other electrolytes. Changes in the plasma chloride concentration usually follow changes in sodium and thus it is more appropriate to interpret the corrected chloride level.

Corrected chloride (mmol/l) =

$$[Cl^-]_{measured} \text{ (mmol/l)} \times \left([Na^+]_{normal} \text{ (mmol/l)} / [Na^+]_{measured} \text{ (mmol/l)} \right)$$

If the corrected chloride level is outside the reference ranges, a true hypo- or hyperchloraemia is present. Potential causes are listed in Figure 10.21.

Hypochloraemia
- Vomiting gastric acid.
- Loop or thiazide diuretic therapy.
- Chronic respiratory acidosis.
- Hyperadrenocorticism.
- Sodium bicarbonate therapy.

Hyperchloraemia
- Diarrhoea.
- Renal failure.
- Renal tubular acidosis.
- Iatrogenic:
o Potassium bromide therapy (interference with assay rather than genuine hyperchloraemia)
o Chloride salt therapy (e.g. KCl)
o Total parenteral nutrition
o Spironolactone
o Salt poisoning.
- Hypoadrenocorticism.
- Diabetes mellitus.

10.21 Causes of hypochloraemia and hyperchloraemia.

Treatment should be directed at the underlying cause.

- Hypochloraemic metabolic alkalosis is the most challenging of these conditions and should be managed by infusion of a fluid high in chloride, such as 0.9% NaCl. Without the administration of chloride this condition will not improve (see Acid–base abnormalities section).
- Symptomatic management is usually effective for treatment of hyperchloraemia.

Magnesium

The majority of the body's magnesium is intracellular. It is present in ionized, protein-bound and complexed forms within the plasma. As with calcium, the ionized fraction is the biologically active portion.

Magnesium has major roles in the cardiovascular and neuromuscular systems. It is absorbed from the gut and controlled and regulated by the kidneys, so renal and gastrointestinal disease are the most common causes of an altered magnesium concentration. Renal disease is also associated with hypermagnesaemia if there is an acute reduction in magnesium excretion.

The clinical importance of hypo- and hypermagnesaemia is unclear. However, therapy of hypomagnesaemia is recommended if a patient is displaying cardiac arrhythmias, has refractory hypokalaemia or increased neuromuscular excitability.

- Magnesium chloride or sulphate can be administered as an intravenous infusion at a dose of 0.375–0.5 mEq/kg/day.
- **Emergency therapy** can be instituted in patients suffering severe cardiac arrhythmias unresponsive to anti-arrhythmic therapy (typically ventricular tachycardia) at a dose of 0.15–0.3 mEq/kg over 5–20 minutes.

PRACTICAL TIP

As magnesium ions are bivalent, 1 mmol is equivalent to 2 mEq.

Acid–base abnormalities

Blood gas analysers are increasingly common in veterinary practices but are, perhaps, not used to their full capability. Acid–base physiology can initially appear to be quite daunting, but understanding a few basic rules will allow appropriate patient management.

Why pH values matter

The pH of a patient's blood is a measurement of the hydrogen ion concentration in the extracellular environment. The pH value is a negative logarithmic scale, which means that:

- As the pH increases, the number of hydrogen ions (and therefore the acidity) decreases
- A one-point difference on the pH scale means a change of 10 times the concentration of hydrogen ions.

This means that small changes in pH can cause large changes in the concentration of hydrogen ions. For example, a decrease in pH from 8 to 7 causes an increase in hydrogen ion concentration from 10 nmol/l to 100 nmol/l. The pH of the extracellular environment is held at around 7.4, which is optimal for physiological function and equates to a hydrogen ion concentration of 40 nmol/l. This is much lower than the concentration of other ions considered to be important in the extracellular fluid; sodium, for example, has a concentration approximately 3.75 million times that of the hydrogen ion concentration.

Deviation from the body's optimum pH of 7.4 leads to changes in enzyme, receptor and ion channel function. This results in abnormalities in a number of organ systems, including the cardiovascular, endocrine and neurological systems.

Simple acid–base disorders

Acid–base disorders are traditionally classified as either metabolic or respiratory in origin:

- Metabolic abnormalities result in alterations in the concentration of bicarbonate (HCO_3^-) or base excess
- Respiratory abnormalities result in alterations in the partial pressure of carbon dioxide (PCO_2).

Bicarbonate is an alkali and CO_2 is an acid. Reference values for pH, venous partial pressure of CO_2, concentration of HCO_3^- and base excess are shown in Figure 10.22.

Mild variation from these values may be expected with different sampling methods and analysers. Arterial samples will tend to have higher pH, lower CO_2 and slightly higher HCO_3^- levels. Although very useful for assessing oxygenation of the blood, arterial samples are not necessary for assessment of acid–base balance. Figure 10.22 also shows the changes in HCO_3^- and CO_2 seen with basic acid–base disturbances,

along with the expected compensatory response.

Simple acid–base disturbances are those with only one abnormal process in the patient's acid–base balance alongside the expected compensation, e.g. a metabolic acidosis with compensatory respiratory alkalosis. It is important to remember that a compensatory response will never have a greater effect on pH than the original disturbance. Therefore, the deviation in pH allows classification of the primary process, i.e. the blood pH in the situation described above would be acidaemic as a result of the primary metabolic acidosis.

Figure 10.23 gives the expected changes in CO_2 and HCO_3^- seen during compensation, which allows calculation of whether an acid–base disturbance is simple or not. It should be noted that different compensatory responses are seen for acute and chronic respiratory acid–base disturbances. This is because metabolic compensation is made up of an immediate intracellular buffering of changes in CO_2 followed by a slower change in acid secretion and HCO_3^- reabsorption by the kidneys. The latter effect takes 2–5 days to reach maximal effect. This is unlike the quick change in respiratory rate leading to changes in CO_2 allowing rapid compensation for metabolic acid–base disturbances.

Figure 10.24 gives a step-by-step guide to assessing simple acid–base disorders.

Base excess

The base excess is often calculated by blood gas analysers. It can be used as an alternative to HCO_3^- concentration to assess whether a metabolic acid–base disturbance is present. It represents the amount of strong acid required to titrate the pH of one litre of blood to 7.4 when temperature and CO_2 levels are held constant at 37°C and 40 mmHg, respectively. This means that the patient's partial pressure of CO_2 does not affect base excess and therefore it is argued to be a better indicator of metabolic disturbances.

Acid–base disorder	pH	HCO_3^- (mmol/l)	Base excess (mmol/l)	PCO_2 (mmHg)
Normal dog	7.35–7.44	20.8–24.2	–2 to +1.5	33.6–41.2
Normal cat	7.28–7.41	18.0–23.2	–4 to +2	32.7–44.7
Metabolic acidosis	↓	↓	↓	↓
Metabolic alkalosis	↑	↑	↑	↑
Respiratory acidosis	↓	↑	↑	↑
Respiratory alkalosis	↑	↓	↓	↓

10.22 Changes in bicarbonate, base excess and carbon dioxide seen with simple acid–base disorders. Primary changes are demonstrated by the red arrows, with compensatory responses demonstrated by the blue arrows. Note that reference values provided are for venous blood (Zweens *et al.*, 1977; Middleton *et al.*, 1981).

Acid–base disorder	Primary change	Compensatory response
Metabolic acidosis	↓ HCO_3^-	0.7 mmHg decrease in PCO_2 for each 1 mmol/l decrease in HCO_3^-
Metabolic alkalosis	↑ HCO_3^-	0.7 mmHg increase in PCO_2 for each 1 mmol/l increase in HCO_3^-
Acute respiratory acidosis	↑ CO_2	1.5 mmol/l increase in HCO_3^- for each 10 mmHg increase in PCO_2
Acute respiratory alkalosis	↓ CO_2	2.5 mmol/l decrease in HCO_3^- for each 10 mmHg decrease in PCO_2
Chronic respiratory acidosis	↑ CO_2	3.5 mmol/l increase in HCO_3^- for each 10 mmHg increase in PCO_2
Chronic respiratory alkalosis	↓ CO_2	5.5 mmol/l decrease in HCO_3^- for each 10 mmHg decrease in PCO_2

10.23 Average compensatory response for simple acid–base disturbances (DiBartola, 2006).

1. Decide if the patient is acidaemic (pH <7.4) or alkalaemic (pH >7.4).

2. Check the bicarbonate level:
   a. If it is *increased*, a **metabolic alkalosis** is present
   b. If it is *decreased*, a **metabolic acidosis** is present.

3. Check the carbon dioxide level:
   a. If it is *increased*, a **respiratory acidosis** is present
   b. If it is *decreased*, a **respiratory alkalosis** is present.

4. Check the pH again:
   a. If it is *increased*, the primary disturbance is an **alkalosis**
   b. If it is *decreased*, the primary disturbance is an **acidosis**.

5. A **compensatory response** may be present which would be in the opposite direction.

6. If both process are alkalotic or acidaemic, a **mixed acid–base** disturbance is present.

7. If the change in the 'compensatory' process is greater than that suggested in Figure 10.23, a **mixed acid–base** disturbance is present.

10.24 Quick guide to assessing acid–base disturbances.

■ A positive base excess indicates that a metabolic alkalosis is present (because acid is required to bring the pH to 7.4).

■ A negative base excess indicates that a metabolic acidosis is present (because a 'negative' amount of acid is required to bring the pH to 7.4, i.e. alkali is required).

Mixed acid–base disorders

Mixed acid–base disturbances should be considered if blood gas analysis reveals that both the respiratory and metabolic components have affected the pH in the same direction (e.g. there is both a respiratory and metabolic acidosis). A mixed disorder should also be suspected if the change in CO_2 or HCO_3^- is greater than that expected by compensation alone, as calculated from the information in Figure 10.23. In these circumstances more than one problem is present. In some cases there can be even more than two acid–base disturbances. A common mixed acid–base disorder is seen in a patient presenting with hypovolaemia and hyperlactataemia leading to metabolic acidosis but with tachypnoea due to fear and pain causing a concurrent respiratory alkalosis.

Metabolic acidosis

Metabolic acidosis is the most common acid–base disturbance seen in cats and dogs. There are many possible causes (Figure 10.25) and it can be useful to differentiate this group into those with a high anion gap and those with a normal anion gap.

Anion gap is sometimes reported on blood gas analysers but can also be simply calculated as:

Anion gap (mmol/l) =
  $([Na^+]_{(mmol/l)} + [K^+]_{(mmol/l)}) - ([HCO_3^-]_{(mmol/l)} + [Cl^-]_{(mmol/l)})$

The 'gap' calculated signifies the anions other than HCO_3^- and chloride in the blood, such as proteins, lactate, ketones, phosphates and sulphates. The usual gap is 12–24 mmol/l in dogs and 13–27 mmol/l in cats.

Metabolic acidosis

Increased anion gap (normochloraemic) metabolic acidosis:
■ Lactic acidosis
■ Diabetic ketoacidosis
■ Uraemic acidosis
■ Acidic toxin ingestion (e.g. ethylene glycol, salicylates).

Normal anion gap (hyperchloraemic) metabolic acidosis:
■ Diarrhoea
■ Rapid administration of high chloride fluids (e.g. 0.9% NaCl)
■ Renal tubular acidosis
■ Drug therapy (e.g. carbonic anhydrase inhibitors, ammonium chloride).

Metabolic alkalosis

■ Vomiting gastric fluid.
■ Diuretic therapy.
■ Hyperaldosteronism.
■ Hyperadrenocorticism.
■ Administration of alkali (e.g. sodium bicarbonate).
■ Volume contraction.
■ Severe potassium or magnesium deficiency.

Respiratory acidosis

■ Respiratory centre depression:
   o Drug-induced (most general anaesthetics and sedatives)
   o Neurological disease.
■ Neuromuscular disease:
   o Spinal cord injury/disease
   o Phrenic nerve injury
   o Drug-induced (e.g. neuromuscular blocking agents)
   o Myasthenia gravis
   o Tetanus
   o Botulism
   o Marked electrolyte abnormalities.
■ Upper/large airway obstruction:
   o Laryngeal paralysis
   o Tracheal collapse
   o Brachycephalic upper airway syndrome
   o Feline allergic airway disease
   o Mass lesion
   o Obstruction of endotracheal tube.
■ Severe pulmonary disease:
   o Severe pulmonary oedema
   o Smoke inhalation
   o Pulmonary thromboembolism
   o Severe pneumonia.
■ Extrapulmonary diseases:
   o Diaphragmatic rupture
   o Pleural space disease (e.g. pneumothorax, pleural effusion)
   o Chest wall trauma/flail chest
   o Pickwickian syndrome.
■ Increased carbon dioxide production with impaired alveolar ventilation:
   o Cardiopulmonary arrest
   o Heatstroke
   o Malignant hyperthermia.

Respiratory alkalosis

■ Hypoxaemia:
   o Decreased inspired oxygen:
      – Anaesthetic machine malfunction
      – High altitude.
   o Pulmonary parenchymal disease
   o Decreased cardiac output
   o Severe anaemia.
■ Centrally mediated hyperventilation.

10.25 Causes of acid–base disturbances. (continues) ▶

Respiratory alkalosis

- Drugs:
  - o Corticosteroids
  - o Salicylates
  - o Progesterone.
- Hyperadrenocorticism.
- Liver disease.
- Central nervous system disease:
  - o Trauma
  - o Neoplasia
  - o Inflammation.
- Exercise.
- Heatstroke.
- Overzealous mechanical/manual ventilation.
- Situations causing pain, fear or anxiety.

10.25 (continued) Causes of acid–base disturbances.

High anion gap acidosis

This is the most common cause of metabolic acidosis and is often due to lactic acidosis. Other causes of high anion gap acidosis include diabetic ketoacidosis, uraemic acidosis and aspirin (salicylate) toxicity.

Lactic acidosis: Lactate is produced from pyruvate as the end product of anaerobic metabolism. In cells with adequate oxygen supplies, pyruvate is transported into the mitochondria and fuels oxidative phosphorylation to produce energy. If inadequate oxygen is present lactate accumulates, leading to metabolic acidosis. Therapy should aim to increase oxygen delivery to the cells, which requires an increase in intravascular volume, an increase in oxygen-carrying capacity or an improvement in function of the cardiovascular system (see Fluid therapy section for further details of management of hypoperfusion).

It can seem confusing that lactate can cause an acidosis in the body when fluids containing lactate, such as Hartmann's, are used to treat patients with metabolic acidosis (see Fluid therapy section). This is because the lactate in such fluids has a sodium ion as its cation, whereas the lactate produced in the body has a hydrogen ion, leading to acidosis.

Lactic acidosis is not always due to hypoxia and can be divided into types A and B (Figure 10.26).

Normal anion gap acidosis

This is normally caused by an increased chloride concentration.

Diarrhoea: Diarrhoea results in normal anion gap metabolic acidosis, as intestinal fluid has a high concentration of HCO_3^- and a lower concentration of chloride. If diarrhoea is profuse it can also lead to hypovolaemia and therefore lactic acidosis worsening the acid–base imbalance. The hypovolaemic patient's losses should be replaced quickly with a fluid containing an HCO_3^- precursor, such as lactate. Hartmann's is the ideal fluid in this situation.

Bicarbonate therapy for metabolic acidosis

In the majority of cases, therapy for metabolic acidosis requires treatment of the underlying disease process and fluid therapy only. Bicarbonate therapy may be required in rare circumstances, such as acute anuric or oliguric renal failure patients with severe uraemic acidosis. Patients must have normal ventilatory function to allow elimination of the carbon dioxide produced. The amount of bicarbonate required can be calculated with the following formula:

Bicarbonate required (mmol/l) =
$$0.15 \times \text{base excess (mmol/l)} \times \text{bodyweight (kg)}$$

This volume can be administered slowly over 15 minutes and then the response assessed. A repeat dose can be given if necessary. Care should be taken, as it is easy to create a metabolic alkalosis if bicarbonate therapy is used inappropriately.

- Sodium bicarbonate should not be administered with calcium-containing fluids, due to the risk of calcium salt precipitation.

Type	Oxygen status	Features

Type A lactic acidosis (most common)	Hypoxic	- Increased oxygen demand:
		  o Severe exercise
		  o Marked struggling during venepuncture (more common in cats)
		  o Seizures
		- Decreased oxygen availability:
		  o Hypoxaemia
		  o Severe anaemia
		  o Hypovolaemia
		  o Distributive abnormalities
		  o Obstruction of venous return
		  o Cardiac output failure
		  o Cardiac arrest

Type B lactic acidosis	Non-hypoxic	- Drugs and toxins:
		  o Ethylene glycol
		  o Salicylates
		- Diabetes mellitus
		- Liver failure
		- Neoplasia
		- Sepsis
		- Hypoglycaemia
		- Renal failure
		- Hereditary defects

10.26 Types of lactic acidosis.

- Sodium bicarbonate therapy is not appropriate for the treatment of respiratory acidosis, as it counteracts acidosis by producing CO_2 to be eliminated, which requires an intact ventilatory response.

Metabolic alkalosis

Potential causes of metabolic alkalosis are listed in Figure 10.25. The most common surgical cause of metabolic alkalosis is loss of gastric acid through vomiting. The loss of hydrogen and chloride ions in gastric acid leads to hypochloraemia and a persistent metabolic alkalosis.

The pathogenesis of this abnormality is complex, and has implications for therapy.

- In health, the kidney reabsorbs sodium and chloride ions together from the renal tubules.
- In patients with gastric acid loss severe enough to result in hypovolaemia, there is a strong requirement for sodium resorption by the kidney in order to retain water.
- In hypochloraemia it is not possible to resorb sodium with chloride and so instead sodium is exchanged for hydrogen ions, resulting in excessive acid loss into the renal tubules, leading to perpetuation of the alkalosis.
- These patients will therefore have an acidic urine pH (so-called paradoxical aciduria).
- Concurrent loss of potassium via gastric acid and in exchange for sodium in the kidneys worsens hypokalaemia, which can contribute to the alkalosis.

In order to restore the acid–base balance, chloride must be provided in high concentrations (i.e. 0.9% NaCl) to replenish the normal pathways for sodium resorption.

- As these patients are usually hypovolaemic, bolus fluid therapy is required initially (see Fluid therapy section above).
- Potassium supplementation is also required and should be supplied in the patient's maintenance fluids once they are cardiovascularly stable.
- The underlying cause of the vomiting should be investigated. These patients often have a surgical cause for their disease (e.g. gastrointestinal obstruction from foreign bodies, intussusceptions or masses). Although the predominant loss of fluid is gastric in origin, the obstruction may be anywhere in the stomach or small intestines.

Respiratory acidosis

Respiratory acidosis is caused by an increase in the partial pressure of CO_2 in the patient's blood. As patients cannot compensate quickly for respiratory acidosis (see Figure 10.23) the change in pH is often pronounced if this is the primary abnormality. Carbon dioxide is usually closely controlled by the ventilatory system and an increased partial pressure infers hypoventilation.

Respiratory acidosis is usually associated with neurological disease or depression of the central nervous system by drugs, but can also be seen with respiratory tract disease. Potential causes of respiratory acidosis are listed in Figure 10.25, including many surgical conditions.

- Management of respiratory acidosis requires treatment of the underlying disease process.
- Temporary or longer term mechanical ventilation may be necessary in some cases, particularly those with neurological disease.
- In all cases, if severe hypercapnia is present it is likely that the patient will also be hypoxaemic and therefore supplemental oxygen should be administered.

General anaesthesia

During anaesthesia, hypoventilation is commonly seen as a result of respiratory depression by anaesthetic and analgesic drugs, typically opioids. In this situation the patient should be provided with intermittent positive pressure ventilation either manually or via a ventilator and the plane of anaesthesia lightened until their respiratory drive returns.

Cervical spinal surgery

Adequate ventilation requires an intact neuromuscular system. Cervical spinal surgery can lead to oedema and bleeding in the region of the nerves supplying the diaphragm and intercostal muscles. Postoperatively these patients need to be monitored closely to assess adequacy of ventilation using capnography or blood gas analysis. If respiratory acidosis develops, mechanical ventilation is required to allow time for the neurological system to recover.

Upper airway disease

Hypoventilation as a result of respiratory disease is particularly associated with upper airway obstructions such as laryngeal paralysis. Exaggerated inspiratory effort increases obstruction through dynamic airway collapse, leading to decreased air movement and hypoventilation. Treatment with sedatives, and cooling if hyperthermia is present, will decrease inspiratory effort and improve air flow, leading to improved ventilation. Induction of general anaesthesia and intubation may be required in rare cases and should be performed before there is fatigue.

Pulmonary parenchymal disease

Pulmonary parenchymal disease, such as pneumonia, very rarely results in respiratory acidosis, as CO_2 is exchanged much more readily between the blood and alveoli compared with oxygen. The increased respiratory drive caused by hypoxia will therefore prevent hypercapnia. In fact, the increased respiratory rate much more commonly results in respiratory alkalosis (see below). If respiratory acidosis is associated with hypoxia and pulmonary parenchymal disease, it suggests that the patient is no longer able to maintain an adequate respiratory rate as a result of muscle fatigue and requires mechanical ventilation.

Trauma

Patients can also develop respiratory acidosis if there is a condition preventing adequate lung expansion. These cases are often surgical (e.g. diaphragmatic rupture or severe chest wall trauma). These patients need to be stabilized (as far as possible) prior to careful general anaesthesia, which almost always requires manual or mechanical ventilation.

Respiratory alkalosis

Any disease process that causes an increase in ventilation will lead to increased CO_2 excretion and therefore a respiratory alkalosis. In general the consequences of respiratory alkalosis are few and treatment is not required, only a search for the potential underlying cause and treatment of that if required. Most importantly, oxygen is vital for patients with a respiratory alkalosis secondary to hypoxia. Potential causes are listed in Figure 10.25 but the most commonly seen cause of a primary respiratory alkalosis in general veterinary practice is hyperventilation secondary to pain, fear, or hypoxaemia. Respiratory alkalosis is also often seen as a compensatory mechanism for a metabolic acidosis.

References and further reading

Adamantos S, Boag A and Hughes D (2005) Clinical use of a haemoglobin-based oxygen-carrying solution in dogs and cats. *In Practice* **27**, 399–405

Alderson P, Bunn F, Li Wan Po A *et al.* (2004) Human albumin solution for resuscitation and volume expansion in critically ill patients. *Cochrane Database of Systematic Reviews* 4

Cohn LA, Kerl ME, Lenox CE *et al.* (2007) Response of healthy dogs to infusions of human serum albumin. *American Journal of Veterinary Research* **68**, 657–663

Day MD, Mackin A and Littlewood J (2000) *BSAVA Manual of Canine and Feline Haematology and Transfusion Medicine.* BSAVA Publications, Gloucester

DiBartola SP (2006) Introduction to acid–base disorders In: *Fluid, Electrolyte and Acid–base Disorders in Small Animal Practice*, ed. SP DiBartola, pp. 229–251. WB Saunders, St Louis

Drobatz KJ and Cole SG (2008) The influence of crystalloid type on acid–base and electrolyte status of cats with urethral obstruction. *Journal of Veterinary Emergency and Critical Care* **18**, 355–361

Francis AH, Martin LG, Haldorson GJ *et al.* (2007) Adverse reactions suggestive of type III hypersensitivity in six healthy dogs given human albumin. *Journal of the American Veterinary Medical Association* **230**, 873–879

Jackson K and Nolan J (2009) The role of hypotensive resuscitation in the management of trauma. *Journal of the Intensive Care Society* **10**, 109–114

King L and Boag A (2007) *BSAVA Manual of Canine and Feline Emergency and Critical Care, 2nd edn.* BSAVA Publications, Gloucester

Langeron O, Doelberg M, Eng-Than A *et al.* (2001) Voluven®, a lower substituted novel hydroxyethyl starch (HES 130/0.4), causes fewer effects on coagulation in major orthopedic surgery than HES 200/0.5. *Anesthesia and Analgesia* **92**, 855–862

Leese T, Holliday M, Watkins M *et al.* (1991) A multicentre controlled clinical trial of high-volume fresh frozen plasma therapy in prognostically severe acute pancreatitis. *Annals of the Royal College of Surgeons of England* **73**, 207–214

Martin LG, Luther TY, Alperin DC *et al.* (2008) Serum antibodies against human albumin in critically ill and healthy dogs. *Journal of the American Veterinary Medical Association* **232**, 1004–1009

Matthews KA and Barry M (2005) The use of 25% human serum albumin: outcome and efficacy in raising serum albumin and systemic blood pressure in critically ill dogs and cats. *Journal of Veterinary Emergency and Critical Care* **15**, 110–118

Middleton DJ, Ilkiw JE and Watson ADJ (1981) Arterial and venous blood gas tensions in clinically healthy cats. *American Journal of Veterinary Research* **42**, 1609–1611

Schenck PA and Chew DJ (2005) Prediction of serum ionized calcium concentration by serum total calcium measurement in dogs. *American Journal of Veterinary Research* **66**, 1330–1336

Trow AV, Rozanski EA, Delaforcade AM *et al.* (2008) Evaluation of use of human albumin in critically ill dogs: 73 cases (2003–2006). *Journal of the American Veterinary Medical Association* **233**, 607–612

Wardrop KJ (1997) Canine plasma therapy. *Veterinary Forum* **14**, 36–40

Weingart C and Kohn B (2008) Clinical use of a haemoglobin-based oxygen carrying solution (Oxyglobin) in 48 cats (2002–2006). *Journal of Feline Medicine and Surgery* **10**, 431–438

Zweens J, Frankena H, van Kampen EJ *et al.* (1977) Ionic composition of arterial and mixed venous plasma in the unanesthetized dog. *American Journal of Physiology – Renal Physiology* **233**, F412–415

Shock, sepsis and SIRS

Andrew J. Brown[†]

Definitions

Shock

Shock is a syndrome that results from inadequate cellular energy production. This arises from an imbalance between oxygen delivery (DO_2) and oxygen consumption (VO_2), and a transition from efficient aerobic to inefficient anaerobic cellular metabolism. Anaerobic metabolism provides a temporary fix for inadequate cellular energy production, but results in lactate accumulation and metabolic acidosis.

DO_2 is dependent on cardiac output and the oxygen content of the blood (C_aO_2) (Figure 11.1).

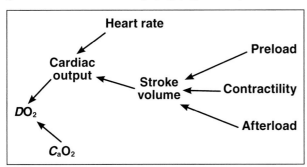

11.1 The delivery of oxygen to tissues (DO_2) is dependent on cardiac output and the oxygen content of arterial blood (C_aO_2).

- Shock commonly results from alterations in tissue perfusion, though severe anaemia or pulmonary dysfunction can result in a significant decrease in C_aO_2 with resultant cellular hypoxia and a switch in energy production to anaerobic metabolism (**hypoxic shock**).
- Alterations in tissue perfusion may result from:
  - A loss of intravascular volume and cardiac preload (**hypovolaemic shock**)
  - Maldistribution of blood flow (**distributive shock**)
  - Cardiac dysfunction (**cardiogenic shock**).
- Additionally, mitochondrial dysfunction, cyanide toxicity and hypoglycaemia may result in a switch to anaerobic metabolism (**metabolic shock**).

The various forms of shock are summarized in Figure 11.2.

Classification	Conditions
Hypovolaemic shock	Haemorrhage Severe dehydration
Distributive shock	Sepsis Anaphylaxis
Cardiogenic shock	Arrhythmias Cardiac tamponade Dilated cardiomyopathy
Hypoxic shock	Anaemia Pulmonary disease Hypoventilation Methaemoglobinaemia Carboxyhaemoglobinaemia
Metabolic shock	Hypoglycaemia Mitochondrial dysfunction Cyanide intoxication

11.2 Classification of shock.

Hypovolaemic shock and **septic shock** (a form of distributive shock) are the two most common forms of shock in the surgical patient.

- Common causes of hypovolaemic shock include:
  - Haemorrhage (trauma, surgical, spontaneous)
  - Gastrointestinal losses (vomiting secondary to gastrointestinal foreign body).
- Common causes of septic shock include:
  - Peritonitis
  - Pyometra
  - Pyothorax.

SIRS

SIRS is the acronym for **systemic inflammatory response syndrome**. It can be triggered by multiple conditions, including infection, trauma, surgery, immune-mediated disease, neoplasia, burns and pancreatitis. Although the definition refers to an 'inflammatory' response, SIRS has both pro- and anti-inflammatory components. Criteria for the diagnosis of SIRS in dogs have been proposed (Hauptman et al., 1997) (Figure 11.3). However, these criteria lack specificity and must be used in conjunction with an interpretation of the clinical picture.

Criterion	Measurement
Temperature (°C)	<38 *or* >39
Heart rate (beats per minute)	>120
Respiratory rate (breaths per minute)	>20
WBC (×10³); % bands	<6 *or* >16; >3%

11.3 Proposed criteria for the diagnosis of SIRS in dogs (two out of four criteria required) (Hauptman *et al.*, 1997).

Sepsis

Sepsis is simply defined as SIRS with infection. This infection may be bacterial, viral, fungal or protozoal.

- **Bacteraemia** is the presence of viable bacteria in the blood.
- **Severe sepsis** is sepsis with evidence of dysfunction of at least one organ.
- **Septic shock** is severe sepsis associated with hypotension, which is unresponsive to appropriate fluid resuscitation.
- **Multiple organ dysfunction syndrome** (MODS) is dysfunction of the endothelial, cardiopulmonary, renal, nervous, endocrine and gastrointestinal systems associated with the progression of systemic inflammation.

Overview and pathophysiology

Hypovolaemic shock

Hypovolaemic shock arises from a depleted effective intravascular volume. Hypovolaemia leads to a decreased cardiac preload (end-diastolic volume) and subsequent reduction in stroke volume.

Hypovolaemic shock (Figure 11.4) can arise from:

- Internal or external blood loss (**haemorrhagic shock**)
- Excessive loss of other body fluids resulting in progressive dehydration and eventual loss of intravascular volume
- Obstruction to venous return (**obstructive shock**).

All these result in a decrease in cardiac preload, decreased stroke volume, decreased cardiac output and clinical signs of shock (see Figure 11.1).

Cause	Source
Haemorrhagic shock	Surgical haemorrhage Trauma Ruptured neoplasm (e.g. haemangiosarcoma) or haematoma Coagulopathy
Interstitial fluid loss	Vomiting Diarrhoea Decreased oral intake Burns Third-spacing Polyuria
Obstructive shock	Gastric dilatation–volvulus (GDV) Intraoperative caval occlusion

11.4 Causes of hypovolaemic shock.

In an attempt to maintain normal tissue perfusion and blood pressure, compensatory mechanisms are activated following a fall in cardiac output.

- An increase in sympathetic activity causes vasoconstriction, tachycardia and an increase in cardiac contractility.
- Vasoconstriction diverts blood to essential organs and the positive inotropic and chronotropic effects increase cardiac output.

Neurohormonal mechanisms are activated in an attempt to return vascular volume to normal:

- A decrease in renal perfusion and glomerular filtration rate (GFR) leads to activation of the renin–angiotensin–aldosterone system (Figure 11.5).
  - Renin is released from the cells of the juxtaglomerular apparatus and converts angiotensinogen to angiotensin I (AT I).
  - AT I in turn is converted to angiotensin II (AT II) by angiotensin-converting enzyme.
  - AT II increases sodium resorption from the proximal tubule of the nephron and stimulates the release of aldosterone from the adrenal gland.
  - Aldosterone increases sodium (and with it water) resorption in the collecting duct in exchange for potassium and hydrogen ions.
  - AT II is also a potent vasoconstrictor and increases GFR.
- In response to severe hypotension, antidiuretic hormone (ADH, also known as vasopressin) is released from the posterior pituitary gland. ADH is a potent vasoconstrictor at the V_1 receptors and increases water resorption in the collecting duct via V_2 receptors.

The net result of these neurohormonal responses is to retain more fluid at the kidney in an attempt to restore normal intravascular volume and cardiac preload.

Sepsis and SIRS

SIRS may be due to infectious (sepsis) or non-infectious causes (Figure 11.6).

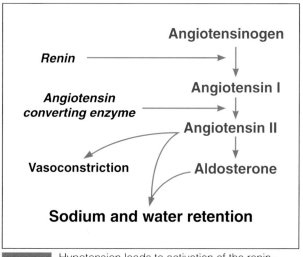

11.5 Hypotension leads to activation of the renin–angiotensin–aldosterone system (RAAS).

Infectious (sepsis)

- Lungs (pneumonia).
- Urinary tract (cystitis, pyelonephritis).
- Abdomen (septic peritonitis).
- Gastrointestinal (e.g. parvoviral entiritis).
- Wounds, incisions.
- Indwelling catheters (catheter-related blood stream infection).
- Surgical implants.
- Heart (infectious endocarditis).
- Pleural space (pyothorax).
- Liver (liver abscess).
- Pancreas (pancreatic abscess).
- Uterus (pyometra).
- Mammary glands (mastitis).
- Prostate (prostatic abscess).
- Joints (septic arthritis).
- Discs (discospondylitis).

Non-infectious

- Immune-mediated haemolytic anaemia.
- Pancreatitis.
- Neoplasia (e.g. lymphoma).
- Trauma (can become septic).
- Burns (can become septic).
- Steroid-responsive meningitis.
- Immune-mediated polyarthritis.

11.6 Causes of SIRS in small animals.

- The most common infectious causes of sepsis in veterinary medicine include septic peritonitis, pyothorax, pyometra, pneumonia and gastrointestinal diseases such as parvoviral enteritis.
- Non-infectious causes include trauma, burns, pancreatitis, surgery, immune-mediated disease and neoplasia.

As medicine has advanced, animals and people have been able to survive multiple conditions that would previously have been fatal. However, although these evolving therapies resulted in patients surviving a specific condition, they did not provide an immediate cure and the body's acute and subacute inflammatory response became apparent. Essentially, the advancement of medicine and successful treatment of a condition has brought to light other problems. Although death from the failure of a single organ has become less common, **multiple organ dysfunction syndrome** (MODS) and **multiple organ failure** (MOF) have become more common.

SIRS represents the body's response to an inciting event (septic or non-septic).

- Following the inciting event, there is a local pro-inflammatory response that leads to an initial systemic response and eventual massive systemic inflammation.
- This is then followed by *excessive* immunosuppression and immunoparalysis.
- In general, the more severe the inciting cause and the longer the duration of the insult, the more likely it is that a patient will develop immunoparalysis.
- If the immunosuppression is self-limited, the patient will usually survive. If not, patients frequently develop secondary infections and die.

This late-stage immunosuppression explains why multiple clinical studies that investigated the blocking of pro-inflammatory mediators in critically ill patients have failed to improve outcome (see Chapter 12 for an in depth discussion of the immune and inflammatory responses to anaesthesia and surgery).

Both Gram-negative and Gram-positive bacteria (Figure 11.7) can initiate the inflammatory response and cause sepsis. Although initiation of the pathway is different, the end result of transcription and release of inflammatory mediators resulting in clinical signs of sepsis occurs in each case.

The clinical and clinicopathological findings seen in sepsis are a result of the systemic inflammation. Unless the clinician is able to remove the inciting cause of the inflammation (e.g. remove the septic focus), the systemic inflammation will continue. Ultimately, untreated or unresponsive sepsis can progress to septic shock.

Gram-negative bacteria

Lipopolysaccharide (LPS) is a key component of the cell wall of Gram-negative bacteria and is a potent initiator of the septic inflammatory cascade. The innate immune response is the first line of defence against invading microbes through activation of transcription factors and generation of cytokines.

- LPS binds to a receptor on macrophages and through cell signalling pathways this ultimately leads to transcription of over 150 genes and the generation and release of pro-inflammatory cytokines.
- The pro-inflammatory cytokines recruit additional cells of the innate immune system to the affected area and cause neutrophils to release reactive oxygen species (ROS), proteases and lysozymes in an attempt to eliminate the invading organism.
- The counter-inflammatory cytokines attempt to limit the pro-inflammatory response and localize tissue destruction.
- Extensive activation occurs with systemic disease (a disproportionate activation of the pro-inflammatory mediators, or a lack of regulatory counter-inflammatory cytokines).

The gastrointestinal (GI) and urogenital (UG) systems are the most common sources of Gram-negative sepsis in veterinary patients. Leakage of GI contents into the abdomen can occur secondary to the ingestion of foreign bodies, enterotomy/biopsy dehiscence, GI neoplasia and perforated ulcers. The leakage of GI contents will result in an extensive inflammatory response and clinical signs resulting from the systemic inflammation.

Gram-positive bacteria

The cell wall of Gram-positive bacteria contains peptidoglycan and lipoteichoic acid, which can activate the inflammatory cascade via toll-like receptor 2 (TLR2). In addition, soluble bacterial exotoxins can activate T-cells, leading to the release of pro-inflammatory cytokines such as tumour necrosis factor (TNF)-α. Sources of Gram-positive sepsis in the surgical patient include wounds and intravenous catheters. *Streptococcus canis* infection can result in toxic shock syndrome and necrotizing fasciitis in the dog.

11.7 Sources and mechanisms of initiation of the inflammatory response to Gram-negative and Gram-positive bacteria.

Septic shock

Septic shock is a form of distributive shock that occurs in response to infectious agents or infection-induced mediators. It is characterized by cardiovascular decompensation, inefficient oxygen delivery and extraction, and resultant cellular dysfunction. A patient with septic shock remains hypotensive despite appropriate fluid resuscitation. The pathophysiology of septic shock is complex and incompletely understood.

Vascular dysfunction

The release of multiple inflammatory mediators in response to infection leads to inappropriate peripheral vasodilatation and altered organ blood flow.

- Nitric oxide (NO) is produced by endothelial cells and cells of the innate immune system by inducible nitric oxide synthase (iNOS) in a calcium-independent manner.
- NO diffuses to the vascular smooth muscle cytosol, and causes vasodilatation through the activation of guanylate cyclase and generation of cyclic guanosine monophosphate (cGMP).
- The vasodilatation leads to altered organ blood flow and hypotension.

Hypotension persists after correction of relative or absolute hypovolaemia due to vasodilatation and vasoplegia.

- There is an attenuated vasoconstrictor response to alpha-adrenergic agonists in sepsis and the dosages of catecholamines needed to increase arterial pressure are higher in septic than normal patients.
- Vasoplegia results from reduced bioactivity of catecholamines, a decrease in associated calcium influx, and alpha-adrenergic receptor internalization.
- Circulating cytokines cause the vasculature to become more permeable. Tight junctions within the vascular endothelium are lost and plasma proteins are able to leak out of the vessel.

Hypoalbuminaemia is also common in septic patients and results in a decreased colloid osmotic pressure (COP).

- As a result of the decrease in COP and the capillary leak, there is increased fluid flux out of the vessels into the interstitium, which results in tissue oedema.
- As more intravenous crystalloids are administered, more leak out of the vessels, with the patient remaining hypovolaemic but becoming severely oedematous.

The aetiology of hypoalbuminaemia in these patients is multifactoral, but mainly results from decreased production by the liver, increased loss, and extravasation through abnormal endothelium. In sepsis the body is in a catabolic state and generation of acute-phase proteins occurs at the expense of albumin. During fluid resuscitation, plasma proteins will be diluted and the albumin concentration will fall further.

Effect on coagulation

Abnormalities in haemostasis are common in septic patients and contribute to the development of organ dysfunction. Coagulation pathways are closely entwined with inflammatory pathways; therefore, systemic inflammation results in activation of the coagulation cascade, with resultant thrombin formation leading to further cytokine production.

- Naturally occurring anticoagulants such as protein C, antithrombin and tissue factor pathway inhibitor (TFPI) are reduced in septic patients.

- The activation of pro-coagulant pathways and loss of anticoagulant pathways lead to a generalized prothrombotic state.
- This leads to the deposition of fibrin and microthrombi in microvascular beds and contributes to the dysregulation of tissue oxygen delivery and subsequent organ dysfunction.
- Coagulation factors and platelets are consumed, resulting in a consumptive coagulopathy and thrombocytopenia.
- This initially can lead to bleeding during an invasive procedure but may ultimately result in spontaneous bleeding. A haemostatic profile is therefore warranted prior to any planned invasive procedure on a septic patient.

The effects of sepsis on the coagulation system are termed **disseminated intravascular coagulation** (DIC). It is important to remember that DIC is a spectrum of abnormalities, and that the patient experiences transition from a hypercoagulable state to a hypocoagulable state during the course of the syndrome.

Cardiac dysfunction

Myocardial dysfunction has been documented in both septic people and dogs. Even during the hyperdynamic phase of septic shock with increased cardiac output, a decrease in ejection fraction has been documented. The decrease in ejection fraction is secondary to a reduction in ventricular compliance, biventricular dilatation and a decrease in contractile function. Myocardial dysfunction peaks within days of the onset of sepsis and typically resolves within 7–10 days in patients who survive.

Low cardiac output is rare in septic patients and is often due to end-stage decompensated myocardial depression. Myocardial depressant factor was thought to be the mediator responsible for sepsis-induced cardiac dysfunction, but it is now believed that a combination of various inflammatory mediators (interleukin (IL)-1, IL-6, TNF-α) is responsible.

Renal dysfunction

Acute renal failure (ARF) is a common sequel to sepsis in humans, but it does not appear to be as common in veterinary medicine. Renal tubular ischaemia secondary to systemic hypotension, afferent arteriole constriction, thromboembolic disease and damage by inflammatory cytokines and reactive oxygen species are thought to contribute to acute tubular necrosis. A decrease in GFR with subsequent elevation in plasma creatinine and urea follows. Urinalysis may reveal tubular casts as a result of the insult.

Pulmonary dysfunction

Systemic inflammation with leucocyte activation, cytokine production and increased vascular permeability can result in loss of normal surfactant and accumulation of protein-rich fluid within the alveoli. This is termed **acute lung injury** (ALI) or **acute respiratory distress syndrome** (ARDS), depending on the severity.

The underlying cause for ALI or ARDS can be sepsis or secondary to any insult that leads to SIRS. Diagnosis is based upon increased respiratory rate/effort, significant hypoxaemia (defined as P_aO_2/F_iO_2 of 200–300 for ALI, and P_aO_2/F_iO_2 of <200 for ARDS), bilateral pulmonary infiltrates on radiographs, evidence of a triggering insult and confirmation of a normal cardiac preload.

Intravenous crystalloids can result in worsening pulmonary oedema due to the decreased COP and increased capillary leak. Care should therefore be taken to avoid fluid overload in these patients. Cats appear to be especially sensitive to ALI/ARDS and are generally more intolerant of intravenous fluids.

Gastrointestinal effects
Hypotension, microthrombi and dysregulation of the regional blood flow can all lead to alterations in GI perfusion. Increased epithelial permeability secondary to the hypoperfusion can result in bacterial translocation into the lymphatics and blood stream. Hypoalbuminaemia can result in bowel oedema. GI signs such as vomiting, diarrhoea, haematochezia and ileus are common.

Hepatic dysfunction
Similar to GI effects, hepatic dysfunction can result from alterations in regional perfusion. Clinical signs can result from icterus, hypoalbuminaemia, hypoglycaemia, hepatic encephalopathy and coagulopathies.

Cardiogenic shock
Cardiogenic shock is inadequate cellular metabolism secondary to cardiac dysfunction when there is adequate intravascular volume. Systolic or diastolic cardiac dysfunction as well as arrhythmias can result in decreased stroke volume, failure of adequate forward flow of blood and cardiogenic shock.

In most cases, the physical examination and history can distinguish between cardiogenic and other causes of shock. On occasion, additional diagnostic tests such as radiography, echocardiography and electrocardiography will help to identify the type of shock. Differentiation from other forms of shock is important, because the patient with cardiogenic shock may not require fluid therapy.

In dogs, systolic dysfunction is most commonly caused by dilated cardiomyopathy and diastolic failure is a result of cardiac tamponade, hypertrophic cardiomyopathy or tachydysrhythmias. Although cardiogenic shock at first appears not to be important to the surgical patient, it must be remembered that surgical patients may have an underlying cardiac disease (e.g. Great Dane with GDV and underlying dilated cardiomyopathy), and many patients develop cardiac dysrhythmias during and following surgery (e.g. post-splenectomy).

Clinical recognition of shock, sepsis and SIRS

History
Diagnosis of shock can be made with physical examination findings alone. However, determining the underlying cause of shock is crucial to being able to direct the diagnostic evaluation and provide definitive therapy. Acquisition of a thorough history may provide the clinician with information to formulate differential diagnoses for the shock. For example, the top differential diagnosis for a dog in septic shock that had a jejunal enterotomy 72 hours previously would be enterotomy dehiscence and subsequent septic peritonitis.

Physical examination
An ability to recognize a patient in shock is an essential skill for any small animal veterinary surgeon (Figure 11.8). A thorough physical examination is crucial to the rapid identification of an animal in shock. The initial evaluation should focus on the cardiovascular system.

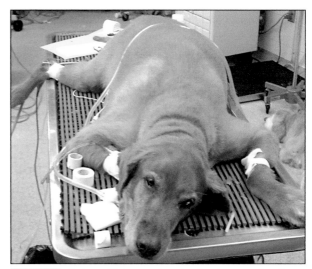

11.8 A dog with hypovolaemic shock secondary to a spontaneous haemoabdomen. The dog is severely depressed, tachycardic, has pale mucous membranes and weak pulses.

Mentation
An assessment of a patient's mentation should include level of consciousness and response to surroundings and manipulation. The brain is the last organ to experience a compromise in blood flow and changes in mentation therefore suggest a significant compromise to perfusion. Decreased mentation secondary to decreased tissue perfusion will resolve following correction of cerebral perfusion.

Mucous membranes
Normal mucous membrane colour is dependent on the presence of oxygen-carrying erythrocytes within the capillaries and a normal level of vasomotor tone. Pale mucous membranes may be secondary to an absolute decrease in red blood cells (anaemia) or peripheral vasoconstriction secondary to hypovolaemia, hypothermia, pain, stress, or various medications.

- A drop in arterial blood pressure secondary to hypovolaemia or sepsis will lead to a baroreceptor-mediated activation of the sympathetic nervous system.
- This will result in vasoconstriction of blood vessels to reduce blood flow to non-essential organs.
- The reduction in blood flow to the capillaries in the mucous membranes will result in membrane pallor.

Capillary refill time is the time it takes (in seconds) for blood to refill the capillary bed following application of digital pressure to the mucous membranes. Blood (and therefore the pink colour) returns in approximately 1–1.5 seconds in the healthy animal. Animals with increased vasomotor tone secondary to hypotension will have a prolonged capillary refill time.

A hyperdynamic state is seen in dogs with early SIRS (especially sepsis) as a result of vasodilatation and increased cardiac output. Mucous membranes are red and capillary refill time is rapid. This hyperdynamic phase is not seen in cats.

Heart rate
Dogs that are hypovolaemic are typically tachycardic with rates over 140 beats per minute. This is an *appropriate* compensatory response to maintain cardiac output in the face of a decreased stroke volume. The increase in heart rate occurs early in the course of the syndrome, and other perfusion parameters such as pulse quality and mucous membrane colour may still be normal. Other differential diagnoses for the tachycardia including pain, hypoxaemia and fever should also be considered.

Cats in septic shock will often have subnormal heart rates of 120–140 beats per minute. Bradycardia is an important presenting sign in cats and should prompt further investigation, including measurement of temperature and blood pressure and a search for the underlying cause.

Pulse
Palpation of peripheral pulse quality provides an assessment of the difference between systolic and diastolic pulse pressures (the height of the pulse wave) and the duration of the pulse waveform (the width). Arteries that are commonly used to assess pulse quality include the femoral, dorsal metatarsal/dorsal pedal, and radial arteries.

- Weak pulses have a decreased pulse pressure but normal width of the waveform, and are commonly identified in hypovolaemic patients.
- Bounding pulses have a large pulse pressure difference and wide waveform, and may be felt in hyperdynamic septic dogs that have increased cardiac output and vasodilatation.

Peripheral pulses should be palpated whilst auscultating the heart to detect pulse deficits.

Core *versus* extremity temperature
Subjective assessment of peripheral perfusion can be obtained by feeling the paws and ears and comparing the temperature with the animal's core. A discernible difference between core and extremity temperatures is consistent with peripheral vasoconstriction and shock.

Physical examination to determine underlying cause
Following evaluation of the cardiovascular system, the history and physical examination should be directed towards identifying the underlying cause of the shock/SIRS. Owners may report lethargy, depression, vomiting, diarrhoea or inappetence, depending on the underlying cause. Duration, progression and any prior treatment should be noted. Some causes of hypovolaemic shock such as trauma-induced blood loss may be evident just from the history.

Body temperature
Hypovolaemic and septic cats are commonly hypothermic. Dogs that are hyperthermic and in shock may be septic or have SIRS. The veterinary surgeon should begin to look for the inciting cause of the SIRS.

Assessment of hydration status
Dogs that have increased gastrointestinal losses and decreased oral intake will become increasingly dehydrated and eventually become hypovolaemic (see Chapter 10). These animals will present with signs of hypovolaemic shock *and* dehydration. However, an animal that has acute blood loss or is suffering from GDV (hypovolaemic or obstructive shock) will be hypovolaemic but *not* dehydrated. Not all hypovolaemic animals are dehydrated and not all dehydrated animals are hypovolaemic.

Loss of interstitial fluid leads to a loss of tissue pliability and lubrication. Dehydration can often be first detected on examination of the mucous membranes, though assessment may be confounded by nausea-induced hypersalivation.

- Physical examination findings may include depression, dry/tacky mucous membranes and a prolonged skin tent.
- Body condition score and age should be considered when assessing skin tenting. Subcutaneous fat provides greater lubrication than lean tissue and the amount of subcutaneous fat decreases with advancing age. As a result, the cranium and axillary region may provide more information about hydration status than the more commonly assessed scruff.
- When the eye of a normal cat is retropulsed, the nictitans immediately slips back into place following release of the eye. In a dehydrated cat the nictitans will stick to the globe and slowly slide back.

Abdominal palpation
A thorough examination of the abdomen should be performed.

- The presence of abdominal pain as well as the severity and localization of the pain should be determined. Pain may be:
  - Focal (e.g. intestinal foreign body)
  - Localized if limited to one organ (e.g. kidney pain)
  - Generalized if disease is widespread (e.g. peritonitis).
- The temperament of the dog and current use of analgesics should be considered. Stoic dogs may give a small reaction to abdominal palpation that would make other dogs yelp.
- Abdominal organs should be identified during palpation and the size and presence of any abnormality should be noted.
- The presence and size of the urinary bladder should be documented.
- Abdominal fluid may be suspected following abdominal ballotment.

Rectal examination
If physically possible, a rectal examination should be performed in all dogs.

- The prostate gland (in male dogs), sublumbar lymph nodes and urethra should be evaluated.
- Size, symmetry and presence/absence of pain on palpation of the prostate gland should be noted.
- The presence or absence of fresh blood or melaena should be documented.

Blood pressure

Patients in shock may be hypotensive. The patient may:

- Be hypovolaemic (hypovolaemic shock)
- Have inappropriate vasodilatation (distributive shock)
- Have impaired cardiac function (cardiogenic shock).

It is common for animals to have components of more than one type of shock (e.g. a dog with septic peritonitis may have a component of hypovolaemic and distributive shock). This may be suspected based upon clinical examination and confirmed by measuring arterial blood pressure, but correction of the hypovolaemic state should not be delayed by attempting to obtain a blood pressure measurement. A diagnosis of hypovolaemic shock should be made based on physical examination, with ancillary tests used to support the diagnosis, tailor therapy and monitor the response.

Blood pressure can be used as a surrogate marker of blood flow to tissues. However, intense vasoconstriction may result in *adequate* blood pressure but with minimal tissue flow. Similarly, different vascular beds may have differing blood flow at the same blood pressure. A mean arterial pressure of <70 mmHg or a systolic arterial pressure of <100 mmHg is considered hypotensive.

Blood pressure can be measured by both direct and indirect methods. Although more accurate, direct blood pressure monitoring is more invasive and more technically demanding. Typically, initial blood pressure is obtained using an indirect technique and an arterial catheter used for ongoing monitoring.

Indirect measurement

Indirect methods include Doppler and oscillometric techniques and rely on the inflation of a cuff to occlude arterial flow, followed by measurement of the pressure at which blood flow returns. Appropriate cuff size selection is important. To select the best cuff, the width of the cuff should be 40% of the circumference of the limb.

Indirect methods are cheap, widely available and can be performed quickly and easily following patient presentation. However, accuracy is limited in the severely vasoconstricted patient.

Direct measurement

Direct blood pressure monitoring using a catheter percutaenously placed into a peripheral artery is considered the gold standard technique.

- Catheterization of the dorsal metatarsal artery is most commonly performed.
- The catheter is connected to non-compliant heparinized saline-filled connection tubing and then to a pressure transducer.
- The pressure transducer converts the mechanical signals induced by pulsatile arterial pressure to electrical signals that are then recorded, quantitated, and displayed graphically.

Emergency database

An emergency database should be obtained in all animals that are in shock. This should include:

- Packed cell volume (PCV)
- Refractometric total solids (TS) or total protein (TP)
- Blood glucose (BG)
- Blood urea nitrogen (BUN)
- Evaluation of a blood smear.

Blood samples can be collected from the hub of an intravenous catheter at the time of placement. During catheter placement, blood can also be collected for additional laboratory tests (venous blood gas and electrolytes, serum biochemistry, complete blood count (CBC) and haemostatic profile). The PCV, TS, dipstick BG, dipstick BUN and blood smear can all be obtained from three heparinized microhaematocrit tubes.

PCV and TS

PCV and TS should be assessed together.

- PCV is used to determine if a patient is anaemic or polycythaemic.
- Refractometric TS allows estimation of serum proteins and a rough estimation of COP. TS is not reliable following the administration of synthetic colloids, since the TS measurement trends towards the TS of the administered colloid.
- An increase in both PCV and TS is consistent with dehydration.
- A decrease in PCV and TS is seen following haemorrhage or after aggressive fluid therapy.
- A decrease in both PCV and TS is not seen immediately following haemorrhage. Initially, TS decrease, due to fluid flux from the interstitium to the intravascular space, but PCV is maintained, due to splenic contraction in an attempt to improve oxygen delivering capacity. Therefore, if an animal is presented in shock and with a low TS yet normal PCV, haemorrhage is the likely diagnosis.
- Low TS may be seen with a normal PCV if there has been protein loss. This loss may be through the kidneys, GI tract or from the vasculature into a body cavity (third-spacing) secondary to inflammation (e.g. peritonitis).
- Normal TS with a low PCV is consistent with enhanced erythrocyte destruction.

Blood glucose

Hypoglycaemia is common in septic patients. If an animal is presented in shock and is hypoglycaemic, sepsis as an underlying cause for the shock needs to be ruled out. Other causes, such as an insulin-secreting tumour and hypoadrenocorticism, should also be considered.

Mild hyperglycaemia is commonly seen in cats following stress. It can also be seen in dogs following head trauma, seizures, and severe hypovolaemia or hypoxaemia.

BUN

BUN can be used as a screening test to identify azotaemic animals. A low dipstick value is accurate, but a high value should be confirmed with additional laboratory tests.

Blood smear evaluation

A blood smear should be performed in all patients in shock. It may aid in differentiating the type of shock, as well as the underlying cause.

- The erythrocytes, leucocytes and platelets should be evaluated, with attention paid to both number and cellular morphology.
  - In a patient with SIRS (septic or non-septic), a leucocytosis may be seen, typically with a left shift and toxic changes to the leucocytes.
  - Septic patients may also be leucopenic as a result of sequestration of the cells at the site of the infection (e.g. pyometra).
- Platelet count should be evaluated. It may be moderately decreased in bleeding or septic patients secondary to consumption, or severely decreased and be the cause of the hypovolaemic shock.

Acid–base and electrolyte status

Acid–base and electrolyte status (see Chapter 10) can be readily evaluated with point-of-care analysers and may aid in determining the cause of the shock.

- A patient in shock will have lactic acidosis secondary to the inadequate delivery of oxygen to tissues and a switch to anaerobic metabolism.
- Although the lactate concentration may give an indication of the severity of hypoperfusion, it should merely support the diagnosis of shock that was made from the physical examination.
- Lactate concentration has also been shown to be of prognostic relevance in dogs with GDV.

Complete blood count, serum biochemistry and haemostatic changes

CBC

Changes to the CBC will vary depending on the underlying cause of shock.

- The most common haematological abnormalities in sepsis include anaemia, leucocytosis (with left shift and toxic neutrophils) or leucopenia, and moderate thrombocytopenia.
- Blood loss, haemolysis and non-regeneration contribute to anaemia and are typically more significant in cats.
- The leucocytosis and left shift occur as a result of systemic inflammation.
- Leucopenia may result from cell sequestration.
- Thrombocytopenia may be present in septic patients as well as animals with hypovolaemic shock secondary to haemorrhage. In both cases thrombocytopenia will result from platelet consumption secondary to activation of the inflammatory and coagulation pathways.

Serum biochemistry

Changes to the serum biochemistry are often reflective of the underlying disease process.

- Animals with septic shock and hypovolaemic shock secondary to haemorrhage are hypoalbuminaemic, which in septic animals is often severe.
- Hyperbilirubinaemia is common in people and in dogs and cats with sepsis. In dogs it is thought to result from an endotoxin-induced defect in hepatocellular transportation of conjugated bile resulting in intrahepatic cholestasis, whereas in cats it is likely a result of haemolysis.

Haemostatic changes

As discussed above, coagulation pathways are activated in conjunction with systemic inflammation. This results in an early prothrombotic state that is not detected with conventional haemostatic profiles (activated partial thromboplastin time (aPTT) and prothrombin time (PT)), but can be detected using thromboelastography.

- Increased fibrin-degradation products (FDPs), D-dimers and decreased antithrombin concentration are consistent with this prothrombotic state.
- As DIC persists, platelet concentration decreases and the haemostatic parameters, aPTT and PT become prolonged as coagulation factors are depleted.

Diagnostic imaging

Although not necessary to diagnose shock or SIRS, radiography and ultrasonography are useful in identifying the underlying cause.

- Soft tissue and orthopaedic structures should be evaluated on radiographs.
- Organ structure and the presence/absence of fluid within a body cavity can be determined with ultrasonography.

Findings from these imaging studies should be interpreted with the history and findings of the physical examination to determine the underlying cause of the shock or SIRS.

Abdominocentesis

The abdomen is commonly the site of the underlying disease which has resulted in shock. If an abdominal effusion is suspected on physical examination or following further diagnostic tests, it is imperative that a sample be obtained for analysis (see Chapter 8). PCV and TS should be obtained from the fluid, as well as cytological evaluation and bacterial culture as necessary.

If abdominal disease is suspected yet no abdominal effusion has been obtained and diagnostic imaging studies have been unremarkable, diagnostic peritoneal lavage can be performed (see Chapter 8).

Bacterial culture

If infection is the suspected underlying condition behind the shock/SIRS, a bacterial culture should be obtained prior to antibiotic therapy. A culture should be taken of any fluid that is suspected of being infected (e.g. blood, urine, synovial fluid). Rapid diagnosis of sepsis followed by appropriate management is essential in maximizing patient survival.

Septic shock

Diagnosis of sepsis is made based on a strong clinical suspicion of infection supported by the combined presence of several of the signs of SIRS.

A source of infection must be rapidly identified so that source control and appropriate antimicrobial therapy can be instituted. When trying to identify a source, the search should initially focus on common sites of infection: lungs, urine, abdomen, wounds and catheters. Pyometra should always be considered in a bitch that has not had an ovariohysterectomy. The search should then move to less common infections, such as pyothorax, endocarditis, discospondylitis and osteomylelitis.

Therapy and monitoring response to therapy

Hypovolaemic shock

Normalization of haemodynamic status is essential to maintain adequate delivery of oxygen to tissues and prevent multiple organ dysfunction syndrome (MODS) and death. In the hypovolaemic patient this is achieved with the use of intravenous fluid therapy and efforts to stop ongoing loss of intravascular volume. In the case of haemorrhagic shock, prevention of ongoing loss of volume is achieved with haemostasis. This may be achieved with correction of a coagulopathy, surgical ex-ploration and ligation of vessels, or a combination of the two.

Haemodynamic support

Recognition of shock and rapid initiation of haemodynamic resuscitation is essential.

PRACTICAL TIP

There is no ideal fluid, no perfect protocol for administering fluids, and therapy should be tailored to each individual patient.

Isotonic crystalloids, hypertonic crystalloids, synthetic colloids and blood products are all therapeutic options that can be utilized in the hypovolaemic patient. Each option has its advantages and disadvantages, and there is no evidence to support one type of fluid over another (see Chapter 10). In practice, a combination of fluid types is often used to achieve haemodynamic stabilization.

When deciding which fluid to use, the clinician should take into consideration the patient's volume status, hydration status and ongoing fluid loss, as well as electrolyte concentration, COP, haemostatic profile and degree of anaemia.

Isotonic crystalloids: Isotonic crystalloids are the initial fluid choice in hypovolaemic patients. They will increase intravascular volume and replace interstitial deficits. A buffered isotonic crystalloid solution (e.g. lactated Ringer's solution) may be a more physiological resuscitation fluid than normal saline. The high concentration of chloride in 0.9% saline may contribute to an existing metabolic acidosis, but the use of 0.9% saline will restore tissue perfusion and is also compatible with blood and blood products.

- Mildly hypovolaemic dogs may only require isotonic crystalloids at 20–30 ml/kg, whereas a dog with evidence of severe hypoperfusion may require isotonic crystalloids at 70–90 ml/kg and the addition of colloids.
- Hypovolaemic cats may respond to a single bolus of an isotonic crystalloid solution at 10–20 ml/kg, or may require a repeated isotonic crystalloid bolus and the addition of a colloid.
- Isotonic crystalloid therapy may prolong coagulation by dilution, worsening of acidosis (if using 0.9% NaCl) and hypothermia (if using fluids at room temperature). This will be more of a problem in a patient with hypovolaemic shock secondary to haemorrhage. Ongoing blood loss leads to consumption of coagulation factors and platelets which is made worse by the fluid therapy.

Hypertonic crystalloids: Hypertonic saline (7.2–7.5% NaCl) can be administered to hypovolaemic patients (dogs: 4–6 ml/kg over 5–10 minutes; cats: 3–4 ml/kg over 5–10 minutes) to achieve a rapid increase in intravascular volume. Infusion of a hypertonic fluid results in a large osmotic gradient that draws water from the interstitial and intracellular fluid compartments and causes rapid expansion of intravascular volume. Uses include resuscitation of dogs with GDV and animals with head trauma.

- Hypertonic saline relies on interstitial fluid for its effect, and as such is not recommended in dehydrated animals.
- The rapid rise in blood pressure that can be attained with only a small volume of hypertonic saline can worsen bleeding. Caution should be exercised in the patient with ongoing haemorrhage.
- The effects of hypertonic saline are diminished within 30 minutes but can be prolonged with the addition of a synthetic colloid. A bolus of 4 ml/kg should be given over 5–10 minutes.

Colloids: Colloids are commonly administered to hypovolaemic patients to provide intravascular volume expansion once TS have decreased to <45 g/l. Options for synthetic colloids include hydroxyethyl starch, dextran and gelatine.

Resuscitation of a hypovolaemic patient typically starts with a 5 ml/kg bolus of a synthetic colloid administered over 15–30 minutes. This can be repeated as necessary, typically to a maximum dose of 20 ml/kg. In the cat, smaller volumes of 3–5 ml/kg should be used.

Synthetic colloids can contribute to a hypocoagulable state. Coagulation factors are diluted to a greater degree with colloids than with crystalloids, since colloids remain in the intravascular space longer. They also cause a reduction in factor VIII activity (greater than through dilution alone), a decrease in plasma levels of von Willebrand factor and inhibition of platelet function and fibrin polymerization. Because of this, limiting the use of synthetic colloids to 20 ml/kg/day is often recommended. If a hypovolaemic patient has received synthetic colloids, a haemostatic profile should be performed if there is a planned invasive procedure.

Blood products: Packed red blood cells (PRBCs) or whole blood may be needed in the bleeding hypovolaemic patient to aid in the restoration of normovolaemia, optimize oxygen-carrying capacity and thus blood oxygen content (Figure 11.9). However, the key is normalization of the intravascular volume; and blood products should not be given at the expense of volume expansion with crystalloids or colloids. Although no specific transfusion trigger exists, failure to achieve normal perfusion parameters following crystalloid and colloid therapy (e.g. persistent tachycardia) and/or an acute drop in haematocrit to <20% would be indications for the provision of PRBCs.

Fresh frozen plasma should be administered if there is prolongation of routine coagulation assays (aPTT and PT) and either there is evidence of clinical bleeding or prior to an invasive procedure. A dose of 10–20 ml/kg should be administered, followed by rechecking of the coagulation assays.

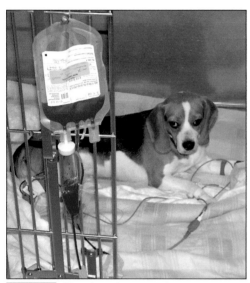

11.9 Blood products may be necessary to stabilize animals with haemorrhagic shock.

Fluid challenge technique: Fluid resuscitation should be performed using a fluid challenge technique.

- A bolus of isotonic crystalloid at 10–30 ml/kg or a synthetic colloid at 3–5 ml/kg should be administered over 15–30 minutes.
- Assessment of endpoints of resuscitation (see below) should be performed following each bolus.
- Fluid administration is continued as long as haemodynamic improvement continues.

Fluid challenges permit a large volume of fluid to be administered over a limited period of time under close monitoring to avoid the development of oedema. Since the patient is hypovolaemic and may have ongoing fluid losses, the volume of fluid administered is typically much greater than output during resuscitation.

Endpoints of resuscitation: Physical examination findings consistent with an improvement in perfusion status (Figure 11.10) and objective endpoints of resuscitation are listed in Figure 11.11.

In the hypotensive patient, fluids should be administered until the central venous pressure (CVP) is >8 mmHg (10.5 cmH$_2$O).

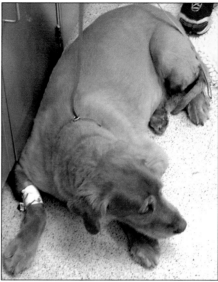

11.10 The dog in Figure 11.8 following fluid resuscitation with intravenous isotonic crystalloids. Mentation has improved, heart rate is normal, pulses are stronger and mucous membranes are pink.

Subjective
- Improved mentation.
- Pink mucous membranes.
- More rapid capillary refill time.
- Stronger pulses.
- Warmer extremities.

Objective
- Decreased heart rate.
- Increased arterial blood pressure.
- Increased urine output.
- Weight gain.
- Decreased blood lactate concentration.
- Increased mixed/central venous oxygen saturation.
- Central venous pressure and pulmonary artery occlusion pressure (can be used as safety endpoints to prevent administration of too much fluid).

11.11 Endpoints of resuscitation.

Hypotensive resuscitation: Hypotensive resuscitation is a technique that aims to reduce ongoing haemorrhage yet permit perfusion of vital organs. By limiting an increase in blood pressure, blood clots are not disrupted and excessive bleeding is reduced.

When performing hypotensive resuscitation, multiple small volumes of fluid should be given by bolus until a systolic pressure of 70–100 mmHg is achieved. Definitive haemostasis must be achieved rapidly by surgical exploration and/or correction of the coagulopathy. Following cessation of haemorrhage, patients should be resuscitated to traditional endpoints.

There have been no studies of hypotensive resuscitation in veterinary patients and the major indication in humans (penetrating trauma) is uncommon in small animals.

Septic shock

In veterinary medicine, the management of a patient with sepsis comprises haemodynamic support, infection control, metabolic support and supportive care (Figure 11.12).

Type of support	Treatment
Haemodynamic support	Fluid therapy Vasopressors
Infection control	Appropriate antimicrobial therapy Source control (removal of infected focus)
Metabolic/endocrine support	Tight glucose control Nutritional support ± Physiological dose of hydrocortisone
Supportive care	Blood products Analgesics Ulcer prophylaxis

11.12 Treatment of septic shock.

Haemodynamic support

Initiation of haemodynamic resuscitation should be instituted without delay. Normalization of cardiovascular function is essential to maintain adequate delivery of oxygen to tissues and prevent multiple organ dysfunction syndrome (MODS) and death. In human medicine it has been documented that early goal-directed resuscitation in patients with septic shock improved patient outcome compared with patients receiving standard treatment (Rivers *et al.*, 2001). This emphasizes the importance of prompt recognition of haemodynamic instability and rapid institution of therapy to attain predetermined endpoints of resuscitation.

Fluid therapy and administration of vasoactive agents are the key components in achieving haemodynamic stabilization. Fluid therapy should be immediately instituted in the septic patient. Crystalloids, synthetic colloids and blood products are all therapeutic options that can be utilized in the septic patient. There is no evidence to support one type of fluid over another and the considerations about which fluid(s) to use are the same as those described above for haemodynamic support of hypovolaemic shock.

Isotonic crystalloids: Isotonic crystalloids are often the initial fluid choice in septic patients. A buffered crystalloid is beneficial, since these animals will typically have lactic acidosis. Isotonic crystalloids will increase intravascular volume and replace interstitial deficits.

- In the healthy dog, only 25% of the isotonic crystalloid solution will remain in the intravascular space after 1 hour.
- In a septic animal with capillary leak and a low COP, even less fluid is likely to remain in the vasculature. As such, it is often not possible to achieve normovolaemia in the septic patient with intravenous crystalloids alone.
- In addition, the extravasated fluid results in oedematous tissues, which may further compromise organ function.

A combination of isotonic crystalloids and synthetic colloids is likely to be necessary for fluid resuscitation of septic patients.

Colloids: Colloids are commonly administered to septic patients to provide intravascular volume expansion and raise COP. Oncotic support can be achieved with both natural and synthetic colloids, with the main synthetic colloids being hydroxyethyl starch, dextran and gelatine.

As described above for hypovolaemic shock, synthetic colloids can contribute to a hypocoagulable state and therefore limiting the use of synthetic colloids to 20 ml/kg/day is often recommended. However, the benefit of colloid support to the septic patient may outweigh the risk of coagulopathy, and it is not uncommon for a postoperative animal with septic peritonitis and severe hypoalbuminaemia to require synthetic colloids at 2 ml/kg/h. In these cases it is prudent to check a haemostatic profile if there is clinical bleeding or if there is a planned invasive procedure. Correction of the coagulopathy with fresh frozen plasma is warranted.

Synthetic colloids are typically prescribed if a septic patient is hypotensive or is oedematous. When resuscitating a hypovolaemic patient, use of a synthetic colloid should be considered once the TS (by refractometry) are less than 45 g/l. Once physical examination findings are consistent with oedema formation, there is often concurrent organ oedema (with resultant organ dysfunction) in the liver, brain, kidneys and gastrointestinal tract. It is important not to wait for obvious signs of decreased oncotic pressure (such as peripheral oedema) before considering its correction.

- If a septic dog is hypotensive, a 5 ml/kg bolus of a synthetic colloid can be administered over 15–30 minutes. This can be repeated as necessary, typically to a maximum dose of 20 ml/kg.
- In the cat, smaller volumes of 3–5 ml/kg are used.
- If a patient has a severely decreased COP, a dose of 1–2 ml/kg/h can be used. The aim is not to return the COP to normal, but to reduce the clinical signs associated with a low COP.

Human serum albumin: Human serum albumin solutions have received much interest in veterinary medicine. Theoretically they have several benefits over synthetic colloids.

- A 5% solution has a COP of 20 mmHg whereas 25% human serum albumin has a COP of approximately 200 mmHg. This compares with hetastarch which has a COP of 33 mmHg.
- The increase in COP is due to the negative charge of albumin and resultant Gibbs–Donnan effect.
  - With a normal endothelial barrier, this increase in COP will oppose fluid exudation from the intravascular space.
  - With an abnormal 'leaky' microcirculatory barrier in conditions associated with vasculitis, such as sepsis or pancreatitis, albumin molecules may be able to traverse the endothelial barrier more easily than the larger particles found in synthetic polydisperse colloid solutions. The negative charge on the albumin may limit this transvascular flow.
- The administration of exogenous human serum albumin will provide a carrier protein for the transport of bilirubin and drugs, thus limiting their toxicity.
- Albumin is also believed to modulate inflammation, ischaemia reperfusion injury and coagulation.

It is known that human serum albumin solutions are not benign and carry considerable risk when administered to a healthy animal (Francis *et al.*, 2007).

Their effect on septic patients is not known and they may still offer some benefit in the dog with septic peritonitis and severe hypoalbuminaemia.

Fluid challenge technique and assessment of resuscitation: As described above for hypovolaemic shock, fluid resuscitation should be performed using a bolus of isotonic crystalloid at 10–30 ml/kg or a synthetic colloid at 3–5 ml/kg, administered over 15–30 minutes. Assessment of endpoints of resuscitation (see above) should be performed following each bolus and the fluid administration should be continued as long as haemodynamic improvement continues.

The fluid challenge technique permits a large volume of fluid to be administered over a limited period of time under close monitoring. With vasodilatation and ongoing capillary leak, many septic patients require continued aggressive administration during the first 24 hours of management. The volume of fluid administered is typically much greater than output during this time.

Animals in septic shock remain hypotensive despite appropriate fluid resuscitation. This is due to peripheral vasodilatation in addition to hypovolaemia. An assessment of *appropriate* fluid resuscitation can be made using a surrogate measure of cardiac preload. This can be achieved by CVP or pulmonary artery occlusion pressure (PAOP; also called pulmonary capillary wedge pressure). Although placement of a pulmonary arterial catheter is necessary for measurement of PAOP and is typically only performed in referral institutions, CVP can be easily measured using a water manometer.

Vasopressors

Vasopressor agents are commonly needed to maintain normal blood pressure in the septic patient (Figure 11.13). They should be started early, even before hypovolaemia has been fully corrected. However, vasopressors should not be used instead of appropriate fluid therapy and normovolaemia must be achieved.

Drug	Dosage
Dopamine	5–20 µg/kg/min i.v.
Noradrenaline	0.1–1.0 µg/kg/min i.v.
Adrenaline	0.005–0.1 µg/kg/min i.v.
ADH	0.5–2.0 IU/kg/min i.v. (dogs)
Dobutamine	5–20 µg/kg/min i.v. (dogs)

11.13 Dosages of vasopressors and positive inotropes.

Dopamine and noradrenaline are the initial vasopressors of choice, though there is no evidence in human medicine to support the use of one over another.

- The aim of administering vasopressors is to cause vasoconstriction and increase arterial blood pressure, but they may also result in excessive vasoconstriction, particularly of the splanchnic circulation. This may lead to gastrointestinal ischaemia and dysfunction. It is therefore important to utilize vasopressors at the lowest dose necessary to maintain arterial blood pressure, and ensure that the animal is normovolaemic.

- The use of vasopressors will also increase the work of the heart. This added workload in combination with septic-induced myocardial depression may require the use of a positive inotrope such as dobutamine.

Noradrenaline: Noradrenaline and dopamine are generally accepted as the first-choice drugs in both human and veterinary medicine. Noradrenaline is a catecholamine with potent alpha-adrenergic but little beta-adrenergic activity. It has pronounced vasoconstrictive effects on the blood vessels at typical doses of 0.1–0.3 µg/kg/min but, due to sepsis-induced vasoplegia, doses often have to be increased.

In a number of open-label trials, noradrenaline has been shown to increase the mean arterial pressure (MAP) in patients who remained hypotensive after fluid resuscitation and dopamine. Because of the intense arterial constriction, there has been concern regarding its effects on the kidneys. However, it has greater vasoconstrictive effects on the efferent than the afferent arteriole, and studies show that noradrenaline may actually optimize renal blood flow and renal vascular resistance. Studies are limited and conclusions on oxygen transport and splanchnic blood flow cannot be made at this time. Despite this, there is evidence to suggest that noradrenaline does improve cardiovascular function in most patients with severe septic shock.

Dopamine: Dopamine is the precursor of noradrenaline and adrenaline and is a transmitter in its own right in the brain and periphery. It has differing dose-dependent effects within the body, with considerable dose overlap.

- At low doses, dopamine stimulates DA_1 and DA_2 receptors and for a long time was used in the prevention of acute renal failure. Following the publication of a large placebo-controlled randomized trial and a meta-analysis of 58 studies, the Surviving Sepsis Guidelines recommend that low-dose dopamine should not be used for renal protection as part of the treatment of severe sepsis (Dellinger *et al.*, 2008).
- At doses of between 5 and 10 µg/kg/min, dopamine exerts predominantly beta-adrenergic effects with resultant positive inotropy and chronotropy. This results in an increase in cardiac output.
- The alpha-adrenergic effects of vasoconstriction (with resultant increase in systemic vascular resistance) occur at doses greater than 10 µg/kg/min, but there is considerable dose overlap, particularly with sepsis-induced vasoplegia.

Dopamine therefore increases the MAP by increasing cardiac output and/or systemic vascular resistance. The dose is often limited by tachyarrhythmias in dogs, which are typically responsive to a dose reduction.

Antidiuretic hormone: ADH is a hormone synthesized in the hypothalamus and released in response to a decrease in blood volume or an increase in plasma osmolality (blood volume takes precedence). Normal physiological concentrations of ADH have little effect on the MAP, but levels rise substantially with hypovolaemia and early septic shock.

- ADH causes vasoconstriction through V₁ receptors that are present on vascular smooth muscle.
- In addition to the direct vasoactive effects of ADH, it increases the responsiveness of the vasculature to catecholamines and inhibits nitric oxide production.
- Although there is a rise in ADH levels during early septic shock, this response soon becomes blunted and patients develop an inappropriately low concentration. This has been described as a *relative ADH deficiency*.

ADH has started to be used in veterinary medicine (Silverstein *et al.*, 2007) but should only be used if a septic patient has failed to respond to noradrenaline and/or dopamine.

Infection control

Antibiotics: Early and appropriate use of antibiotics is essential. All necessary samples for bacterial culture (e.g. blood, urine, abdominal effusion, pleural effusion, wound, fluid from endotracheal wash) should be obtained prior to administration of antibiotics, but there should be no delay in starting antibiotics if it is not possible to obtain all of the fluid samples immediately. Septic human patients who received antibiotics within 1 hour of documented hypotension had increased survival rates (Kumar *et al.*, 2006). It is now recommended that intravenous antibiotic therapy be administered as early as possible and within the first hour of recognition of septic shock.

Empirical therapeutic antibiotics should be started in a septic patient whilst waiting for the culture and sensitivity test results. In one veterinary retrospective study, dogs that did not receive appropriate antibiotic therapy for septic peritonitis had a decreased likelihood of survival compared with those who did receive appropriate empirical antibiotic therapy (Beal and Pashmakova, 2008).

The choice of initial intravenous therapeutic antibiotic should be made based on the likely infectious agent and the local patterns of susceptibility. For example, good choices for a septic abdomen include a second-generation cephalosporin, such as cefuroxime, or a combination of ampicillin and enrofloxacin. Metronidazole may also be given, in addition to other antimicrobials, if large intestinal contamination is suspected.

Changes can be made to the protocol following identification of the organism and the antimicrobial sensitivity.

Source control: Following identification of infection (Figure 11.14), the source should be removed or dealt with.

- If there is suspicion of a catheter-related blood stream infection (CRBSI), the catheter should be removed immediately.
- Wounds should be explored, debrided, lavaged and permitted to drain.
- Septic peritonitis and pyothorax are common causes of sepsis in small animals, and surgical exploration, removal of the septic focus, lavage of the cavity and placement of drainage catheters is essential.

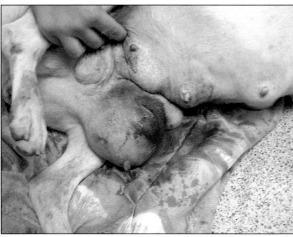

11.14 A source of infection in the septic patient should be readily identified and treated. In this example, mastitis has progressed to signs of septic shock.

- Surgical removal of the septic focus should be performed immediately following identification and patient resuscitation.
- Samples of infected fluid/tissue should be collected and submitted for bacteriological culture and antibiotic sensitivity testing.

Metabolic/endocrine support

Glucose control: Septic patients are commonly hypoglycaemic and will typically require dextrose supplementation.

- An intravenous bolus of dextrose at 0.5 g/kg can be administered over 5–10 minutes.
- Supplementation of maintenance fluids with 2.5% or 5% dextrose may then be necessary.

Despite the high incidence of hypoglycaemia in septic patients, avoidance of hyperglycaemia has also become increasingly appreciated in the critically ill patient. One study in a human cardiac surgical intensive care unit (ICU) demonstrated a reduction in mortality and length of hospitalization with intensive intravenous insulin to a target blood glucose level (van den Berghe *et al.*, 2001). Efforts should therefore be made to avoid both hypo- and hyperglycaemia in the septic patient.

Corticosteroids: High-dose corticosteroids were historically administered to patients with sepsis or septic shock, due to their anti-inflammatory effects and reports of an ability to stabilize membranes. Two large prospective studies and one large meta-analysis in human medicine concluded that high-dose corticosteroid therapy is ineffective or harmful in people with severe sepsis or septic shock. As a result, it is recommended that high-dose corticosteroid therapy is *not* prescribed to patients with severe sepsis or septic shock.

Intravenous corticosteroids are, however, recommended for adult septic shock patients after it has been confirmed that their blood pressure is poorly responsive to fluid resuscitation *and* vasopressor therapy. This is not the historical high dose but a more physiological dose for relative adrenal gland insufficiency associated with sepsis. There is no direct clinical evidence in veterinary medicine to support the use of low-dose steroid supplementation. The author has used intravenous hydrocortisone at 1 mg/kg every 6 hours, and continued until the patient has been weaned from vasopressor therapy.

Nutrition: Nutritional support is important in all critically ill animals. The approach to nutrition should be proactive in septic animals: 'waiting to see if a patient eats' is not acceptable practice.

Benefits of enteral over parenteral nutrition are well documented in people, but many septic patients will not tolerate enteral feeding. Use of the GI tract should be avoided in those patients that are hypotensive or require vasopressors; and total parenteral nutrition (TPN) should be prescribed. Enteral nutrition via a nasoenteric (oesophageal, gastric or jejunal) or surgically placed feeding tube should be considered in all septic patients that can tolerate enteral feeding, have no contraindication to the placement of a feeding tube and are not meeting their resting energy requirements (RER). Chapter 15 gives a detailed description of nutritional support in critically ill patients.

Supportive care

Analgesia: All septic patients should be assessed for their analgesic need. It is likely that these patients are in pain secondary to the inflammation, in addition to any surgical procedures that may have occurred. The effect of an analgesic on GI perfusion, renal perfusion, level of consciousness and GI tract should be considered prior to administration. For example, non-steroidal anti-inflammatory drugs (NSAIDs) compromise renal perfusion and can result in GI ulceration and as such should be avoided in septic patients. Analgesics are covered in more detail in Chapter 14.

Ulcer prophylaxis: Ulcer prophylaxis using an H_2 blocker (e.g. ranitidine) or proton pump inhibitor (e.g. pantoprazole) is recommended in people with severe sepsis to prevent upper GI bleeding. However, no study has looked at the use of ulcer prophylaxis specifically in people with severe sepsis, although trials have confirmed a benefit of reducing upper GI bleeds in general ICU populations. Despite a similar lack of evidence to support this recommendation in veterinary patients, ulcer prophylaxis is commonly instituted in septic animals.

Use of blood products in sepsis: Disorders of coagulation and fibrinolysis are common in septic patients. In addition, septic patients are hypoalbuminaemic. Unfortunately, fresh frozen plasma (FFP) is a poor source of albumin and large volumes have to be given to have any effect on plasma albumin concentration. In addition, FFP is known to have immunological effects and, as such, current recommendations state that the use of FFP in septic people should be limited to those in which there is active bleeding or a planned invasive procedure (Dellinger *et al.*, 2008).

Optimal transfusion triggers in septic patients remain unclear but are likely to vary between patients and for different disease processes. The decision to administer a blood transfusion should be made based on patient signalment, clinical signs, underlying disease and chronicity of the anaemia, not on a number.

The clinician should weigh up the benefits of providing an increased oxygen-carrying capacity against the known potential risks of transfusion.

Septic animals are likely to benefit from maintaining the haematocrit above 20%, with a higher haematocrit recommended prior to anaesthesia. It should also be remembered that anaemia is not tolerated as well in older or severely ill patients, particularly those with cardiac, respiratory or cerebrovascular disease.

Prognosis

Treatment of septic shock requires a combination of the above therapies tailored to the individual case. For example, haemodynamic support, infection control, metabolic care and supportive care are all essential in the postoperative cat with septic shock secondary to septic peritonitis (Figure 11.15).

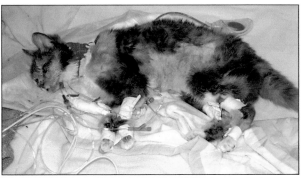

11.15 Haemodynamic support, infection control, metabolic care and supportive care are essential in this postoperative cat with septic shock secondary to septic peritonitis.

The prognosis of a patient in shock is dependent on the underlying cause and the response to therapy. An animal with hypovolaemic shock secondary to a GI obstruction that responds to intravenous crystalloid therapy has a much better prognosis than a dog with septic peritonitis and severe septic shock.

Prospective clinical trials of dogs and cats with shock do not exist. Quoted survival rates are based on outdated retrospective data and expert opinion, and do not reflect an accurate picture of veterinary critical care medicine in the 21st century.

- If an animal presents in hypovolaemic shock, responds to therapy and where a complete cure is possible, prognosis is good.
- If an animal has sepsis and the source is identified and treated without the patient developing septic shock, the prognosis is good.
- Patients in septic shock have a poor prognosis, and those that have septic shock and multiple organ failure have a guarded prognosis.

References and further reading

Beal MW and Pashmakova MB (2008) Empirical antibiotic therapy in canine septic peritonitis (2000–2007). *Journal of Veterinary Emergency and Critical Care* **18**, 409–431

Dellinger RP, Levy MM, Carlet JM *et al.* (2008) Surviving Sepsis Campaign: International guidelines for management of severe sepsis and septic shock: 2008. *Intensive Care Medicine* **34**, 17–60

Francis AH, Martin LG, Haldorson GJ *et al.* (2007) Adverse reactions suggestive of type III hypersensitivity in six healthy dogs given human albumin. *Journal of the American Veterinary Medical Association* **230**, 873–879

Hauptman JG, Wakshaw R and Olivier NB (1997) Evaluation of the sensitivity and specificity of diagnostic criteria for sepsis in dogs. *Veterinary Surgery* **26**, 394–397

Kumar A, Roberts D, Wood KE *et al.* (2006) Duration of hypotension before initiation of effective antimicrobial therapy is the critical determinant of survival in human septic shock. *Critical Care Medicine* **35**, 1589–1596

Rivers E, Nguyen B, Havstad S *et al.* (2001) Early goal-directed therapy in the treatment of severe sepsis and septic shock. *New England Journal of Medicine* **345**, 1368–1377

Silverstein DC, Waddell LS, Drobatz KJ *et al.* (2007) Vasopressin therapy in dogs with dopamine-resistant hypotension and vasodilatory shock. *Journal of Veterinary Emergency and Critical Care* **17**, 399–408

van den Berghe G, Wouters P, Weekers F *et al.* (2001) Intensive insulin therapy in critically ill patients. *New England Journal of Medicine* **345**, 1359–1367

The immune and inflammatory response to anaesthesia and surgery

12

Elizabeth Armitage-Chan and Stephen J. Baines

Introduction

It is assumed that, in immunocompetent patients, the immune response will allow a normal inflammatory response to tissue trauma. However, alterations in immune system function may be seen in the surgical patient, which can have an adverse effect on recovery in the postoperative period.

The main causes of alteration of the immune response are tissue injury, either intentional (e.g. surgery) or accidental (e.g. trauma), and haemorrhage. Although not commonplace in veterinary medicine, cardiopulmonary bypass also causes immunological aberrations by direct contact activation of the immune system following exposure of the blood to foreign surfaces, ischaemia reperfusion injury to vital organs and systemic endotoxaemia from gut translocation of endotoxins.

The effects of these stimuli are twofold: activation of the inflammatory response and depression of cell-mediated immunity, usually in that order. The function of the inflammatory response is to promote wound healing and prevent wound infection, and a normal balanced well controlled immune response results in an uneventful recovery. However, some patients (for instance, those with pre-existing diseases such as chronic respiratory disease, renal failure or diabetes mellitus) may be unable to mount an appropriate inflammatory response. Other patients develop an exaggerated or insufficient inflammatory response, resulting in increased morbidity. Increased morbidity and mortality in the surgical patient is most likely in animals with pre-existing immunosuppression or those already at risk of postoperative infection.

The immune response

The function of the immune system is to recognize pathogens and eradicate them from the host. The immune system is divided into an early innate and a later adaptive response.

- The first line of defence against invading microorganisms is the epithelial (epidermal or mucosal) barrier, augmented by antimicrobial enzymes and immunoglobulin A (IgA).

- Microorganisms that invade this barrier or that gain entry after traumatic disruption to this barrier, including surgery, are recognized by components of the innate immune system, leading to activation of immune cells, cytokine secretion, activation of the complement and coagulation cascades and secretion of acute-phase proteins and neuroendocrine mediators.

- Later, the adaptive immune response, which is concerned with antigen presentation and expansion of antigen-specific lymphocytes, is invoked, which leads to specific immunological memory for the pathogens, in the form of antibody-secreting plasma cells and cytotoxic T cells.

Elements of the immune response are set out in Figure 12.1.

Cytokines are molecules produced by cells involved in inflammation and immunity, which can affect their own growth and behaviour or that of other cell types. They include interleukins, interferons, tumour necrosis factor (TNF) and growth factors. They are messengers in the immune system and can be broadly divided into:

- Pro-inflammatory
- Anti-inflammatory.

Lymphocytes are white blood cells of the adaptive immune system that are responsible for specific immunity. Major types of lymphocyte are B cells and T cells.

- **B lymphocytes**, also known as **B cells**, play a large role in humoral immune responses and produce circulating antibodies.
- **T lymphocytes**, also known as **T cells**, are primarily responsible for cell-mediated immune responses.

T lymphocytes bear antigen-specific receptors on their cell surface to recognize foreign pathogens. They are also a major source of cytokines. There are two main T lymphocyte subsets: those that express CD4+ surface molecules and those that express CD8+ surface molecules (CD is the internationally recognized abbreviation for 'cluster of differentiation').

- CD4+ subset = **Helper T cells (Th)**.
- CD8+ subset = **Cytotoxic T cells (TC)** or cytotoxic T lymphocytes (CTL).

12.1 Some elements of the immune response. (continues) ▶

Helper T cells (Th) are the most prolific cytokine producers. They are T lymphocytes of the CD4+ subset that provide 'help' in the form of interleukins to other lymphocytes, allowing them to differentiate and perform their immune effector functions.

T helper cells can be divided into two polarized responses against pathogens:

- **Th1**-type cytokines tend to be ***pro-inflammatory*** – they produce inflammation to kill foreign pathogens and are effective against ***intracellular*** pathogens. The main Th1-type cytokine is interferon (IFN)-γ
- **Th2**-type cytokines tend to be ***anti-inflammatory*** – counteracting Th1 effects to some extent. They are effective against ***extracellular*** pathogens. The main Th2-type cytokines are interleukins (IL) -4, -5 and -13, associated with promotion of IgE, and IL-10.

Ideally, there should be a balance between Th1 and Th2 types within the body.

- **Interferons** have antiviral activity.
- **Interleukins** influence the differentiation of T lymphocytes or other cells, including division, activation and proliferation of B cells.
- **Immunoglobulins** are antibodies against specific antigens.

12.1 (continued) Some elements of the immune response.

Normal immune response to trauma and anaesthesia

Protective immunity critically depends on an adequate Th1/Th2 immune response, an intact monocyte/T-cell interaction and an appropriate cytokine response. The local inflammatory response includes chemotaxis and activation of immune cells, release of cytokines (such as IL-6 and TNF-α) and other inflammatory mediators, vasodilatation and increased vascular permeability.

Aberrant immune response to tissue trauma, haemorrhage and anaesthesia

The immune response to tissue injury may be influenced by:

- Severity of the tissue trauma
- Presence and severity of haemorrhage
- Presence of sepsis
- Gender.

As the extent of the trauma and tissue damage increases, the magnitude of this response increases and moves from a local to a systemic reaction, leading to generalized vasodilatation and vessel leakage. This is termed the **systemic inflammatory response syndrome** (SIRS) (see Chapter 11) and is responsible for organ failure and mortality after major trauma and surgery.

Conversely, in patients with a *suppressed* immune response, or a depleted immune system following prolonged illness, the outcome may be compromised organ function requiring exogenous support, known as **multiple organ dysfunction syndrome** (MODS).

Although the traditional view of SIRS involves a massive upregulation of the inflammatory response, a second compensatory anti-inflammatory response is now recognized that is equally damaging. Originally believed to be a modulator of the pro-inflammatory response, important in preventing the development of SIRS, this second wave of the immune response to surgery is believed to be *immunosuppressive*, increasing

the risk of postoperative and hospital-acquired infections and the development of sepsis. Markers of this response include activated regulatory T lymphocytes and increased levels of anti-inflammatory cytokines (such as IL-10 and IL-1 receptor antagonists), which lead to a state of immune paralysis and therefore inhibit the ability of the immune system to fight infection.

The determinants of whether the pro-inflammatory or anti-inflammatory arm of the immune response dominates after a major surgery are not fully understood. However, factors that almost certainly have modulatory influences that may augment or attenuate either the pro-inflammatory or anti-inflammatory pathway are listed in Figure 12.2. Some of these (e.g. surgery, general anaesthesia) cannot be avoided, while for others their potential deleterious effects are outweighed by the harmful effects of avoiding them (e.g. possible adverse effects of analgesics are negligible compared with the effects of pain; immune-suppressive effects of blood transfusions are less of a threat than those posed acutely by severe anaemia and hypovolaemia). By examining the immunological effects of these factors in more detail, it may be possible to alter the way in which patients are managed to improve the direction and magnitude of the postoperative immune response. This may have implications in the development of SIRS, organ failure, surgical site infections and sepsis after major surgery.

- Pain.
- Stress.
- Surgery.
- General anaesthesia.
- Analgesic agents.
- Haemorrhage.
- Blood transfusion.

12.2 Factors affecting inflammatory pathways.

Of particular importance are any interventions that may influence the pathway of the immune response in high-risk patients, such as those with pre-existing immune suppression or sepsis, those that have suffered major trauma, and those that are undergoing multiple or extensive surgeries.

Specific immune aberrations in the surgical patient

Cardiovascular responses after trauma and blood loss

Trauma and blood loss result in altered cardiac output and organ blood flow, with consequent decreased tissue perfusion and oxygen delivery. A reduction in vascular endothelium-derived nitric oxide leads to excessive vasoconstriction and compromised perfusion, increased microvascular permeability, increased platelet aggregation and increased neutrophil infiltration.

Macrophage function after tissue injury and haemorrhage

Depressed cell-mediated immunity is found immediately after trauma and haemorrhage. Macrophages secrete less IL-1, IL-6 and TNF-α in response to appropriate stimuli and this effect may persist for up to 7 days after trauma. The presence of a fracture induces a more prolonged response than soft tissue trauma alone (Wichmann *et al.*, 1996). This depression in macrophage function renders the patient more susceptible to postoperative infectious complications. Recovery of the pro-inflammatory, but not the anti-inflammatory, response is associated with survival from sepsis.

Antigen presentation may also be depressed in surgical patients as reduction in expression of major histocompatibility complex (MHC)-II and co-stimulatory molecules may be identified, which results in poorer stimulation of effector T cells. Recovery from sepsis is more likely and more rapid in those patients where this lesion is reversible.

Lymphocyte function after tissue injury and haemorrhage

Decreased lymphocyte function is found after tissue injury, both as a primary defect within the lymphocytes and as a result of reduced macrophage/T-cell interactions. Reduction in Th1 cytokines (e.g. IL-2, IFN-γ) and an increase in Th2 cytokines (e.g. IL-10) may also be seen.

Circulating inflammatory and anti-inflammatory mediators

Postoperative immune depression is associated with increased concentrations of various inflammatory cytokines, reflecting the presence of activated immunocompetent cells in the patient. In this respect, the depressed immune response seen in the surgical patient reflects hyporesponsiveness to a second stimulus after initial massive activation *in vivo*.

- Typically there is an elevation in pro-inflammatory cytokines (IL-1, IL-6, TNF-α).
- This is then modulated by:
  - The anti-inflammatory effects of IL-6
  - The secretion of IL-1 receptor antagonists and TNF receptors, which bind their respective cytokines
  - Secretion of the immune suppressants prostaglandin E_2 (PGE_2) and IL-10.

Measurement of the plasma cytokine concentration provides some insight into the presence and magnitude of the inflammatory response, but, since this is only one part of the immune response and since the plasma concentration may not reflect the concentration in other body compartments, this should be interpreted with caution.

Specific therapies directed at cytokine-mediated immune dysfunction, such as antibodies to IL-10, are being investigated, though no clear benefit has been noted to date.

Factors affecting the postoperative immune response

Patient-specific factors

The inherent immune competence of the patient and the presence of pre-existing disease may influence the response of an individual patient to a given level of tissue injury. One factor of note is the gender of the patient. Numerous studies have documented a gender-specific immune response after trauma and haemorrhage. In female animals, macrophage and lymphocyte-mediated immune responses tend to be maintained or even enhanced after tissue injury or trauma. This effect is mediated via sex hormones, such that male sex hormones tend to be immunosuppressive, whereas female sex hormones tend to be immunoprotective. The effect in females is more marked in pro-oestrus and the effects seen in both sexes are abolished by neutering.

Effect of surgery on the immune response

The magnitude of the response to surgery and trauma depends on the extent of the tissue damage. Non-invasive surgical techniques, for example laparoscopy and thoracoscopy, are therefore associated with a reduced inflammatory response, lower morbidity and a reduced risk of postoperative SIRS and infection, compared with open surgeries.

In addition, the number of surgical procedures, as well as the surgical trauma per procedure, has an effect. Patients undergoing multiple surgeries, or surgery following a traumatic injury, display a greater inflammatory response than those undergoing the same surgery as an isolated procedure. Known as the 'second hit phenomenon', this illustrates how an inflammatory response to tissue injury primes the immune system for a greater reaction to subsequent tissue damage. Evidence suggests that the response to the second injury is more likely to take the immune suppressive pathway, increasing the risk of infection and tumour metastasis.

This would suggest that the best method of managing patients with multiple injuries is to repair all the surgical lesions at once. However, surgical and total anaesthesia time also influence outcome, with longer procedures being associated with a poorer outcome, greater inflammatory complications and an increased risk of infection.

Since tissue injury and blood loss are major stimuli of an immune response after surgery, this underscores the importance of basic surgical principles in the prevention of an adverse immune response. It is important to adhere to Halsted's principles in order to minimize tissue trauma, prevent tissue ischaemia, minimize blood loss and prevent tissue contamination.

Effect of anaesthetic agents on the immune response

Although the severity and extent of surgical trauma has the greatest impact on the magnitude and nature of the postoperative inflammatory response, there is a large volume of literature devoted to the potential immunomodulatory effects of anaesthetic and analgesic agents.

Many pro-inflammatory and anti-inflammatory effects of anaesthetic and analgesic agents can be identified, particularly *in vitro*. However, it is important to emphasize that the clinical importance of these is often unknown, and is probably most relevant to critically ill patients that are at high risk of septic and inflammatory complications. In addition, in many cases it can be difficult to ascertain whether the observed changes are beneficial or detrimental. For example, if a given agent decreases inflammatory cytokine production, will this agent be of use in the prevention of SIRS, or will it have immunosuppressive effects and increase the risk of postoperative infections? Changes in clinical outcome are difficult to demonstrate, not least because it is hard to distinguish the relatively minor effects of anaesthesia from those of surgery. Despite this uncertainty, there is some evidence that certain anaesthetic and analgesic agents may have the ability to prevent an adverse inflammatory response to surgery and improve overall patient outcome.

Propofol

Propofol has been repeatedly associated, in people and in dogs, with an increased risk of surgical site infection (Heldmann *et al.*, 1999). Initially this was attributed to bacterial contamination caused by inappropriate handling of propofol vials (including failure to discard within 6 hours of opening), but more recently an immunomodulatory contribution has been proposed. The use of propofol has been shown to increase the release of anti-inflammatory cytokines and decrease release of pro-inflammatory mediators, inhibit lymphocyte proliferation and decrease neutrophil function, thus providing mechanistic evidence supporting an immunosuppressive role for this agent (Galley *et al.*, 2000). It is currently unclear whether this is a pharmacological function of propofol itself, or a property of the lipid solvent, the immunomodulatory effects of which have also been demonstrated.

Ketamine

Ketamine appears to have beneficial effects on immune function. Administration of ketamine has been associated with blunting of surgery- and endotoxaemia-associated increases in IL-6 and TNF-α in horses (Lankveld *et al.*, 2005), dogs (DeClue *et al.*, 2008) and people (Beilin *et al.*, 2007). These cytokines are known to be instrumental in the pathogenesis of SIRS, and high levels are a negative prognostic indicator in diseases associated with a systemic inflammatory response. Because of the subtle nature of this effect, improvements in clinical outcome will be difficult to demonstrate. However, in people at high risk of postoperative SIRS-associated cardiovascular derangement, administration of preoperative ketamine not only attenuated surgery-induced cytokine release, but also resulted in improved postoperative cardiac function (Bartoc *et al.*, 2006). Despite the anti-inflammatory effects demonstrated, there appears to be no evidence of an increase in postoperative infection risk, and thus incorporation of ketamine into anaesthetic protocols may be protective in patients at risk of inflammatory complications.

Local anaesthetics

There is widespread evidence for potent anti-inflammatory effects of local anaesthetics (Hollmann and Durieux, 2000). Intravenous infusions of lidocaine (1.5–3 mg/kg/h) are used frequently during general anaesthesia in endotoxaemic dogs and horses, not only to help reduce requirements for volatile anaesthetic agents, but also in an attempt to ameliorate the adverse inflammatory process in these patients. In cats, intravenous use of lidocaine produces unacceptable levels of cardiac depression and therefore this drug is not recommended in this species. Use of local anaesthetics during surgery attenuates surgery-induced increases in both pro-inflammatory and anti-inflammatory cytokines, while also improving postoperative pain management and intestinal function (Kuo *et al.*, 2006).

Isoflurane and sevoflurane

Although *in vitro* studies suggest that the exposure of inflammatory cells to volatile anaesthetics results in alterations in cytokine production and chemotaxis, there is little evidence that these agents have significant beneficial or detrimental immunomodulatory effects in clinical patients.

Opioids

Agonists at the mu opioid receptor (which include morphine, methadone, pethidine and fentanyl) are frequently selected in the anaesthetic management of critically ill patients, because of their minimal cardiovascular effects and volatile anaesthetic-sparing properties. They are therefore frequently used in high doses in patients at risk of septic and inflammatory complications. However, recent studies suggest that anaesthetic protocols based on high doses of opioids result in an impaired cell-mediated immune response (particularly decreases in natural killer cell activity and phagocytosis of pathogens). High doses of fentanyl appear to have particularly pronounced effects (Yardeni *et al.*, 2008).

Effect of postoperative analgesia on the immune response

Since opioids appear, at least experimentally, to have detrimental effects on the immune response following surgery, possibly leading to increased surgical infection risk, it is pertinent to explore other options, but bearing in mind the following:

- Opioids are the most potent analgesics available and they have many advantages over other analgesic agents in the postoperative patient (for example, compared with the nephrotoxic and ulcerogenic effects of non-steroidal anti-inflammatory agents (NSAIDs) in high-risk patients, and the profound cardiovascular effects of alpha-2 agonists)
- Not only is it unethical to withhold analgesics from patients after surgery, but pain and distress during this period lead to increased levels of stress hormones, which themselves suppress the immune response and increase the risk of postoperative infection
- Pain has its own immunomodulatory effects, which most likely outweigh those incited by opioid administration. Nonetheless, if alternative analgesic agents with more favourable inflammatory effects (such as ketamine and local anaesthetics) can be incorporated into a multimodal analgesic regimen, resulting in reduced opioid requirements and improved pain management, this may have the additional advantage of reducing the detrimental immunological effects associated with high-dose opioid use.

An alternative strategy for reducing the immunological response to opioid administration is to administer the opioid agent via a local or regional route, instead of systemically. As with multimodal analgesic techniques, this has the dual advantages of decreasing the total dose of opioid administered and reducing postoperative pain. In addition, by administering the opioid at a peripheral site, the receptors responsible for immunological effects (thought to be in the brain) are not activated. When compared with systemic use, epidural administration of opioids has repeatedly been associated with a less pathological inflammatory response (Beilin *et al.*, 2003; Ahlers *et al.*, 2008). The inflammatory response to surgery is attenuated when opioids are administered in this way, including blunting of cortisol and adrenaline responses and prevention of surgery-induced depression of T cell function. This route of administration therefore has great potential in reducing postoperative immunosuppression and surgical infection rates.

With all these studies, it is difficult to ascertain whether the improvements observed are the result of reduced systemic opioid administration or caused by improved pain management, as invariably pain scores are better in patients receiving multimodal or epidural-based analgesia. The inclusion of a local anaesthetic with epidural opioids confers additional benefits, although again this could be explained by improvements in pain management, reductions in systemic opioid requirements, or by the direct effect of the local anaesthetic agent. Whatever the underlying physiology of this response, the evidence for the benefits of epidural and (to a lesser extent) multimodal analgesia are amongst the most conclusive when examining ways of positively manipulating the immune response to surgery.

Effect of perioperative immune dysfunction on the surgical patient

In contrast to the large number of publications reporting alterations in immune cell function caused by surgery and anaesthesia, there are very few data describing changes in patient outcome. This reflects the complexity of the pathogenesis of postoperative infection, sepsis and SIRS, and the outcome for such patients is determined by many factors. In spite of these challenges, there is emerging evidence not only for the importance of the direction of the immune response in determining outcome, but also for the potential for alterations in patient management to have a direct impact on survival.

The state of immune paralysis is a direct contributor to postoperative infection and tumour metastasis, and there is much interest in modulating this response to prevent postoperative immunosuppression (Hotchkiss *et al.*, 2009). Ketamine has been shown to decrease mortality in experimental models of sepsis, an effect attributed to its immunomodulatory properties (Taniguchi *et al.*, 2003). During the pro-inflammatory response to surgery and sepsis, IL-6 elevations are correlated with increased disease severity and mortality in people (Mokart *et al.*, 2002), dogs (Rau *et al.*, 2007) and horses (Barton and Collatos, 1999), and it is therefore probable that interventions that reduce the IL-6 response to surgery (such as administration of ketamine and use of local anaesthetics) will have beneficial effects on patient outcome. Improving analgesia, by administering systemic or epidural morphine prior to surgery, has been shown to decrease tumour metastasis in various

models of abdominal neoplasia (Page *et al.*, 1998; Wada *et al.*, 2007), and this represents an important focus for the improved outcome of critically ill patients.

Minimizing immune dysfunction following anaesthesia and surgery

Changes in patient management to reduce the impact of a dysfunctional immune response may confer benefits in those patients at greatest risk of sepsis, SIRS, postoperative infection and tumour metastasis. A summary of the strategies that may reduce the impact of the inflammatory response on post-surgical outcome is given below.

Identifying patients at risk

Identification of patients at risk of an adverse immune response in the postoperative period is essential if interventions designed to ameliorate this response are to have an effect on overall outcome. Risk factors are listed in Figure 12.3.

- Immunosuppressive drugs.
- Immunosuppression from malnutrition or chronic disease.
- Cancer.
- Severe trauma.
- Invasive surgery.

12.3 Risk factors used to identify those patients in danger of experiencing an adverse immune response in the postoperative period.

Recommendations for anaesthetic management

Recommendations for reducing the adverse effects of surgery and anaesthesia on the immune response, while limiting any potential adverse effects of the anaesthetic and analgesic agents themselves, are listed in Figure 12.4.

- Use effective pre-medication.
- Maintain normothermia.
- Use a high FiO_2 (fraction of inspired oxygen).
- Maintain tissue oxygenation.
- Treat hyperglycaemia.
- Consider epidural analgesia.
- Treat postoperative pain effectively.
- Use NSAIDs when possible.

12.4 Recommendations for reducing the adverse effects of surgery and anaesthesia on the immune response.

Immunomodulation as a therapeutic option

Immunomodulatory strategies usually aim to block an overwhelming inflammatory response. This strategy risks impairing host defences in animals already at risk of infection; hence a more rational course of action is to modulate the immune response more specifically. The following drugs are currently being investigated for their ability to modulate the immune reponse.

Granulocyte colony-stimulating factor

The administration of granulocyte colony-stimulating factor (G-CSF), which stimulates the release of new monocytes, ameliorates some of the detrimental immune responses by preventing monocyte deactivation, conserving the Th1/Th2 ratio and alleviating some of the acute-phase response.

Corticosteroids

Corticosteroids are strong immune suppressants and can reduce the secretion of inflammatory cytokines. However, their various side effects, such as impaired wound healing, increased risk of postoperative infection and metabolic consequences (e.g. hyperglycaemia), outweigh any potential clinical benefit.

Aprotinin

Aprotinin, an inhibitor of serine proteases (e.g. trypsin, chymotrypsin, kallikrein), suppresses the release of IL-8, activates both coagulation and fibrinolysis and results in a better recovery from tissue ischaemia. Formal trials are needed to assess the usefulness of this drug.

Pentoxifylline

Pentoxifylline, a phosphodiesterase inhibitor, is a vasodilator with positive inotropic and bronchodilator activities. It also improves blood rheology and has an immunomodulatory action, with reductions in IL-6, IL-8 and IL-10 secretion.

Steroid hormones

The relatively depressed immune responses seen in males may be improved by administration of exogenous oestrogens. Dehydroepiandrosterone, which has oestrogenic effects but lacks the prothrombotic effects of oestradiol, is a known long-term immune-enhancing drug in humans and might provide useful therapy for immune depression in surgical patients.

The relative immune depression seen in male animals is abolished by castration, but may be recapitulated by administration of exogenous testosterone. Flutamide, an androgen-receptor blocker, is associated with improved survival in experimental models of sepsis after haemorrhage.

Other immunomodulatory strategies

Immuno-enhancing diets and the use of hypertonic saline in resuscitation may also be strategies to reduce the rate of septic complications in surgical patients.

Conclusion

The inflammatory response to anaesthetized (e.g. surgery) or non-anaesthetized (e.g. trauma) injury is a predictable and well orchestrated adaptive set of events that have evolved to optimize the healing potential of an organism. A normal, balanced, well controlled inflammatory response in previously healthy patients usually results in an uneventful recovery, but the development of an exaggerated or insufficient response may lead to SIRS and MODS, respectively. The surgeon should be aware of this phenomenon, be able to recognize patients at risk of these events and do whatever possible to avoid, or enhance the triggers of, this aberrant immune response.

References and further reading

Ahlers O, Nachtigall I, Lenze J *et al.* (2008) Intraoperative thoracic epidural anaesthesia attenuates stress-induced immunosuppression in patients undergoing major abdominal surgery. *British Journal of Anaesthesia* **101**, 781–787

Angele MK and Chaudry IH (2005) Surgical trauma and immunosuppression: pathophysiology and potential immunomodulatory approaches. *Langenbecks Archives of Surgery* **390**, 333–341

Angele MK and Faist E (2002) Immunodepression in the surgical patient and increased susceptibility to infection. *Critical Care* **6**, 298–305

Bartoc C, Frumento RJ, Jalbout M *et al.* (2006) A randomized, double-blind, placebo-controlled study assessing the anti-inflammatory effects of ketamine in cardiac surgical patients. *Journal of Cardiothoracic and Vascular Anesthesia* **20**, 217–222

Barton MH and Collatos C (1999) Tumor necrosis factor and interleukin-6 activity and endotoxin concentration in peritoneal fluid and blood of horses with acute abdominal disease. *Journal of Veterinary Internal Medicine* **13**, 457–464

Beilin B, Rusabrov Y, Shapira Y *et al.* (2007) Low-dose ketamine affects immune responses in humans during the early postoperative period. *British Journal of Anaesthesia* **99**, 522–527

Beilin B, Shavit Y, Trabekin E *et al.* (2003) The effects of postoperative pain management on immune response to surgery. *Anesthesia and Analgesia* **97**, 822–827

DeClue AE, Cohn LA, Lechner ES, Bryan ME and Dodam JR. (2008) Effects of subanesthetic doses of ketamine on hemodynamic and immunologic variables in dogs with experimentally induced endotoxemia. *American Journal of Veterinary Research* **69**, 228–232

Galley HF, Dimatteo MA and Webster NR (2000) Immunomodulation by anaesthetic, sedative and analgesic agents: Does it matter? *Intensive Care Medicine* **26**, 267–274

Heldmann E, Brown D and Shofer F (1999) The association of propofol usage with postoperative wound infection rate in clean wounds: a retrospective study. *Veterinary Surgery* **28**, 256–259

Hollmann M and Durieux ME (2000) Local anesthetics and the inflammatory response: A new therapeutic indication? *Anesthesiology* **93**, 858–875

Hotchkiss RS, Coopersmith CM, McDunn JE and Ferguson TA (2009) The sepsis seesaw: tilting towards immunosuppression. *Natural Medicine* **15**, 496–497

Kohl BA and Deutschmann CS (2006) The inflammatory response to surgery and trauma. *Current Opinion in Critical Care* **12**, 325–332

Kuo CP, Jao SW, Chen KM *et al.* (2006) Comparison of the effects of thoracic epidural analgesia and i.v. infusion with lidocaine on cytokine response, postoperative pain and bowel function in patients undergoing colonic surgery. *British Journal of Anaesthesia* **97**, 640–646

Lankveld DP, Bull S, Van Dijk P, Fink-Gremmels J and Hellebrekers LJ (2005) Ketamine inhibits LPS-induced tumour necrosis factor-alpha and interleukin-6 in an equine macrophage cell line. *Veterinary Research* **36**, 257–262

Lenz A, Franklin GA and Cheadle WG (2007) Systemic inflammation after trauma. *Injury* **38**, 1336–1345

Lin E, Calvano SE and Lowry SF (2000) Inflammatory cytokines and cell response in surgery. *Surgery* **127**, 117–126

Mayers I and Johnson D (1998) The non-specific inflammatory response to injury. *Canadian Journal of Anaesthesia* **45**, 871–879

Page GG, McDonald JS and Ben-Eliyahu S (1998) Preoperative versus postoperative administration of morphine: impact on the neuroendocrine, behavioural and metastatic-enhancing effects of surgery. *British Journal of Anaesthesia* **81**, 216–223

Rau S, Kohn B, Richter C *et al.* (2007) Plasma interleukin-6 response is predictive for severity and mortality in canine systemic inflammatory response syndrome and sepsis. *Veterinary Clinical Pathology* **36**, 253–260

Taniguchi T, Takemoto Y, Kanakura H, Kidani Y and Yamamoto K (2003) The dose-related effects of ketamine on mortality and cytokine responses to endotoxin-induced shock in rats. *Anesthesia and Analgesia* **97**, 1769–1772

Wada H, Seki S, Takahashi T *et al.* (2007) Combined spinal and general anesthesia attenuates liver metastasis by preserving TH1/TH2 cytokine balance. *Anesthesiology* **106**, 499–506

Wichmann MW, Zellweger R, Williams C *et al.* (1996) Immune function is more compromised following closed bone fracture and haemorrhagic shock than haemorrhage alone. *Archives of Surgery* **131**, 995–1000

Yardeni IZ, Beilin B, Mayburd E, Alcalay Y and Bessler H (2008) Relationship between fentanyl dosage and immune function in the postoperative period. *Journal of Opioid Management* **4**, 27–33

Postoperative management

Arthur House and Robert Goggs

Introduction

The goals of the immediate postoperative period are to:

- Recover the patient from anaesthesia
- Prevent and manage postoperative complications
- Provide ongoing treatment for pre-existing disease
- Identify new problems rapidly and treat them appropriately
- Support the patient's physiology effectively, promoting rapid recovery
- Ensure patient welfare.

To achieve these goals, close patient monitoring and regular assessment are required to alert the clinician to changing patient needs and permit timely intervention. The completion of a surgical procedure never constitutes the conclusion of a patient's veterinary care.

Repeated physical examination

The aims of the physical examination are to:

- Identify major body system abnormalities
- Assess the other body systems (particularly those known to be abnormal or those directly affected by surgery)
- Review the appearance of all surgical wounds
- Monitor for the occurrence of post-surgical complications.

In the postoperative patient, a full physical examination should be conducted by the surgeon at least twice daily, though the frequency of assessment should be tailored to the individual patient's needs. A single 'snapshot' assessment of a patient provides limited insight into postoperative progress. Repeated physical examination ensures that significant alterations in patient status are rapidly identified and permits evaluation of response to therapy.

Following completion of the physical examination, the patient's medical record should be thoroughly reviewed to put the physical examination findings in context and permit a better interpretation of any changes in patient status. The first physical examination of the day should be performed before daily treatment orders are written, to allow adjustment of ongoing fluid therapy or analgesic plans.

If the veterinary surgeon cannot examine the patient with the desired frequency, other members of staff must be able to assess patients with clear written guidance regarding when to contact the clinician or initiate interventions. This is best accomplished by a well designed medical record that specifies assessment parameters and sets limits for clinician notification or therapeutic intervention (Figure 13.1).

Physical examination should begin with assessment of the major body systems: cardiovascular, respiratory and neurological. The primary cause of death in the postoperative period is failure of these systems and they should therefore receive particular attention. Any clinically important anomalies (particularly novel) in these systems should be investigated and treatment initiated prior to completion of the remainder of the physical examination.

Cardiovascular system

Reliable assessment of cardiovascular function cannot be based on a single parameter but should include evaluation of:

- Heart rate and rhythm
- Pulse rate, rhythm character and synchronicity
- Mucous membrane colour
- Capillary refill time.

Descriptions of pulse quality such as 'thready' or 'poor' should be avoided, since their meaning is not universal. It is preferable to describe the pulse trace palpated using descriptors such as normal, tall and narrow, or short and narrow (Figure 13.2a). A useful rule-of-thumb is that metatarsal artery pulses typically become undetectable when mean arterial blood pressure falls below 60mmHg.

Shock

Detection of inadequate tissue perfusion (shock) is a primary concern. Shock is best defined as inadequate cellular energy generation, most commonly due to inadequate tissue oxygen delivery (see Chapter 11). In dogs, the onset of shock follows a similar pattern regardless of the inciting cause.

RVC
Queen Mother Hospital for Animals
Royal Veterinary College

✳ DEA 1.1 POSITIVE ✳
ICU Treatment Sheet

Label		

PROBLEM LIST

RTA 14/04
PNEUMOTHORAX / SUB-CUTANEOUS EMPHYSEMA
RIB FRACTURES (L) / PULM. CONTUSIONS
L FEMORAL FRACTURE
— REPAIRED 18/04
DEGLOVING INJURY DISTAL L HL
— WET-TO-DRY DRESSINGS PLACED
R MILA CHEST DRAIN PLACED 17/04
O' TUBE PLACED 17/04
PRBC TRANSFUSION 17/04

Date: 19/04/09   Weight: am 24.9 kg pm:

Clinician: ARTHUR HOUSE   Signature: _Hou_

Clinician tel: ▓▓▓   Bleep: 17

Student:

P

Catheter site R JUG / R CEPH	Date placed 17/04 / 18/04
Checked ☑ KH ☑ KH	Code status R (DNR)

DAILY ORDERS

GA REDRESS WOUNDS   1100 ☑

✱ NOTIFY CLINICIAN IF CHEST ✱
DRAIN AIR VOL > 10 ml/kg
DURING ANY 4HR PERIOD

Ṽ VISIT
1500 ☑

DIAGNOSTIC TESTS

CBC ☑

CHEST FLUID CYTOLOGY
— IN HOUSE ☑

Weight 6am | **24.6** kg |

	6	7	8	9	10	11	12	13	14	15	16	17	18	19	20	21	22	23	0	1	2	3	4	5	6	7	8
MM / CRT / PULSES / HR Q6h					/				✓	✓							✓						✓	✓		✓	
RR / EFFORT Q4h					/				✓			✓					✓				✓				✓		
Temp Q12h					/												✓										
PCV / TS Q12h					/												✓										
Nova Q12h					/												✓										
CSL 2ml/kg/hr CRI																											▷
MLK CRI (see protocol in file) 25ml/hr																											▷
DRAIN R CHEST DRAIN Q4h					/				✓			✓					✓				✓				✓		
DRAIN URINE BAG & RECORD UOP/USG Q4h					/				✓			✓					✓				✓				✓		
ROPIVACAINE 1.5mg/kg IP Q8h					/							✓					✓				✓						
CO-AMOXY-CLAV 20mg/kg Q8h					/							✓					✓				✓						
NIBP Q6h					/				✓								✓						✓				
O' TUBE FEEDING (see protocol in file)	✕	✕	✕	✕					✓								✓						✓				
TURN Q4h					R				L			S					R				L				S		
~~Walk / Carry / Hoist / Trolley~~ check bed																											
Food OFFER IN ADDITION TO O'TUBE PROTOCOL	✕	✕	✕						✕NI								✓50%						✓25%				
Water AD LIB																											➤
Notify >		150	50														2.5	200									
Notify <							20							4.0								0.5ml/kg/h		70				

TIME	T	P	R	MM	CRT	PCV	TS	Na	K	BG	Lac	Creat	UOP	MAP
10.15	38.1	110	32			26	54	145.2	3.62	6.58	0.7	122	0.7	90
1400			28										2.2	
16:00		100	28											86
18:20			34										1.0	
22:00	38.3	115	30			24	52	147.3	3.65	5.54	0.5	127	1.9	94
0210			26										0.9	
04:00		130	30											77
0615			28										0.4	

M080795

a

13.1   **(a)** A detailed complete intensive care unit sheet from a patient's medical record. Note the extensive problem list, list of therapeutic procedures with scheduled administration times and the use of clinician notification parameters towards the bottom of the sheet. (continues) ▶

b

Time	CVP	OSCILL ~~DOPPLER~~ NIBP	RH Cuff Size	~~IBP~~
10:00		131/69 (90)	3	
16:20		119/70 (86)	3	
22:10		100/68 (74)	3	
0405		127/81 = 95	3	

URINE OUTPUT

Time	Volume (ml)	SG	Total	ml/kg/hr
10:15	68	1·015	68	0·68
14:05	220	1·019	288	2·21
1820	102	1·022	390	1·02
22:00	185	1·020	575	1·86
0210	89	1·014	664	0·39
0605	40	1·037	704	0·40

LEFT   CHEST   ASPIRATES

TIME	DESCRIPTION	FLUID (ml)	AIR (ml)	Total ml/kg/hr
TOTAL				

RIGHT   CHEST   ASPIRATES

TIME	DESCRIPTION	FLUID (ml)	AIR (ml)	Total ml/kg/hr
10:00	serosang.	2	10	
14:00	"	2	53	
18:15	serosang	10	45	
22:00	"	5	60	
0205	—	0	10	
0600	—	0	61	
TOTAL				

URINALYSIS

Glucose:	1+		
Bilirubin:	—		
Ketones:	—		
Blood:	1+		
pH:	6		
Protein:	1+		
SG:	1·015		
Sediment:			

Time	Food Intake	Food Type	Water Intake	Urination	Defaecation

13.1 (continued) **(b)** The sheet should also facilitate recording of all 'ins and outs', i.e. urine output, faecal production and drain effusion volumes.

- In early shock, sympathetic nervous system stimulation permits compensation via increases in heart rate and peripheral vascular tone. Consequently physical examination findings in this phase are characterized by tachycardia, tall and narrow pulses and a brisk capillary refill time.
- With the progression of shock, the physical examination findings deteriorate to persistent tachycardia and reductions in pulse pressure amplitude.
- With further deterioration, inappropriate bradycardia may occur accompanied by short and narrow pulses, pale or grey mucous membranes and a sluggish capillary refill time.
- With improving cardiovascular function (in response to therapy) a reversal of the trend shown in Figure 13.2b should be appreciated.

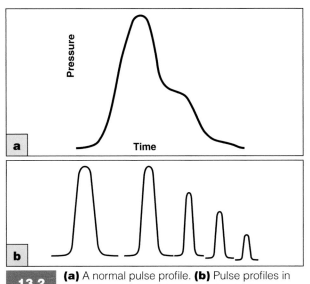

13.2 **(a)** A normal pulse profile. **(b)** Pulse profiles in hypovolaemia. In early shock, physical examination findings are characterized by tachycardia, tall and narrow pulses and a brisk capillary refill time. With clinical deterioration, inappropriate bradycardia may occur accompanied by short and narrow pulses, pale or grey mucous membranes and a sluggish capillary refill time.

In the cat, the initial tachycardic response may not be present and some feline patients in shock only demonstrate inappropriate bradycardia.

If progressive deterioration in cardiovascular function is recognized, identifying the inciting cause is critical. Since postoperative haemorrhage and infection are universal complications, these two possibilities must be considered first. The surgical wound should be evaluated. Shock in patients following body cavity surgery necessitates assessment of these areas by auscultation or palpation, combined with diagnostic imaging if necessary.

Respiratory system
Monitoring respiratory function is based on the assessment of multiple parameters, including:

- Respiratory rate and effort
- Breathing pattern
- Patient posture
- Assessment of chest wall compliance
- Thoracic auscultation.

Initial observations of rate, effort and pattern should be made from a distance prior to handling. Regularly checking resting respiratory rate can be a sensitive tool for detecting deterioration in pulmonary function. With progressive loss of respiratory function, subtle increases in respiratory rate and effort can progress to the patient recruiting extrathoracic muscles to augment ventilation. These include:

- The scalene and sternomastoid muscles of the neck increasing the craniocaudal thoracic dimension
- The alae nasae dilating the external nares
- The muscles of the abdominal wall contracting during active expiration.

Clinicians may observe flared nostrils and abdominal effort in such patients. In dogs, this is often combined with an orthopnoeic stance as well as elbow abduction and neck extension, designed to minimize the work of breathing. In feline patients, severe respiratory distress typically manifests as open-mouth breathing and recumbency (Figure 13.3). Such patients should be considered critical and at risk of a respiratory arrest.

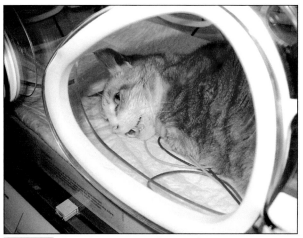

13.3 A cat in severe respiratory distress demonstrating characteristic open-mouth breathing and anxiety. The patient is in a paediatric incubator being monitored with telemetric ECG. Oxygen is being supplemented via tubing visible in the background. (Courtesy of H Wilson)

PRACTICAL TIP

If increased respiratory effort is observed, attempts should be made to differentiate between patients with:
- Increased inspiratory effort – classically secondary to upper airway obstruction
- Both increased inspiratory and expiratory effort – classically due to reduced lung compliance.

Any upper airway noise should be evaluated in order to localize the site of origin. For example:

- Stertor (snoring) results from an overlong soft palate or nasal obstruction
- Stridor (sawing/whistling) is typically laryngeal or tracheal in origin.

Complete thoracic auscultation for assessment of respiratory function should evaluate ventral and dorsal lung fields bilaterally, both cranially and caudally.

- Pleural space disease is frequently characterized by dull lung sounds with muffled cardiac sounds.
- Typically with pleural effusion, lungs sounds are dull ventrally and harsh dorsally; whilst with pneumothorax they may be dull dorsally first before becoming generally reduced.
- A 'sprung' or excessively expanded thoracic cavity is indicative of severe pneumothorax.
- Patients with pleural space disease typically adopt a rapid, shallow respiratory pattern, in contrast to the deeper, slower pattern associated with parenchymal disease.

PRACTICAL TIPS

- Lower airway disease is challenging to diagnose but auscultation of wheezes may aid identification.
- Parenchymal disease typically produces harsh lung sounds, which may progress to crackles (like crinkling foil crisp packets) when significant alveolar disease is present.
- The identification of gastrointestinal sounds within the thoracic cavity indicates herniated abdominal organs and is frequently accompanied by paradoxical abdominal movement (abdominal wall moving in during inspiration rather than out).

Neurological system

A full neurological assessment is rarely required as a component of repeated physical examination. In most postoperative patients, repeated assessment of mentation is sufficient. If concerns exist, further evaluation of cranial nerves, proprioception, segmental reflexes and peripheral sensation should be conducted. Patients undergoing neurological surgery may require focused or more complete neurological assessment for determination of progress.

Monitoring

Careful detailed patient monitoring is the essence of critical care, but monitoring can only improve outcome if the information is used to initiate or alter treatment and it is never a substitute for thorough and regular physical examinations. The data obtained must therefore be integrated with knowledge of the patient's history and disease pathophysiology and with accurate physical examination and clinicopathological information.

Cardiovascular system

Electrocardiography

Continuous electrocardiography is a valuable monitoring tool for post-surgical patients, particularly those with pre-existing rhythm disturbances or disease processes that predispose to arrhythmias, such as gastric dilatation–volvulus (GDV). Intermittent recording is of limited value in this setting, because important rhythm disturbances may go unnoticed.

Ideally, patient electrocardiograms (ECGs) should be monitored continuously, either on a patient-side monitor (Figure 13.4a) or telemetrically via a central station (Figure 13.4b). A lead II ECG recording is most frequently displayed to aid interpretation. Notes must be made in the medical record about the nature of any rhythm disturbances identified and personnel able to interpret and act on ECG abnormalities should be available.

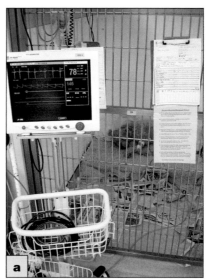

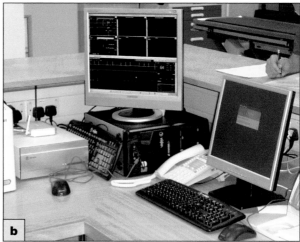

13.4　**(a)** Monitoring the post-surgical patient with a bedside ECG monitor. The multiparameter monitor is also displaying a direct arterial blood pressure tracing. **(b)** A telemetric ECG monitoring screen mounted within the intensive care unit nurses station.

Blood pressure

Mean arterial pressure (MAP) is the set-point for homeostatic regulation of the cardiovascular system. As such it is a critical monitoring value but one that is a late marker of cardiovascular dysfunction.

Both hypo- and hypertension may be identified in the post-surgical patient.

- Hypotension may be due to a reduction in effective circulating volume, myocardial failure, drug therapy or inappropriate vasodilatation due to sepsis or systemic inflammatory response syndrome (SIRS, see Chapter 11).

■ Hypertension may be seen secondary to pain, drug therapy or underlying diseases, including renal insufficiency.

Blood pressure monitoring can be performed non-invasively or directly and may help to guide fluid therapy and use of vasopressors or inotropes.

Non-invasive monitoring: Non-invasive blood pressure monitoring is easy, cheap and safe to perform, but only provides intermittent data and is less accurate than invasive measurement, particularly at the extremes of pressure or patient size or in those with rhythm disturbances. Non-invasive blood pressure monitoring can be performed using a Doppler flow probe and a sphygmomanometer (Figure 13.5) or using a proprietary oscillometric blood pressure monitor, which may be a stand-alone device or a component of a multiparameter monitor.

Accuracy of non-invasive measurements is best assured by correct cuff sizing and placement.

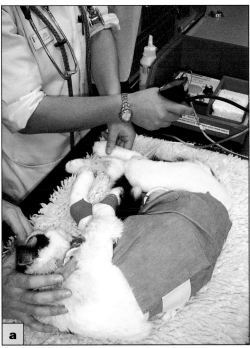

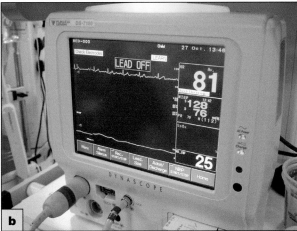

13.5 **(a)** A blood pressure recording being taken by Doppler sphygmomanometry from the plantar metatarsal artery in a cat following thoracotomy. **(b)** Oscillometric blood pressure reading from a dog using a multiparameter monitor.

With all non-invasive blood pressure techniques, corrective action should only be taken if the measured values are repeatedly abnormal.

Oscillometric blood pressure machines measure systolic, mean and diastolic pressure by alternately inflating and deflating the cuff and detecting cuff pressure oscillations due to pulses in the constricted limb. Oscillometric devices frequently do not work in very small patients, patients with rhythm disturbances and those who will not sit still. For these patients, the Doppler method may be more suitable. The Doppler method provides only a single value, likely representing the systolic arterial pressure (SAP) in dogs but probably closer to the MAP in cats (Caulkett *et al.*, 1998).

Invasive monitoring: Invasive blood pressure monitoring is the gold-standard method but requires placement of an indwelling arterial catheter, typically in the dorsal metatarsal artery. The catheter is then connected to a fluid line and the pressure in the fluid column is measured using an electronic pressure transducer. Invasive blood pressure monitoring (Figure 13.6a) is useful because it can provide serial measurements automatically without needing an operator present.

Frequency of monitoring: Blood pressure should be measured routinely at least once in all postoperative patients soon after their return to the recovery room, intensive care unit (ICU) or surgical ward. Repeated

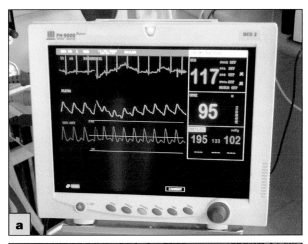

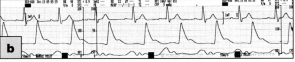

13.6 **(a)** Direct arterial blood pressure monitoring in a postoperative patient. **(b)** Simultaneous paper tracings of ECG, direct arterial blood pressure and central venous pressure from a patient following cardiopulmonary bypass surgery.

measurement may not be required in stable patients with ASA classifications I or II (see Chapter 8). Unstable patients with high ASA classifications, patients with previously documented hypotension, significant intraoperative fluid losses or those with disease processes predisposing to hypotension such as sepsis must have their blood pressure monitored more frequently.

PRACTICAL TIPS

- Assessment of blood pressure every 4–6 hours may be appropriate in sick but stable animals.
- Critical patients should be monitored more frequently or continuously via an arterial catheter.

Hypo- and hypertension: Patients with systolic blood pressure consistently <100 mmHg or MAP <60 mmHg may require cardiovascular support via plasma volume expansion or administration of positive inotropes or vasopressors, depending on the underlying pathophysiology.

In contrast to hypotension, which is common, hypertension rarely requires direct therapeutic intervention in the post-surgical patient. Anti-hypertensive therapy should only be initiated if end-stage organ damage is present or highly likely to occur, and if systolic blood pressure is consistently >180 mmHg (Brown *et al.*, 2007). Pain should be assessed and managed appropriately before vasoactive drugs are used to control hypertension.

Central venous pressure

Central venous pressure (CVP) is the pressure within the intrathoracic portion of the cranial or caudal vena cava and is determined by the interaction of cardiac function and venous return. CVP measurement requires a central venous catheter. A jugular catheter is most commonly used, but a long saphenous catheter whose tip lies in the caudal vena cava can also be used.

CVP is typically measured using an electronic pressure transducer to display a CVP waveform that can be viewed directly on the monitor or printed out with other waveforms (see Figure 13.6b). CVP is measured relative to an arbitrary reference level: the midpoint of the right atrium. In small animals in lateral recumbency, the manubrium is used as a corresponding reference point, whilst in sternal recumbency, this point is approximately level with the glenohumeral joint.

Fluid challenge: CVP measurement may be used to optimize cardiac preload and improve cardiac output via the Frank–Starling mechanism (Figure 13.7). Using CVP, a fluid challenge can be performed to determine volume responsiveness, i.e. whether an increase in CVP leads to improved cardiac output. It is vital that the fluid challenge is administered rapidly. An intravenous fluid bolus (10 ml isotonic crystalloid/kg) should be administered over 5 minutes whilst the CVP is monitored. In a euvolaemic animal with normal cardiac function this should result in an increase in CVP of 2–4 mmHg, which returns to the baseline within 15 minutes.

- Minimal or no increase in CVP with little change in heart rate or pulse quality implies hypovolaemia.

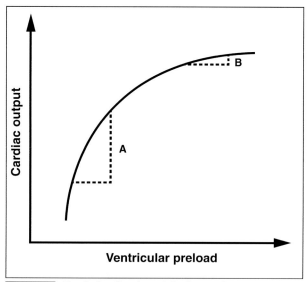

13.7 Frank–Starling law of the heart, demonstrating the curvilinear relationship between ventricular preload and cardiac output. A hypovolaemic patient, represented by A, is likely to be volume-responsive, i.e. a small increase in ventricular preload leads to a large increase in cardiac output. In contrast, a patient with high filling pressures consistent with heart failure, represented by B, is not likely to be volume-responsive, i.e. a large increase in ventricular preload produces a minimal increase in cardiac output.

- A rise in CVP with a rapid return to the baseline (<5 minutes) also implies reduced intravascular volume.
- Large increases in CVP (>4 mmHg) imply reduced cardiac compliance or increased intravascular volume or both.
- A prolonged return to the baseline (>30 minutes) also suggests hypervolaemia relative to cardiac function.

Fluid challenges should be performed with caution in patients with pre-existing cardiac disease.

Respiratory system

Pulse oximetry

Pulse oximeters estimate arterial haemoglobin oxygen saturation (S_pO_2) and are potentially valuable for assessing pulmonary function in the postoperative patient.

- Pulse oximeters only provide information about S_pO_2 in the tissue bed examined and do not provide any information about cardiac output or tissue oxygen delivery.
- Unfortunately, many probes designed for human fingers or ears are not suitable for small animals and are prone to interference from extraneous light or movement.
- Values from pulse oximeters are only reliable if the signal is strong, the tracing pulsatile and clear, and the rate and rhythm match that of the patient.
- Pulse oximeters are of limited value in patients breathing supplemental oxygen because in this situation abnormally low S_pO_2 values are only displayed once a patient's lung function is seriously impaired.

- In contrast, pulse oximeters provide more useful estimates of lung performance if patients are breathing room air since any deterioration in lung function will register as desaturation.

Oxygen saturation should be checked in any tachypnoeic postoperative patient to aid diagnostic and therapeutic decision-making.

- Identification of S_pO_2 <95% ($P_aO_2 \approx$ 80 mmHg) should prompt oxygen therapy and investigation of the underlying cause.
- S_pO_2 <90% equates to a P_aO_2 of 60 mmHg and necessitates *urgent intervention*.

Blood gases

Blood gas analysis in the postoperative patient is often performed in combination with assessments of electrolytes, metabolites and packed cell volume (PCV)/total solids (TS). Following respiratory tract or thoracic surgery, patients must have their oxygenation and ventilation status checked at least once daily. Oxygenation may be crudely assessed with a pulse oximeter, but for the full picture arterial blood gas analysis should be performed.

Clinically, arterial blood gas analysis is the measurement of the partial pressures of oxygen (P_aO_2) and carbon dioxide (P_aCO_2) in arterial blood (Figure 13.8). Blood gas analysers measure pH, P_aO_2 and P_aCO_2 and then calculate bicarbonate (HCO_3^-), base excess and haemoglobin saturation. Blood gas analysis permits evaluation of ventilation, oxygenation and acid–base status (see Chapter 10).

Parameter	Normal arterial values	Normal venous values
pH	7.35–7.45	7.30–7.40
P_aO_2	90–105 mmHg	50–60 mmHg
P_aCO_2	37–42 mmHg	40–45 mmHg
HCO_3^-	18–23 mmol/l	20–25 mmol/l
Base excess	+2 to -2 mmol/l	+2 to -2 mmol/l
Lactate	<2.0 mmol/l	0.6–2.5 mmol/l

13.8 Normal reference intervals for arterial and venous blood gas analysis in dogs.

Blood gas evaluation is now readily available to the general practitioner using inexpensive portable point-of-care units and many modern machines also measure electrolytes, glucose and lactate.

- Arterial blood is typically collected from the dorsal metatarsal or femoral artery using a heparinized syringe and a 25 gauge needle.
- Venous blood samples provide information about pH and P_vCO_2 and are particularly useful for assessing acid–base status, but should not be used to assess oxygenation.

Neurological system

Mentation scoring following neurological surgery is of value for assessing response to surgical intervention, for monitoring for post-surgical complications or deterioration and for prognostication. The Modified Glasgow Coma Scale (Platt *et al.*, 2006) may be of value for this purpose, particularly since it will often comprise part of the initial presurgical assessment of neurologically impaired patients, allowing direct comparison with presurgical values.

Other parameters

Electrolytes and metabolites

Routine laboratory evaluations including PCV, TS, glucose and urea should be performed at least daily in postoperative patients until considered stable.

- Metabolic parameters most often abnormal in the postoperative patient include glucose, electrolytes, urea, creatinine and acid–base status.
- Frequent monitoring of serum glucose is warranted for animals prone to hypoglycaemia, including toy breeds, neonates and patients with sepsis or liver dysfunction.
- Electrolytes may change rapidly as a result of surgery and fluid losses and should be checked at least daily in stable patients and more regularly in critical patients with significant fluid fluxes (see also Chapter 10).

Urine output and urine specific gravity

Urine output is technically easy to measure and provides useful information about renal perfusion. Patients with altered fluid balance, and third-space fluid losses or recumbent patients unable to urinate voluntarily should have an indwelling urinary catheter placed and maintained with a closed collection system.

- Urinary catheters must be inserted using aseptic technique and removed as soon as possible, since any indwelling catheter causes mechanical urethritis and allows bacterial colonization of the urinary tract, increasing the risk of acquiring a nosocomial urinary tract infection.
- Urine production should be measured hourly in unstable patients, decreasing to every 4 hours once more stable.
- Urine production should be at least 0.5 ml/kg/h. Normal urine output is 1–2 ml/kg/h but the measured value must be assessed in light of current fluid therapy and integrated with physical examination findings and understanding of other fluid losses.

Urine specific gravity (USG) must be measured whenever urine output is assessed. USG is typically measured using a refractometer as a surrogate for urine osmolality.

> **PRACTICAL TIPS**
>
> - Healthy animals can have a wide range of USG (1.001–1.065).
> - Normal canine USG is >1.030.
> - Normal feline USG is >1.035.

USG measurements in post-surgical patients must be related to assessments of hydration status and fluid balance. One potential confounder of the use of USG in the postoperative patient is the use of colloid fluid therapy, which artificially increases USG for up to 24 hours post-administration (Smart *et al.*, 2009).

- Patients with low urine output, clinical dehydration and hypersthenuria require more fluid.
- Patients with high urine output and hyposthenuria (USG <1.008) are likely receiving an excessive fluid volume.
- Patients with renal insufficiency will typically have isosthenuria. These patients are less able to deal with high sodium and fluid loads and are at greater risk of volume overload and oedema formation.

Temperature

Hypothermia is common postoperatively, particularly in small patients. Hypothermia reduces the metabolism of anaesthetic agents, prolongs recovery time and in-creases the risk of organ dysfunction and coagulopathy.

Rectal temperature should be measured frequently in hypothermic postoperative patients until normal. This can be performed intermittently or via an indwelling rectal temperature probe to improve patient comfort. Skin temperature measurement and a comparison between skin and core temperature may allow assessment of the adequacy of circulation.

- Normal patients should have a rectal to peripheral temperature gradient of <5°C.
- Values greater than this suggest hypoperfusion.

Pyrexia

Pyrexia is not a universal feature of sepsis, particularly when hypoperfusion is present. Conversely, pyrexia is not solely associated with infection and may result from any inflammatory process. Consequently mild to moderate pyrexia is frequently observed in the postoperative patient, typically as a result of surgical trauma. If a patient's rectal temperature is persistently high or increases over time, concern for postoperative infection should heighten.

Fluid production

Many patients will undergo drain placement during surgery. Monitoring the volume, type, cytological and biochemical nature of the fluid produced from wounds or body cavities is vital following surgery. This information will guide fluid therapy, enable decision-making regarding drain removal and potentially direct further investigation, or repeat surgery.

Packed cell volume and total solids

The volume of fluid and its gross appearance should be noted whenever drains are emptied. If the fluid is sanguineous the PCV and TS must be checked at every drainage interval and the values compared both with previous readings and with those of the patient's peripheral blood. This will enable trends to be identified that may promote drain removal or warrant further investigation for the site and cause of haemorrhage if the PCV of the fluid is high or is rising. Emptying of drains must be performed using sterile gloves and aseptic technique to minimize the risk of acquiring a nosocomial wound infection.

For patients with infected wounds, septic peritonitis or pyothorax, the biochemical and cytological nature of the drained fluid should also be assessed.

- Decreasing cellularity and a reduction in bacterial number suggest that therapy is succeeding and will prompt drain removal in due course.

- An increase in nucleated cells (particularly degenerate neutrophils) and/or the continued or renewed presence of bacteria (particularly intracellular bacteria) warrants continuation of the current therapy or potentially a change in therapy (e.g. change in antibiotic therapy and/or repeat surgery).

Drain removal

In many cases, the most difficult decision facing clinicians is when to remove the drain. Most drains can be removed within 2–5 days. The decision should be guided by a reduction in drainage volume to a small consistent plateau volume. Since drains themselves are foreign bodies, they incite fluid production simply by their presence and thus fluid production is unlikely ever to fall to zero.

Thoracostomy tubes are assumed to induce 0.5–2.0 ml of pleural fluid/kg/day and it is suggested they be maintained until fluid production has dropped to <2.0 ml/kg/day (Tillson, 1997). A more recent study suggested that removing drains in some patients whilst fluid production is above this limit (as high as 10 ml/kg/day) may not prolong hospitalization (i.e. does not have an adverse effect) (Marques *et al.*, 2009). In addition, the fluid PCV and TS should be stable and low, and fluid cytology must be benign with no evidence of worsening inflammation or infection.

> **PRACTICAL TIP**
>
> Drains should be left in place for the minimum amount of time required for them to accomplish the desired task.

Coagulation

Post-surgical patients may manifest both hypo- and hypercoagulable syndromes due to the underlying disease process or therapeutic intervention. The most common postoperative disorders are coagulopathies due to consumption and dilution of coagulation factors and thrombocytopenia. Hypercoagulable syndromes do occasionally occur in surgical patients, typically secondary to underlying disease processes such as sepsis. Thrombotic complications of recumbency and orthopaedic procedures are rare in comparison with human medicine.

Coagulation assays, including clotting times and a platelet count, should be evaluated in any post-surgical patient with evidence of haemorrhage.

- Postoperative coagulation assessment is best performed bedside with point-of-care assays to facilitate decision-making.
- All coagulation assays test particular facets of clotting, which may not accurately represent *in vivo* cell-based haemostasis. As such these tests may be insensitive to clinically relevant haemostatic abnormalities.
- All *in vitro* tests are conducted at 37°C, which may mask a clinically relevant coagulopathy due to hypothermia.
- The most widely used assays are the prothrombin time (PT), a test of the Tissue-Factor/Factor-VII (TF–FVII) pathway, and the activated partial thromboplastin time (aPTT) and activated clotting time (ACT), which test the contact activation (intrinsic) pathway.

Platelet number

Estimation of platelet number can be rapidly performed by examination of a stained thin blood film.

1. A stained thin blood film from a sample anticoagulated with EDTA is first scanned under low power to identify any platelet clumps, typically present in the feathered edge.
2. If present, these will falsely decrease the platelet count and a fresh smear should be examined.
3. The monolayer behind the feathered edge should then be examined and the number of platelets in several oil immersion fields counted.
4. Each platelet in a × 100 field represents approximately 15×10^9 platelets/litre. Values below 50×10^9/l confer the risk of spontaneous haemorrhage.
5. If the platelet count appears adequate but there remains suspicion of a primary haemostatic disorder, a buccal mucosal bleeding time (BMBT) test should be performed.

Buccal mucosal bleeding time

The BMBT is the time taken for bleeding from a standardized superficial incision to cease and should only be performed in patients with adequate platelets (>100 × 10^9/l).

1. A BMBT test is performed with the animal minimally restrained in lateral recumbency.
2. The upper lip is folded back and held in place by a gauze bandage.
3. An incision is made in a non-vascular area of the mucosa with a spring-loaded cutting device (see Chapter 8).
4. The edge of filter or blotting paper is used to absorb the blood, but must not be allowed to disturb the developing clot.
5. The time from making the incision to the cessation of bleeding is recorded.

Normal BMBT values range from 1 to 4 minutes in the dog and 1 to 3 minutes in the cat. Prolonged bleeding times are seen with von Willebrand's disease (vWD) and other causes of thrombocytopathia.

Hypercoagulable syndrome tests

Hypercoagulable syndromes are relatively uncommon in veterinary post-surgical patients. This may be because of a truly low incidence, or potentially due to difficulties in identifying anything other than catastrophic thrombotic complications. Few tests exist that will identify a hypercoagulable syndrome.

Thromboelastography is one such test but is not widely available, though there is now a substantial number of related publications in the veterinary literature. As experience of this technology grows it may become more widely available, particularly if the capital costs fall.

D-dimers are produced following enzymatic degradation of cross-linked fibrin (Stokol, 2003). As such, D-dimers indicate that physiological or pathological thrombus formation has occurred, though some assays are potentially confounded by haemorrhage (Griffin *et al.*, 2003). D-dimers are specific for fibrinolysis following thrombus formation but do not necessarily imply a hypercoagulable state.

Bodyweight

Patients should be routinely weighed at least once daily. Knowing an accurate weight is a requisite for administration of almost all medications and monitoring bodyweight can also be valuable for two other reasons. Bodyweight in combination with body condition scoring (see Chapter 8) may be a useful guide for nutritional supplementation.

Acute changes in bodyweight in a hospitalized patient are not likely to be due to changes in muscle mass or body fat but in total body water. Therefore repeated bodyweight measurements may be particularly valuable in assessing overall fluid balance in patients on fluid therapy, with multiple drains or catheters and in those with abnormal and unquantifiable losses such as those with exudative wounds or with vomiting or diarrhoea. Provided that the patient's bodyweight remains stable and physical examination confirms no changes in hydration status and no oedema, the fluid therapy plan is likely to be adequate for the patient's requirements.

Bodyweight may actually be a better guide to fluid gains and fluid requirements than physical examination assessments (Hansen and DeFrancesco, 2002).

PRACTICAL TIPS

- Acute gains in weight suggest third-space fluid shifts – ascites, or peripheral oedema in particular.
- Acute falls in weight, particularly associated with increases in PCV/TS and skin turgor, are consistent with a hydration deficit.

Pain scoring

Since pain itself can be detrimental, recognition of pain is a key component of post-surgical patient assessment (see Chapter 14). Accurate assessment can be challenging in stoical patients or where a particular focus of pain cannot be identified.

PRACTICAL TIPS

- Persistent tachycardia in the absence of other clinical evidence of shock is suggestive of pain, particularly if accompanied by hypertension.
- Uncomplicated surgical wounds should not elicit a response on gentle palpation when analgesia is adequate.

Various pain scoring systems have been described and validated for use in dogs and cats, ranging from simple visual analogue scales to more complex scores requiring assessor–patient interactions. The formalization of pain scoring through use of these scales serves several purposes:

- Employing a scale and writing pain scoring up as an order on the medical record forces the clinician to make serial assessments of a patient's pain and should improve analgesia provision
- Pain scores allow objective adjudication of whether a patient requires more analgesia, which can both inform and substantiate a decision to alter medication type or dosage

- Pain scales permit clinicians and nursing staff with various levels of training and experience to evaluate patients using the same criteria and help to improve standardization of assessment where multiple staff care for the patient.

Postoperative use of clinical pathology

Packed cell volume and total solids

Changes in PCV and TS may indicate changes in hydration status or blood or protein loss (see Chapter 10). The colour of the serum in the haematocrit tube should be observed for signs of icterus (yellow) or haemolysis (red). The buffy coat may be examined for a crude appraisal of the white blood cell (WBC) count.

Lactate

Lactate is very useful for assessing illness severity and response to therapy in both humans and small animals. Studies in critically ill dogs have identified hyperlactataemia in up to 95% of patients and demonstrated significantly higher lactate concentrations in non-survivors *versus* survivors or controls (Lagutchik *et al.*, 1998). Serial lactate measurements should be performed in the postoperative period and used to guide fluid therapy or other forms of cardiovascular support.

Hyperlactataemia and lactic acidosis occur commonly in critically ill post-surgical patients. Hyperlactataemia is most frequently due to tissue hypoperfusion, but it can also result from sepsis, neoplasia or liver failure, drug administration or mitochondrial defects (Allen and Holm, 2008) (Figure 13.9).

- All 'type A' causes of hyperlactataemia are due to inadequate tissue oxygen delivery, leading to an increase in anaerobic metabolism to ensure continued adenosine triphosphate (ATP) generation, with consequent increased lactate production.
- 'Type B' causes are not due to hypoperfusion but arise due to a derangement in normal cellular metabolism.

Some of the disease processes described as B1 may also give rise to a type A hyperlactataemia. In the postoperative patient, hyperlactataemia should be assumed to be perfusion related until proven otherwise and efforts must be directed at restoring normal perfusion in the first instance. If the clinician is confident that no perfusion abnormality exists, the hyperlactataemia may be due to a type B process.

Provided that no contraindications exist, hyperlactataemia in the postoperative patient may be treated with a fluid challenge and reassessed. If hyperlactataemia fails to respond to attempts to improve perfusion, or if the patient appears stable, a type B hyperlactataemia may be responsible.

Careful ongoing monitoring of such patients is essential to avoid missing the development of hypoperfusion.

Haematology and serum biochemistry

Complete blood cell counts

Complete blood cell counts in the postoperative patient are valuable for monitoring inflammatory and haemopoietic responses to surgery and for investigating whether thrombocytopenia may be contributing to postoperative haemorrhage. Much of this information can be gained from routine in-house blood film examination, which provides information immediately without the delay of submission to an external laboratory. Absolute leucocyte counts and confirmation of the leucocyte appearance and degree of regeneration provide valuable additional information in sick postoperative patients.

Serum biochemistry

Serum biochemistry profiles also provide important monitoring information in the post-surgical patient. Greater availability of in-house biochemical analysers provides a mechanism for short turnaround times, allowing fluid therapy strategies to be tailored to changing patient requirements and for further investigations to be performed if significant abnormalities such as hyperbilirubinaemia are identified.

Hypoalbuminaemia: Hypoalbuminaemia has been associated with increased mortality in humans (Knaus *et al.*, 1991; Goldwasser and Feldman, 1997) and small animal surgical patients (Hardie *et al.*, 1995; Papazoglou *et al.*, 2002; Ralphs *et al.*, 2003) and appears to be an independent risk factor as well as

Type A	
Common causes	**Uncommon causes**
- Shock (global hypoperfusion) - Regional hypoperfusion - Severe anaemia (PCV typically <10%) - Severe hypoxaemia (P_aO_2 typically <50 mmHg)	- Seizures - Carbon monoxide intoxication - Exercise

Type B		
B1: Underlying diseases	**B2: Drugs/toxins**	**B3: Mitochondrial disorders**
- Diabetes mellitus - Liver disease - Neoplasia - Renal failure - Sepsis	- Carbon monoxide - Adrenaline - Ethylene glycol - Paracetamol - Propylene glycol - Salicylates	- Congenital - Acquired

13.9 Causes of hyperlactataemia in dogs and cats.

being a marker of disease severity. As such, it is vital that serum albumin concentrations are measured frequently to monitor disease severity and progression. It is unclear whether support of colloid osmotic pressure (a major function of albumin) or exogenous replacement of albumin with an allogeneic transfusion of plasma or use of human serum albumin solutions improve outcome (Alderson *et al.*, 2004; Trow *et al.*, 2008).

Fluid analysis

Cytological and biochemical analysis of fluid in the postoperative period is just as valuable as in the preoperative assessment and diagnosis. Aims of postoperative fluid analysis include:

- Monitoring response to surgical intervention for disorders such as chylothorax
- Identifying post-surgical complications such as septic peritonitis following enterectomy
- Monitoring fluid type to identify post-surgical haemorrhage.

Fluid samples may be obtained directly from body cavities by paracentesis or from drains. Caution must be exercised if interventions are planned on the basis of examination of fluid from drain reservoirs, since such fluid may not be representative of the process occurring within the drainage site.

Basic in-house cytological analysis can readily be performed using rapid Romanowsky stains. Indeed, if sepsis is suspected following surgery, it is imperative that this is identified as rapidly as possible, since in the presence of septic shock each hour of delay in achieving administration of effective antibiotics is associated with an increase in mortality (Kumar *et al.*, 2006). Bacterial sepsis can be definitively diagnosed by identifying neutrophilic inflammation with intracellular bacterial organisms (Figure 13.10a).

If the cytological picture is indistinct, biochemical fluid analysis may aid decision-making.

- Abdominal fluid from patients with septic peritonitis typically has higher concentrations of hydrogen ions (low pH), carbon dioxide and lactate, and lower concentrations of glucose and oxygen than peripheral blood (Figure 13.10b).
- Assessment of the gradient between the fluid and blood may help to improve sensitivity and specificity of fluid analysis (Bonczynski *et al.*, 2003).
- Assessment of biochemical gradients between the fluid and blood may also aid identification of chylothorax, bile peritonitis or uroperitoneum (Fossum *et al.*, 1986; Ludwig *et al.*, 1997; Schmidt *et al.*, 2001).

It should be remembered that non-infectious inflammatory conditions, such as pancreatitis, may produce similar cytological and biochemical results to sepsis (Swann and Hughes, 1996). If the evidence for postoperative sepsis following fluid analysis is equivocal, careful re-evaluation of the whole case – including physical examination findings and other clinicopathological data – is warranted in order to estimate the likelihood of sepsis. Ultimately, repeat surgery may be necessary if uncertainty remains.

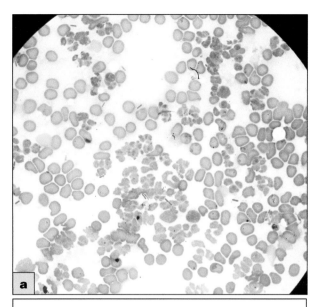

a

PATIENT LOCATION					
icu					
SAMPLE TYPE					
SAMPLE INFORMATION					
Time Analyzed		5/5/2009 01:04 PM			
PAT. TEMP. °C		37.0			
FIO2%		20.9			
BAROMETER:		757.62 mmHg			
Analyzed by:		novaservice			
Released by:		novaservice			
Errors					
Hct Low Range					
Hb Dependency					
Comments					

			Test Ranges		
Test	**Results**	**Units**	**Low**	**High**	**flags**
BLOOD GAS					
pH	7.082		7.360	7.470	<
pCO2	54.1	mmHg	33.0	52.0	>
pO2	15.5	mmHg	28.0	61.0	<
Hct	10	%	37	55	<<<
Hb		g/dL	12.0	18.0	E
CALCULATED					
A	84.2	mmHg			
HCO3-	16.3	mmol/L			
BEecf	-14.0	mmol/L			
BEb	-13.4	mmol/L			
SO2%	11.6				
SBC	12.8	mmol/L			
CHEMISTRY					
Na+	141.5	mmol/L	140.0	153.0	
K+	4.10	mmol/L	3.60	4.60	
Cl-	124.0	mmol/L	106.0	120.0	>
Ca++	1.23	mmol/L	1.13	1.33	
Mg++	0.48	mmol/L	0.35	0.55	
Glu	0.87	mmol/L	4.20	6.60	<
Lac	12.1	mmol/L	0.6	2.5	>
Urea	5.0	mmol/L	3.0	10.0	
Creat		umol/L	50	140	UC
CALCULATED CHEMISTRY					
TCO2	17.9	mmol/L			
Gap	1.3	mmol/L			
Osm	278.1	mOsm/kg			
Reported by		Time:			
Notes					

b

13.10 **(a)** In-house cytology of abdominal fluid from a patient with septic peritonitis. Multiple rod-shaped bacterial organisms are visible and there are a large number of degenerate neutrophils. Erythrocytes are also visible in the background. (X 400 original magnification, rapid Romanowsky staining). **(b)** Blood gas, electrolyte and metabolite analyses performed on the fluid demonstrated a very low pH, low P_aO_2 and low glucose concentration with high P_aCO_2 and high lactate concentration.

Urinalysis

Urinalysis in the postoperative period may provide valuable information about the functional integrity of the kidneys and renal perfusion. Urine sediment examination may provide an early warning of renal injury secondary to anaesthetic-induced hypotension or drug-related nephrotoxicity before changes in urea or creatinine occur. Urinalysis can also be used to identify urinary tract infections (UTIs).

Samples collected by cystocentesis provide the most robust information. Although cystocentesis is safe, it is invasive and should be performed with caution in patients with bladder disease. Samples collected by free-catch or via a urinary catheter will provide adequate information for most tests, apart from bacterial culture.

Urine sediment examination should be performed using specific sediment stains (e.g. SediStain) to enhance contrast.

■ Normal urine contains very few red blood cells.
■ High erythrocyte numbers may indicate infection, inflammation, a bleeding disorder or trauma from catheterization, surgery or cystocentesis itself.
■ Pyuria (>5 WBCs per high power field) indicates the presence of urinary tract inflammation, most commonly due to bacterial UTI. Normal urine is free of bacteria and the presence of bacteria in combination with pyuria is diagnostic of UTI.

Modified Wright's-stained urine samples are superior for identification of bacterial UTI compared with traditional wet-mounts (Swenson, 2004). Bacterial UTIs are quite common in patients post-surgery, due to urinary retention, dilute urine and the use of indwelling urinary catheters. Frequent urinalysis should be performed in patients at risk and bacterial culture and sensitivity requested if bacteriuria is identified.

Occasionally, yeast or fungal hyphae may be seen in a urine sample and often represent contamination. True fungal UTIs are rare but may occur in patients on prolonged antibiotic or immunosuppressive therapy or with long-term cystostomy catheters.

Casts

Casts comprising matrix mucoprotein with or without cells may form in the renal tubular lumen. Up to two casts per low power field is normal.

■ Cast formation more commonly occurs with acidic, highly concentrated urine and a low glomerular filtration rate (GFR).
■ Cylindruria may be induced by hypoxia and does not necessarily indicate renal disease.
■ Hyaline casts are protein precipitates commonly associated with proteinuria.
■ The presence of any cellular cast is abnormal.
■ Casts containing renal epithelial cells indicate acute renal tubular injury, but can be difficult to distinguish from those containing leucocytes.
■ White cell casts typically contain neutrophils and occur in bacterial pyelonephritis.
■ Red cell casts indicate tubular haemorrhage, but are rare.
■ Granular casts contain debris associated with tubular cell necrosis and usually indicate tubulointerstitial disease.

Management of drains, tubes and catheters

Intravenous catheters

Intravenous catheters are vital for vascular access, but their use increases risk of local and systemic infectious complications. In human medicine the majority of serious catheter-related infections are associated with central venous catheters. A prevalence survey found that 42.3% of bloodstream infections in English medical hospitals were central line-related (Humphreys *et al.*, 2008).

Central venous access is frequently used for extended periods, during which time the catheter may be manipulated multiple times per day for the administration of fluids and drugs or to obtain blood samples for laboratory analysis. Such manipulations increase the potential for contamination and subsequent clinical infection. Extensive guidelines for preventing catheter-related bloodstream infection exist and can be obtained from the UK Department of Health (www.dh.gov.uk) and the American Centers for Disease Control (www.cdc.gov) websites.

Prevention of catheter-related infections

The key aspects of catheter management relate to the insertion of the catheter and its ongoing care. Recommendations adapted from human public health sources are given in Figures 13.11 and 13.12.

Feeding tubes

Management of feeding tubes focuses on prevention of tube dislodgement or obstruction and preventing local and systemic infectious complications. For naso-oesophageal and oesophagostomy feeding tubes a component of tube placement is to ensure that the tube does not extend beyond the oesophageal hiatus, as this can result in gastric reflux, oesophageal ulceration and potentially stricture formation. Prevention of tube dislodgement is best achieved using a Chinese finger-trap suture pattern (Figure 13.13) (Song *et al.*, 2008). To prevent the patient standing on or chewing the tube, a bandage that incorporates the tube is required (Figure 13.14).

To prevent obstruction of the tube, flushing it with water before and after feeding (using a volume appropriate for the size of the tube, e.g. 5 ml for a 14 Fr oesophagostomy tube or 10 ml for a 19 Fr tube) is recommended. If tubes become obstructed, a small volume of a carbonated soft drink may be used to unblock them. The narrow diameter of naso-oesophageal and jejunostomy tubes frequently necessitates the use of a constant rate infusion in order to achieve the required volume of nutrition and minimize the chance of tube obstruction.

Recommendations to reduce the risk of local and systemic infectious complications include:

■ Effective hand hygiene prior to tube handling
■ Wearing of examination gloves to manipulate a tube
■ Daily inspection of the exit site and early treatment of redness or exudate
■ Swabbing of the exit site for bacterial culture if there is any suspicion of infection
■ Consideration of topical therapy (e.g. 10% povidone–iodine ointment) for treatment of an infected exit site.

Action	Recommendations
Education and training	■ Healthcare workers should be educated and trained in correct catheter insertion and maintenance ■ Insertion and maintenance of intravascular catheters by inexperienced staff may increase risk of catheter colonization and local and systemic infectious complications
Aseptic technique	■ Use correct hand hygiene procedure ■ For peripheral venous catheters, good hand hygiene before catheter insertion combined with proper aseptic technique during catheter manipulation provides protection against infection. Appropriate aseptic technique does not necessarily require sterile gloves; a new pair of disposable non-sterile gloves can be used ■ For central venous catheters, use aseptic technique including cap, mask, sterile gown, sterile gloves and large sterile sheet
Skin preparation	■ Carefully remove hair using clean well maintained clippers. Skin abrasions will increase bacterial colonization of the skin ■ Use 2% chlorhexidine gluconate in 70% isopropyl alcohol. Allow to dry before insertion ■ If patients are sensitive to chlorhexidine, use povidone–iodine product
Catheter material	■ Teflon® or polyurethane catheters are associated with fewer infectious complications than those made of polyvinyl chloride or polyethylene ■ Use central venous catheter with minimum number of ports or lumens essential for management of patient ■ Consider antimicrobial-impregnated central venous catheters if dwell times expected to exceed 5 days and risk of bacterial infection high (e.g. leucopenia) (Veenstra *et al.*, 1999)
Technique	■ For peripheral catheters, use of non-sterile gloves acceptable if access site not touched after application of skin antiseptics ■ Do not routinely use venous cut-down procedures as a method to insert catheters
Dressing	■ For peripheral catheters, use sterile semi-permeable transparent dressing (e.g. Opsite) or standard sterile gauze and tape dressing to allow observation of insertion site. Chlorhexidine-impregnated sponge (Biopatch™) might reduce catheter colonization and catheter-related bloodstream infections (Garland *et al.*, 2002) ■ For central catheters, use sterile semi-permeable transparent dressing (e.g. Opsite) over insertion site
Documentation	■ Record date of insertion in medical record

13.11 Recommendations for the insertion of intravenous catheters.

Action	Recommendations
Hand hygiene	■ Observe hand hygiene before/after palpating catheter insertion sites and before/after replacing, accessing, repairing or dressing intravascular catheter
Continuing clinical indication	■ Ensure all intravenous catheters and associated devices still indicated. Remove intravenous catheters once no longer required
Site inspection	■ Monitor catheter sites visually or by palpation through intact dressing daily ■ If patients have tenderness at insertion site, fever without obvious source, or other manifestations suggesting local or systemic infection, remove dressing to allow thorough examination of site
Dressing	■ An intact dry adherent dressing should be present ■ Replace catheter-site dressing when it becomes damp, loosened or soiled or when inspection of site is necessary ■ Replace dressings on central catheters sites every 2 days, except when risk of dislodging catheter outweighs benefit of changing dressing
Cannula access	■ Use 2% chlorhexidine gluconate in 70% isopropyl alcohol, 70% alcohol or an iodophor on i.v. injection ports ■ Allow antiseptics to dry prior to accessing the cannula
Anticoagulant flush	■ Use anticoagulant flush (1 IU heparin/ml of 0.9% saline) every 6–8 hours to prevent thrombi and fibrin deposits on catheters that might serve as nidus for microbial colonization
Administration set replacement	■ Immediately after administration of blood products ■ All other fluid sets after 72 hours ■ Replace tubing used to administer propofol infusions every 6–12 hours
Routine cannula replacement	■ Replace peripheral venous catheters every 72–96 hours. Based on a clinical trial in human medicine (Widmer, 2003), replacing peripheral catheters only when clinically indicated does not appear to increase incidence of phlebitis or catheter-related infections when compared with routine replacement at 72 hours. However, this has not been adopted as policy by medical authorities ■ When adherence to aseptic technique cannot be ensured (e.g. catheters inserted during medical emergencies) all catheters should be replaced as soon as possible ■ In patients with limited venous access or in neonates, leave peripheral venous catheters in place until intravenous therapy is completed, unless complications occur ■ Do not routinely replace central venous catheters ■ Do not remove central venous catheters on the basis of fever alone. Use clinical judgement regarding appropriateness of removing catheter if infection present elsewhere or if non-infectious cause of fever suspected

13.12 Ongoing care actions for intravenous catheters.

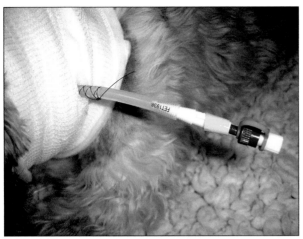

13.13 A finger-trap suture securing an oesophagostomy tube in a dog.

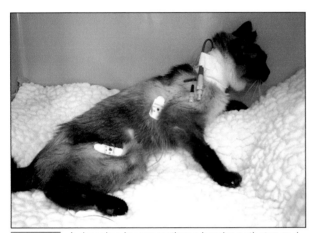

13.14 A dressing incorporating a jugular catheter and an oesophagostomy tube in a post-surgical feline patient.

Removal of feeding tubes

Naso-oesophageal and oesophagostomy feeding tubes can be removed at any time after insertion. Gastrostomy and jejunostomy tubes should not be removed until 10 days after placement to ensure adequate adhesions have formed. Naso-oesophageal, oesophagostomy, jejunostomy and some gastrostomy tubes (surgically placed dePezzer tubes) are removable by traction. Generally, feeding tubes are removed from the conscious patient and rarely is sedation required. Gastrostomy tubes that cannot be removed by traction generally require endoscopic retrieval.

Following gastrostomy tube removal, the stoma should not be sutured and will typically close within 48 hours. Some gastric contents may leak from the stoma. Emptying the stomach via the tube beforehand may minimize this.

Urinary catheters

In the UK, UTIs account for approximately 20% of all human hospital-acquired infections (Emmerson *et al.*, 1996). The presence of a urinary catheter and the duration of its use contribute to the development of UTIs. Guidelines for preventing urinary catheter-associated UTIs are divided into recommendations for insertion and ongoing care (Figures 13.15 and 13.16).

Action	Recommendations
Need for catheter	▪ Avoid if possible
Cleaning prior to insertion	▪ Clean urethral meatus prior to insertion with 4% chlorhexidine diluted 1:10 ▪ Use sterile lubricant
Drainage system	▪ Use sterile closed drainage system
Hand hygiene	▪ Use correct hand hygiene procedure before and after each patient contact
Aseptic technique	▪ Use sterile gloves and sterile catheter

13.15 Recommendations for the insertion of urinary catheters.

Action	Recommendations
Hand hygiene	▪ Use correct hand hygiene procedure before and after each patient contact
Urine sampling	▪ Perform aseptically
Drainage bag position	▪ Above floor, but below bladder level, to prevent reflux or contamination
Catheter manipulation	▪ Wear examination gloves to manipulate catheter
Catheter removal	▪ Remove catheter as soon as possible

13.16 Ongoing care of urinary catheters.

Chest drains

Complications associated with chest drains can lead to significant morbidity and mortality. Chest drains in veterinary patients require 24-hour monitoring, since pneumothorax secondary to dislodgement or patient interference with the tube can be fatal.

- Like feeding tubes, chest drains are best secured using a Chinese finger-trap suture pattern.
- Additionally a bandage that incorporates the tube is required.
- All adaptors should be inserted firmly with at least three ridges of the connector within the tube or encircled with cerclage wire for additional security.
- If the chest drain is not attached to a continuous suction system, a minimum of two forms of tube security should be fitted. Typically this includes a clamp and a three-way tap with injection port bungs securing the openings (Figure 13.17).

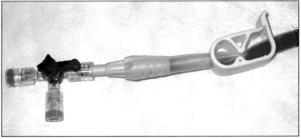

13.17 All adaptors should be inserted firmly with at least three ridges of the connector within the chest drain or encircled with cerclage wire for additionally security. A minimum of two forms of tube security should be fitted. Typically this includes a clamp and a three-way tap with injection port bungs securing the openings.

Chest tubes are usually drained intermittently. Continuous suction may be necessary in patients with persistent large-volume pneumothorax, but this is uncommon. Continuous suction requires additional equipment (suction machine, disposable integrated three-bottle drainage system) and constant monitoring to minimize the chance of disconnection. Figure 13.18 gives guidelines for the ongoing management of chest drains.

Surgical drains

Surgical drains are typically placed to facilitate drainage of fluid that cannot be entirely removed at surgery, or to manage surgical dead space and prevent seroma formation. Drains are either passive (e.g. Penrose drains) or active (e.g. Jackson–Pratt drains). For further information see Chapter 17.

The primary complications associated with surgical drains are ascending infection and dislodgement. Rare complications including intestinal perforation (for abdominal drains), haemorrhage, fistula formation and vascular compromise of tissue flaps are all associated with the location and choice of drain rather than the ongoing care. To minimize the risk of dislodgement, tubing associated with drains should be secured with a Chinese finger-trap suture, if possible, in addition to a bandage. Figure 13.19 gives guidelines for the ongoing management of surgical drains.

Respiratory care

Assessment of pulmonary function

The lungs have two principle functions: ventilation and oxygenation.

- Ventilation is the removal of carbon dioxide from the blood by the lungs and P_aCO_2 is directly proportional to minute ventilation.
  - Hypoventilation causes increased P_aCO_2 and respiratory acidosis.
  - Hyperventilation reduces P_aCO_2 and causes respiratory alkalosis.
- Hypoventilation in the post-surgical patient may be due to:
  - Depression of the respiratory centre by drugs or neurological disease
  - Excessive dead space whilst intubated or less commonly secondary to airway obstruction
  - Respiratory muscle failure due to neuromuscular disease, fatigue, flail chest or diaphragmatic rupture.
- Hyperventilation in the post-surgical patient may occur:
  - Due to pain
  - Due to anxiety
  - As compensation for a metabolic acidosis
  - Secondary to hypoxaemia.

Action	Recommendations
Inspection	■ All aspects of the chest drainage system should be inspected at least daily
Flushing	■ To ensure patency, small-bore drains should be flushed regularly with normal saline
Hand hygiene	■ Use correct hand hygiene procedure before and after each patient contact
Dressings	■ Change dressings regularly (minimum daily) to enable insertion site to be monitored for signs of infection
Infection control	■ Swab chest drain site for bacterial culture if any suspicion of infection
Analgesia	■ Adequate regular analgesia must be prescribed: indwelling chest drains can be painful
Drain removal	■ Remove chest drains as soon as possible ■ Decision to remove should be made on basis of volume of fluid or air aspirated, cytology of fluid aspirated and disease process for which tube was placed ■ 0.5–2 ml/kg/day frequently cited as volume of pleural fluid induced by presence of chest drain but tube removal can be justified in patients with pleural effusions as high as 10 ml/kg/day ■ Following removal, wound should be closed using a previously placed purse-string suture or pressure, and appropriate dressing applied

13.18   Ongoing management of chest drains.

Action	Recommendations
Insertion site	■ Cover insertion site with sterile dressing. This is important for passive (e.g. Penrose) and active tube drains
Hand hygiene	■ Use correct hand hygiene procedure before and after each patient contact
Drain manipulation	■ Wear examination gloves to manipulate a drain
Dressings	■ For active drains, dressings should be changed regularly to enable insertion site to be monitored for signs of infection ■ For passive drains, frequency of dressing changes is based on volume of effusion. Dressings should be changed if strikethrough observed. Effusion volumes can be estimated by weighing dressings prior to application and on removal
Inspection	■ All aspects of drainage system should be inspected at least daily
Infection control	■ Swab surgical drain insertion site if any clinical signs of acquired infection
Drainage	■ Accurately measure and record drainage output at least twice daily
Monitoring	■ Monitor changes in character or volume of fluid
Drain removal	■ See Monitoring section above (Drain removal)

13.19   Ongoing management of surgical drains.

Hypoxaemia

Hypoxaemia (P_aO_2 <80 mmHg) in the postoperative patient is most likely to be due to hypoventilation or ventilation/perfusion mismatch.

P_aO_2:F_iO_2 ratio: Evaluation of hypoxaemia is aided by calculation of the P_aO_2:F_iO_2 ratio, where P_aO_2 is the partial pressure of oxygen in arterial blood and F_iO_2 is the fraction of inspired oxygen (which varies between 0.21 and 1.0). The calculation assesses whether the P_aO_2 is significantly different from that expected for a given F_iO_2, and is a useful measure of the severity of hypoxaemia and can be used in patients breathing supplemental oxygen.

■ P_aO_2 is measured by arterial blood gas analysis, whilst F_iO_2 is measured with a calibrated oxygen sensor or is estimated:
  ● At sea level F_iO_2 is assumed to be 0.21
  ● At higher altitudes, it should be measured.
■ If the P_aO_2:F_iO_2 ratio is more than 400, pulmonary function is normal.
■ Any ratio below 400 is abnormal.
■ A ratio below 300 is potentially consistent with acute lung injury.
■ A ratio below 200 is a criterion for the diagnosis of acute respiratory distress syndrome in humans.

Alveolar/arterial (A–a) gradient: The A–a gradient is a slightly more cumbersome calculation (Figure 13.20) which is used to assess the degree of hypoxaemia but also accounts for the influence of ventilation on oxygenation. It is only meaningful for patients breathing room air. The formula determines the difference between the predicted alveolar partial pressure of oxygen and the measured P_aO_2. Large differences between these values (i.e. a large A–a gradient) suggest a clinically relevant defect in oxygenation. If the A–a gradient is normal (<15 mmHg) in a hypoxaemic patient, the hypoxaemia is due to hypoventilation.

Capnography

Capnography is the measurement and graphical display of the amount of carbon dioxide in a patient's exhaled breath over time, whilst capnometry is simply the measurement of the end-tidal carbon dioxide

---

A–a gradient = A – a

where:

$a = P_aO_2$

$A = F_iO_2 (P_{atm} - PH_2O) - (P_aCO_2/R) + F$

Simplified:

$A = 150 - (1.1 \times P_aCO_2)$

Symbols:	
a	arterial oxygen
A	alveolar oxygen
P_aO_2	Measured partial pressure of oxygen in arterial blood
F_iO_2	Fraction of inspired oxygen (0.21–1.0)
P_{atm}	Atmospheric pressure (mmHg)
PH_2O	Water vapour pressure (~47 mmHg at 37°C)
P_aCO_2	Measured partial pressure of carbon dioxide in arterial blood
R	Respiratory quotient
F	Correction factor of ~2 mmHg ($F - P_aCO_2 \times F_iO_2 \times 1 - R/R$)

13.20 Calculation of the A–a gradient.

($ETCO_2$) value. Capnography is of much greater value, since the waveform combined with numerical data allows evaluation of perfusion, ventilation and metabolism as well as anaesthetic and ventilator equipment.

Capnography is typically performed in intubated patients, but nasal catheters may also be used to provide this information (Pang *et al.*, 2007).

■ In the postoperative patient, capnography may only be required until a patient is recovered from anaesthesia and is extubated.
■ In patients with respiratory disorders, or following neurological surgery, continued capnography may be useful, particularly for identifying hypoventilation (defined as $ETCO_2$ >55 mmHg; normal range 35–45 mmHg).

The $ETCO_2$ value should closely approximate the P_aCO_2. Significant differences between these values suggest ventilatory or perfusion abnormalities that warrant investigation.

Capnography produces continuous data and thus may be useful as a trending monitor as it will provide immediate notification of significant changes in ventilatory status.

Oxygen supplementation

Hypoxaemia in post-surgical patients is common, due to prolonged recumbency, atelectasis and hypoventilation secondary to an underlying disease process or drug therapy. Short-term administration of supplementary oxygen is indicated in any post-surgical patient at risk of hypoxaemia, or in patients in whom hypoxaemia is suspected or demonstrated.

Methods of delivery

Oxygen therapy can be delivered by one of several methods, including:

■ Flow-by
■ Oxygen mask
■ Oxygen hood
■ Nasal prongs
■ Nasal catheter(s)
■ Transtracheal catheter
■ Oxygen kennel
■ Endotracheal intubation.

The most appropriate technique for individual patients is dependent on equipment availability, likely duration of therapy, F_iO_2 required and the nature of the patient.

The aim of oxygen supplementation is to maintain P_aO_2 ≥60 mmHg (S_pO_2 ≥90%) with the lowest possible inspired oxygen concentration.

■ Haemoglobin is almost fully saturated at a P_aO_2 of 100 mmHg and although further increases in F_iO_2 and P_aO_2 will marginally increase blood oxygen content this also increases the risk of oxygen toxicity.
■ The aim should be to keep F_iO_2 below 0.6 (60%) if oxygen supplementation is likely to be required for more than 24 hours, since continuous exposure to >60% oxygen for >24 hours may be detrimental.
■ If adequate oxygenation cannot be produced with F_iO_2 ≤0.6, mechanical ventilation may be necessary.

All oxygen supplies should be humidified to minimize drying of the respiratory mucosa, which increases the viscosity of airway secretions, reduces mucociliary function, produces inflammation and may increase risk of infection. Humidification is particularly important in techniques that bypass parts of the upper respiratory tract, such as nasal catheters.

Face masks and flow-by: Face masks and flow-by oxygen are temporary measures that provide an F_iO_2 ≤0.3. Face masks are poorly tolerated in most conscious patients, but may be useful in recumbent postoperative patients.

Oxygen kennels: Specifically designed, dedicated oxygen kennels potentially provide an F_iO_2 ≤0.9 but not all models available provide such high levels of oxygen supplementation. A disadvantage of oxygen kennels is that they isolate patients from caregivers, limiting interactions and access for repeated assessment. Entry into the kennel reduces F_iO_2 and large amounts of oxygen are required to fill the cages, so they can be expensive to use. Only purpose-built oxygen kennels allow independent control of temperature, humidity and F_iO_2 and remove carbon dioxide. Air in adapted kennels typically becomes hot, humid and laden with CO_2 and can only achieve F_iO_2 values ≤0.5. If a specifically designed kennel is not available, other methods of oxygen supplementation may be preferable.

Nasal catheters and prongs: Nasal oxygen is generally well tolerated and, following placement of the catheter, is easily administered. It is particularly useful when longer term oxygen therapy or frequent access to the patient is required. Placement of a nasal oxygen catheter is illustrated in Technique 13.1.

TECHNIQUE 13.1
Placement of a nasal oxygen catheter

1 A 5–8 Fr catheter or feeding tube is premeasured from the external nares to the medial canthus of the eye.

2 Local anaesthetic drops (e.g. proxymetacaine) are instilled into the nostril.

3 After a couple of minutes, the nasal planum is elevated dorsally and the lubricated catheter is gently inserted in a ventromedial direction.

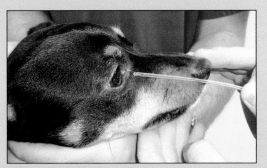

4 Once inserted up to the mark, it is secured to the nose, muzzle and head with tape butterflies and sutures or superglue.

5 Oxygen should be humidified to limit irritation of the nasal mucosa by passing it through a bubble humidifier.

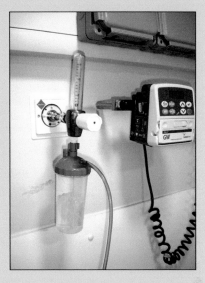

6 A maximum of 100 ml/kg/min can be passed through a single nasal catheter before it becomes irritating. A second catheter should be placed if higher flow rates are required.

Nasal catheters produce an F_iO_2 of up to 0.6 (Dunphy *et al.*, 2002). They also allow measurement of $ETCO_2$, which can be useful for continuously monitoring an extubated patient in whom hypoventilation is a concern.

Nasal prongs are a quick and easy alternative to nasal catheters, though they typically achieve an F_iO_2 ≤0.4. Despite their soft flexible construction, nasal prongs are poorly tolerated and frequently become displaced.

Monitoring and weaning
The response to oxygen therapy should be monitored by repeated physical examination and serial blood gases or pulse oximetry if appropriate. As lung function improves, F_iO_2 can be reduced until the patient is breathing room air. Weaning should be performed gradually and the response to reductions in F_iO_2 monitored via blood gas analysis or pulse oximetry.

Positive pressure ventilation
Positive pressure ventilation of veterinary patients for longer than an hour or so is infrequently undertaken in practice, due to high costs and the expense and time involved in nursing ventilated patients. Short-term ventilation, however, may be all that is necessary for some patients to overcome a transient problem or for temporary stabilization prior to definitive intervention.

Temporary positive pressure ventilation can be easily accomplished with an anaesthetic machine, breathing system and a willing operator. The indications for ventilation include:

- Severe hypoxaemia (P_aO_2 <60 mmHg) despite supplemental oxygen
- Hypoventilation, defined as P_aCO_2 >60mmHg
- Excessive work of breathing, which causes respiratory muscle fatigue and typically hypoventilation and hypoxaemia.

> ### WARNING
>
> If an animal is unable to sleep and will not lie down it is likely to be at risk of respiratory muscle fatigue and respiratory arrest. Referral to a critical care centre will be necessary for patients that require long-term ventilation provided that the owners are emotionally and financially committed.

Positioning

Specific positioning of postoperative patients may be used to improve ventilation/perfusion and prevent atelectasis. For animals with unilateral lung disease, lying the animal with the affected side down can maximize remaining lung capacity. Alternatively, sternal recumbency may improve arterial oxygenation and provide time for resolution of complicating atelectasis and oedema in the dependent lung.

Pulmonary diagnostic tests

Thoracic radiography may be required to assess patients who develop respiratory distress or in whom pulmonary function is impaired postoperatively.

- Radiographs should only be taken if the patient is sufficiently stable and if a thorough physical examination suggests lower airway or pulmonary parenchymal disease.
- Thoracic radiographs should not be taken to confirm a pleural effusion; ultrasonography is the preferred technique and positioning such a patient in lateral recumbency for radiography risks decompensation.

Further diagnostic tests such as bronchoscopy, transtracheal washes or bronchoalveolar lavage should be based on physical examination, clinicopathological data and radiographic findings.

Empirical therapy without further testing may be necessary in an unstable patient.

Care of the recumbent patient

Attentive, proactive and compassionate nursing care is as important as ongoing medical therapy in post-surgical patients. Nursing care in the postoperative period aids recovery and a rapid return of function through tender physical interactions, close monitoring, prevention of postoperative complications and through an organized programme of rehabilitation.

Proactive rehabilitation should begin as soon as the patient is stable, to limit complications associated with prolonged hospitalization. Recovery time will be shortened with the application of simple techniques such as massage, cold-packing and passive range of motion exercises.

Time

Time spent with patients when no treatments are being administered is sometimes difficult to achieve in a busy practice, but this time is particularly valuable in nurturing the bond between staff and patients and in providing the care and attention that animals would normally receive from their owners. Nursing staff are likely to spend the most one-to-one time with post-surgical patients and thus are well placed to identify changes in patient demeanour and to flag up alterations in patient parameters.

> ### PRACTICAL TIPS
>
> - Recumbent postoperative patients and in particular large patients, those with multiple drains, catheters or monitors and those with exudative wounds present the greatest nursing challenges.
> - Bedding should be checked and changed frequently to prevent complications associated with decubital ulceration, urine scald or faecal soiling.
> - Prevention of pressure sores and urine scald is easier and more cost-effective than attempting to manage these complications after they occur.

Pressure sores

Debilitated animals, older heavier patients, those with sensory perception deficits or impaired mobility and patients in negative energy balance are at greater risk of developing pressure sores. These are most likely to form over bony prominences and the skin in these areas should be inspected frequently to detect early signs of pressure sores. Preventive strategies for at-risk patients include frequent changes in position, the use of soft bedding or air mattresses and avoiding re-positioning or moving patients by dragging them.

Positioning

Specific positioning of postoperative patients may be used to improve respiratory function, reduce dependent peripheral oedema, aid patient comfort and prevent decubital ulcer formation. Typically this involves alternating patient position between sternal recumbency and left or right lateral recumbency every 2–4 hours, and the use of supports such as foam wedges, pillows or blankets.

Passive range of motion exercises

Passive range of motion (PROM) exercises consist of therapeutic movement about a joint to maintain musculoskeletal integrity. PROM exercises may be combined with stretching to lengthen shortened tissue and to decrease muscle stiffness. In postoperative recumbent patients, PROM exercises should be initiated as soon as the patient will tolerate them.

- All appendicular joints should undergo multiple slow gentle flexion and extension cycles.
- Joints should be flexed for 10–15 seconds then slowly moved through the range of motion until in an extended position.
- The extended position should be held for 10–15 seconds.
- Each cycle should be repeated 10–15 times.
- PROM exercises should be repeated 2–3 times a

day and are ideally performed after the joints are warmed with hot packs.

- Extra attention should be focused on joints in which motion appears to be restricted.

PROM exercises do not prevent muscle atrophy and should only be the first step in a more extensive rehabilitation programme including massage, facilitated standing and assisted walking (see *BSAVA Manual of Canine and Feline Rehabilitation, Supportive and Palliative Care* for case examples).

References and further reading

Alderson P, Bunn F, Lefebvre C *et al.* (2004) Albumin Reviewers. Human albumin solution for resuscitation and volume expansion in critically ill patients. *Cochrane Database of Systematic Reviews* **4**, CD001208

Bandt C, Rozanski EA, Chan DL *et al.* (2005) Characterization of fluid retention in critically ill dogs with peripheral edema. *Journal of Veterinary Emergency and Critical Care* **15** (3), S2

Bonczynski JJ, Ludwig LL, Barton LJ, Loar A and Peterson ME (2003) Comparison of peritoneal fluid and peripheral blood pH, bicarbonate, glucose, and lactate concentration as a diagnostic tool for septic peritonitis in dogs and cats. *Veterinary Surgery* **32**, 161–166

Brown S, Atkins C, Bagley R *et al.* (2007) Guidelines for the identification, evaluation, and management of systemic hypertension in dogs and cats. *Journal of Veterinary Internal Medicine* **21**, 542–558

Caulkett NA, Cantwell SL and Houston DM (1998) A comparison of indirect blood pressure monitoring techniques in the anesthetized cat. *Veterinary Surgery* **27**, 370–377

Chan DL, Rozanksi EA, Freeman LM *et al.* (2004) Retrospective evaluation of human albumin use in critically ill dogs [abstract]. *Journal of Veterinary Emergency and Critical Care* **14**, S8

Dunphy ED, Mann FA, Dodam JR *et al.* (2002) Comparison of unilateral versus bilateral nasal catheters for oxygen administration in dogs. *Journal of Veterinary Emergency and Critical Care* **12**, 245–251

Emmerson AM, Enstone JE, Griffin M, Kelsey MC and Smyth ET (1996) The Second National Prevalence Survey of infections in hospitals – overview of the results. *Journal of Hospital Infection* **32**, 175–190

Fossum TW, Jacobs RM and Birchard SJ (1986) Evaluation of cholesterol and triglyceride concentrations in differentiating chylous and nonchylous pleural effusions in dogs and cats. *Journal of the American Veterinary Medical Association* **188**, 49–51

Garland JS, Alex CP, Mueller CD *et al.* (2001) A randomized trial comparing povidone–iodine to a chlorhexidine gluconate-impregnated dressing for prevention of central venous catheter infections in neonates. *Pediatrics* **107**, 1431–1436

Goldwasser P and Feldman J (1997) Association of serum albumin and mortality risk. *Journal of Clinical Epidemiology* **50**, 693–703

Griffin A, Callan MB, Shofer FS and Giger U (2003) Evaluation of a canine D-dimer point-of-care test kit for use in samples obtained from dogs with disseminated intravascular coagulation, thromboembolic disease, and hemorrhage. *American Journal of Veterinary Research* **64**, 1562–1569

Guyton AC, Granger HJ and Taylor AE (1971) Interstitial fluid pressure. *Physiological Reviews* **51**, 527–563

Hansen B and DeFrancesco T (2002) Relationship between hydration estimate and body weight change after fluid therapy in critically ill dogs and cats. *Journal of Veterinary Emergency and Critical Care* **12**, 235–243

Hardie EM, Jayawickrama J, Duff LC *et al.* (1995) Prognostic indicators of survival in high-risk canine surgery patients. *Journal of Veterinary Emergency and Critical Care* **5**, 42–49

Humphreys H, Newcombe RG, Enstone J *et al.* (2008) Hospital Infection Society Steering Group. Four country healthcare associated infection prevalence survey 2006: risk factor analysis. *Journal of Hospital Infection* **69**, 249–257

Knaus WA, Wagner DP, Draper EA *et al.* (1991) The APACHE II prognostic system. Risk prediction of hospital mortality for critically ill hospitalized adults. *Chest* **100**, 1619–1636

Kumar A, Roberts D, Wood KE *et al.* (2006) Duration of hypotension prior to initiation of effective antimicrobial therapy is the critical determinant of survival in human septic shock. *Critical Care Medicine* **34**, 1589–1596

Ladlow J (2009) Surgical drains in wound management and reconstructive surgery. In: *BSAVA Manual of Canine and Feline*

Wound Management and Reconstruction, 2nd edn, ed. J Williams and A Moores, pp. 54–68. BSAVA Publications, Gloucester

Lagutchik MS, Ogilvie GK, Hackett TB *et al.* (1998) Increased lactate concentrations in ill and injured dogs. *Journal of Veterinary Emergency and Critical Care* **8**, 117–127

Ludwig LL, McLoughlin MA, Graves TK and Crisp MS (1997) Surgical treatment of bile peritonitis in 24 dogs and 2 cats: a retrospective study (1987–1994). *Veterinary Surgery* **26**, 90–98

Lund T, Onarheim H, Wiig H *et al.* (1989) Mechanisms behind increased dermal imbittion pressure in acute burn edema. *American Journal of Physiology* **256**, H940–H948

Marques AIDC, Tattersall J, Shaw DJ and Welsh E (2009) Retrospective analysis of the relationship between time of thoracostomy drain removal and discharge time *Journal of Small Animal Practice* **50**, 162–166

Moore LE and Garvey MS (1996) The effect of hetastarch on serum colloid osmotic pressure in hypoalbuminemic dogs. *Journal of Veterinary Internal Medicine* **10**, 300–303

Pang D, Hethey J, Caulkett NA and Duke T (2007) Partial pressure of end-tidal CO2 sampled via an intranasal catheter as a substitute for partial pressure of arterial CO2 in dogs. *Journal of Veterinary Emergency and Critical Care* **17**, 143–148

Papazoglou LG, Monnet E and Seim HB (2002) Survival and prognostic indicators for dogs with intrahepatic portosystemic shunts: 32 cases (1990–2000). *Veterinary Surgery* **31**, 561–570

Platt SR, Radaelli ST and McDonnell JJ (2001) The prognostic value of the modified Glasgow Coma Scale in head trauma in dogs. *Journal of Veterinary Internal Medicine* **15**, 581–584

Ralphs SC, Jessen CR and Lipowitz AJ (2003) Risk factors for leakage following intestinal anastomosis in dogs and cats: 115 cases (1991–2000). *Journal of the American Veterinary Medical Association* **223**, 73–77

Reine NJ and Langston CE (2005) Urinalysis interpretation: how to squeeze out the maximum information from a small sample. *Clinical Techniques in Small Animal Practice* **20**, 2–10

Schmiedt C, Tobias KM and Otto CM (2001) Evaluation of abdominal fluid: peripheral blood creatinine and potassium ratios for diagnosis of uroperitoneum in dogs. *Journal of Veterinary Emergency and Critical Care* **11**, 275–280

Smart L, Hopper K, Aldrich J *et al.* (2009) The effect of hetastarch (670/0.75) on urine specific gravity and osmolality in the dog. *Journal of Veterinary Internal Medicine* **23**, 388–391

Smiley LE and Garvey MS (1994) The use of hetastarch as adjunct therapy in 26 dogs with hypoalbuminemia: a phase two clinical trial. *Journal of Veterinary Internal Medicine* **8**, 195–202

Song EK, Mann FA and Wagner-Mann CC (2008) Comparison of different tube materials and use of Chinese finger trap or four friction suture technique for securing gastrostomy, jejunostomy, and thoracostomy tubes in dogs. *Veterinary Surgery* **37**, 212–221

Stokol T (2003) Plasma D-dimer for the diagnosis of thromboembolic disorders in dogs. *Veterinary Clinics of North America, Small Animal Practice* **33**, 1419–1435

Swann H and Hughes D (1996) Use of abdominal fluid pH, pO2, (glucose), and (lactate) to differentiate bacterial peritonitis from non-bacterial causes of abdominal effusion in dogs and cats. *Proceedings, International Veterinary Emergency and Critical Care Society, San Antonio, TX*, p. 884

Swenson CL, Boisvert AM, Kruger JM *et al.* (2004) Evaluation of modified Wright-staining of urine sediment as a method for accurate detection of bacteriuria in dogs. *Journal of the American Veterinary Medical Association* **224**, 1282–1289

Taylor AE (1990) The lymphatic edema safety factor: the role of edema dependent lymphatic factors (EDLF). *Lymphology* **23**, 111–113.

Tillson DM (1997) Thoracostomy tubes. Part II. Placement and maintenance. *Compendium on Continuing Education for the Practicing Veterinarian* **19**, 1331–1338

Trow AV, Rozanski EA, Delaforcade AM and Chan DL (2008) Evaluation of use of human albumin in critically ill dogs: 73 cases (2003–2006). *Journal of the American Veterinary Medical Association* **233**, 607–612

Veenstra DL, Saint S, Saha S, Lumley T and Sullivan SD (1999) Efficacy of antiseptic-impregnated central venous catheters in preventing catheter-related bloodstream infection: a meta-analysis. *Journal of the American Medical Association* **281**, 261–267

Widmer AF, Witschi A, Graber P and Frei R (2003) Routine replacement of peripheral intravenous catheter does not prevent phlebitis or infection: a randomized, controlled clinical trial. Infection Control Team; Interscience Conference on Antimicrobial Agents and Chemotherapy (43rd: 2003: Chicago, Ill.). *Abstracts Interscience Conference on Antimicrobial Agents and Chemotherapy Sep 14–17 2003* **43**, K-2041

Principles and practice of analgesia

14

Verónica Salazar and Elizabeth A. Leece

Introduction

Pain is not just a sensation, but rather an 'experience' that includes both sensory–discriminative and motivational–affective components. The International Association for the Study of Pain (IASP) defines pain as:

'an unpleasant sensory and emotional experience associated with actual or potential tissue damage, or described in terms of such damage'.

Molony and Kent (1997) proposed a further definition of pain more specific to animals:

'Pain is an aversive sensory and emotional experience representing awareness by the animal of damage or threat to the integrity of its tissues ... producing a change in physiology and behaviour directed to reduce or avoid the damage, reduce the likelihood of recurrence and promote recovery.'

Classifications of pain

Nociception is the neural response *only* to noxious or traumatic stimuli. **Therefore, all nociception produces pain, but not all pain results from nociception.** This concept leads to a differentiation of pain into two categories:

- **Acute pain** due entirely to nociception
- **Chronic pain** in which behavioural and psychological factors play a major role, even though nociception may have been involved initially.

Pain can also be classified according to its pathophysiology:

- **Nociceptive pain** due to activation of nociceptors
- **Neuropathic pain** due to acquired abnormalities or injury of peripheral or central neural structures.

Other terms frequently used in pain management are summarized in Figure 14.1.

Acute pain

Acute pain is caused by noxious stimulation due to injury or a disease process. It is usually due entirely

Term	Definition
Analgesia	Absence of pain perception
Anaesthesia	Absence of all sensation
Allodynia	Perception of a non-noxious stimulus as pain
Hyperalgesia	Increased response to noxious stimulation
Hyperaesthesia	Increased response to mild stimulation
Neuralgia	Pain in the distribution of a nerve or group of nerves
Paraesthesia	Abnormal sensation perceived without an apparent stimulus
Radiculopathy	Functional abnormality of one or more nerve roots

14.1 Frequently used terms in pain management.

to nociception and as such has the evolutionary role of detecting, localizing and limiting tissue damage. It is usually self-limiting and evolves into chronic pain if unresolved. The most common examples are postoperative pain, post-traumatic pain, or pain associated with medical conditions such as biliary obstruction or pancreatitis.

There are two types of acute pain: somatic and visceral, depending on origin and other characteristics.

- **Somatic pain** is due to injury or a disease process affecting structures innervated by the somatic system, such as bone, muscles or tendons.
- **Visceral pain** is due to injury or a disease process of an internal organ or its covering (e.g. peritoneum, pericardium or pleura) and can be further subdivided into the following categories:
  - **Localized visceral pain** (dull and diffuse, associated with autonomic nervous system activation leading to cardiovascular and haemodynamic changes, nausea, sweating etc.)
  - **Localized parietal pain** (sharp stabbing sensation localized to the affected area)
  - **Referred pain** to cutaneous areas, sometimes even distant from the affected area (this phenomenon is the result of characteristic

patterns of embryological development and of migration of tissues that lead to the convergence of both somatic and visceral afferent input into the central nervous system).

All types of acute pain share a common neurophysiological process constituted by four distinct phases: transduction, transmission, modulation and perception (see below).

Chronic pain

Chronic pain is a pain persisting beyond the usual course of injury or disease process, resulting from perpetuation of pain that is nociceptive and/or neuropathic in origin. In chronic pain environmental factors and psychological mechanisms both play a fundamental role.

Physiology of nociception

The neurophysiological process of nociception takes place in four different phases: transduction; transmission; modulation; and perception.

Transduction

Transduction occurs at the sensory nerve endings (nociceptors) present in the skin and deep tissues, and is the process by which a noxious stimulus is converted into an electrical impulse.

- Some nociceptors only respond to one stimulus (**thermal**, **mechanical** or **chemical** nociceptors).
- Others respond to more than one stimulus (**polymodal** nociceptors).
- Others do not respond to any stimuli and are called **silent** nociceptors. Under normal circumstances these receptors are relatively insensitive to any stimuli. However, if inflammation occurs, the associated mediators will allow activation of silent nociceptors by thermal and mechanical stimuli.

Transmission

Transmission is the conduction of this electrical impulse to the central nervous system along the axons of the nociceptive afferent neurons. These axons enter the spinal cord through the dorsal nerve roots and may be:

- A-δ fibres (1–5 μm diameter, myelinated, fast conducting, associated with sharp and pricking pain)
- C fibres (0.2–1.5 μm, unmyelinated, slow conducting, associated with slow and burning pain).

Modulation

Modulation occurs at both central (spinal and supraspinal) and peripheral (at the nociceptor site) levels within the nervous system. It is the process by which inhibitory and excitatory mechanisms alter this electrical impulse transmission through endogenous descending analgesic systems (opioid, serotonergic, noradrenergic). Pain modulation by these endogenous systems can occur at any point along the nociceptive pathway where synaptic transmission occurs (peripheral and/or central modulation).

Sensitization

Sensitization can occur following repeated stimulation at both peripheral and central levels. It manifests as an enhanced response to noxious stimulation or a newly acquired responsiveness to a wider range of stimuli that includes non-noxious stimuli.

- **Peripheral sensitization** occurs when nociceptors are sensitized. It results in a decrease in threshold, an increase in the frequency response to the same stimulus intensity, a decrease in response latency and spontaneous firing even after cessation of the stimulus.
- **Central sensitization** occurs when activated N-methyl-D-aspartate (NMDA) receptors increase excitability of secondary afferent neurons in the dorsal horn. This results in an increase in input from peripheral C-fibres, which changes the subsequent response of these neurons to future input. This phenomenon can also be called **central wind-up**, and is responsible for an abnormal interpretation of information from low-threshold sensory fibres whose input is interpreted as pain. This phenomenon has two main consequences:
  - Pain is more difficult to manage and higher doses and multiple drugs need to be administered
  - Due to the altered interpretation of stimuli, pain is perceived as greater by the patient.

Perception

Perception occurs at the level of the thalamus, with the cerebral cortex helping to discriminate specific sensory experiences, such as onset, location, intensity and character of the noxious stimuli.

Systemic responses to pain

The systemic responses differ between acute and chronic pain.

Acute pain

Acute pain typically elicits a neuroendocrine stress response that is proportional to pain intensity. Sympathetic activation increases both visceral sympathetic tone and catecholamine release from the adrenal gland. The endocrine response results from hypothalamically mediated reflexes and increased sympathetic tone. Figure 14.2 lists the most common systemic effects of acute pain, which are wide-ranging.

Thus, treatment of acute pain should be a priority in the postoperative period, not only for ethical reasons, but also to minimize its negative influence on postoperative morbidity and mortality.

Chronic pain

The neuroendocrine stress response is absent or attenuated in most cases of chronic pain. If present, it usually affects those patients that suffer from central pain associated with paraplegia or those that have recurring peripheral nociceptive stimulation.

System affected	Side effects
Cardiovascular	Tachycardia Hypertension ↑ Myocardial irritability ↑ Cardiac output (but ↓ if ventricular insufficiency) Myocardial ischaemia (due to increased myocardial oxygen demand)
Respiratory	↑ Minute ventilation (due to increased total body oxygen consumption and CO_2 production) ↑ Work of breathing ↓ Tidal volume and functional residual capacity (due to guarding) Atelectasis, intrapulmonary shunting, hypoxaemia, hypoventilation ↓ Vital capacity Impaired coughing and clearing of secretions
Gastrointestinal	Ileus ↑ Sphincter tone ↑ Gastric acid secretion Stress ulceration Nausea, vomiting, constipation Abdominal distension leading to decreased lung volume
Urinary	Urinary retention
Endocrine	↑ Release of catabolic hormones (catecholamines, cortisol, glucagon) ↓ Release of anabolic hormones (insulin, testosterone) Negative nitrogen balance, increased lipolysis Sodium retention, water retention, oedema
Haematological	↑ Platelet adhesiveness Hypercoagulability ↓ Fibrinolysis
Immune	Leucocytosis with lymphopenia

14.2 Systemic effects of acute pain.

Recognition of pain

The morbidity associated with acute and chronic pain and associated welfare aspects have led to multiple attempts to create efficient and comprehensive tools to recognize and assess animal pain qualitatively and, to some extent, quantitatively.

Recent surveys of the perioperative provision of analgesia to small animals suggest that the use of analgesic drugs in small animal veterinary practice could be improved (Capner *et al.*, 1999). Difficulties in recognizing pain was cited as one of the major reasons for withholding analgesic treatment, suggesting that the development of a pain assessment tool for a practice setting should help to improve pain management.

The recognition of pain in animals is problematic. In people, the self-reporting of pain is the gold standard for the assessment of pain. In veterinary medicine, the recognition and subsequent assessment of animal pain has a number of limitations. The recognition of pain relies uniquely on interpretation of the animal's behaviour by an observer. Observers have to learn to interpret the signs of pain, which involve both behavioural and physiological responses.

- Analgesia should not be withheld just because it may be difficult to recognize pain in an animal.
- Veterinary surgeons must be proactive in looking for signs of pain in postoperative patients.
- If there is uncertainty about whether a post-operative patient is in pain, administering analgesia and assessing response to treatment is recommended.

Among the factors that influence physiological and behavioural responses to pain, species specificity is important but the effects of gender, age, breed, individual temperament and environment should not be underestimated. Species specificity is mainly linked to the species' evolutionary survival mechanism; for example, prey animals such as small rodents and rabbits tend to hide signs of injury or pain. For maximal reliability, the pain assessment tool should be species-specific. A degree of variability is still present within the same species and there may be some breed specificity.

The presence or absence of additional stressors such as fear, anxiety or debilitating disease should not be forgotten. ***Reducing patient anxiety is a very important aspect of pain management and it should not be underestimated.*** Environmental factors should not be forgotten either, as an animal in pain in a hospital environment is not going to have the same behavioural response as a pet in pain in its familiar domestic environment. Considering all of these complex aspects, the development of a reliable tool for pain assessment that can be used in practice is not an easy task.

Pain scales

Initial attempts to create an effective tool to assess and recognize pain were based on objective and measurable physiological variables such as heart rate, respiratory rate, pupil size, plasma cortisol and β-endorphin levels. However, these parameters have been found to be inconsistent and unreliable objective measures. Changes in wound tenderness have proven to correlate well with visual analogue scales in cats. Force-plate gait analyses have also shown successful results in evaluating the degree of lameness in dogs and cats subjected to a number of surgical procedures and analgesic treatments.

A number of pain scales have been developed:

- Simple Descriptive Scale (SDS)
- Numerical Rating Scale (NRS)
- Visual Analogue Scale (VAS) and Dynamic and Interactive Visual Analogue Scale (DIVAS)
- Composite Scale (CS).

Glasgow Composite Measure Pain Scale (GCMP)

The GCMP is the most vigorously validated animal pain scoring scale. It is a behaviour-based composite scale developed to assess acute pain in dogs. It takes the form of a structured questionnaire completed by an observer while following a standard protocol that includes the assessment of spontaneous and evoked behaviours, interactions with the animal and clinical observations.

There are seven behavioural categories:

- Posture
- Comfort
- Vocalization
- Attention to the wound
- Demeanour and response to humans
- Mobility
- Response to touch.

It is the first scale designed for use in dogs in which the validity of the categorization and assignment of expression within each category was assessed statistically. Since pain is not a static process, frequent assessments are necessary, which can become quite time-consuming in a busy practice. This is the GCMP's biggest drawback. The behaviours and interactions listed in the GCMP will vary with the nature and temperament of the animal; therefore, it is sensible to perform a baseline pain scale assessment prior to surgery, especially in patients presented following trauma or with painful disease conditions.

Short Form of the GCMP: The Composite Measure Pain Scale – Short Form (CMPS-SF) (Figure 14.3) is a modified shorter version of the GCMP and should only take a few minutes to perform (Reid *et al.*, 2007).

It has been designed as a clinical decision-making tool and was developed for dogs in acute pain. It includes 30 descriptor options within six behavioural categories, including mobility. Within each category, the descriptors are ranked numerically according to their associated pain severity and the person carrying out the assessment chooses the descriptor within each category that best fits the dog's behaviour or condition. It is important to carry out the assessment procedure as described on the questionnaire, following the protocol closely.

The pain score is the sum of the rank scores. The maximum score for the six categories is 24, or 20 if mobility is impossible to assess. The total CMPS-SF score has been shown to be a useful indicator of analgesic requirement and the recommended analgesic intervention level is 6/24 or 5/20.

Pain scoring and analgesia

One of the most basic ways of assessing pain is to administer analgesia and then re-evaluate the patient. When incorporating a pain scoring system for postoperative pain, it should be repeated as a method of deciding whether the appropriate level of analgesia is being provided, whether the dose given is appropriate or whether a different analgesic modality is required.

The introduction of simple pain assessment scores within practices results in more interaction with the patients, better nursing care and improved knowledge and provision of analgesia. From the veterinary surgeon's point of view, it provides a written assessment of the animal, enabling better planning of analgesia for future cases as well as knowledge of how that individual animal has responded.

Multimodal and pre-emptive analgesia

The term analgesia has been defined as the absence of pain perception. In the clinical setting,

only a reduction in the intensity of pain perceived can be achieved (with the exception of local anaesthetic administration through local blocks). Analgesia is achieved by interrupting the nociceptive pathway at one or more points between the peripheral nociceptor and the cerebral cortex. All four of the neurophysiological phases of nociception can be altered pharmacologically:

- **Transduction** can be obtunded using of local anaesthetics administered in a number of ways: infiltrated at the site of injury or incision, intravenously, intrapleurally, intra-articularly or intraperitoneally. Non-steroidal anti-inflammatory drugs (NSAIDs) can also reduce transduction by reducing the production of endogenous algogenic substances (substances that cause pain) at the site of injury
- **Transmission** of the noxious stimulus can be interrupted by local anaesthetics, administered either by peripheral nerve blockade or by epidural or subarachnoid injection
- **Modulation** can be enhanced by opioids and/or alpha-2 agonists administered by epidural or subarachnoid injection
- **Perception** can be abolished by the administration of general anaesthetics or by systemic administration of opioids and alpha-2 agonists, either alone or in combination with tranquillizers and sedatives.

This introduces the concept of **multimodal analgesia**, which results from the administration of different analgesic drugs in combination and at multiple sites in order to alter more than one part of the nociceptive process. It therefore relies on the additive or synergistic effects of two or more analgesic drugs working at different levels of the nociceptive pathway. This approach to analgesia may allow the doses of individual drugs to be reduced, thereby reducing the potential for any drug to induce adverse effects.

The concept of **pre-emptive analgesia** is also extremely important. It has been proven that not only is the choice of drug administered of clinical importance, but also the timing of administration. It refers to the application of multimodal analgesic techniques prior to exposing the patient to the initial painful stimuli. By using this approach to analgesia, the spinal cord is not exposed to the barrage of afferent nociceptive impulses that lead to central hypersensitivity, also known as central wind-up (see Sensitization, above). As a result, intra- and postoperative analgesic requirements are significantly reduced. Providing effective pre-emptive analgesia for surgical patients will not only reduce postoperative pain, it will also form part of a balanced anaesthesia plan leading to a potential reduction in induction and maintenance agent requirements, allowing for a smoother plane of anaesthesia and dramatically improving recovery characteristics.

PRACTICAL TIP

Giving analgesia *prior* to surgery will reduce analgesic requirements during and after surgery and result in a smoother postoperative recovery.

SHORT FORM OF THE GLASGOW COMPOSITE PAIN SCALE

Dog's name: _____

Hospital number: **Date**   /   /   **Time**

Surgery: **Yes/No** (delete as appropriate)

Procedure or condition: _____

_____

In the sections below please circle the appropriate score in each list and sum these to give the total score

A. Look at dog in Kennel

Is the dog?

(i)		(ii)	
Quiet	0	Ignoring any wound or painful area	0
Crying or whimpering	1	Looking at wound or painful area	1
Groaning	2	Licking wound or painful area	2
Screaming	3	Rubbing wound or painful area	3
		Chewing wound or painful area	4

> In the case of spinal, pelvic or multiple limb fractures, or where assistance is required to aid locomotion do not carry out section **B** and proceed to **C**
> *Please tick if this is the case* ☐ then proceed to **C**.

B. Put lead on dog and lead out of the kennel.

C. If it has a wound or painful area including abdomen, apply gentle pressure 2 inches round the site.

When the dog rises/walks is it?

Does it?

(ii)		(iv)	
Normal	0	Do nothing	0
Lame	1	Look round	1
Slow or reluctant	2	Flinch	2
Stiff	3	Growl or guard area	3
It refuses to move	4	Snap	4
		Cry	5

D. Overall

Is the dog?

Is the dog?

(v)		(vi)	
Happy and content or happy and bouncy	0	Comfortable	0
Quiet	1	Unsettled	1
Indifferent or non-responsive to surroundings	2	Restless	2
Nervous or anxious or fearful	3	Hunched or tense	3
Depressed or non-responsive to stimulation	4	Rigid	4

Total score (i + ii + iii + iv + v + vi) = _____

14.3 The Short Form of the Glasgow Composite Measure Pain Scale (CMPS-SF), which measures pain score quickly and reliably in a clinical setting. (© University of Glasgow)

Analgesic plans and drug groups

Analgesic drugs are those whose primary effect is to suppress pain or induce analgesia. In small animal medicine these drugs usually belong to one of the following groups:

- Opioids
- NSAIDs
- Local anaesthetics
- NMDA antagonists
- Alpha-2 agonists
- Anticonvulsants.

When creating an analgesic plan for a surgical patient, the likely tissue trauma and resulting pain should be considered, along with a means of assessing the effectiveness of the analgesic plan. The basic analgesic plan should follow the simple structure in Figure 14.4.

The first line of analgesia is usually opioid-based and then analgesia is built on in a multimodal manner using NSAIDs and local anaesthetic techniques wherever possible. If analgesia is insufficient, the dose or choice of opioid may be altered and additional modes of therapy considered.

The following outlines of drugs used in a basic analgesia plan for the surgical patient provide practical information for each type of agent. Their relevance to perioperative pain is highlighted and situations where particular agents may be of benefit discussed. More comprehensive information can be found in the *BSAVA Manual of Canine and Feline Anaesthesia and Analgesia.*

Opioids

The term **opiate** refers to all naturally occurring substances with morphine-like activity, while **opioid** refers only to those synthetic substances that have an affinity for opioid receptors. Opioid analgesic agents play a primary role in all perioperative pain management and ideally should be used pre-emptively as part of a good preanaesthetic medication plan. Opioids can be administered by intravenous, intramuscular or subcutaneous injection and are generally well absorbed via the latter routes. There are differences in bioavailability and onset times for the different routes, with intravenous being the most reliable.

Mechanism of action

Opioids exert their analgesic and side effects through action on the different opioid receptors (mu, delta and kappa) and the analgesia produced is beneficial for all surgical patients. The effects are dose-dependent within the clinical dose ranges used in small animal patients. Drugs acting on opioid receptors are classified as agonists, partial agonists, agonist/antagonists and antagonists (Figure 14.5).

Systemic side effects

Central nervous system: Opioid-induced excitatory effects can occur in any species, but are uncommon when administered to cats or dogs in pain, or in combination with sedatives/tranquillizers. Opioids usually result in sedation in small animal patients.

Respiratory: Both the sensitivity of the brainstem to carbon dioxide and its response to hypoxic stimuli are

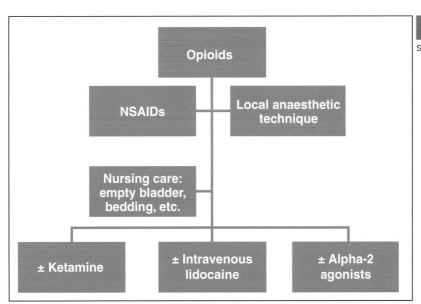

14.4 Structure for the basic approach to analgesia of the surgical patient.

Category	Opioid receptor	Relationship with receptor	Drugs
Agonist	mu (μ)	High affinity and high intrinsic activity	Morphine, hydromorphone, oxymorphone, methadone, fentanyl, sufentanil, alfentanil
Partial agonist	μ	High affinity and low intrinsic activity	Buprenorphine
Agonist/ antagonist	kappa (κ), μ	High affinity and high intrinsic activity for κ High affinity and no intrinsic activity for μ	Butorphanol
Antagonist	μ	High affinity and no intrinsic activity	Naloxone

14.5 Classification of opioids according to their affinity and intrinsic activity with opioid receptors.

reduced. The respiratory rate is decreased, more so than the tidal volume, and the coughing reflex is also suppressed. In healthy pain-free dogs, panting is frequently observed due to alteration of the central thermoregulation set-point rather than due to direct respiratory effects.

Cardiovascular: Different degrees of bradycardia due to a reduction in sympathetic tone are observed. However, no direct myocardial or systemic blood pressure effects are commonly seen. Hypotension as a result of histamine release (e.g. with intravenous pethidine) may be observed.

Gastrointestinal: Gastric emptying time and intestinal peristalsis are decreased and constipation may be observed after opioid administration. Vomiting may occur, particularly after intramuscular administration. The incidence appears lower with intravenous injection and if acepromazine has been previously administered.

Ocular: Opioids can produce miosis in dogs and mydriasis in cats. Due to mydriasis, cats that have received opioids should be handled carefully.

Urinary: Opioids have been reported to decrease detrusor muscle contractility and to increase urethral sphincter tone. Ureteric tone also seems to be increased and voiding reflex inhibition has been described. Therefore, short-term urinary retention may be seen.

Thermoregulation: In dogs, opioids decrease the thermoregulatory set-point in the CNS, causing hypothermia and/or panting. In cats, postoperative hyperthermia is sometimes seen after administration of pure mu agonists.

Auditory sensitivity: Hyperacusia can be observed after administration of certain opioids, such as fentanyl.

Choice of opioid
Opioids are subject to strict legal regulation and appropriate guidelines must be followed for their use. The doses of commonly used opioids in small animal patients are shown in Figure 14.6.

The choice of opioid and dosage used will depend on the type of surgery. In general, increasing the dose will increase the effect as well as the duration of analgesia. An agonist is used in the preanaesthetic medication to provide pre-emptive analgesia and also sedation.

Fentanyl: The shorter acting potent opioid analgesic agents (fentanyl, alfentanil, remifentanil) can be administered intraoperatively by intravenous continuous rate infusion (CRI). Fentanyl administered as a CRI results in constant and reliable plasma levels that not only provide excellent analgesia, but also help to spare inhalant agents and thus help to minimize the related cardiovascular and haemodynamic effects of the inhalant agent. It is particularly useful in patients that need profound analgesia but may benefit from a significant reduction in inhalant concentration, such as patients undergoing thoracotomy or other extensive soft tissue surgical procedures. Fentanyl CRI is well suited to intraoperative analgesia, because any respiratory depression is easily managed by ventilating the patient and because its short duration of action means that it can be stopped just before the end of surgery with no systemic effects lasting into the postoperative period. However, to ensure adequate postoperative analgesia, it is important to administer a longer acting analgesic agent at least 30 minutes before discontinuing the infusion.

One method of avoiding repeated injections is the use of fentanyl patches. These should be applied to

Drug	Class of opioid	Dose (dog)	Dose (cat)	Duration of effect after bolus
Morphine	mu (µ) agonist	0.1–1 mg/kg s.c., i.m., i.v. CRI: 0.1–0.2 mg/kg/h i.v. Epidural: 0.1–0.2 mg/kg	0.1–0.4 mg/kg s.c., i.m., i.v. CRI: 0.1–0.2 mg/kg/h i.v. Epidural: 0.1–0.2 mg/kg	3–6 hours
Pethidine	µ agonist	2–5 mg/kg s.c., i.m.	2–5 mg/kg s.c., i.m.	1–2 hours
Methadone	µ agonist	0.1–0.5 mg/kg i.m., i.v.	0.1–0.3 mg/kg i.m., i.v.	4 hours
Hydromorphone	µ agonist	0.05–0.1 mg/kg s.c., i.m., i.v.	0.05–0.1 mg/kg s.c., i.m., i.v.	4–6 hours
Fentanyl	µ agonist	5–20 µg/kg i.v. CRI: 5 µg/kg bolus followed by 0.3–0.7 µg/kg/min i.v.	5–10 µg/kg i.v. CRI: 5 µg/kg bolus followed by 0.3–0.6 µg/kg/min i.v.	20–30 minutes
Sufentanil	µ agonist	3–5 µg/kg followed by CRI 2.6–3.4 µg/kg/h	Not determined in this species	10–20 minutes
Alfentanil	µ agonist	CRI: 0.5–1 µg/kg/min i.v.	CRI: 0.5–1 µg/kg/min i.v.	10–20 minutes
Remifentanil	µ agonist	CRI: 0.3–0.6 µg/kg/min i.v.	CRI: 0.3–0.6 µg/kg/min i.v.	4 minutes
Tramadol	µ agonist	2–5 mg/kg orally q8h 2 mg i.v., s.c.	2–4 mg/kg orally q8h 1–2 mg/kg i.v., s.c.	6–12 hours
Butorphanol	kappa (κ) agonist µ antagonist	0.2–0.5 mg/kg s.c., i.m., i.v.	0.2–0.5 mg/kg s.c., i.m., i.v.	1–2 hours
Buprenorphine	Partial µ agonist	0.01–0.02 mg/kg i.m., i.v.	0.01–0.02 mg/kg i.m., i.v.	6–8 hours
Naloxone	µ antagonist	0.002–0.04 mg/kg s.c., i.m., i.v.	0.002–0.04 mg/kg s.c., i.m., i.v.	30–60 minutes

14.6   Doses of commonly used opioids in dogs and cats. Increasing the dose will increase the duration and the effect.

dry skin and held for a few minutes after application to allow adhesion. At a dose of 5 µg/kg/h, analgesia can be provided for several days, though the amount of analgesia is unpredictable, meaning that pain assessment and provision of additional opioid analgesia will still be necessary. Plasma levels can take 12–24 hours in dogs and up to 24 hours in cats to develop, so patches should be placed the day before surgery. Additional analgesia will still be required in the immediate postoperative period. A pure mu agonist can be used during this time, but buprenorphine has also been used for this purpose. Fentanyl patches can be useful for patients that are predicted to need prolonged opioid administration, but should never be relied upon alone.

Morphine: Morphine is also suited to intraoperative use in dogs and cats. An intravenous infusion of morphine will de-crease the minimum alveolar concentration (MAC) of inhalational anaesthetic agents and provide additional analgesia during the operative period, but this may be associated with some sedation.

Buprenorphine: Buprenorphine is a partial mu receptor agonist. It shows a higher receptor affinity than a pure mu agonist; as a result it can displace these from the mu receptor if administered concurrently, and its reversal by naloxone is difficult. Its receptor binding properties are also responsible for its characteristic dose–response curve. Early studies showed that a bell-shaped dose–response curve was elicited by the administration of increasing doses, i.e. the administration of higher doses led to a reduced analgesic effect. However, more recent studies have proven that the doses that result in reduction of analgesic efficacy are significantly higher than those used clinically. Therefore, the administration of buprenorphine at doses within the clinical range may only elicit a plateau effect, in which administration of increasing doses will not produce further increases in analgesic efficacy.

Buprenorphine is characterized by a very convenient long duration of action (6–8 hours) compared to other commonly used mu receptor agonists (e.g. morphine or methadone). However, regular pain assessments must be performed and if further analgesia is required an additional dose is given. Its analgesic effects have been proven to be moderate compared to pure mu agonists such as morphine or methadone. As a consequence, buprenorphine may not be the drug of choice for the management of severe pain (e.g. very invasive orthopaedic procedures or thoracotomies). In addition, the onset time of analgesia is longer compared with other opioids such as morphine or methadone, although analgesia may happen more quickly in some animals.

Buprenorphine has poor and unpredictable analgesic effects when administered subcutaneously and therefore does not have authorization for this route of administration in dogs and cats. Oral transmucosal administration of preservative-free buprenorphine has been shown to be as effective as the intravenous route in cats, providing a simple non-invasive method of administration for provision of analgesia for approximately 6 hours. This offers more flexibility and improved nursing care for cats in the postoperative period and avoids repeated injections. Enteral administration is not often used in the immediate perioperative period but may be implemented 24 hours after surgery.

Tramadol: This drug has agonist properties at all opioid receptors, but particularly at mu receptors. Additionally it inhibits the re-uptake of noradrenaline and serotonin, and stimulates presynaptic serotonin release. Its analgesic potency is one-tenth that of morphine, and the resulting respiratory depression and constipation are milder than those seen with morphine. Its use is contraindicated in seizure-prone patients and those with hepatic insufficiency.

Tramadol is an excellent postoperative analgesic drug to prescribe to patients that are ready to be downstaged on to oral analgesic medication following a surgical procedure. It is particularly useful in patients where NSAIDs alone would be insufficient, or where NSAIDs are contraindicated. It is worth keeping small animals in the hospital whilst pain requires opioid administration, although in some circumstances oral drugs such as tramadol may allow the patient to return home sooner. Its main advantage remains the fact that, unlike most opioids, it is not a Controlled Drug, making it an excellent option for pain management at home once the patient is discharged. It can be administered orally at 2–4 mg/kg q8h for 3–5 days.

Non-steroidal anti-inflammatory drugs

NSAIDs are used widely to treat mild to moderate pain and also to reduce opioid consumption in the perioperative period. They possess a much lower therapeutic index than opioids and are not reversible: they exert anti-inflammatory properties as well as analgesia.

The duration of anti-inflammatory action is considerably longer than the measured plasma half-life, since NSAIDs tend to accumulate at the site of inflammation. Cats have a limited ability to metabolize some NSAIDs through glucuronidation. NSAIDs should be avoided in patients with severe hepatic or renal disease due to reduced metabolism and excretion, and also in critical patients that initially present with hypovolaemia, dehydration and hypotension (see side effects and contraindications below).

> **WARNING**
>
> The half-life of some NSAIDs is prolonged in cats, increasing the risk of toxicity in this species.

However, NSAIDs should be used in all animals where no contraindication is found, as part of multimodal analgesia. Figure 14.7 describes the commonly used NSAIDs in dogs and cats. The authors use meloxicam or carprofen over other NSAIDs for routine perioperative use in most small animal patients, because both drugs are licensed for this use in dogs and cats, have a low risk of side effects and provide reliable clinical efficacy.

Many injectable NSAIDs are not authorized for enteral use following perioperative injection. Although such use is commonplace to provide postoperative analgesia, such off-license protocols should be discussed with the appropriate pharmaceutical manufacturer. The combination of paracetamol at 33 mg/kg

Drug	COX selectivity	Dose (dog)	Dose (cat)	Adverse effects
Carprofen	COX-2 selective	1–4 mg/kg i.v., s.c., orally q12–24h	0.3 mg/kg s.c. OR 0.2 mg/kg s.c. followed by 0.05 mg/kg orally 24 hours later	Impaired gastrointestinal protection
Meloxicam	COX-2 selective	Initial dose: 0.2 mg/kg s.c., orally (if given as a single preoperative injection, effects last for 24 hours). Can be followed by a maintenance dose of 0.1 mg/kg orally q24h	Initial dose: 0.2 mg.kg s.c. (if given as a single preoperative injection, effects last for 24 hours). To continue treatment for up to 5 days, may be followed 24 hours later by oral suspension at a dose of 0.05 mg/kg	Impaired gastrointestinal protection
Ketoprofen	Not COX-2 selective	1–2 mg/kg s.c. q24h	1–2 mg/kg s.c. q24h (not licensed for cats in USA)	Impaired gastrointestinal protection Impaired platelet aggregation
Tolfenamic acid	COX-2 preferential	1–4 mg/kg s.c., i.m., orally q24h for 3 days, 4 days off, then repeat cycle	1–4 mg/kg s.c., i.m., orally q24h for 3 days, 4 days off, then repeat cycle	Impaired gastrointestinal protection Impaired platelet aggregation
Deracoxib	COX-2 selective	1–2 mg/kg orally q24h	N/A	Impaired gastrointestinal protection Impaired platelet aggregation Hepatotoxicity
Firocoxib	COX-2 selective	5 mg/kg orally q24h	N/A	Impaired gastrointestinal protection Impaired platelet aggregation Hepatotoxicity
Robenacoxib	COX-2 selective (very short plasma half-life but accumulation in inflamed tissues)	1 mg/kg orally q24h 1 mg/kg i.v. 30 minutes prior to surgery	1 mg/kg orally q24h (only 6 days) 1 mg/kg i.v. 30 minutes prior to surgery	Yet to be fully assessed

14.7   Doses of commonly used NSAIDs in dogs and cats.

with codeine at 0.75 mg/kg (Pardale V) is authorized for analgesia in dogs but may not provide as effective analgesia as tramadol at the given dose.

> **WARNING**
>
> Never give paracetamol to cats as it is toxic, even at low doses.

Mechanism of action

NSAIDs inhibit the enzyme cyclo-oxygenase (COX), thereby preventing the production of thromboxanes, prostacyclin and prostaglandins from membrane phospholipids. COX exists as two isoenzymes, COX-1 and COX-2, whose main structural difference lies in the substitution of one amino acid that allows access to a hydrophobic side pocket which acts as an alternative specific binding site for drugs. By inhibiting COX enzymes, most NSAIDs have been shown to divert arachidonic acid towards the pathway catalysed by 5-lipoxygenase (5-LOX), which constitutes the initial step towards leucotriene biosynthesis. Some leucotrienes (e.g. leucotriene B4, LTB) can be potent mediators of inflammation, and therefore excessive production can lead to NSAID-induced ulcers. However, the LOX pathway is not only pro-inflammatory, it can also lead to an anti-inflammatory pathway.

COX-1: COX-1 is the constitutive form; it is involved in the synthesis of thromboxane, as well as prostacyclin and prostaglandins, which are themselves responsible for the control of renal blood flow and for the formation of the protective gastric mucosal barrier. A variant of COX-1 (derived from the same gene as COX-1) is **COX-3**, which is involved in the initiation of pyrexia.

COX-2: COX-2 is the inducible form; it is synthesized in response to tissue damage and it facilitates the inflammatory response. In addition, it has been proven that abnormally upregulated COX-2 expression is directly implicated in the pathogenesis of a number of carcinomas. COX-2 is also involved in prevention and promotion of healing of mucosal erosions, as well as playing a role in renal maturation and protection. COX-2 mediates synthesis of prostacyclin in vascular endothelium; as a result, inhibition of COX-2 could alter the fine balance between thromboxane and prostacyclin towards platelet aggregation, vasoconstriction and thromboembolism.

Systemic side effects

Gastrointestinal: Prostaglandins are involved in the maintenance of many elements that play a key role in gastric and intestinal protection, such as the mucous layer, bicarbonate secretion, rapid cell turnover and adequate blood supply. With prolonged or excessive use of NSAIDs, gastric and intestinal protection is impaired. Although experimentally NSAIDs may reduce mucosal blood flow, there is no clear evidence to support the withholding of these drugs in uncomplicated gastrointestinal surgery, i.e. in patients without pre-existing ulcers, erosions or other significant gastrointestinal compromise.

The coxib group of NSAIDs were originally marketed as being more sparing of gastrointestinal side effects when compared with other less COX-1-sparing NSAIDs. However, more recent findings have indicated that coxib NSAIDs do not necessarily guarantee gastroprotection with chronic use. In fact, the most common side effects after chronic administration are vomiting and diarrhoea.

Respiratory: COX inhibition causes more arachidonic acid conversion to leucotrienes, which may provoke bronchospasm.

Hepatic: A rise in serum transaminase levels may be observed after prolonged or excessive use of NSAIDs.

Renal: Inhibition of prostaglandins produced by the kidneys can impair maintenance of adequate renal perfusion when the level of circulating vasoconstrictors is high, potentially leading to acute renal failure.

Cartilage: Side effects are controversial and depend on the specific NSAID. Studies investigating the effects of either meloxicam or carprofen administered at therapeutic doses have shown no adverse pharmacological or toxicological action on cartilage proteoglycan metabolism. Additionally, meloxicam has been shown to exert an anti-inflammatory effect at inflamed sites in the joints of patients suffering from osteoarthritis.

Platelet function: The inhibition of thromboxane A_2 formation, by inhibiting COX-1, will reduce haemostasis by impairing platelet aggregation and vasoconstriction. Non-selective COX inhibitors are not recommended for use preoperatively, and their use should be withdrawn 10–14 days before elective surgical procedures. COX-2 preferential inhibitors have a minimal effect on platelet function, but inhibition of COX-2 can also alter the balance between thromboxane and prostacyclin towards excessive platelet aggregation, vasoconstriction and thromboembolism.

Reproductive: Inhibition of prostaglandins can impair normal labour, ovulation, embryo implantation and closure of the ductus arteriosus in the neonate.

Contraindications
The use of NSAIDs is not recommended in patients that present with the following conditions:

- Hypovolaemia or dehydration
- Coagulopathies
- Gastrointestinal ulcers
- Impaired renal function
- Impaired hepatic function (including portosystemic shunts)

- Breeding, pregnant or lactating
- Are less than 6 weeks old
- Already receiving corticosteroids or other NSAIDs.

Local anaesthetics
Local anaesthesia is the only effective way of blocking nerve conduction and providing complete analgesia. Local anaesthetics may be administered perineurally to produce nerve conduction blockade, but they can also be administered systemically (orally or intravenously) to supplement analgesia. When administered perineurally, transmission of nociception is blocked and this will minimize central sensitization for the duration of the blockade. Local anaesthetics are normally employed for specific nerve blocks, but they can be used in many different ways. Figure 14.8 describes the pharmacology and intravenous toxic doses of commonly used local anaesthetic drugs.

Mechanism of action
The main mechanism by which local anaesthetics exert their action is the blockage of sodium channels. The non-ionized lipid-soluble drug passes through the cell membrane into the cell, where it is ionized and binds to the internal surface of the sodium channel.

Systemic side effects

Central nervous system: Local anaesthetics are capable of penetrating the brain rapidly and exert a biphasic effect. Initially, inhibitory interneurons are blocked, resulting in excitatory phenomena such as visual disturbances, tremors, dizziness and eventually convulsions. Finally, all central neurons are depressed, leading to coma and apnoea. Consequently, close monitoring for signs of neurological toxicity should be implemented during and after administration. Clinical signs such as twitching, tremors, agitation and nausea may indicate that lidocaine toxicity is occurring.

Cardiovascular: Both lidocaine and bupivacaine block cardiac sodium channels and decrease the maximum rate of increase of phase 0 of the cardiac action potential. They also exert direct myocardial depressant properties. The PR and QRS intervals are increased and the refractory period prolonged. The fact that bupivacaine takes ten times longer than lidocaine to dissociate from the sodium channels results in a longer persistent cardiac depression with bupivacaine, which can lead to re-entrant arrhythmias and ventricular fibrillation.

Intravenous lidocaine
Despite lacking full understanding of its mechanism of action, clinical evidence supporting the use of intravenous lidocaine infusions to manage intraoperative

Drug	Recommended dose	Onset (minutes)	Duration (hours)	Approximate intravenous toxic doses
Lidocaine	1–4 mg/kg	5–15	1–2	Cats: 11 mg/kg Dogs: 20 mg/kg
Bupivacaine	1–2 mg/kg	10–20	4–6	Cats: 3.8 mg/kg Dogs: 4 mg/kg
Ropivacaine	1–2 mg/kg	10–20	4–6	Dogs: 4.9 mg/kg

14.8 Pharmacology and toxic doses of commonly used local anaesthetic drugs in dogs and cats.

pain is increasing. In human medicine, several studies have shown that lidocaine infusions are associated with decreased postoperative pain, reduced opioid consumption, improved bowel function, shortened hospital stays, and earlier rehabilitation in patients undergoing major abdominal surgery. In veterinary medicine, different studies have documented both the safety (Valverde *et al.*, 2004) and isoflurane MAC reductions (McDougall *et al.*, 2009) associated with intravenous lidocaine. Doses for cats and dogs are shown in Figure 14.9.

Although these studies suggest that lidocaine infusions seem to be safe in isoflurane-anaesthetized dogs and that they may be valuable anaesthetic adjuncts, they do not address the issue of analgesia directly. Lidocaine appears to provide good analgesia for pain associated with inflammatory states and can be a useful addition in pain management for cases with conditions such as pancreatitis or peritonitis.

In cats, investigations of the effects of lidocaine in isoflurane-anaesthetized patients have documented significant dose-dependent isoflurane MAC reductions with intravenous lidocaine infusions, but these MAC reductions were associated with a greater degree of cardiovascular depression than the equipotent dose of isoflurane alone. One study (Pypendop *et al.*, 2007) evaluated the effects of lidocaine infusions on a model of thermal antinociception in this species and it failed to prove any beneficial effects, despite documenting moderate plasma lidocaine levels.

Dogs	Cats
1–4 mg/kg i.v. followed by CRI 25–80 µg/kg/min	0.2 mg/kg i.v. followed by CRI 1–10 µg/kg/min

14.9   Doses of lidocaine for intravascular administration in small animal patients. Blood pressure should be monitored during the infusion; if hypotension occurs, the infusion should be discontinued.

Topical application

Topical local anaesthetics may be employed for ocular surgeries, but repeated use should be avoided as this may result in problems with corneal healing. The use of a eutectic mixture of local anaesthetic (EMLA) cream prior to venepuncture has been suggested to decrease pain and discomfort during venepuncture. Clinically this certainly appears to be the case, but more data are required to determine efficacy and timing of application.

Patch application

Lidocaine 5% patches are receiving veterinary attention for application alongside wounds where there appears to be allodynia. In human patients these patches provide local analgesia, but not local anaesthesia, i.e. nociception is diminished whilst sensation is maintained. The author has found these to be effective for large reconstructive wounds. In cats, low systemic absorption has been demonstrated coupled with high local lidocaine concentrations in the skin, suggesting that their use may be warranted. Low plasma levels were also detected in dogs, suggesting that any analgesia seen following placement is most likely due to the local effect rather than a systemic effect.

Local infiltration

Local infiltration can be used before, during and at the end of surgery. When nerves are to be transected (e.g. amputation) local anaesthetic can be applied directly over the nerve prior to transection. Infiltration of tissues around the distal extremities using local anaesthetic may be used to produce a ring block and the same technique may be used for the removal of cutaneous masses. Infiltration may be useful during procedures such as bone marrow and nasal biopsy. Ideally infiltration should be performed prior to surgery; however, splash blocks can also be employed whilst closing surgical wounds (Figure 14.10). It is important to apply the local anaesthetic at various levels during wound closure.

Local anaesthetic may also be injected adjacent to the wound during closure (bupivacaine 1 mg/kg). This has been shown to reduce pain postoperatively and reduce opioid requirements following laparotomy.

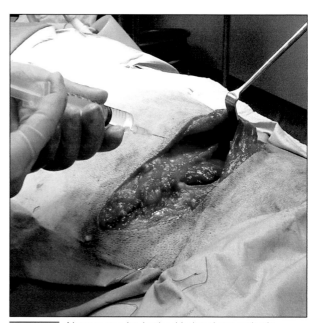

14.10   Nerves can be bathed in local anaesthetic during surgery, prior to transection for procedures such as amputation; or local anaesthetic can be splashed on to the muscle layers during closure to augment postoperative analgesia.

Intra-articular administration

Pre- and postoperative intra-articular local anaesthetic injections have been found to provide similar analgesia to extradural local anaesthetic and morphine following tibial plateau levelling osteotomy (TPLO) and this is probably the most common application of this technique.

Intraperitoneal administration

It has been suggested (Carpenter *et al.*, 2004) that the combination of intraperitoneal bupivacaine before surgery with subcutaneous wound infiltration with bupivacaine postoperatively provides improved analgesia, based on lower numbers of dogs requiring rescue analgesia compared with groups receiving lidocaine and saline in a similar manner following ovariohysterectomy. Prior to laparoscopy in human patients, intraperitoneal lidocaine has been shown to be beneficial.

Intrapleural administration

Intrapleural local anaesthetic may be administered via chest drains to provide analgesia in a variety of pleural conditions and after thoracotomy. Following drainage of the chest, a 0.25% solution of bupivacaine (1.5 mg/kg) should be injected slowly via the drain and if any discomfort is noted the administration should be stopped. The bupivacaine is then flushed through the drain into the pleural cavity by injecting enough saline to fill the chest drain. Usually this technique will provide approximately 6 hours of analgesia, but it can depend on the position of the drain. The pleural cavity can still be drained every hour if necessary without affecting the efficacy of analgesia. It is a good idea to administer local analgesia immediately before removing the drain.

Neutering

Local anaesthetic may be used during routine neutering. There is little published work examining the efficacy of intratesticular local anaesthetic in dogs and cats during castration (McMillan *et at.*, 2011), but it appears to be helpful in the clinical situation. Benefits have been identified in horses. The author injects 1–5 ml of lidocaine into the testicle prior to castration (Figure 14.11). There was minimal benefit from local anaesthesia of the mesovarium during ovariohysterectomy in dogs based on autonomic variables and isoflurane requirements intraoperatively, although postoperative analgesia was not assessed (Bubalo *et al.*, 2008).

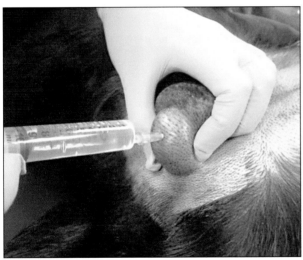

14.11 Intratesticular local anaesthetic injection appears to improve analgesia clinically. Always aspirate prior to injection to avoid intravascular injection.

Wound soaker catheters

Wound diffusion catheters, otherwise known as wound soaker catheters, should be placed at different depths of the wound to exit the area dorsally. They should be placed aseptically at the end of surgery, exit the skin remotely from the incision and be secured in place with a Chinese finger-trap suture. Fears of increased wound infection or breakdown are unfounded and the incidence of these complications appears to be the same in dogs where wound soaker catheters are not placed (Abelson *et al.*, 2009). Wound drains and wound soaker catheters can be placed during the same surgery, but it is important to label the wound soaker catheter and to handle it separately using appropriate aseptic technique.

> **PRACTICAL TIP**
>
> ### Nasogastric tube as wound soaker catheter
>
> A soft nasogastric tube can be made into a wound soaker catheter:
>
> 1. Different lengths of catheter can be made by cutting the end of the catheter at the appropriate length using a flame to seal the end.
> 2. An insulin needle can then be used to make perforations in the catheter approximately 5–10 mm apart for the length of infiltration required.
> 3. The catheters can then be re-sterilized (or the catheters can be made at the time of surgery).
> 4. Each catheter should be checked to ensure that, when saline is injected, each hole has flow through it. If the holes are too big or not evenly distributed, the local anaesthetic will tend to leave the catheter at one site and not along the length of the catheter.

Custom-made wound soaker catheters

Custom-made wound soaker catheters of various lengths may also be used. They are extremely useful for extensive surgeries, such as amputation, tumour resection, mastectomy, thoracic surgery and abdominal surgery, and can be used in both cats and dogs (Figure 14.12). They are well tolerated and, if placed properly, can decrease opioid requirements and improve patient comfort postoperatively in combination

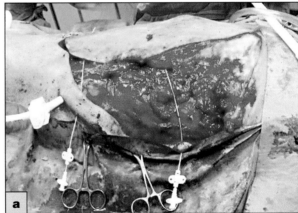

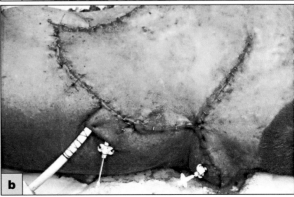

14.12 **(a)** Custom-made wound catheters placed during wound closure to ensure maximum coverage. **(b)** The wound catheters exit remotely from the wound closure and are secured in place with a Chinese finger-trap suture. Wound catheters should be clearly marked to avoid confusion with wound or chest drains.

with NSAIDs. In some cases, opioids may no longer be required following the immediate postoperative period and so pain assessment is important to plan appropriate additional analgesia.

The end of the catheter should be sealed with a catheter bung and local anaesthetic injected through it (bupivacaine 1–2 mg/kg q6–8h). Lidocaine has also been administered by infusion at 2 mg/kg/h but this can be associated with catheter disconnection, since these patients tend to be more mobile. One case of possible lidocaine toxicity has been reported where the catheter was placed adjacent to the brachial plexus (Abelson *et al.*, 2009) and so if this technique is used patients should be carefully monitored. The catheters can be removed at 48 hours or remain in place for longer (up to 72 hours) as required.

Occasionally the catheters may fail to provide analgesia for the full extent of the surgical site and this may be due to incorrect placement, uneven distribution of local anaesthetic or blockage of the catheter. It is a good idea to instil local anaesthetic prior to removing the catheter and to wait for the appropriate length of time for the drug used (e.g. 5–15 minutes for lidocaine and 10–20 minutes for bupivacaine).

Local nerve blocks

Local anaesthetic nerve blocks can be an easy and inexpensive way to provide effective analgesia in veterinary patients but they still tend to be overlooked. Practising the techniques will allow veterinary surgeons to provide the most effective analgesia, decreasing anaesthetic and analgesic costs and allowing client and veterinary satisfaction. Detailed information on how to perform the nerve blocks described here can be found in the *BSAVA Manual of Canine and Feline Anaesthesia and Analgesia*. A summary of some of the nerve blocks that can be used for head and limb surgery is provided in Figures 14.13 and 14.14. Some limb nerve blocks, such as epidural and the brachial plexus block, can be performed easily. For some of the other more specific nerve blocks, the use of a nerve locator (Figure 14.15) can greatly increase success rates.

Retrobulbar nerve block: A retrobulbar nerve block may be employed during enucleation or orbitectomy to provide excellent surgical conditions and good postoperative analgesia. This block will also result in a central eye (central pupil) and so can be useful for corneal and intraocular surgery.

Initial reports suggest that intraocular pressure is decreased, despite the injection of a volume of drug behind the eye, due to relaxation of the periorbital muscles. A retrobulbar block has the potential to increase bleeding due to vasodilation, but this does not appear to be a clinical problem. It also carries the risk of subarachnoid injection, intravascular injection, haemorrhage and globe puncture, and so aspiration of the needle should always be performed prior to injection. These complications are extremely rare in small animals as long as the procedure is performed correctly. It is a good idea to use this block for enucleations initially until the technique has been fully mastered.

Nerve block	Area of desensitization	Ease of block	Potential uses
Retrobulbar	Globe and retrobulbar space	+++	Enucleation, corneal and intraocular surgery
Infraorbital	Teeth of upper arcade rostral to premolars, nose	+++	Dental, nasal and muzzle surgery, pre-maxillectomy
Maxillary	Upper dental aracade, nose, soft and hard palates	+++	Dental, nasal surgery, nasal biopsy, maxillectomy
Mental	Lower dental arcade and mandible rostral to injection site	++	Dental
Inferior alveolar	Lower dental arcade, mandible, tongue	+++	Dental, mandibular fracture
Auriculotemporal and great auricular	Inner surface of auricular cartilage, external ear canal	++	Total ear canal ablation, ear examination

14.13 Nerve blocks to the head in dogs and cats. (+++ indicates the easiest block)

Nerve block	Area of desensitization	Ease of block	Potential uses
Brachial plexus	Thoracic limb distal to elbow (up to shoulder if nerve locator used)	+++	Surgery distal to elbow (if nerve locator used, area of blockade can be increased to shoulder)
Radial, ulnar, median and musculocutaneous nerves (RUMM)	Thoracic limb distal to elbow	++	Surgery distal to elbow (nerve locator required for consistent blockade)
Saphenous, common peroneal and tibial nerves	Pelvic limb distal to stifle	+	Surgery distal to stifle
Epidural analgesia	Pelvic limbs, perineum, caudal abdomen (level depends on volume of local anaesthetic injected)	++	Surgery of pelvic limb, perineum, abdomen
Digital nerve blocks	Digits	+++	Surgery to digits
Intravenous regional analgesia (IVRA)	Area below level of tourniquet placement	+++	Surgery to distal limb following tourniquet placement. Postoperative analgesia is minimal

14.14 Nerve blocks to the limbs in dogs and cats. (+++ indicates the easiest block)

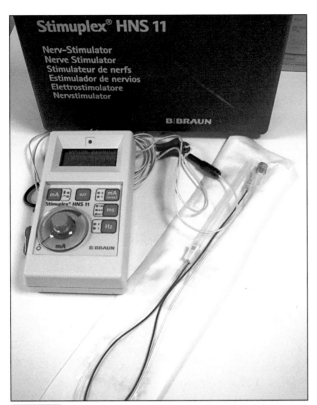

14.15 Nerve locator used in a number of limb blocks to locate motor nerves and allow placement of smaller volumes of local anaesthetic immediately adjacent to the nerves.

The block can be achieved by introducing a needle at the lateral canthus and directing it towards the opposite temporomandibular (TM) joint or by introducing the needle at the dorsal point of the orbit and following it ventrally. Currently, the author uses either a spinal needle which is curved to follow the outline of the globe, or a custom-made retrobulbar needle. With one finger deflecting the globe ventrally, the needle is introduced at the dorsal aspect under the orbital rim and directed behind the globe (Figure 14.16). The globe is seen to deflect dorsally when the needle reaches the muscle cone and, following aspiration to check that the tip has

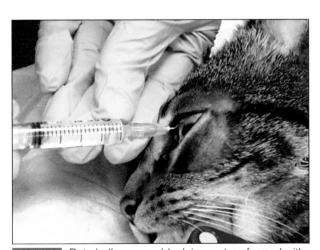

14.16 Retrobulbar nerve block in a cat performed with a curved needle introduced via the conjunctiva and guided around the globe. The needle should be aspirated to check for blood prior to injection of local anaesthetic. Alternatively, a spinal needle can be curved and introduced in the same way. The globe should rotate centrally once the local block takes effect.

not penetrated a blood vessel, 0.5–2.5 ml of local anaesthetic is injected.

Extradural/epidural analgesia

Epidural techniques can provide analgesia for perineal or pelvic limb surgery, using local anaesthetics or morphine (0.1 mg/kg) or both. A similar combination can be used at a higher volume (0.2 mg/kg) to provide analgesia for abdominal procedures. Morphine alone (0.1–0.3 mg/kg with volume made up to 0.25 ml/kg with sterile saline) can be used to provide additional analgesia for thoracic surgery or thoracic limb amputations.

A combination of long-acting local anaesthetic drugs and morphine are most commonly used, due to their prolonged duration. A brief summary of drugs used epidurally is given in Figure 14.17.

Analgesia can be induced by injecting drugs such as morphine and local anaesthetic into the epidural space, usually at the lumbosacral junction. In adult dogs the spinal cord normally terminates at the level of the caudal lumbar vertebrae, whereas it extends further back to the mid-sacrum in cats. In young dogs, termination may also be caudal to L7.

Drug	Dose	Duration of action	Possible side effects
Morphine (preservative-free)	0.1–0.3 mg/kg	Up to 24 hours	Pruritus, urinary retention
Lidocaine	1–4 mg/kg	45–90 minutes	Self-limiting paresis Splanchnic vasodilation (avoid in hypovolaemic animals)
Bupivacaine 0.5%	1 mg/kg	120–360 minutes	As for lidocaine
Ropivacaine	1 mg/kg	90–420 minutes	As for lidocaine
Medetomidine	5 µg/kg	120–240 minutes	Additive effect when combined with opioids

14.17 Drugs administered via the epidural route in dogs and cats.

Technique: The technique is easy to perform and time should be taken to ensure identification of the landmarks in the various breeds.

- The cranial edge of the wings of the ilium are used to locate the spinous process of the last lumbar vertebra.
- Caudal to this process, a depression can be palpated in the midline overlying the lumbosacral space.
- Further caudal to this the fused sacrum can be palpated.
- The injection needs to be given into the midline at the centre of the depression between the spinous process of L7 and the sacrum.

The technique can be performed with the patient in sternal or lateral recumbency, with the legs pulled forward, following aseptic preparation.

TECHNIQUE 14.1
Epidural injection

1 Place the needle in the centre of the depression, in the midline, directed perpendicular to the skin. An increase followed by a decrease in resistance to the advancement of the needle is often reported as the needle passes through the ligamentum flavum and enters the epidural space. This may not be easy to detect when using a spinal needle (shown at top) but is easier with the Tuohy needle (below).

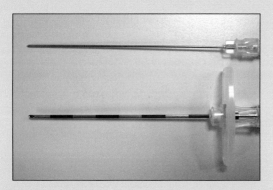

2 First, determine whether the tip of the needle is correctly placed in the epidural space.

A A small amount of air or sterile saline is injected. If it can be injected without encountering resistance, correct placement is confirmed. A loss-of-resistance syringe can be used. The plunger will spring back if any resistance is encountered during injection. These syringes are much more sensitive than normal syringes and can also be used to inject the drugs.

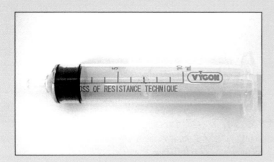

Following injection of air into the extradural space, air bubbles may persist for 24 hours. If too much air is introduced, the bubbles created may lead to displacement of the local anaesthetic solution and cause a 'patchy' blockade. If resistance is encountered, the needle should be repositioned and re-tested.

B If the stylet is removed from the needle before advancement into the extradural space, a bleb of sterile saline or local anaesthetic can be placed in the needle hub. When the tip of the needle reaches the extradural space, the bleb will be 'sucked' into the needle as loss of resistance is encountered, confirming correct placement. The placement should still be tested as above to ensure it is correct. This 'hanging drop' technique works well in sternal but not in lateral recumbency and can result in false negatives. Some authors have also looked at measuring the pressure to identify the epidural space.

C If bone is encountered during placement of the needle it may be possible that the extradural space has been missed and the ventral floor of the spinal canal has been encountered. The needle should be gradually retracted and loss of resistance re-tested every 0.5 mm until the epidural space is encountered. Using this technique increases the likelihood of penetrating blood vessels, but should not cause any significant problems.

3 Inject the drug. An air bubble can be used during injection to check correct placement. As the plunger is depressed, the air bubble should retain its shape. If resistance is encountered, the air bubble will be compressed.

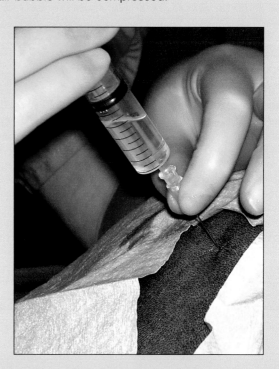

WARNING

Contraindications to epidural injection include:

- Skin infections over the injection site
- Coagulopathies
- Low platelet count
- Systemic sepsis
- Pelvic/sacral fractures if the space cannot be palpated.

Complications of epidural injection: Problems that may be encountered include the following:

■ Lack of or slow hair regrowth of the patch of hair clipped for epidural injection may occur in some dogs, and owners should be warned of this before the block is performed

■ Depending on which drugs are used, hindlimb function may be lost for a variable duration of time. Occasionally, the duration of blockade lasts longer than 24 hours, but this is rare. If loss of hindlimb function is not desirable following the surgical procedure, morphine alone should be used. Occasionally, hyperaesthesia can occur after epidural blockade and chewing of the hindlimbs may be encountered, but this complication is extremely rare

■ Bladder function should be monitored following epidural morphine administration, since urinary retention may occur. Manually expressing the bladder once is usually enough to manage this problem.

Extradural/epidural catheters

For certain procedures or conditions, longer term epidural analgesia may be preferable and an epidural catheter may be placed to allow repeated administration of analgesia. For example, conditions such as pancreatitis or extensive hindlimb/pelvic or abdominal surgeries may benefit from this technique. Epidural catheters may also be useful for extensive thoracic surgeries (e.g. median sternotomy), depending on the other local anaesthetic techniques employed. Epidural catheters can remain in place for prolonged periods if managed with strict asepsis.

An epidural catheter may be placed at the lumbosacral junction. A Tuohy needle is used to introduce the catheter into the extradural space. Needle placement is similar to that for extradural injection, but the needle needs to be introduced into the extradural canal at a shallower angle so that the catheter is then fed down into the extradural space without any kinking. Before placement of an extradural catheter, the procedure should be practised using a cadaver to get an idea of the degree of resistance usually encountered while feeding the catheter through the Tuohy needle.

1. Once the needle has been placed and tested for correct placement, the catheter is fed through the needle into the epidural space. Injection of a small amount of lidocaine through the Tuohy needle before catheter insertion has proved helpful for advancement of the catheter in humans.
2. The distance of insertion into the canal beyond the length of the needle should be estimated prior to placement so that the tip of the catheter can be positioned at the correct location.
   • For pelvic limb procedures, catheters can be placed at the level of the caudal lumbar vertebrae at L4.
   • For abdominal procedures, the tip should lie at L1–2.
   • For thoracotomies the tip may be placed more cranially at T5–6.

• Radiography or fluoroscopy should be used to verify correct placement. A positive response, seen as improved patient comfort, to administration of analgesic agents may also demonstrate correct positioning in the conscious patient.
3. A filter is connected to the catheter, which is then secured in place using a Chinese finger-trap suture along with butterfly tape and sutures. Since dislodgement of catheters is the most common complication of epidural catheter use in dogs, it is important to ensure good stabilization at the outset.

Drugs are administered in smaller volumes to provide segmental analgesia and can be given to effect in many cases. Intermittent administration of analgesic drugs can be given, or an infusion provided using a syringe driver. Preservative-free morphine (0.1 mg/kg) can be administered every 12–24 hours, whilst bupivacaine (0.06–0.12 mg/kg) can be administered intermittently as required. Infusions of morphine at 0.0125 mg/kg/h and bupivacaine at 0.03 mg/kg/h have been reported (Hansen, 2001). If motor blockade is excessive, the infusion is temporarily stopped and the bupivacaine diluted further (0.125–0.25%). The administration of analgesia can be adjusted, depending on the patient's needs.

Intravenous regional analgesia (IVRA)

Local anaesthetic agents such as lidocaine may be administered intravenously via a limb vein distal to a tourniquet to allow surgery of the distal limb, such as toe amputation. Lidocaine is used as it has a rapid onset of action and systemic intravenous use carries few risks at recommended dose rates.

■ IVRA relies on the presence of a tourniquet to keep the local anaesthetic in the area distal to the tourniquet. Analgesia is maintained until shortly following tourniquet release and therefore does not provide postoperative analgesia.

■ IVRA with lidocaine has been used in the dog at recommended dose rates of 0.5–5 mg/kg. The technique has also been used experimentally in cats, with 3 mg/kg providing analgesia for up to 20 minutes following removal of the tourniquet.

It is important to remember that postoperative analgesia is not a feature of this technique and perhaps specific digital nerve blocks would be more useful, or could be used in conjunction with this technique. Drugs such as bupivacaine, which are extensively protein-bound, are not ideally suited for this technique, but recent work suggests that they may provide a more long-term effect due to extensive tissue binding. Alpha-2 agonists have also been used in human practice to provide more profound analgesia.

The easiest way to perform this technique is to place a small-gauge intravenous catheter in a vein distal to the predicted tourniquet placement and then wrap the catheter to secure it in place while the tourniquet is placed in the normal fashion. Once the tourniquet has been secured, lidocaine at 1–2 mg/kg can be injected and the catheter removed (Figure 14.18).

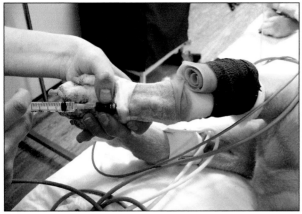

14.18 Intravenous regional analgesia (IVRA). Following placement of an intravenous catheter, an Esmarch bandage is placed and secured. The lidocaine is injected through the catheter to provide analgesia distal to the tourniquet until its release. The catheter is removed following injection.

NMDA antagonists
NMDA glutamate receptor plays a key role in central nervous system sensitization and hyperalgesia in pain syndromes. The use of NMDA antagonists may help in reducing the development of central sensitization following surgery and may also be of particular benefit for surgical procedures resulting in nerve damage.

Mechanism of action
Although these agents belong to a group of drugs called dissociative anaesthetics, they are used at sub-anaesthetic doses for analgesia. A number of mechanisms of action have been proposed apart from the antagonism at the NMDA receptor site, such as:

- Depression of acetylcholine receptors
- Prolongation and enhancement of gamma-aminobutyric acid (GABA$_A$) receptors
- Depression of nociceptive neurons in the reticular formation and in laminae I and V of the dorsal horn
- Action on voltage-dependent sodium, potassium and calcium channels.

Tissue trauma causes continuous nociceptive stimulation of C fibres that activate NMDA receptors in the central nervous system. This causes a decrease in the threshold for glutamate in the nociceptive pathways, making these receptors even more receptive to stimuli. Central wind-up may subsequently develop, which will amplify postoperative pain.

NMDA antagonists undergo significant hepatic biotransformation. Metabolism of these agents is slower in animals that suffer from any kind of hepatic dysfunction.

Systemic side effects

Central nervous system: Cerebral vasodilation and elevated systemic blood pressure lead to significant increases in cerebral blood flow, intracranial pressure and cerebrospinal fluid pressure. Abnormal behaviour may occur; head bobbing is commonly seen if excessive doses are administered, but more serious side effects such as nystagmus and seizures can occur.

Cardiovascular: NMDA antagonists cause cardiovascular stimulation via sympathetic activation.

Respiratory: Salivation and increased respiratory tract secretions occur with extensive doses.

Thermoregulation: At higher doses hyperthermia may be seen.

Ketamine
In veterinary medicine, use of bolus injections or low-dose ketamine infusions for adjunctive analgesia has become common practice in the perioperative setting (e.g. orthopaedic procedures, hemilaminectomies for treatment of intervertebral disc disease, amputations).

A number of studies that have investigated the MAC-sparing properties of ketamine clearly suggest that ketamine may contribute to balanced anaesthesia protocols in dogs and cats, but they do not address the question of postoperative analgesia *per se*. At present, there are very few studies that evaluate the analgesic effects of ketamine in the perioperative period in dogs. The results available so far demonstrate that ketamine administration decreases pain scores, rescue analgesic requirements and postoperative wound hyperalgesia. Suggested doses for ketamine use in dogs and cats are given in Figure 14.19.

Dogs	Cats
0.25–1 mg/kg i.v. followed by CRI 5–10 µg/kg/min	0.25–1 mg/kg i.v. followed by CRI 5–10 µg/kg/min
Postoperatively use at a rate of 5 µg/kg/min, add 75 mg ketamine to 500 ml fluid bag to administer at 2 ml/kg/h	Postoperatively use at a rate of 5 µg/kg/min, add 75 mg ketamine to 500 ml fluid bag to administer at 2 ml/kg/h

14.19 Suggested doses for ketamine in dogs and cats.

Alpha-2 adrenoreceptor agonists
Although not considered first-line analgesics like opioids or NSAIDs, alpha-2 agonists are commonly used as adjunctive analgesics. Because their mechanism of action is similar to that of opioids, co-administration of these two classes of drugs is thought to produce synergistic analgesic effects.

Mechanism of action
Analgesia seems to be the result of both cerebral and spinal effects, possibly in part mediated by serotonin and the descending endogenous analgesia system. In addition, alpha-2 adrenergic receptors and opioid receptors seem to be able to interact, though the mechanism of this interaction is still not fully understood.

Systemic side effects

Cardiovascular: The effect is biphasic, with an initial peripheral phase of vasoconstriction, hypertension and reflex bradycardia and a subsequent central phase of decreased sympathetic tone. Atricoventricular (AV) block can occur. Cardiac output decreases due to the decreased heart rate and increased vascular resistance, but blood flow to essential organs is maintained by redistribution of flow from less vital organs and tissues.

Respiratory: Respiratory rate and minute ventilation decrease after administration, but this seems to be related to a decrease in carbon dioxide production.

Gastrointestinal: Nausea and vomiting are described at higher doses.

Renal: Alpha-2 agonists interfere with the action of antidiuretic hormone on the renal tubules and collecting ducts, which causes an increase in urine production and a decrease in urine specific gravity.

Urogenital: Myometrial contractility is increased and alpha-2 agonists are contraindicated in the last trimester of pregnancy.

Endocrine: Preoperative administration attenuates the stress response associated with the surgical trauma, and catecholamine and cortisol concentrations are reduced postoperatively. The release of insulin is temporarily inhibited, resulting in hyperglycaemia, which may contribute to polyuria.

Thermoregulation: Hypothermia is observed. It is caused by a number of factors, including depression of the thermoregulatory centre, muscle relaxation and reduced shivering.

Medetomidine and dexmedetomidine
Of the available alpha-2 agonists, medetomidine is currently the one most commonly used for adjunctive analgesia in veterinary medicine. Dexmedetomidine is the pharmacologically active enantiomer found in the racemic mixture of medetomidine.

Medetomidine and dexmedetomidine may be used as adjunctive analgesics in a variety of clinical settings. It is noteworthy that the analgesic effects of these drugs are of shorter duration than the sedative effects. Perhaps most commonly, medetomidine is used in combination with an opioid before inducing general anaesthesia in dogs and cats.

Routes of administration
CRI techniques using alpha-2 agonists are suitable for pain management both intra- and postoperatively. A recent study demonstrated that a dexmedetomidine CRI was equally as effective as a morphine CRI in providing postoperative analgesia, with no clinical adverse reactions observed (Valtolina et al., 2009). Patients receiving such treatment typically appear sedated but are easily rousable, which is advantageous if postoperative inactivity is desired (e.g. spinal trauma). In the situations described above, the alpha-2 agonist is always used at a low dose (Figure 14.20) in a patient that is cardiovascularly stable, and is perhaps most useful for patients that require anxiolysis in addition to analgesia.

As well as systemic administration, alpha-2 agonists may be administered by other routes. The spinal site of action seems to be important in mediating alpha-2 agonist-induced analgesia. It has been demonstrated that incorporation of a low dose of medetomidine into an epidural protocol in dogs produces additive or synergistic analgesic effects when combined with standard doses of opioids or local anaesthetics. Medetomidine is lipophilic and rapidly cleared from cerebrospinal fluid. Consequently, when the total dose administered approaches that which would otherwise be given systemically, the specificity of the regional analgesic effect may be lost. Recommended doses of alpha-2 agonists for use by the above routes are provided in Figure 14.20.

In addition to the epidural route, alpha-2 agonists may be administered by other peripheral routes to supplement analgesia. For example, alpha-2 adrenergic receptors have been identified intra-articularly and perineurally, where they seem to contribute to analgesia by inhibition of noradrenaline release. There are currently no veterinary studies evaluating medetomidine administered by these routes.

Drug	Dose (dogs)	Dose (cats)	Duration of effect after bolus
Medetomidine	1–5 µg/kg s.c., i.m., i.v. CRI: 0.5–2 µg/kg/h	1–5 µg/kg s.c., i.m., i.v. CRI: 0.5–2 µg/kg/h	1–2 hours (dose-dependent)
Dexmedetomidine	0.5–3 µg/kg s.c., i.m., i.v. CRI: 0.25–1 µg/kg/h	0.5–3 µg/kg s.c., i.m., i.v. CRI: 0.25–1 µg/kg/h	1–2 hours (dose-dependent)

14.20 Doses of medetomidine and dexmedetomidine in dogs and cats.

Anticonvulsants
Neuromodulating drugs, such as anticonvulsants, have become the mainstay of treatment for neuropathic pain in human patients in the last decade. Both pregabalin and gabapentin have been shown to have a similar mechanism of action, mediated via the $\alpha_2\delta$ subunit of voltage-gated calcium channels, which are upregulated in the dorsal root ganglia and spinal cord after a noxious insult.

Mechanism of action
The exact mechanism by which these drugs produce their analgesic effects is still not fully understood. Although they are structurally related to GABA, they do not bind directly to this receptor. They are believed to bind selectively to the $\alpha_2\delta$ subunit of the voltage-gated calcium channels, reducing the calcium influx into the presynaptic nerve terminal and thereby inhibiting the release of excitatory neurotransmitters involved in pain transmission, such as glutamate and substance P.

Systemic side effects
Dizziness, sleepiness and headache are the most commonly reported side effects in human patients. Weight gain and peripheral oedema have also been described, but definitions of weight gain varied and oedema was not accompanied by evidence of cardiac and renal dysfunction. In veterinary medicine, when used as an anticonvulsant in dogs, the side effects are minimal and are restricted to mild sedation and pelvic limb ataxia.

Clinically used anticonvulsants
Anticonvulsants can be administered either during the perioperative period, as analgesic adjuvants, or long term for the treatment of chronic pain of a neuropathic nature. However, at the time of publication, only a limited number of veterinary publications on their use are available.

Gabapentin: The use of gabapentin as an adjunctive analgesic agent has increased significantly in veterinary medicine over the past few years. Gabapentin is a useful oral analgesic agent for potential neuropathic pain states and can be a useful adjunct following spinal surgery, pelvic trauma, amputation or whenever nerve damage is suspected. Gabapentin can be given orally preoperatively to decrease postoperative pain scores. It has anecdotally been used to treat chronic neuropathic pain, chronic cancer pain, chronic osteoarthritis pain and, increasingly lately, perioperative pain in dogs and cats. A recent study supports the routine preoperative use of gabapentin to provide postoperative analgesia in dogs undergoing spinal surgery (Cashmore *et al.*, 2009).

Dosing guidelines in veterinary medicine have been largely based on human recommendations, despite some key species differences in pharmacokinetics. In dogs, gabapentin is known to undergo significant hepatic metabolism to *N*-methyl-gabapentin before renal elimination. Gabapentin disposition has not been studied to date in cats. Based on collective clinical experience, doses in the range of 5–10 mg/kg orally q8–12h are recommended initially, and most regimens typically require adjustments to achieve the desired analgesic effect without significant sedation.

Pregabalin: Pregabalin is the developmental successor of gabapentin, and as such it was designed to present a higher potency and a linear pharmacokinetic profile. In human medicine, the analgesic efficacy of pregabalin has been studied extensively. It has been proven effective for neuropathic pain and also when administered perioperatively for various soft tissue surgical procedures. Several large clinical trials substantiate its safety and efficacy for each of these indications.

Analgesic effects of pregabalin have not been investigated in veterinary species to date. At the time of publication, the only pharmacokinetic study in dogs suggested that oral administration of pregabalin at 4 mg/kg q12h is appropriate.

Summary and planning of rational multimodal analgesia

There is no point having elaborate analgesic protocols without the use of pain scoring systems that can assess the standard of analgesia provided. Simple systems can be adapted for use in the practice setting and they have many advantages.

Analgesia should always be administered prior to the surgery whenever possible. Such pre-emptive analgesia has been shown to improve pain management during the postoperative period in animals.

If using an opioid in the preanaesthetic medication, it should be administered so that the peak effect is seen during surgery (usually 30–60 minutes before induction of anaesthesia). This will help to provide a smooth induction, maintenance and recovery period. It must be remembered that one dose may not be sufficient and some animals will require a further top-up of opioid either intraoperatively or before recovery, when analgesic requirements will be highest. Good pre-emptive analgesia is paramount for ensuring smooth recoveries and will not delay recovery time.

Opioids are the first drugs used for surgical pain but a multimodal approach should be taken in all patients (see Figure 14.4). NSAIDs should be administered pre-emptively where there is no contraindication. In animals where hypovolaemia has not been corrected fully prior to surgery and where there is a risk of hypotension, NSAIDs should be withheld until blood volume has been corrected in the postoperative period. Robenacoxib may need to be administered at the time of induction, as it has a short plasma half-life but will concentrate in inflamed tissues including tissues inflamed as a result of surgical trauma.

For the majority of surgeries, the use of a combination of opioids and NSAIDs will be sufficient if their administration is timed correctly and a suitable dose is used. For opioids, a higher dose or a subsequent top-up may be required for more invasive surgeries. In addition to opioids and NSAIDs, local anaesthetic techniques should be employed wherever possible to prevent intra- and postoperative nociception.

If an opioid proves insufficient, an additional dose should be administered. If this needs to be repeated frequently or a high dose is required, adjunctive analgesic agents should be administered depending on the procedure.

- Intravenous infusions (or single bolus doses) of ketamine may be administered if a neuropathic component to the pain is suspected.
- Intravenous lidocaine can be useful if there is marked inflammatory pain (e.g. abdominal surgery) and can also be used when neuropathic pain is suspected.
- Alpha-2 adrenoceptor agonists can be administered as a bolus, particularly for patients exhibiting poor recoveries, to provide sedation and analgesia whilst a further dose of opioid is administered, or as a an intravenous infusion to provide mild sedation and analgesia.

Simple nursing care steps can also allow the animal to recover in a more comfortable environment. For example, the bladder should be emptied at the end of surgery if possible and warm, comfortable bedding provided. Non-slip bedding is particularly useful for orthopaedic patients. If recumbency is predicted, an indwelling urinary catheter should be placed at the time of surgery.

References and further reading

Abelson AL, McConn EC, Shaw S *et al.* (2009) Use of wound soaker catheters for the administration of local anesthetic for post-operative analgesia: 56 cases. *Veterinary Anaesthia and Analgesia* **36**, 59–60

Boscan P, Pypendop BH, Solano AM and Ilkiw JE (2005) Cardiovascular and respiratory effects of ketamine infusions in isoflurane-anesthetized dogs before and during noxious stimulation. *American Journal of Veterinary Research* **66**, 2122–2129

Bubalo V, Moens YP, Holzmann A and Coppens P (2008) Anaesthetic sparing effect of local anaesthesia of the ovarian pedical during ovariohysterectomy in dogs. *Veterinary Anaesthesia and Analgesia* **35**, 537–542

Buber T, Saragusty J, Ranen E *et al.* (2007) Evaluation of lidocaine treatment and risk factors for death associated with gastric dilation and volvulus in dogs: 112 cases (1997–2005). *Journal of the American Veterinary Medical Association* **230**, 1334–1339

Capner CA, Lascelles BDX and Waterman-Pearson AE (1999) Current British veterinary attitudes to peri-operative analgesia for dogs. *Veterinary Record* **145**, 95–99

Carpenter RE, Wilson DV and Evans AT (2004) Evaluation of intraperitoneal and incisional lidocaine or bupivacaine for analgesia following ovariohysterectomy in the dog. *Veterinary Anaesthesia and Analgesia* **31**, 46–52

Cashmore RG, Harcourt-Brown TR, Freeman PM *et al.* (2009) Clinical diagnosis and treatment of suspected neuropathic pain in three dogs. *Australian Veterinary Journal* **87**, 45–50

Hansen BD (2001) Epidural catheter analgesia in dogs and cats: technique and review of 182 cases (1991–1999). *Journal of Veterinary Emergency and Critical Care* **11**, 95–103

MacDougall LM, Hethey JA, Livingston A *et al.* (2009) Antinociceptive, cardiopulmonary, and sedative effects of five intravenous infusion rates of lidocaine in conscious dogs. *Veterinary Anaesthesia and Analgesia* **36**, 512–522

McMillan M, Seymour C and Brearley J (2011) Effect of intratesticular lidocaine on isoflurane requirements and postoperative pain in dogs undergoing elective castration. *BSAVA Congress Scientific Proceedings: Veterinary Programme*, p.488 [abstract]

Molony V and Kent JE (1997) Assessment of acute pain in farm animals using behavioral and physiological measurements. *Journal of Animal Science* **75**, 266–272

Muir WW 3rd and Hubbell JA (1988) Cardiopulmonary and anesthetic effects of ketamine and its enantiomers in dogs. *American Journal of Veterinary Research* **49**, 530–534

Ngo LY, Tam YK, Tawfik S *et al.* (1997) Effects of intravenous infusion of lidocaine on its pharmacokinetics in conscious instrumented dogs. *Journal of Pharmaceutical Science* **86**, 944–952

Pascoe PJ, Ilkiw JE, Craig C and Kollias-Baker C (2007) The effects of ketamine on the minimum alveolar concentration of isoflurane in cats. *Veterinary Anaesthesia and Analgesia* **34**, 31–39

Pypendop BH and Ilkiw JE (2005a) Assessment of the hemodynamic effects of lidocaine administered IV in isoflurane anesthetized cats. *American Journal of Veterinary Research* **66**, 661–668

Pypendop BH and Ilkiw JE (2005b). The effects of intravenous lidocaine administration on the minimum alveolar concentration of isoflurane in cats. *Anesthesia and Analgesia* **100**, 97–101

Pypendop BH, Ilkiw JE and Robertson SA (2006) Effects of intravenous administration of lidocaine on the thermal threshold in cats. *American Journal of Veterinary Research* **67**, 16–20

Reid J, Nolan AM, Hughes JML *et al.* (2007) Development of the short-form Glasgow Composite Measure Pain Scale (CMPS-SF) and derivation of an analgesic intervention score. *Animal Welfare* **16**(S), 97–104

Seymour C (2010) Acute pain: assessment and management. In: *BSAVA Manual of Canine and Feline Rehabilitation, Supportive and Palliative Care*, ed. S. Lindley and P. Watson, pp.7–18. BSAVA, Gloucester

Solano AM, Pypendop BH, Boscan PL and Ilkiw JE (2006) Effect of intravenous administration of ketamine on the minimum alveolar concentration of isoflurane in anesthetized dogs. *American Journal of Veterinary Research* **67**, 21–25

Steagall PV, Teixeira Neto FJ, Minto BW *et al.* (2006) Evaluation of the isoflurane-sparing effects of lidocaine and fentanyl during surgery in dogs. *Journal of the American Veterinary Medical Association* **229**, 522–527

Valtolina C, Robben JH, Uilenreef J *et al.* (2009) Clinical evaluation of the efficacy and safety of a constant rate infusion of dexmedetomidine for postoperative pain management in dogs. *Veterinary Anaesthesia and Analgesia* **36**, 369–383

Valverde A, Doherty TJ, Hernández J and Davies W (2004) Effect of lidocaine on the minimum alveolar concentration of isoflurane in dogs. *Veterinary Anaesthesia and Analgesia* **31**, 264–271

Wagner AE, Walton JA, Hellyer PW *et al.* (2002) Use of low doses of ketamine administered by constant rate infusion as an adjunct for postoperative analgesia in dogs. *Journal of the American Veterinary Medical Association* **221**, 72–75

Principles of nutritional support

Daniel L. Chan

Introduction

Appropriate nutritional support has long been considered essential for the recovery of postoperative, critically ill and injured human patients. Whilst there is convincing evidence of the deleterious effects of malnutrition in people, the optimal nutritional strategies for critically ill and postoperative animals remain controversial and are largely unknown.

Despite the lack of definitive answers, it must be emphasized that recommendations for nutritional support of critically ill animals are based on current understanding of the metabolic response to injury and the limited clinical information available. This should not discourage the implementation of nutritional support for critically ill or injured animals. In fact, with proper patient selection, sound nutritional planning and careful monitoring, nutritional support can be an integral part in the successful recovery of many critically ill animals (see *BSAVA Manual of Canine and Feline Rehabilitation, Supportive and Palliative Care* for case examples).

Metabolic responses

The metabolic responses to illness or severe injury are complex and place critically ill animals at high risk for malnutrition and its deleterious effects. These effects, which may result in significant morbidity, include alterations in energy and substrate metabolism, depressed immune function and impaired wound healing, all of which have important implications for surgical patients.

Ebb and flow phases

Whilst generalizations tend to oversimplify complex systems, the concept of 'ebb/flow' offers a basic description of the metabolic response to critical illness and severe injury. According to this model, there is an initial hypometabolic response (**ebb phase**), followed by a period of a more prolonged course of hypermetabolism (**flow phase**).

Ebb phase

The ebb phase is usually a period of haemodynamic instability associated with:

- Decreased energy expenditure
- Hypothermia
- Mild protein catabolism
- Decreased cardiac output
- Poor tissue perfusion.

Without stabilization, this may progress to a state of refractory or irreversible shock characterized by severe lactic acidosis, decreased tissue perfusion, multiple organ failure and death. Nutritional intervention at this stage carries a greater risk of complications such as electrolyte abnormalities, which may result in further detrimental effects in some critically ill animals.

Flow phase

Following successful resuscitation, patients enter the flow phase, during which profound metabolic alterations occur. Hallmarks of this response include:

- Increased energy expenditure
- Increased glucose production
- Increased insulin and glucagon concentrations
- Increased cardiac output
- Profound protein catabolism.

Provision of nutritional support during this stage of illness can attenuate and sometimes reverse the detrimental effects of malnutrition.

Body protein catabolism

One of the major metabolic alterations associated with critical illness involves body protein catabolism, in which protein turnover rates may become markedly elevated.

- Healthy animals primarily lose fat when deprived of sufficient calories (**simple starvation**).
- Sick or traumatized patients catabolize lean body mass when they are not provided with sufficient calories (**stressed starvation**).

In the healthy state:

- During the initial stages of fasting, glycogen stores are used as the primary source of energy

- Within days, a metabolic shift occurs towards the preferential use of stored fat depots, sparing catabolic effects on lean muscle tissue.

In diseased states:

- The inflammatory response triggers alterations in cytokine and hormone concentrations and rapidly shifts metabolism towards a catabolic state
- Glycogen stores are quickly depleted, especially in strict carnivores such as the cat, and this leads to an early mobilization of amino acids from muscle stores
- As cats undergo continuous gluconeogenesis, the mobilization of amino acids from muscle is more pronounced than that observed in other species
- With continued lack of food intake, the predominant energy source is derived from accelerated proteolysis (muscle breakdown), which in itself is an energy-consuming process
- Muscle catabolism that occurs during stress provides the liver with gluconeogenic precursors and other amino acids for glucose and acute-phase protein production.

The resulting negative nitrogen balance or net protein loss has been documented in critically ill dogs and cats. One study estimated that 73% of hospitalized dogs (including postoperative patients) evaluated in four different veterinary referral centres were in a negative energy balance (Remillard *et al.,* 2001).

The consequences of continued lean body mass losses include negative effects on wound healing, immune function, strength (both skeletal and respiratory muscle strength), and ultimately on overall prognosis. In the context of postoperative patients, this could lead to greater risk of surgical wound dehiscence and postoperative infections. Due to the metabolic alterations associated with critical illness, and in part due to an inability or reluctance of many critically ill and postoperative dogs and cats to take in sufficient calories, this patient population is at increased risk for rapid development of malnutrition.

Given the serious sequelae of malnutrition, preservation or reversal of deteriorating nutritional status via nutritional support is very important. Nutritional support is therefore aimed at minimizing the impact of malnutrition and enhancing rate of recovery.

Identifying the need for nutritional support

The ideal approach in the treatment of postoperative patients would be to ensure adequate nutrient intake in all cases. However, from a practical point of view this is not feasible in many cases (e.g. short-term hospitalization or concurrent problems such as nausea or severe vomiting). Therefore the aim of performing nutritional assessment (see below) is to identify those patients where nutritional intervention is likely to have the most beneficial effect.

Risk factors

Currently, identification of overt malnutrition in animals can be challenging because there are no established criteria of malnutrition in companion animals. However, there are some proposed risk factors in dogs and cats that should prompt immediate consideration for implementing nutritional support (Figure 15.1).

- In dogs, a period as short as 3 days of anorexia has been documented to produce metabolic changes consistent with those seen associated with starvation in people. These dogs would not necessarily exhibit any easily detectable abnormalities on clinical assessment suggestive of being malnourished. Dogs with overt signs suggestive of malnutrition (Figure 15.2) usually have a more protracted period (usually weeks to months) of disease progression.

Factor	Examples
Bodyweight	Loss of at least 10% since onset of clinical signs
Physical signs	Non-healing wounds Poor haircoat and skin quality Muscle wasting
Food intake	Prolonged inadequate intake, defined as consuming <75% of resting energy requirement (RER) for >5 days
Catabolic processes	Chronic infection High glucocorticoid condition (endogenous or exogenous) Burns Neoplasia Chronic inflammatory conditions
Dietary deficiencies	Long-term use of unbalanced diets deficient in macro- and/or micronutrients
Chronic malabsorptive digestive disease	Chronic diarrhoea Steatorrhoea Exocrine pancreatic insufficiency Lymphangiectasia Inflammatory bowel disease Infiltrative neoplasia
Large protein-wasting processes	Draining wounds Exudative processes resulting in severe hypoalbuminaemia

15.1 Proposed risk factors for malnutrition in animals.

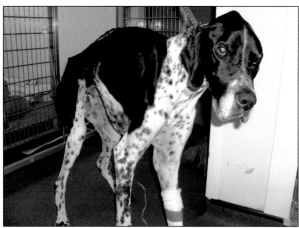

15.2 Dog with overt signs of malnutrition showing marked muscle wasting.

- In cats, detectable impairment of immune function can be demonstrated in healthy cats subjected to acute starvation by day 4 and so recommendations to institute some form of nutritional support in any ill cat with inadequate food intake for more than 3 days have been made.
- In both dogs and cats, there is some consensus that there is an urgent need to implement nutritional intervention (e.g. place feeding tube, commence parenteral nutrition) when the animal has not eaten for more than 5 days.

Therapeutic goals

Regardless of the severity of malnutrition, the immediate goals of therapy in any critically ill patient should focus on cardiovascular resuscitation, stabilization of vital signs and identification of primary disease process.

As steps are taken to address the primary disease, formulation of a nutritional plan should strive to prevent (or correct) overt nutritional deficiencies and imbalances. Where adequate energy substrates, protein, essential fatty acids and micronutrients are provided, the body can support wound healing, immune function and tissue repair.

A major goal of nutritional support is to minimize metabolic derangements and the catabolism of lean body tissue. During hospitalization, recovery of normal bodyweight is not the top priority, as this should occur once the animal is discharged from the hospital and completes its recovery at home.

Nutritional assessment

Since all nutritional support techniques carry some risk of complications, appropriate patient selection is crucial in ensuring the full benefits of nutritional support. Subjective clinical assessment remains the predominant method of identifying malnourished patients that require nutritional support (see Figure 15.1) and determining how best to provide that nutritional support, taking into consideration the animal's specific needs.

Formulation of a nutritional plan should address:

- Which patient requires nutritional support
- How that nutrition should be delivered
- The form or type of support
- The duration of administration.

Nutritional assessment should also identify factors that can affect the nutritional plan, such as electrolyte abnormalities, hyperglycaemia, hypertriglyceridamia, hyperammonaemia, or concurrent illnesses (e.g. renal or hepatic failure). For example, a malnourished dog with hepatic encephalopathy would not be a candidate for aggressive nutritional support predominantly composed of protein. Similarly, a cat with severe uraemia would not be a good candidate for an energy-dense high-protein, and therefore high-phosphate, food.

Finally, nutritional assessment takes into consideration all factors that are likely to affect how the animal responds to or tolerates nutritional intervention. Factors to be considered when performing nutritional assessment are summarized in Figure 15.3.

- Is the patient showing overt signs of malnutrition?
- Does the patient have risk factors for the development of malnutrition?
- How urgently does the patient need nutritional support?
- Does the patient have a contraindication to being fed enterally?
- If the patient cannot be fed enterally, can it be safely fed parenterally?
- Are there abnormalities that will complicate the nutrition plan (e.g. hyperglycaemia, hypertriglyceridaemia, severe uraemia, hepatic failure)?

15.3 Factors to be considered when performing nutritional assessment.

Nutritional plan

The key to successful nutritional management of critically ill patients lies in the proper diagnosis and treatment of the underlying disease. Another crucial factor is the selection of the appropriate route of nutritional support.

Providing nutrition via a functional digestive system is the preferred route of feeding and particular care should be taken to evaluate whether the patient can tolerate enteral feeding. Even if the patient can only tolerate small amounts of enteral nutrition, this route of feeding should be used and supplemented with parenteral nutrition only if deemed necessary to meet the patient's nutritional needs.

On the basis of the nutritional assessment, the anticipated duration of nutritional support and appropriate route of delivery (i.e. enteral or parenteral), a nutritional plan is formulated to meet the patient's nutritional needs, which for the majority of patients is the provision of its resting energy requirement (RER). Some animals will require more than their RER, but the initial target for most animals should be to meet the RER in a couple of days and only to increase this amount if after reassessment the animal continues to lose weight.

The first steps in instituting nutritional support include:

- Restoring proper hydration status
- Correcting electrolyte or acid–base disturbances (see Chapter 10)
- Achieving haemodynamic stability.

Commencing nutritional support before these abnormalities are addressed can increase the risk of complications and, in some cases, further compromise the patient.

It should be emphasized that this is *not* counter to the concept of 'early nutritional support', which has been documented to result in positive effects in several animal and human studies (Lewis *et al.*, 2001; Bisgaard *et al.*, 2002). Early nutritional support advocates feeding as soon as feasible (usually within 48 hours from admission, or within 48 hours after surgery) after achieving haemodynamic stability, rather than delaying nutritional intervention by several days. Previously, nutritional support in both animals and people did not begin until after 10 days of poor food intake.

Implementation of the nutritional plan should be gradual, with the goal of reaching target levels of nutrient delivery in 48–72 hours.

Nutritional requirements

Protein

Whereas the protein requirements of critically ill and postoperative human patients have been determined based on nitrogen balance studies, nitrogen balance is not commonly measured in critically ill animals.

One method of estimating the extent of amino acid catabolism is to measure urinary urea nitrogen content. Whilst measurement of urinary urea nitrogen in critically ill and postoperative dogs has been shown to be a feasible tool in assessing nitrogen balance, further studies are warranted to identify the specific protein requirements of critically ill animals.

Currently, many authors recommend that:

- Hospitalized dogs should be supported with at least 4–6 g of protein/100 kcal (15–25% of total energy requirements)
- Hospitalized cats should be supported with 6–8 g of protein/100 kcal (25–35% of total energy requirements).

These targets are in excess of the minimal required amounts for the maintenance of healthy dogs and cats as described in guidelines published by the National Research Council and the European Pet Food Industry Federation (FEDIAF). No specific recommendations have been made with regards to the protein requirements of veterinary postoperative patients, but guidelines for critically ill animals are thought to be adequate. Patients with protein intolerance (e.g. those with hepatic encephalopathy or severe uraemia) should receive reduced amounts of protein.

Other nutrients

Patients with hyperglycaemia or hyperlipidaemia may also require decreased amounts of these nutrients. Other nutritional requirements will depend upon the patient's underlying disease, clinical signs and laboratory parameters.

Glutamine and arginine: A number of recent human studies have evaluated the modulation of disease with nutrients such as such as glutamine, arginine, and omega-3 fatty acids.

Glutamine is a primary energy source for enterocytes and cells of the immune system and its supplementation may prevent increased gastrointestinal permeability and improve overall immune function. In certain populations of critically ill people, supplementation with either enteral or parenteral glutamine has been

shown to reduce infectious complications and improve survival. Studies in dogs and cats have failed to demonstrate clear benefits of glutamine supplementation but these trials did not evaluate outcome variables or incidence rates of complications. Nevertheless, it is increasingly evident that the requirements of specific nutrients during critical illness may be considerably different from those during a healthy state.

Arginine is another example of a nutrient that can be depleted in certain patients and supplementation may bring positive effects (e.g. improved surgical healing, reduced rate of postoperative infection, fewer complications).

Conditionally essential nutrients: When an animal is unable to synthesize adequate amounts of a nutrient and must rely on dietary sources, that nutrient is qualified as being 'essential'. During certain conditions, such as critical illness, the demands for a normally non-essential nutrient (which the animal would otherwise synthesize enough of to meet metabolic demands) increase significantly and must be supplemented in the diet to avoid a relative deficiency. These nutrients have been termed 'conditionally essential' and glutamine is a good example (at least in people). Future studies are warranted to evaluate whether this phenomenon actually occurs in animals.

Formulating the nutritional plan

Ideally, nutritional support should provide ample substrates for gluconeogenesis, protein synthesis and energy production necessary to maintain homeostasis. Ensuring that enough calories are being provided to sustain critical physiological processes, such as immune function, wound repair and cell division and growth, would necessitate the measurement of the patient's actual total energy expenditure. However, precise measurements of energy expenditure (calorimetry) in clinical patients are still in the developmental phases.

Calorimetry

The basic premise of calorimetry is to measure the total heat lost by an animal, as a reflection of total energy produced by metabolism.

- With direct calorimetry, the animal is placed in an airtight insulated chamber and precise thermal measurements are made of the chamber. This method is only suitable in an experimental setting, as clinical patients could not be managed in this type of condition or environment.
- Indirect calorimetry is more commonly employed in human hospitals and by veterinary clinical researchers to extrapolate energy requirements.

Indirect calorimetry provides a non-invasive means of estimating energy expenditure (heat production) by measuring the rate of oxygen consumption and the rate of carbon dioxide production and applying the obtained values to a mathematical equation known as the Weir formula (O'toole *et al.*, 2004). As consumption of oxygen and production of carbon dioxide can be directly related to glucose, protein and fat metabolism, energy expenditure can be calculated from the measured variables. This requires specialized equipment, so-called metabolic carts, making it available only to a few sites. Oxygen and carbon dioxide exchange is measured with a hood, canopy or expiratory collection device. These systems are portable and easier to use in clinical situations.

Energy formulae: RER and IER

Whilst a few studies have used indirect calorimetry to estimate energy expenditure in certain groups of clinical patients, currently the use of mathematical formulae remains the most practical means of estimating a patient's energy requirement (Figure 15.4).

RER (resting energy requirement) is defined as: *the number of calories required for maintaining homeostasis at rest in a thermoneutral environment whilst the animal is in a post-absorptive state.*

> **RER** (kcal/day) = 70 × (current bodyweight in kg)$^{0.75}$

Or for animals weighing between 2 and 30 kg:

> **RER** (kcal/day) = (30 × current bodyweight in kg) + 70

- To convert kcal to kilojoules (kJ), multiply the number of kcal by 4.185.
- Some patients with more severe diseases that have resulted in >5 days of poor food intake should be initially fed 33–55% of their RER and gradually increased to the full RER.
- Some animals will require significantly more than the RER to maintain weight, but the RER should be the initial goal of nutritional support.
- Some animals that develop metabolic complications such as hyperglycaemia, hyperbilirubinaemia and azotaemia may need to be fed less than the RER.

15.4 Calculation of the RER and estimation of energy needs.

Results of indirect calorimetry studies in dogs support the recent trend of formulating nutritional support to meet the RER as a starting point, rather than the more generous illness energy requirement (IER), which requires multiplying the resting or even the maintenance energy requirement (MER) by an illness factor.

Until recently, it was recommended that the RER should be multiplied by an illness factor between 1.0 and 2.5, yielding an IER, to account for increases in metabolism associated with different diseases and injuries. However, less emphasis is now being placed on such subjective and extrapolated factors and the current recommendation is to use more conservative energy estimates (i.e. start with the animal's RER), to avoid overfeeding (feeding in excess of nutritional needs). Overfeeding can result in metabolic and gastrointestinal complications, hepatic dysfunction and increased carbon dioxide production.

It should be emphasized that these general guidelines should be used as starting points, and animals receiving nutritional support should be closely monitored for tolerance of nutritional intervention. Complications such as vomiting, regurgitation, abdominal pain or diarrhoea are indicative that the animal is not tolerating feeding. Continual decline in bodyweight or body condition should prompt reassessment and perhaps modification of the nutritional plan (e.g. increasing the number of calories provided by 25%).

Nutritional requirements in special cases

There is much that remains unclear regarding the nutritional requirements of surgical patients or critically ill animals in general. In certain circumstances

assumptions are made that nutritional requirements in animals are similar to those for people afflicted with similar diseases. However, it is important to recognize that there may be significant species and disease differences that make direct comparisons or extrapolations less applicable.

Thermal burns

Experimental data suggest dramatic changes in energy requirements in animals with thermal burns, but there are virtually no clinical data to support this notion. In experimental models, dogs with thermal burns experienced increased energy requirements, accelerated gluconeogenesis, glucose oxidation, lipolysis and increased amino acid oxidation. In the absence of definitive data to suggest otherwise, current recommendations are to start nutritional support as soon as it is deemed safe and initially to target the RER but to reassess the patient continually, as energy requirements may exceed 2 × the RER. The goal of nutritional support is to optimize protein synthesis and preserve lean body mass. Feeding at least 6–7 g protein/100 kcal (25–35% of total energy) may be necessary. It is unknown whether nutrients such as glutamine and arginine would provide extra benefits in this patient population.

Perioperative nutrition

As malnutrition is a well recognized comorbidity in people with surgical disease, the concept of perioperative nutrition has arisen, whereby surgical intervention is delayed until the nutritional status of the patient improves following commencement of some form of nutritional support. The delay may only be a few days, but could be extended to weeks to reduce the risk of postoperative complications. This approach has not been well described in dogs or cats, but could be considered. Cases where this approach may be sensible include patients with gastrointestinal neoplasia that have become severely debilitated. In these patients an argument could be made that some form of nutritional support should be provided before performing major surgery.

Sepsis

Animals with sepsis are perhaps another population for which nutritional requirements may be altered. The intense inflammatory response, coupled with changes in substrate handling, are likely to alter the metabolic rate and nutrient requirements. Experimental data in dogs suggest that energy expenditure may increase by 25% during the early phase of sepsis and this appears to be accompanied by an increase in oxidation of free fatty acids and triglycerides.

However, it is also recognized that energy expenditure can be quite variable in sepsis and may even decrease in septic shock. Depending on the type of sepsis, protein requirements may also dramatically increase. For example, nutritional recommendations for animals with septic peritonitis may involve initially feeding at the RER with 35% of total calories derived from protein, 40% from fats and 25% from carbohydrates. Further studies are warranted to determine whether these recommendations are optimal for clinical patients with sepsis. The number of calories provided may be increased upon reassessment of bodyweight and body condition score, or conversely decreased if metabolic complications such as hyperglycaemia or hyperlipidaemia develop following the initiation of nutritional support.

Modes of nutritional support

Oral feeding

Ideally, animals recovering from surgical disease should eat, voluntarily and without any coaxing, sufficient amounts of food to enable a full recovery. Voluntary food intake may be problematic in many critically ill and recovering postoperative patients, and common strategies to overcome this problem include enticing the patient with very palatable food items (e.g. cooked chicken, fish, rice), hand-feeding (Figure 15.5), syringe-feeding and the use of appetite stimulants (especially in cats; Figure 15.6).

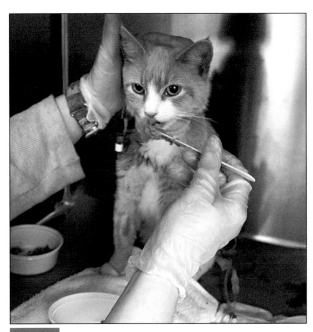

| **15.5** | Coaxing a cat to eat by hand-feeding.

In the recovering postoperative patient a possible reason for poor appetite could be related to nausea, ileus and drug side effects. Many antibiotics and analgesic agents used in postoperative patients can affect gastrointestinal motility or induce nausea.

The strategies mentioned above are largely ineffective at meeting the patient's RER. If a patient fails to consume a reasonable amount of food orally (at least 50% of the calculated RER) for more than 3–4 days, strong consideration for placement of a feeding tube should be given.

Enteral tube feeding

Enteral nutrition is safer and less expensive than parenteral nutrition, and helps to maintain intestinal structure and function. Even in patients not eating voluntarily, the enteral route for providing nutritional support is usually preferred. Patients with feeding tubes can easily be discharged for homecare with good owner compliance. Contraindications to using the enteral route include persistent vomiting, severe malabsorptive conditions and an inability to guard the airway.

The majority of complications with feeding tubes involve tube occlusion or localized irritation at the tube exit site. More serious complications include infection at the exit site or, rarely, complete tube dislodgment and peritonitis if the tube in question was a gastrostomy or jejunostomy tube. Complications can be avoided by using the appropriate tube, securing the tube correctly, proper food selection and preparation and careful monitoring.

Choice of feeding tube

Feeding tubes commonly used in dogs and cats include naso-oesophageal, oesophagostomy, gastrostomy and jejunostomy tubes (more detailed discussion about the indications, contraindications and techniques are covered in the *BSAVA Manual of Canine and Feline Emergency and Critical Care*).

Choosing which feeding tube is best to achieve the nutritional plan depends on several factors.

Drug	Dose	Comments
Cyproheptadine	0.1–0.5 mg/kg orally q8–24h	A serotonin antagonist and antihistamine that can cause sedation and lower the seizure threshold
Diazepam	0.5–1.0 mg/kg i.v. once	No longer recommended in cats because of reported cases of fatal hepatic necrosis associated with repeated oral use (Center et al., 1996). A single intravenous injection may be safe but the owner should be warned of the potential serious side effects. The effect is very rapid and short-lived, so a food bowl should be available immediately when the drug is injected
Midazolam	0.05–0.1 mg/kg i.v.	No reports of hepatotoxicity to date
Mirtazapine	3.75 mg/cat orally every 3 days Can also be used in dogs (dose depends on bodyweight): <10 kg: 3.75 mg/dog orally q24h 10–15 kg: 5–7.5 mg/dog orally q24h 15–20 kg: 7.5 mg/dog orally q24h 21–60 kg: 15 mg/dog orally q24h >60 kg: 30 mg/dog orally q24h The dose may be increased from these starting points id no response id seen in 24–48 hours; **maximum** 0.6 mg/kg orally q24h	Antidepressant (alpha-2 antagonist) that increases CNS noradrenaline and serotonin; reported to increase appetite in humans as side effect. Anecdotally reported as effective as an appetite stimulant in dogs and cats and rapidly becoming the preferred agent in these species, but only recently used so no extensive pharmacokinetic and safety data available. Significant renal and hepatic clearance; avoid in renal/hepatic disease or use with caution and at 30% of usual dose. Serotonin syndrome (increased heart rate, shivering, dilated pupils, high blood pressure) potential side effect if CNS serotonin levels get too high, but this should only occur if combined with serotonin-increasing medications such as tramadol, tricyclic antidepressants (e.g. clomipramine) and monoamine oxidase inhibitors (e.g. selegiline)

| **15.6** | Potential appetite stimulants for use in cats. Note that these are of limited usefulness and none is authorized for this use in the UK.

- The chosen tube should utilize as much of the functional gastrointestinal tract as possible. For example:
  - An animal with a broken jaw (Figure 15.7) should be supported with an oesophagostomy tube

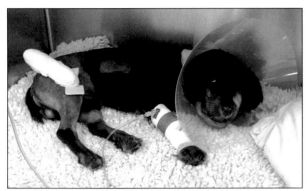

15.7 Dog with broken jaw requiring placement of an oesophagostomy feeding tube to enable adequate nutritional support.

- A dog with a hiatal hernia should be supported with a gastrostomy tube.
- Another consideration is the anticipated duration of tube feeding:
  - Animals requiring very short-term nutritional support (<3–4 days) could be managed with a naso-oesophageal tube
  - Patients requiring longer-term support could be managed with an oesophagostomy or gastrostomy tube
  - In the context of surgical patients, it is vitally important to have considered in advance whether a patient requires placement of a feeding tube, as this is best achieved when the patient is already anaesthetized for the primary surgical procedure.
- The next consideration relates to risk of complications:
  - Patients with severe catabolic and debilitating conditions are at high risk of dehiscence and therefore not good candidates for gastrostomy or jejunostomy tube placement, as leakage results in life-threatening septic peritonitis
  - With oesophagostomy tubes, the major complication is wound infection, but this is easily treated and in many cases the tube can remain in place and be used for feeding whilst the infection is treated medically.
- The final consideration is what food can be used with the tube:
  - Patients with naso-oesophageal and jejunostomy tubes usually require completely liquid diets
  - Placement of larger tubes such as oesophagostomy and gastrostomy tubes means there is a greater choice of diets that can be used
  - Some of these diets require significant modification, such as liquidizing with additional water (Figure 15.8), and this will tend to dilute the caloric density of the diet.

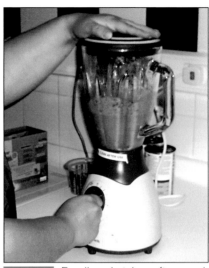

15.8 Feeding via tubes often requires liquidizing the diet with additional water.

Once the desired feeding tube is in place, radiography should be performed to confirm satisfactory tube placement. For naso-oesophageal and oesophagostomy tubes, the tip of the tube should lie in the distal oesophagus.

Prevention of premature removal of tubes can be accomplished by using an Elizabethan collar and by bandaging the tube securely. Care should be taken to avoid wrapping too tightly as this could lead to patient discomfort and even compromise proper ventilation.

Choice of diet

Based on the type of feeding tube and the disease process being treated, an appropriate diet should be selected. For example, naso-oesophageal tubes require true liquid diets, whilst larger tubes such as oesophagostomy and gastrostomy tubes can accommodate thicker gruel diets with high caloric density (for greater details for appropriate diet selection, refer to Michel, 1998).

Feeding plan

With information such as the desired caloric content of the diet and the RER of the patient, the amount of food required is calculated and a specific feeding plan should be devised. Important points for the feeding plan are as follows.

PRACTICAL TIPS

- Feedings should be administered every 4–6 hours.
- Feeding tubes should be flushed with 5–10 ml of water after each feeding to minimize clogging of the tube.
- By the time of hospital discharge, the number of feedings should be reduced to 3–4 times/day to facilitate owner compliance.
- Generally speaking, a volume of 5–10 ml/kg per individual feeding is well tolerated but this may vary with the individual patient.
- As enteral diets are mostly composed of water (for example, most canned foods are already >75% water) the amount of fluids administered parenterally should be adjusted accordingly to avoid volume overload.

Parenteral nutrition

Parenteral nutrition (PN) is more expensive than enteral nutrition and is usually only available in certain referral centres. Indications for PN include:

- Protracted vomiting
- Acute pancreatitis
- Severe malabsorptive disorders
- Severe ileus.

There are generally two major types of PN.

- **Total parenteral nutrition** (TPN) (Figure 15.9) is typically delivered via a central venous (jugular) catheter and provides all of the energy requirements of the patient.
- With **partial parenteral nutrition** (PPN) only a portion (40–70%) of the animal's energy requirements are met.

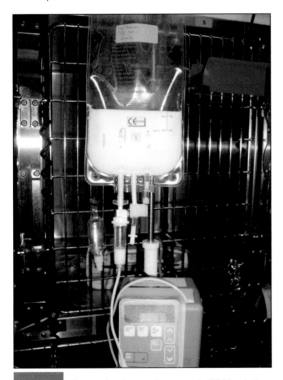

15.9 Example of a custom-made TPN solution.

The one advantage of PPN is that the solution is made with less concentrated components, allowing the osmolarity of the solution to be tolerated in a large peripheral vein such as the lateral saphenous vein in dogs and the femoral vein in cats.

Because PPN provides no more than a portion of the patient's requirements, it is only intended for short-term use in a non-debilitated patient with average nutritional requirements.

Catheters

Regardless of the exact form of PN, intravenous nutrition requires catheters that are placed specifically for nutrition using strict aseptic technique. Multi-lumen catheters (in which up to three different solutions can be administered via separate ports) are often recommended for parenteral nutrition because they can remain in place for longer periods of time as compared with normal jugular catheters and provide other ports for blood sampling and administration of additional fluids and intravenous medications. Suitable materials for these catheters include silicone and polyurethane.

> **PRACTICAL TIP**
>
> With both TPN and PPN, the catheter and lines must be handled with aseptic technique to avoid complications.

PN solutions

Most PN solutions are composed of:

- A carbohydrate source (e.g. 5% and 50% dextrose)
- A protein source (e.g. 8.5% and 11% amino acids)
- A fat source (e.g. 20% lipids).

Vitamins and trace metals can also be added.

Osmolarity: When compounding parenteral nutrition, components with the highest osmolarity are added first to specially made fluid bags intended for parenteral nutrition. These special bags limit the oxidation of components, preserving the quality of the product. Typically, amino acid solutions are the first component to be added to these bags, followed by dextrose and finally lipids. Other fluids can be added to adjust the osmolarity of the solution.

As precise volumes of each component must be aseptically measured and mixed into the bags, the use of special equipment such as a TPN compounder is considered the best way to prepare parenteral nutrition. For these reasons, PN solutions are not feasible in most practices and using TPN compounding services at human hospitals may be an alternative.

- Due to the high osmolarity of the TPN solution (usually 1100–1500 mOsm/l), it must be administered through a central venous (jugular) catheter. Administering a solution with very high osmolarity may increase the risk of thrombophlebitis.
- PPN is formulated to have a lower osmolarity (<1100 mOsm/l) so that it can be administered through a peripheral catheter but, because it is more dilute, it can only provide a portion of the patient's energy requirements.

Commercial preparations: Commercial ready-to-use preparations of glucose and amino acids are available for peripheral use (Figure 15.10) but these only provide <70% of the required calories (when administered at maintenance fluid rate) and should only be used for short-term or interim nutritional support.

- The great advantages of these solutions are that they are already mixed and require no specialized equipment other than fluid infusion pumps.
- The major disadvantage is that they cannot be tailored to the patient's needs, as the components are fixed in proportion.
- Another problem is that these solutions often already contain 16–20 mmol of KCl per litre and therefore administering at higher than maintenance fluid rates (>4 ml/kg/h) is likely to result in hyperkalaemia.

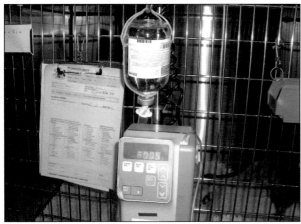

15.10 Example of a ready-made commercially available PPN solution.

Feeding plan

As with enteral nutrition, PN should be instituted gradually over 48–72 hours. Most animals are given 33–55% of their RER on the first day of PN and the delivery of calories (not necessarily volume) is increased so that by 72 hours 100% of the RER is provided.

Other intravenous fluids should be adjusted accordingly for the amount of PN fluid being administered to avoid volume overload.

Complications of providing nutrition in the critically ill

Bodyweight should be monitored daily with both enteral and parenteral nutrition. The use of the RER as the patient's caloric requirement is merely a starting point. The number of calories provided may need to be increased to keep up with the patient's changing needs, typically by 25% if well tolerated. In patients unable to tolerate the prescribed amount, the clinician should consider reducing the amount of enteral feeding and supplementing the nutritional plan with PPN.

Enteral nutrition

Possible complications of enteral nutrition include:

- Mechanical complications, such as clogging of the tube or early tube removal
- Septic complications, such as infection at the feeding tube exit site (Figure 15.11)

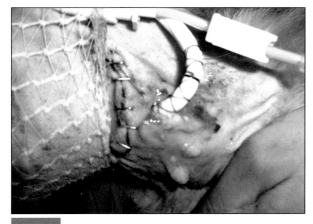

15.11 Infected gastrostomy tube site.

- Metabolic complications, such as electrolyte disturbances, hyperglycaemia, volume overload and gastrointestinal signs (e.g. vomiting, diarrhoea, cramping, bloating).

Monitoring parameters for patients receiving enteral nutrition include:

- Daily bodyweight
- Serum electrolytes
- Tube patency
- Appearance of tube exit site
- Gastrointestinal signs (e.g. vomiting, regurgitation, diarrhoea)
- Signs of volume overload or pulmonary aspiration.

Parenteral nutrition

Possible complications of PN include:

- Sepsis
- Mechanical complications of the catheter and lines
- Thrombophlebitis
- Metabolic disturbances such as hyperglycaemia and electrolyte shifts.

Avoiding serious consequences of complications associated with PN requires early identification of problems and prompt action.

- Vital signs should be monitored at least twice a day.
- Catheter-exit sites should be checked daily.
- Routine biochemistry panels should be checked daily.

With continual reassessment, the clinician can determine when to change the patient from assisted feeding to voluntary consumption of food. The discontinuation of nutritional support should only begin when the patient can consume approximately its RER without much coaxing. In patients receiving TPN, the transition to enteral nutrition should occur over the course of at least 12–24 hours, depending on patient tolerance.

Summary

- Nutritional support of critically ill and postoperative patients should be considered an essential part of the overall treatment plan.
- Metabolic responses to illness or severe injury place critically ill patients at high risk for development of malnutrition.
- Consequences of malnutrition include altered substrate metabolism, compromised immune function, impaired wound healing and potentially increased mortality.
- Energy expenditure in critically ill animals may vary considerably depending on the patient, underlying disease and illness severity; therefore, initial nutritional support should target the RER.
- Specific nutritional requirements for critically ill dogs and cats have not been determined, but recommended levels of protein provision include feeding 6–7 g protein/100 kcal or 25–35% of total calories derived from protein.
- Before implementation of nutritional support, patients must be cardiovascularly stable and have

any hydration, acid–base and electrolyte abnormalities addressed.

- Monitoring of patients receiving nutritional support is extremely important, as this population is prone to various metabolic complications.
- Upon reassessment, nutritional support may be increased, decreased or discontinued, depending on patient response and disease progression.
- With appropriate patient selection, accurate nutritional assessment and careful execution of the nutritional plan, nutrition can play an instrumental role in the successful recovery of many critically ill patients undergoing surgery.

References and further reading

Biolo G, Toigo G, Ciocchi B *et al.* (1997) Metabolic response to injury and sepsis: changes in protein metabolism. *Nutrition* **13**, 52S–57S

Bisgaard T and Kehlet H (2002) Early oral feeding after elective abdominal surgery – what are the issues? *Nutrition* **18**, 944–948

Center SA, Elston TH, Rowland PH *et al.* (1996) Fulminant hepatic failure associated with oral administration of diazepam in 11 cats. *Journal of the American Veterinary Medical Association* **209**, 18–25.

Conejero R, Bonet A, Grau T *et al.* (2002) Effect of a glutamine-enriched enteral diet on intestinal permeability and infectious morbidity at 28 days in critically ill patients with systemic inflammatory response syndrome: a randomized, single-blind, prospective, multicenter study. *Nutrition* **18**, 716–721

Heyland DK (2000) Enteral and parenteral nutrition in the seriously ill, hospitalized patients: a critical review of the evidence. *Journal of Nutritional Health & Aging* **1**, 31–41

Lewis SJ, Egger M, Sylvester PA *et al.* (2001) Early enteral feeding versus 'nil by mouth' after gastrointestinal surgery: systematic review and meta-analysis of controlled trials. *British Medical Journal* **323**, 773–776

Michel KE (1993) Prognostic value of clinical nutritional assessment in canine patients. *Journal of Veterinary Emergency and Critical Care* **3**, 96–104

Michel KE (1998) Nitrogen metabolism in critical care patients. *Veterinary Clinical Nutrition* **5** (Suppl.), 20–22

Michel KE (1998) Interventional nutrition for the critical care patient: optimal diets. *Clinical Techniques in Small Animal Practice* **13**, 204–210

Michel KE, King LG and Ostro E (1997) Measurement of urinary urea nitrogen content as an estimate of the amount of total urinary nitrogen loss in dogs in intensive care units. *Journal of the American Veterinary Medical Association* **210**, 356–359

O'toole E, Miller GW, Wilson BA et al. (2004) Comparison of the standard predictive equation for calculation of resting energy expenditure with indirect calorimetry in hospitalized and healthy dogs. *Journal of the American Veterinary Medical Association* **225**, 58–64.

Remillard RL, Darden De, Michel KE *et al.* (2001) An investigation of the relationship between caloric intake and outcome in hospitalized dogs. *Veterinary Therapeutics* **2**, 301–310

Walton RS, Wingfield WE, Ogilvie GK *et al.* (1996) Energy expenditure in 104 postoperative and traumatized injured dogs with indirect calorimetry. *Journal of Veterinary Emergency and Critical Care* **6**, 71–79

Watson P and Chan DL (2010) Principles of clinical nutrition. In: *BSAVA Manual of Canine and Feline Rehabilitation Supportive and Palliative Care: Case Studies in Patient Management*, ed. S Lindley and P Watson, pp. 42–59. BSAVA Publications, Gloucester

Wernerman J and Hammarqvist F (1999) Glutamine: a necessary nutrient for the intensive care patient. *International Journal of Colorectal Diseases* **14**, 137–142

Wray CJ, Mammen JM and Hasselgren P (2002) Catabolic response to stress and potential benefits of nutrition support. *Nutrition* **18**, 971–977

Aseptic technique

Tim Hutchinson

Introduction

The aim of aseptic technique is to ensure that surgery can be performed with minimal risk of contamination by microorganisms. The patient itself is a major source of contaminating organisms; however, any wound open to the atmosphere will become contaminated and with time those contaminant organisms may colonize the wound and establish an infection. The longer a wound is open, the greater the risk of contamination and, potentially, infection. Prophylactic antimicrobials are recommended for certain surgical procedures (see Chapter 18), but use of antimicrobial agents will not eliminate problems relating to poor aseptic technique.

During surgery a wound will be exposed to:

- The environment of the operating theatre
- The animal's own bacterial flora
- Theatre personnel, equipment and instruments.

Whilst instruments can be sterilized and hard inert surfaces treated with disinfectants, the reduction of the bacterial flora of the patient and the operating personnel must be balanced with the potential damage to their tissues that removing these bacteria may cause.

Most procedures that are performed as part of aseptic technique have arisen through their development in the human field. The veterinary field, whilst similar in its aim, may differ from human hospitals, not least from the difference in patients, but also in scale, ranging from a large veterinary referral hospital with dedicated theatre suites and personnel, to a small clinic with one or two veterinary surgeons, in which surgical procedures may need to be slotted in between consulting sessions and performed in rooms in an adapted building.

It is important for every practice, regardless of its size, to establish strict protocols (local rules) aimed at minimizing the risk of surgical wound contamination and to enforce them. This chapter focuses on the ideal standard, but the principles of aseptic technique are relevant to all practices. Hopefully it will act as a stimulus to any practice to review their current procedures and identify areas that can be improved.

Preparation of the patient and surgical site

The patient is the major source of contamination of the surgical wound: endogenous staphylococci and streptococci from the skin are the most frequently cultured organisms from wound infections.

- **Transient microorganisms** are usually easy to remove from the skin through physical scrubbing and can be almost completely eliminated with effective antiseptics.
- **Resident organisms** are more complex, in that bacteria that are present within an animal's tissues for a significant time form complicated biofilms, rather than existing as single free-moving (planktonic) organisms or groups (Paulson, 2005).

Clinically significant biofilms occur when resident bacteria attach to tissue or implants (e.g. sutures, metallic items or drains), adhere and attract other similar organisms to form a biofilm matrix. Such infections pose a challenge to the surgeon because:

- Normal skin residents do not immediately trigger an immune response, so the infection is not readily identified
- The efficient metabolism of bacteria within a biofilm matrix means that their uptake of antimicrobial agents is reduced and doses greater than the normal minimum inhibitory concentration (MIC) for a longer period of time may be required.

It is of paramount importance, therefore, that the surgical team makes every effort to ensure that exposure of the wound to contaminating microorganisms is kept to an absolute minimum, through careful clipping, thorough skin preparation and appropriate draping.

Urination and defecation

The inappropriate voiding of urine and faeces in the operating theatre is a hazard that should be minimized. Owners should be encouraged to take dogs for a short toilet walk prior to admission and kennel staff should ensure that dogs have adequate opportunity to defecate and urinate before premedication. Cats pose more of a problem in that they will have been confined to the house for at least 12 hours before admission and may be reluctant to use a litter tray.

Once the animal is anaesthetized, a full bladder may be gently emptied manually, or by catheterization. Whilst urine itself is usually free of significant numbers of microorganisms, if an animal urinates during surgery the urine will soak into the fur and may lead to bacterial strikethrough. In animals with a full rectum, the manual extraction of faeces and/or placement of a purse-string suture may be required.

For surgical procedures carried out in the perineal region, manual evacuation and a purse-string suture are preferable to the administration of an enema, as the latter tends to result in liquid faeces that are more likely to leak.

Hair removal

Hair acts as a filter, trapping bacteria and dirt, and creates a microclimate at the skin level. The volume of hair vastly increases the surface area for the attachment of microorganisms and particulate matter, so it is essential to remove hair from a wide area around the proposed incision site.

For routine procedures clients should be encouraged to present their animals in a clean state: bathing with a mild shampoo at least 24 hours prior to surgery might be appropriate in some cases (though should be discouraged closer to the time of surgery, as a damp coat will increase evaporative heat losses during the anaesthetic). Toileting on the morning of surgery should be away from muddy fields and other areas of gross soiling.

Hair should be removed over a wide enough area to allow draping of the proposed surgical site and extension of the incision, should it be required during the procedure. In general, a 15 cm border of clipped skin should be present around the proposed incision site. The hair should be removed using electric clippers. The use of razor blades causes damage to the skin, resulting in colonization by bacteria and superficial infections. Hair removal creams may also be associated with cutaneous reactions.

Clippers

Clippers are recommended for hair removal, but poor clipping technique and lax maintenance of clippers will lead to skin abrasion ('clipper rash'), small nicks and even lacerations. Bacteria from deeper layers of the skin and hair follicles are then exposed and rapidly colonize these lesions. Additionally, the irritation to the animal results in licking and self-mutilation of the area around the incision and there may be wound infection and dehiscence. Clipper rash is easily avoided provided basic rules are followed.

Clipping technique: Unless already extremely short, hair should always be removed with a two-stroke technique (Figure 16.1).

- The bulk of the hair is removed by clipping in the direction of the lie of the hair.
- A closer clip is achieved by shaving against the direction of the hair.

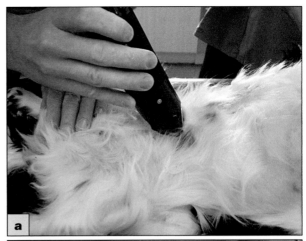

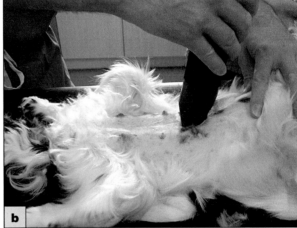

16.1 Hair should be removed in a two-stage process: **(a)** first clipping with the lie of the hair; **(b)** a second cut against the lie of the hair to achieve the close surgical clip, but with minimal skin trauma.

Different blades may be used for these different clips, reserving very fine blades for the final clip and using coarse blades for the bulk of the hair removal. When long hair is clipped with a single stroke against the lie of the hair, the hair tends to drag the surrounding skin up into the blades of the clippers, leading to abrasions (Figure 16.2).

During clipping, one hand should be used to pull the skin taut to avoid creases of skin catching in the blades. For extremities, an assistant might be required to take the weight of the limb to allow both hands to be used for clipping.

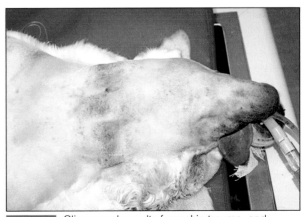

16.2 Clipper rash results from skin trauma, and traumatized skin may be colonized by bacteria. (Courtesy of S Baines)

When clipping large areas the blades will become hot, and proteins and lipoproteins from the skin and hair will coagulate and bind to the cutting edges of the blades. This effectively dulls the cutting surface and reduces the efficiency of the cut, allowing hair to snag on the blades, resulting in clipper rash. Blades should therefore be changed or cooled during clipping if they become hot or a sense of dragging is perceived.

Cleaning: Blades should be cleaned between each patient to avoid the transmission of one animal's microflora to another. Hair should be removed from the blades and the head of the clipper with a fine brush, taking care to ensure that hair is not trapped between the blades (preventing their close contact). The blades must have any tissue debris removed to restore the fine cutting edge. This is not easily removed with water (and may lead to rusting of the blades), and so a proprietary solvent-based solution (e.g. Oster Blade Wash) is recommended.

The most effective cleaning technique is to dip the tips of the oscillating blades in a dish of this solution, brushing as required. The blades should then be dried, before the application of a thin film of lubricating oil. Blades that have not been cleaned or lubricated effectively will perform poorly and lead to clipper rash.

Blade maintenance: Thorough and correct cleaning will extend the working life of clipper blades, but they will require sharpening. The design of the blades is such that there is a fixed guard blade against which a cutting blade oscillates. Each blade has V-shaped cutting edges, which sever the hair shafts with a scissor action. The cutting blade is intentionally shorter than the guard blade, so that the sharp oscillating metal points do not contact the skin.

With repeated sharpening two problems may occur. Firstly, the distance between the tips of the points of the cutting and guard blades reduces (Figure 16.3) and if this distance becomes too small the oscillating blade will begin to contact the skin during the hair-clip, resulting in clipper rash. Secondly, the tips of the guard blade lose their rounded ends and develop sharp points. These then dig into the skin and, with careless clipping technique, can cause lacerations.

PRACTICAL TIP

A clipper blade has a finite life and should be discarded when:

- The points of the guard blade become excessively sharp
- The gap between the tip of the guard and cutting blades is significantly reduced
- There is gross damage, such as broken teeth.

Clipper blades should therefore be inspected regularly. When sharpening is required, it is worth investing in a premium service that will dismantle the blades, sharpen each one separately and try to minimize the problems noted above.

Hair disposal

To minimize the risk of hair particles contaminating the surgical field, hair removal should always be carried

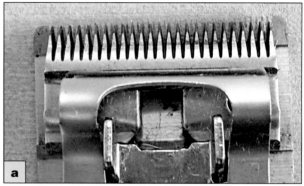
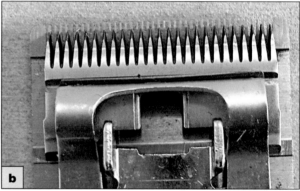

16.3 With repeated sharpening, the distance between the tips of the clipper guard and cutting blades reduces. The blades in **(a)** have been sharpened too many times and the tips of each blade are so close together that trauma to the skin is likely. In **(b)** there is still an appropriate gap between the two rows of tips.

out in a room separate from the sterile preparation and operating theatre. The bulk of the shaved hair can easily be gathered and disposed of, but a vacuum cleaner should be used to remove smaller remnants and loose hair from the animal. The floor of the preparation area should also be kept free from hair, to prevent it drifting into the theatre. A vacuum cleaner with a fine-particulate filter should be used if possible, to reduce aerosols, and the filters should be changed regularly.

Draping out

If access to the limb but not the foot is required during surgery, it is better and less traumatic to drape out the foot from the surgical field rather than clipping it (Figure 16.4). The foot should first be covered by an

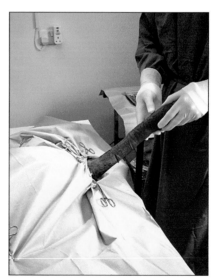

16.4 Rather than clipping all the hair from a foot, it can be draped out of the surgical field by the use of a sterile impervious layer and sterile cohesive bandage.

impervious layer, e.g. a latex glove, held in place by tape or a cohesive bandage. During draping this can then be covered by a sterile cover, such as a glove or cohesive bandage, allowing the foot to be held to manipulate the limb during surgery. It has been shown that the incorporation of a sterile impervious layer is essential to prevent bacterial strikethrough (Vince *et al.*, 2008).

Preoperative antiseptic preparation

Before the animal is moved into the operating theatre, initial skin preparation should be performed. The aim of this treatment is to remove gross dirt and loose skin squames, eliminate transient microorganisms and begin the reduction in the level of the animal's resident bacterial flora. The ideal skin scrub should:

- Be lathering (to remove dirt and grease)
- Have broad-spectrum bactericidal, virucidal, fungicidal and sporicidal properties
- Kill microorganisms with minimal contact time
- Be non-irritating to the skin and any other tissues
- Be economical.

Commonly used scrub solutions and their properties are listed in Figure 16.5. In practice, the two most frequently used are based on chlorhexidine or iodophors. Chlorhexidine has superior residual activity due to the fact that it binds to keratin. Irrespective of the compound used, contact time is the most significant factor relating to the reduction of the number of microorganisms.

Cotton wool, sponges or swabs may be used for this initial scrub, beginning at the site of the proposed incision and working away from it in a circular pattern (Figure 16.6). Whilst the removal of dirt and loose skin is important to expose bacteria that may be trapped beneath, excessive scrubbing that damages the skin surface should be avoided as such abrasions will be colonized by bacteria postoperatively.

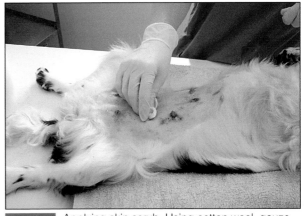

16.6 Applying skin scrub. Using cotton wool, gauze swabs or sponges, the skin is cleaned gently, working from the site of the incision to the periphery with a circular motion.

For male dogs undergoing abdominal procedures, the prepuce should be flushed with an antiseptic solution; likewise the vulva of bitches undergoing perineal surgery. Dilute chlorhexidine solution (one part chlorhexidine to 50 parts water) is recommended for this purpose (Neihaus *et al.*, 2010).

Patient positioning

The position of the patient on the operating table will depend on the procedure to be performed. Detailed description is beyond the scope of this chapter and the reader is referred to the appropriate chapter of other surgical texts. However, some general points are given here.

- The animal should be moved into theatre in such a way that the initially prepared surgical field is not contaminated.
- All anaesthetic monitoring aids and extension lines are attached, diathermy ground plates placed and warm-air blankets positioned prior to the sterile scrub and draping.

Antiseptic	Mechanism of action	Properties	Examples
Iodophors (e.g. povidone–iodine)	Iodophors are stable solutions of iodine that are able to penetrate the cell wall of bacteria. Bacterial death is the result of oxidation and replacement of intracellular molecules with free iodine	Broad spectrum (broader than chlorhexidine), including fungi, viruses and some spores. Activity reduced by presence of organic material. Greater contact time required than with chlorhexidine. May be more likely to cause skin irritation than chlorhexidine	Medidine; Pevidine; Vetasept povidone–iodine
Bisdiguanides (e.g. chlorhexidine gluconate)	Precipitate intracellular proteins after disruption of cell wall and membrane	Broad spectrum, but less effective against Gram-negative than Gram-positive bacteria. Virucidal. Low activity against fungi. Good residual action through binding to keratin. Less inhibited by organic matter than iodophors	Hibiscrub; Medihex; Vetasept chlorhexidine
Alcohol	Denatures cell wall proteins, DNA, RNA and lipids	Broad spectrum, including fungi and viruses. Rapid onset of action	70% Isopropyl alcohol
Alcohol-based solutions	Synergistic effect through combining 70% isopropyl alcohol with an antiseptic (e.g. chlorhexidine)	Broad spectrum due to combining different agents with different modes of action	Actiprep (ethanol + zinc pyrithione); Exidine (isopropyl alcohol and chlorhexidine)

16.5 Comparison of different skin-scrub solutions.

■ Knowledge of the procedure will be required in order to anticipate access to parts of the body, positioning of the surgeon and assistant, and location of the instrument trolleys.

Positioning aids

To minimize cross-contamination, positioning aids should be easily cleaned, dedicated to the theatre and not used in other parts of the building. Various aids are available.

■ Troughs are a good way of keeping patients in dorsal recumbency and are ideal for positioning for work on the extremities, but limit access to the thorax and may compromise abdominal surgery.
■ More versatile are clean sandbags or towels rolled into a trough shape (Figure 16.7).
■ Wipe-clean beanbags, which conform to the animal's shape and then maintain that position by removal of air from the bag by suction, can be very useful, but limit repositioning of the animal during a procedure and may be punctured.
■ Extension arms for the table to support the patient's limbs are preferred by some surgeons.

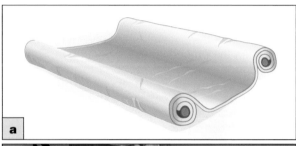

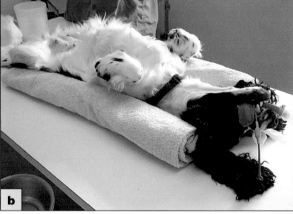

16.7 Rolled towels make versatile positioning aids.

Sterile skin preparation

Preoperative skin preparation should have removed all dirt and transient organisms and suppressed the animal's resident flora. The sterile preparation augments this, using the same antiseptic agent as for the initial skin scrub, but applied with sterile gauze/sponges and sterile forceps or a sterile gloved hand. There should be a similar pattern of application, working from the incision site to the periphery.

Finally the skin is coated with a solution of the antiseptic, which may be in an alcohol solution. Alcohol alone is an effective antimicrobial agent, but has no residual activity and may dilute the residual activity of the previously applied chlorhexidine and

especially povidone–iodine. Rinsing with 70% isopropyl alcohol after a 4% chlorhexidine scrub is less effective than rinsing with saline (Osuna *et al.*, 1990), but chlorhexidine has a synergistic effect with alcohol (Hibbard, 2005).

Two techniques have been suggested:

■ Scrubbing with povidone–iodine, followed by the application of (non-lathering) 10% povidone–iodine solution, either sprayed or painted on to the area
■ Scrubbing with chlorhexidine, followed by the application of a chlorhexidine/alcohol solution.

Povidone–iodine has been reported to have a greater incidence of tissue irritation than chlorhexidine.

Blue dye can be incorporated into the final spray so that it is clear which areas of the skin have been treated, though the entire clipped area should be prepared. Care should be taken to ensure that solutions do not pool in depressions such as the inguinal region.

Draping

Surgical drapes function as a physical barrier to prevent microorganisms from the unprepared parts of the patient and operating table gaining access to the surgical field. All parts of the patient, apart from the surgical field, should be draped out. This barrier must be maintained throughout the procedure, for instance if the drape becomes wet with blood or lavage fluid, or the patient requires repositioning. Draping material must therefore be:

■ Strong, but flexible
■ Readily conformable to the patient
■ Able to be cut (if the surgeon desires a fenestrated single drape rather than a four field pattern), while resisting tearing
■ Water-resistant
■ Easy to sterilize
■ Economical to use.

Draping material

There is no ideal single draping material that will satisfy all the above criteria, so draping techniques will frequently use different materials to achieve different aspects of the overall requirement.

As for whether to use reusable cloth drapes or disposable non-woven types, the same considerations apply as for the choice of materials for surgical gowns (see below). In general, cloth drapes should be avoided in any area subject to wetting, because once wet they offer no barrier to bacterial strikethrough. Cloth drapes should always therefore be covered by an impervious layer. Contamination can be in the form of strikethrough from those parts of the patient that have not been clipped and prepared, or from the resident microflora deep within the hair follicles of the prepared skin. Scrubbed skin should not be viewed as sterile.

Draping techniques

The technique used for draping will vary according to the procedure to be performed and the location of the surgical site, with the aim being to choose the technique that best prevents contamination.

Initially the clipped and prepared skin should be isolated from the surrounding hair and skin either by placing a single large drape, fenestrated to the required size (Figure 16.8a), or by draping with four field drapes (Figure 16.8b). With the latter technique:

■ Four separate drapes are used, one at each of the four edges of the prepared skin
■ The edge of the drape is folded inwards and the drapes are overlapped before securing at each corner of the field with Backhaus towel forceps.

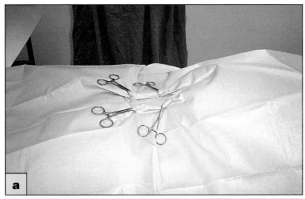

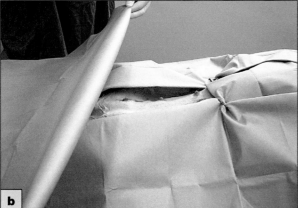

16.8 **(a)** A single large drape is placed over the entire animal, fenestrated to expose the limit of the proposed skin incision. **(b)** Four drapes are placed with a folded leading edge and fastened securely with Backhaus towel clips, to define the limit of the scrubbed area.

Cloth drapes may be used for these field drapes, as they conform to the patient better than disposable drapes, which may help to maintain the sterile field especially if the animal's position is adjusted during the procedure. Cloth drapes should always be covered by an impervious layer to prevent strikethrough when wetting occurs.

With the above draping patterns the only skin that is left exposed is the area into which the incision is to be made. However, there is still a risk of contamination of the wound from resident bacteria deep in the hair follicles, if they are disturbed during surgery. There is much debate about how best to exclude this final potential source of contamination.

■ One technique is to suture the edges of the drape into the skin incision or clip skin towels to the edge of the skin incision so that, during surgery, the cut skin edge is contiguous with the sterile drape.
■ A quicker alternative is to use transparent incise drapes (these may be impregnated with iodine), which adhere to the skin and the incision is made directly through the drape.

Incise drapes: Incise drapes often adhere less well to animal skin than to human skin, and a recent study (Owen *et al.*, 2009) confirmed findings from similar human studies that the use of incise drapes does not affect the rate of bacterial contamination of surgical wounds in clean procedures. However, these drapes are useful in preventing fluids from seeping under the edges of the drapes and may also increase the efficacy of forced-air warmers by preventing the escape of warm air through the edges of the drapes.

Hanging leg preparation: For limb surgery that does not involve the foot, the foot may be draped out of the field using a sterile impervious layer held in place by a sterile cohesive dressing (see Figure 16.4). For such procedures it may be useful to perform a hanging leg preparation, where the limb is suspended from a drip stand during the skin preparation and field-draping before the final sterile layers are placed on the foot. For fracture repairs in which a hanging limb is maintained throughout the procedure, the foot can be covered with a sterile layer whilst still suspended from the stand.

Preparation of the surgical team

The surgical team can potentially contaminate the patient both directly (by contact from the surgeons and the scrub nurse) and indirectly (through increasing the level of airborne bacteria in the theatre environment).

The level of bacteria in the theatre air is directly proportional to the number of personnel and their movement. The number of personnel involved with a procedure should therefore be kept to a minimum and traffic in and out of the theatre should be restricted. Advance planning for a technique is important to ensure that all necessary equipment and theatre disposables are at hand.

Various methods can be employed by the team to minimize contamination and bacterial shedding (detailed below). The degree to which they are utilized will depend on the procedure to be performed. For instance, scrubbed hands and sterile gloves might suffice for the biopsy of a cutaneous mass or feline orchidectomy, but this would obviously be inadequate preparation for more invasive surgery.

General theatre clothing

Scrub suits
Scrub suits should be considered mandatory for all personnel in the surgery suite. Apart from their obvious function to reduce bacterial contamination, they help to differentiate the surgical team from other members of clinical staff (Figure 16.9) and instil an inherent discipline to follow good theatre practice.

Clean suits should be worn at the start of each theatre session and changed if they become soiled. If a member of theatre staff is required to leave the theatre suite, they should change into normal clothing. It may be acceptable on occasion to cover their suit with a white coat to reduce contamination, but this should be avoided.

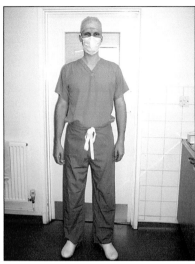

16.9 Dedicated theatre clothing is inexpensive, helps to enforce the discipline of theatre protocols and is a valuable component of the whole aseptic technique. A theatre hat is arguably as important as a sterile gown.

Scrub suits are generally made from a woven polyester/cotton-blend fabric to provide comfort, durability and easy laundering, and their tight weave forms a barrier to microorganisms. This barrier is significantly reduced when the fabric becomes wet and, additionally, bacteria are shed from the open sleeves and trouser legs. The tunic should therefore be worn tucked into the drawstring trousers.

Laundering damages the fibres of the fabric, increasing the size of the holes in the weave and reducing the barrier to microorganisms. Following routine laundering, bacteria may remain on the fabric, so periodic sterilization may be used. Scrubs should be regularly inspected for signs of wear and replaced as required.

Footwear
The level of bacteria on theatre floors is no different whether standard or specially designed theatre shoes are worn (Mangram *et al.*, 1999) and the use of theatre shoes has no effect on the incidence of surgical infection. However, the use of dedicated footwear or shoe covers when out of the theatre suite does reinforce discipline and may help to reduce the transference of hair and other particulate matter.

Theatre hats and head covers
Hair is a significant carrier of bacteria. The head is often positioned directly over the surgical site and shedding from hair has been shown to increase the surgical infection rate. All hair should therefore be covered by all members of the surgical team. It should be considered essential that if a procedure justifies the use of sterile gloves and gown, hair should also be covered.

Good-quality cheap disposable theatre hats are most commonly used, but cloth caps are available and if used they should be laundered, inspected and treated like scrub suits. Theatre hoods, made from similar fabric, are available for those with facial hair.

Masks
Of all the standard items of theatre wear, the mask is probably the most iconic but arguably the least valuable component. Masks rapidly become saturated, which reduces their resistance to the passage of microorganisms considerably. Additionally, microorganisms will pass around the sides of the mask during exhalation.

The primary function of the mask is to prevent direct expulsion of larger contaminated droplets from the mouth and nose of theatre personnel during talking, coughing and sneezing. Masks should be close-fitting, using the wired seam to contour the face, and they should be worn by all personnel in theatre.

Surgical scrub
As for the preparation of the patient's skin, the aims of the surgeon's scrub are to:

- Remove dirt and grease
- Eliminate transient microorganisms
- Reduce the resident microflora to as low a level as possible for as long as possible.

The same considerations regarding time, efficiency, tolerance and economy apply as for the patient's skin scrub. Gross soiling should be washed off with soap first.

The traditional approach to scrubbing-up, using an antiseptic solution and bristle brush (either by time or by counted brush-stroke methods – see below), is based on convention rather than stringent research and there is no definitive technique, with each surgical textbook offering a variation. Recently this traditional approach has been questioned. The physical action of the brush aids in the removal of dirt and transient bacteria and is especially useful around and under the nails (Figure 16.10). However, repeated brushing dries and damages the skin through the removal of the surface layers, leading to dermatitis and bacterial colonization, which, as with clipper rash, acts as a source of infection. It is probably acceptable to limit the use of the brush to the tips of the fingers/nails or to use a nail-pick and to apply antiseptic to the hands and arms manually without scrubbing.

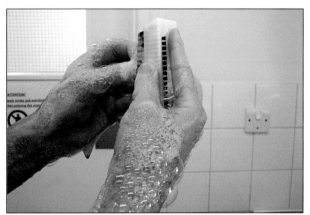

16.10 The scrubbing brush is still a valuable tool for cleaning the nails, but its role on the skin of the hands and arms is now being questioned.

Alternative approaches have been suggested, including brushless techniques (often employing the use of alcohol-based antiseptic solutions) and a nail-pick to remove debris trapped beneath the nails. They are less damaging and irritating to the skin and several recent studies suggest that they may be more effective than traditional chlorhexidine or povidone–iodine scrubs. The use of these techniques is gaining popularity in the United States and some UK medical centres.

Irrespective of the technique employed, it is important to ensure that all parts of the hands and forearms are treated, paying particular attention to the nails, backs of hands and the areas between the fingers. The aim is to ensure that the fingers and hands are the cleanest, so the hands should always be held raised above the level of the elbows, allowing liquid to run down the forearms and drop from the point of the elbow. Hands should not be shaken to disperse water or the scrub solution.

Before scrubbing, all jewellery should be removed. It is important to keep nails short and in good condition. Nail varnish should be discouraged, since worn or chipped varnish may harbour bacteria.

Timed technique

This is probably the most common technique employed (and the most varied), using timed scrubbing of anatomical sections of the hands and forearms. The scrub technique recommended by the World Health Organization is shown in Figure 16.11.

This scrub is used for the first procedure of the day. Provided that no gross soiling occurs, subsequent scrubs need only be of 3 minutes in duration.

Steps before starting surgical hand preparation

1. Keep nails short and pay attention to them when washing your hands – most microbes on hands come from beneath the fingernails.
2. Do not wear artificial nails or nail polish.
3. Remove all jewellery (rings, watches, bracelets) before entering the operating theatre.
4. Wash hands and arms with a non-medicated soap before entering the operating theatre area or if hands are visibly soiled.
5. Clean subungual areas with a nail file. Nailbrushes should not be used as they may damage the skin and encourage shedding of cells. If used, nailbrushes must be sterile and single use, although reusable autoclavable nail brushes are on the market.

Protocol for surgical scrub with a medicated soap

6. Start timing.
7. Scrub each side of each finger, between the fingers, and the back and front of the hand for 2 minutes.
8. Proceed to scrub the arm, keeping the hand higher than the arm at all times. This helps to avoid recontamination of the hands by water from the elbows and prevents bacteria-laden soap and water from contaminating the hands.
9. Wash each side of the arm from wrist to the elbow for 1 minute.
10. Repeat the process on the other hand and arm, keeping hands above elbows at all times. If the hand touches anything at any time, the scrub must be lengthened by 1 minute for the area that has been contaminated.
11. Rinse hands and arms by passing them through the water in one direction only, from fingertips to elbow. Do not move the arm back and forth through the water.
12. Proceed to the operating theatre holding hands above elbows.
13. Once in the operating theatre, hands and arms should be dried using a sterile towel and aseptic technique before donning gown and gloves.

At all times during the scrub procedure, care should be taken not to splash water on to surgical attire.

16.11 The scrub technique as recommended by the World Health Organization.

Counted brush-stroke technique

With this technique, the hands and arms are washed and lathered as before but, instead of timing the scrub section, brush strokes are counted. Tips of the fingers are treated as one unit and each finger and arm is considered to have four units: dorsal, palmar, axial and abaxial sides (the dorsal and palmar aspects of the fingers and thumb and the outer sides of the little finger and thumb are scrubbed from tip to wrist). This creates 25 anatomical regions on each hand and arm, all of which should receive an equal number of brush strokes – recommended to be between 20 and 30 strokes, with a stroke consisting of a full back-and-forth motion.

Brushless scrub technique

The recommended protocol will vary according to the manufacturer of the individual scrub solution. The following is an example of the method for Exidine™ (Scrub Care™) 2% chlorhexidine brushless surgical scrub.

1. Rinse hands for 30 seconds with warm running water.
2. Clean finger nails using a nail-pick.
3. Scrub for 90 seconds with the solution, without a brush, paying particular attention to nails, cuticles and the skin between the fingers.
4. Rinse thoroughly for 30 seconds.
5. Scrub for a further 90 seconds and rinse for 30 seconds.

Drying

Once the scrub has been completed the surgeon should move to the gowning area. The sterile pack containing gown and towel should be placed on a dry surface away from the operating table and instrument trolley and opened by a theatre assistant. The hands and forearms should be dried using a 'four-corner' technique: one corner of the towel is used in turn for each hand and forearm, taking care not to touch the parts of the towel once it has been used to dry a part of the body.

Gowns

Types of gown

Two types of gown are available: reusable woven gowns; and disposable gowns made from non-woven material.

Reusable gowns: Reusable gowns are usually woven from cotton or a polyester/cotton-blend. High-quality fabrics of up to 270 fibres per square inch are becoming standard and have better barrier properties than standard 140 muslin when dry.

Reusable cotton gowns are adequate for routine use, but do require care and regular inspection. With age and repeated laundering, areas of gross damage develop, especially around the seams and junctions of the cuffs to the sleeves. Laundering causes thinning of the fabric and, irrespective of the type of cloth used, widening of the pores in the fabric, reducing the barrier to microorganisms. Cotton and polycotton blends, of whatever fabric density, will lose their barrier effect when wet and it is vital that this is considered when using reusable gowns for procedures where significant wetting is likely. Cloth gowns are available that have been treated with a water-repellent fluorochemical. Gore-Tex reusable gowns may have the best barrier properties.

The common models of bench-top autoclaves are unreliable for sterilizing bulky cloth items in sealed packages and even vacuum models only recommend one gown per load, making routine sterilization laborious unless large porous-load autoclaves or ethylene oxide are available.

Increased duration of the surgical procedure will increase stretching of the gown and contamination with blood and other fluids, thereby increasing the risk of strikethrough. Disposable gowns should be used for all procedures in which there is a significant risk of contamination with fluids.

Disposable gowns: Non-woven disposable gowns are not made directly from yarn, but from cellulose or synthetic fibres closely bonded together to increase the barrier effect compared with woven materials, especially in the presence of moisture. This material can be reinforced to provide additional barrier protection to the lower sleeves and gown-front with impervious material.

Disposable gowns are now available pre-packed and pre-sterilized, including hand-towels. Cost is no longer prohibitive, especially if bought in bulk, when the hidden cost of laundering and sterilizing (electricity, labour and environmental factors) of reusable gowns is considered. The purchase price of disposable gowns is now less than a fifth of the cost of standard reusable gowns and a tenth of the cost of treated fabric gowns.

Gowning technique

Gowning technique is shown in Technique 16.1.

TECHNIQUE 16.1
Gowning

1 Gowns should be folded such that the body of the gown (but not the sleeves) is inside-out. The sterile pack should be opened on a surface away from the operating table.

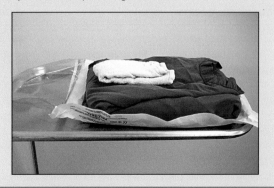

2 After drying their hands, the scrubbed surgeon should grasp the gown by the inside of the neck and allow the rest of the gown to fall.

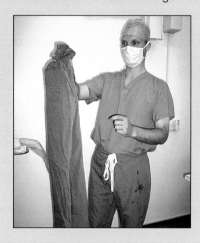

3 Touching only the inside surface of the gown, the arms are inserted into the sleeves, keeping the hands covered (see Gloving techniques).

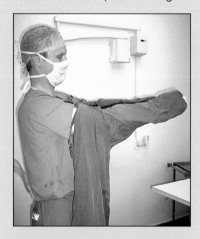

4 An assistant then pulls the gown over the shoulders (touching the inside surface of the gown only) and fastens the rear ties. With hands still within the sleeves, the surgeon passes the waist tie to the side, allowing the tip of the tie to dangle for the unscrubbed assistant to grasp. If wrap-around disposable gowns are used, they are tied by the surgeon after donning gloves.

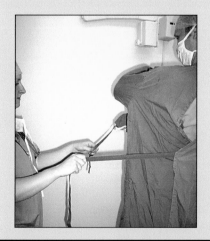

Gloves

The elastic properties of latex gloves allow them to conform to the shape of the surgeon's hands and stretch comfortably with movement. Gloves should be snug-fitting to reduce the possibility of undetected trauma to baggy pouches around the fingers.

Latex gloves form a very effective barrier, but there may be small holes in up to 1.5% of them before use (quality control standard) and gloves may be punctured in up to 13% of surgical procedures, so they are not a substitute for a thorough skin scrub technique. Double-gloving decreases the risk of complete accidental perforation, but reduces the surgeon's sensitivity which, as well as potentially compromising technique, makes the surgeon less aware that the glove has been punctured. Damaged gloves should be changed during surgery (see below). It may be useful to wear two pairs of gloves for draping the animal, so that the outer pair can be removed prior to starting the surgery, thereby eliminating the risk of accidental contamination.

Latex allergy

Gloves made solely from latex are extremely difficult to put on, so a lubricating agent is required. Traditionally this has taken the form of a powder, usually talcum or cornstarch, but there is concern over the potential for irritation of surgical wounds by the powder from gloves. Additionally, these powders play a significant role in the development of latex glove allergy, as they act as haptens, raising the antigenicity of the tiny latex particles. Type I (acute), type IV (delayed) and non-allergic irritant contact dermatitis are reported reactions to latex gloves (Figure 16.12).

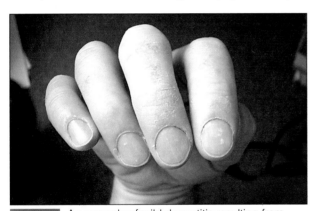

16.12 An example of mild dermatitis resulting from type IV (delayed) latex allergy.

Powder-free gloves coated with an adherent hydrogel should therefore be used for all latex allergy sufferers and, given the rise in latex allergy, should be considered for all staff. Powdered gloves have now been withdrawn from UK hospitals. Further information about latex allergy is available from www.bad.org.uk//site/1029/default.aspx and www.hse.gov.uk/latex/about.htm

Gloving technique

There are three techniques for donning gloves: closed gloving, open gloving and assisted gloving.

Closed gloving: The closed gloving technique is illustrated in Technique 16.2. This technique ensures that the scrubbed hands always remain in the sleeves

of the gown until covered by the sterile gloves. Ungloved hands never touch the outside of the gown or the gloves, so it is the most reliable way of maintaining asepsis and is therefore the technique of choice prior to surgery.

TECHNIQUE 16.2
Closed gloving

1 The inside surface of the cuff of the left glove is grasped by the left hand through the fabric of the gown, so that the fingers remain covered at all times.

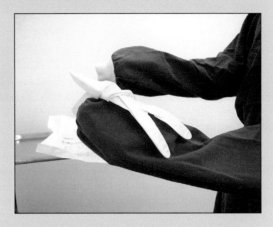

2 The right hand (which remains inside the sleeve) is used to draw the cuff over the left hand.

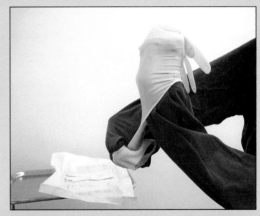

3 The fingers of the left hand are allowed through the sleeve of the gown and into the glove.

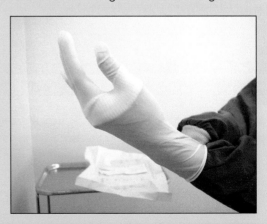

4 The process is repeated for the right glove.

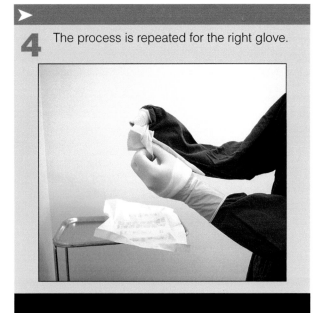

Open gloving: The open gloving technique is illustrated in Technique 16.3. Here, the hands are exposed, but only touch the inside of the glove. Because the hands are exposed the maintenance of a strict aseptic technique is less reliable and this technique is therefore suitable for a minor procedure when a sterile gown is not worn.

TECHNIQUE 16.3
Open gloving for a gownless procedure

1 Touching only the inner surface of the glove, the fingers of one hand are inserted.

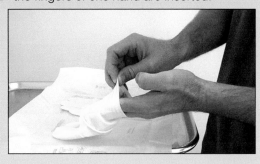

2 The thumb remains within the cuff.

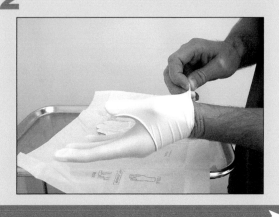

3 The opposite glove can then be picked up in such a way that outer surfaces do not contact inner surfaces.

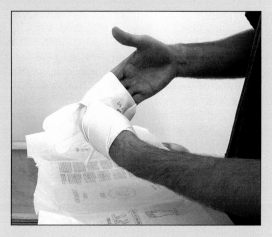

4 The opposite hand is then inserted into the glove.

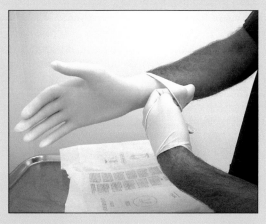

5 The gloves are pulled over the wrists.

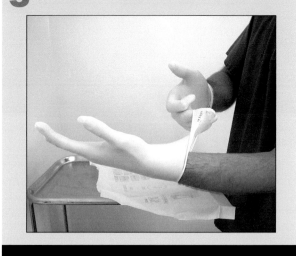

Assisted gloving: Assisted gloving relies on the presence of a previously scrubbed, gowned and gloved assistant to stretch open the cuff of the glove so that the surgeon can plunge the hand into it. The surgeon's hand is exposed prior to insertion in the glove and there is an increased risk of accidental contact with the outside of the glove and also the potential to push the cuff of the gown too far up the forearm. This is not recommended for veterinary practice.

Glove changing during surgery: If gloves have to be changed during surgery, a non-sterile assistant should be used to assist in removing the glove by pulling on the glove and cuff of the gown so that the surgeon can retract the hand back into the sleeve of the gown. The surgeon should then replace the glove in a closed manner.

Maintenance of aseptic technique during surgery

Provided the above procedures have been followed, the surgical team should be able to approach the draped scrubbed patient with clean dry sterile gowns and gloves. However, attention to detail and discipline are required to maintain the integrity of the sterile surgical field.

The sterile field consists of:

- The properly prepared and draped patient
- The surgeons in sterile gowns
- Instrument trolleys completely covered in sterile impervious drapes.

Instruments

Only personnel in sterile gowns and gloves should lay out instrument trolleys. Instrument trolleys should be laid out completely with all the instruments and implants that may be required before the first incision is made, with the exception of some items that are not required until the end of the procedure (e.g. skin staplers).

PRACTICAL TIPS

- When additional items are brought into the sterile field, the assistant should take care to pass instruments in such a way that they do not contact edges of packaging or bring ungloved hands or unopened packets directly over sterile drapes.
- Scrubbed personnel should remove sterile items from the packaging with gloved hands and items should not be tipped on to the surgical table by unscrubbed theatre personnel.

Personnel

Scrubbed personnel should consider that only the front of the gown is sterile, from the level of the chest to the height of the table. The neckline, axillae and cuffs will collect moisture, which will allow bacterial strikethrough and so are not sterile.

PRACTICAL TIPS

- Hands should remain in front of the surgeon at all times, between waist and shoulder height. Hands should either be clasped, or allowed to rest on the draped area, but arms should not be folded.
- No scrubbed member of the team should touch or approach a non-sterile surface.
- All scrubbed members should face the surgical field at all times.
- Only in exceptional circumstances should a member of the team enter or leave the room.

Contamination

If a glove becomes contaminated, the gloves should be changed (a stock of spare gloves should be maintained in theatre) away from the surgical field. If an incident of gross contamination occurs, it may be necessary for a surgeon or assistant to change gown and gloves completely and in this case it may be prudent to start a short scrub again.

References and further reading

Arrowsmith VA, Mauder JA, Sargent RJ and Taylor R (2001) Removal of nail polish and finger rings to prevent surgical infection. *Cochrane Database of Systematic Reviews* **4**, CD003325

Hibbard JS (2005) Analyses comparing the antimicrobial activity and safety of current antiseptic agents: a review. *Journal of Infusion Nursing* **28**, 194–207

Hsieh HF, Chiu HH and Lee FP (2006) Surgical hand scrubs in relation to microbial counts: a systematic literature review. *Journal of Advanced Nursing* **55**, 68–78

Mangram AJ, Horan TC and Pearson ML (1999) Guidelines for prevention of surgical site infection. *Infection Control and Hospital Epidemiology* **20**, 250–278

Mulberry G, Snyder AT, Heilman J, Pyrek J and Stahl J (2001) Evaluation of a waterless, scrubless chlorhexidine gluconate/ethanol surgical scrub for antimicrobial efficacy. *American Journal of Infection Control* **29**, 377–382

Neihaus SA, Hathcock T, Boothe DM and Goring RL (2010) A comparison of the antiseptic efficacy of chlorhexidine diacetate and povidone-iodine for presurgical preparation of the canine preputial cavity. *Veterinary Surgery* **39**, 46

Osuna DJ, DeYoung DJ and Walker RL (1990a) Comparison of three skin preparation techniques in the dog: experimental trial. *Veterinary Surgery* **19**, 14–19

Osuna DJ, DeYoung DJ and Walker RL (1990b) Comparison of three skin preparation techniques in the dog: clinical trial in 100 dogs. *Veterinary Surgery* **19**, 20–25

Owen LJ, Gines JA, Knowles TG and Holt PE (2009) Efficacy of adhesive incise drapes in preventing bacterial contamination of clean canine surgical wounds. *Veterinary Surgery* **38**, 732–737

Paulson DS (2005) Efficacy of pre-operative antimicrobial skin preparation solutions on biofilm bacteria. *AORN Journal* **81**, 492–501

Pereira LJ, Lee GM and Wade KJ (1997) An evaluation of five protocols for surgical hand washing in relation to skin condition and microbial counts. *Journal of Hospital Infection* **36**, 49–55

Tanner J, Swarbrook, S and Stuart J (2008) Surgical hand antisepsis to reduce surgical site infection. *Cochrane Database of Systematic Reviews* **23**, CD004288

Vince KJ, Lascelles BDX, Mathews KG, Altier C and Roe SC (2008) Evaluation of wraps covering the distal aspect of pelvic limbs for prevention of bacterial strike-through in an *ex vivo* canine model. *Veterinary Surgery* **37**, 406–411

Healing of elective surgical wounds

Davina Anderson

Introduction

The initial responses of a tissue to injury are highly predictable: there is bleeding and haemostasis, inflammation, swelling and oedema, heat and pain. This tissue response to injury then progresses to healing, and the process of normal tissue healing is also predictable: inflammation and debridement lead to regeneration and repair. Different tissues achieve these goals in different ways and timescales vary according to the injury and the tissue, and even with the species, but healing should progress with these basic processes.

Phases of wound healing

The phases of wound healing are illustrated in Figure 17.1 and are described below (see also Chapter 1 of the *BSAVA Manual of Canine and Feline Wound Management and Reconstruction*).

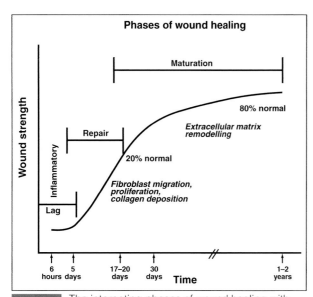

17.1 The interacting phases of wound healing with inflammation, followed by proliferation and finally repair, regeneration and remodelling of the scar tissue. (Reproduced from *BSAVA Manual of Canine and Feline Wound Management and Reconstruction, 2nd edn*)

Inflammatory phase (0–48 hours)

At the time of the initial injury (i.e. the incision):

- There is a small amount of haemorrhage, which triggers clot formation as the vessel wall is plugged with platelets
- The cytokine release that occurs on vessel wall damage, together with platelet activation, triggers an inflammatory response in the tissue:
  - The immediate response is vasoconstriction, which contributes to haemostasis
  - Within minutes, the inflammatory response causes vasodilatation, which is characterized clinically by the classic signs of heat, redness/erythema, swelling and pain.

The cellular processes are complex and a vast array of inter-reacting cells and cytokines are responsible for the early changes in injured skin.

- The coagulation response triggers chemotaxis of large numbers of neutrophils and macrophages, which kill bacteria and remove contaminants or necrotic material, including foreign bodies and dead cells.
- Epithelial cells also respond to this environment and within 12 hours of injury epithelial cells are preparing to proliferate and migrate.
- The inflammatory phase is initiated within hours of injury (Figure 17.2), and in normal circumstances

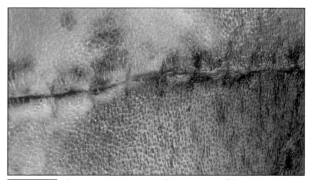

17.2 A wound 24 hours after surgery. The skin edges have been accurately apposed and there is a thin clot between the edges. Inflammation is already receding and there is a seal on the wound, but the skin edges can still be easily peeled apart. (© DM Anderson)

should only last 2–3 days after injury. If there are factors that perpetuate the inflammatory response:

- This phase persists
- The wound does not progress to the next phase
- Healing is delayed or halted.

Proliferative phase (2–5 days)

As the environment becomes more conducive to fibroblast and epithelial cell activity:

■ The macrophages and neutrophils decrease in number

■ Fibroblasts, endothelial and epithelial cells dominate the wound and migrate into the area, proliferate and proceed with regeneration and repair

■ This results in the establishment of granulation tissue, providing a matrix on to which cells adhere and migrate.

The appearance of granulation tissue in open wounds is obvious (Figure 17.3). It also occurs, in a very thin layer, between the apposed skin edges of a surgical incision. This thin layer establishes very quickly and the progression to sealing the wound and providing wound strength is rapid in wounds that are correctly apposed with sutures.

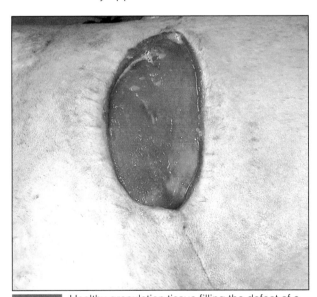

17.3 Healthy granulation tissue filling the defect of a dehisced surgical wound, prior to reconstruction. Granulation tissue is established in the proliferative phase of wound healing and consists of large amounts of extracellular matrix laid down by macrophages and fibroblasts. There are loops of immature capillaries that give it the very vascular and granular appearance. (© DM Anderson)

Granulation tissue consists of an extracellular matrix of proteins, including collagen and fibronectin. These proteins stimulate the cells and bind and present growth factors to provide positive feedback of the regeneration and repair process.

Myofibroblasts are also seen in the wound at this stage. These cells are contractile and, as the collagen matrix is laid down, they can pull the wound edges together using the collagen fibres. In large open wounds, these cells can contribute up to 30% of the wound closure. In surgical wounds, the contraction

force serves to pull the skin edges even closer together. Ultimately the epithelial surface is restored as the epithelial cells proliferate and migrate over the surface of the granulation tissue.

Remodelling phase

Finally the extracellular matrix and vascular bed slowly mature underneath the epithelial surface to form scar tissue and provide functional strength to the repair. The duration of this phase is determined by how much repair is necessary: in elective surgical wounds closed primarily, this phase is relatively brief (a few weeks). The collagen that is laid down initially is remodelled by the remaining fibroblasts and in large wounds it can be many months before the wound reaches its maximum strength. Wounds of the linea alba, which are required to be very strong, may take a longer time than the overlying skin to reach functional strength (Figure 17.4).

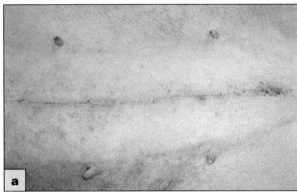

a

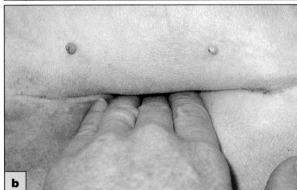

b

17.4 **(a)** Ventral abdomen of a Lurcher that had had sutures removed from a coeliotomy wound 5 days previously. The skin appears to have healed well and there is no sign of persistent inflammation or lack of healing. **(b)** The owner had noticed that the ventral abdomen was sometimes bulging. Deep palpation of the midline revealed that the underlying linea alba had not healed and there was an incisional hernia. Despite the appearance of fully healed skin, this dog was at great risk of evisceration as the skin wound would still not have been strong enough to withstand the weight of the abdominal contents had the dog been very active or straining. (© DM Anderson)

PRACTICAL TIP

Wounds that heal by second intention heal largely by the process of granulation, contraction and epithelialization, but the time frame to repair depends on the size of the wound and its management.

Species differences

Recent research has shown that there are differences in the healing of wounds between dogs and cats, and even between horses and ponies. Dogs appear to be able to mount a brisk and effective inflammatory response to skin wounds even if the subcutaneous tissue has been removed. Cats are unable to do this, and dehiscence of sutured wounds over a deficit of subcutaneous tissue is common (e.g. axillary wounds). Ponies have a good inflammatory response compared with horses; wounds in ponies are more likely to heal normally and less likely to develop poorly vascularized chronic granulation tissue.

Delayed healing

There is a huge body of research regarding the ideal conditions for healing processes. Normal healing is essentially very efficient: there are many redundancies built in that make it difficult to improve on the rate of normal healing.

What is known is that it is very easy for human interventions to hamper this process and to slow the rate of healing. Research on wounds that are failing to heal has produced interesting results regarding factors that delay healing.

- Exudate from acute wounds stimulates angiogenesis, fibroblast proliferation and collagen synthesis, whereas exudate from chronic wounds is fundamentally inhibitory to these cellular responses.
- Chronic wounds have also been shown to contain high levels of matrix metalloproteinases that degrade growth factors, inhibit cell function and break down extracellular matrix, thus preventing the progression of normal healing.
- Wounds that fail to epithelialize may have senescent epithelial cells at the margins in response to a poor granulation tissue bed, which has become biochemically chronic. This means that it is possible for a wound to fail to heal because of the wound fluid itself. It is on this basis that the recommendation to lavage chronic wounds is founded – removing this inhibitory 'soup' will help the normal healing processes to be reinstated.

Healing of surgical incisions

Surgical incisions made with a sharp blade create minimal trauma and the inflammatory response to injury should be relatively mild and of short duration. Thus, in a healthy surgical wound that has been accurately sutured, the stages are as follows.

- There is a short period where the wound is slightly swollen, red and painful, which generally reduces by 48 hours postoperatively. At this stage, the wound is sealed and the proliferative phase of healing causes the skin edges to start to heal as the granulation tissue fills the gap.
- By 5–7 days postoperatively, the wound edges are firmly adherent.
- Sutures are not usually removed until there is some strength in the wound, i.e. when the collagen fibres are remodelled and realigned according to the tension lines of the skin. At this stage (7–10 days

after the incision), there is no sign of inflammation and the wound is considered healed.
- In animals with poor collagen remodelling (see later), the wound may take several more weeks before the scar has regained strength approaching that of normal tissue.

Electroscalpel and laser incisions

Electroscalpel incisions create wounds with a much greater inflammatory response, due to the charred tissue at the edge of the incision. This charred rim each side of the incision (regardless of how narrow it is) will also have to be debrided at a cellular level in order for healing to proceed. It is generally accepted that incisions made with an electroscalpel take a few days longer to gain the strength required for suture removal and sutures are often removed 2–3 days later than when a scalpel blade is used.

The other end of the scale is the laser incision, which is associated with little inflammation and a relatively small coagulatory stimulus, resulting in a very brief inflammatory response. There is very little tissue damage and the debridement of damaged cells is completed quickly. Healing is usually rapid, and sutures may be removed 2–3 days *earlier* than with scalpel incisions.

PRACTICAL TIPS

- Surgical incisions heal using the same mechanisms as in wound healing, but the process is much faster.
- The inflammatory phase should have ceased within 2–3 days and at that point there is a thin layer of granulation tissue between the skin edges.
- This granulation tissue lasts a very short time before it is remodelled into scar tissue between the skin edges.

Clinical expectation of surgical wound healing

The elective surgical wound is created in an aseptic manner, with minimal damage to the skin edges, and is accurately apposed using sutures (Figure 17.5). Under these circumstances, there is minimal debridement necessary, no infection, no trauma or bruising and good haemostasis.

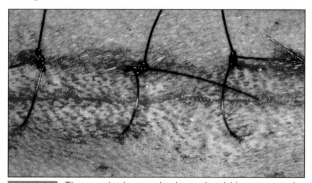

17.5 The surgical wound edges should be apposed with no tension on the sutures, which should be slightly loose at the time of placement to allow for postoperative swelling. This also makes them less irritating for the patient and easier to remove. (© DM Anderson)

The inflammatory phase is very short. Thus, the redness and swelling of the surgical wound should be largely resolved within 24–48 hours after the surgery. At this stage, the wound is not painful and is smooth and dry with no exudation.

Thereafter, the process is largely proliferative; the oedema, vasodilatation and pain should resolve and the cells involved secrete growth factors, rather than inflammatory mediators. Matrix is laid down to replace the thin layer of blood clot between the apposed skin surfaces and this is quickly converted to collagen and then to mature scar tissue. The epithelialization starts over the top of the clot within hours and is complete within 24 hours, providing a seal to the surface of the wound.

Factors affecting surgical wound healing

The healing process is much slower in circumstances where the skin edges separate or there is a prolonged inflammatory phase (e.g. where the wound is infected, the animal licks at the wound or there has been rough tissue handling during surgery). The skin edges may even start to separate as the inflammatory fluid seeps out, preventing the sealing of the edges with granulation tissue and the repair of the skin. The cardinal signs of a problem with wound healing are fluid seeping through the wound, redness and swelling of the wound edges, and continued pain associated with the skin surface beyond that expected in the initial 24–48 hours postoperatively.

Endogenous factors (local and systemic)

Any factor that affects the duration of the inflammatory phase will delay the progression of the wound towards healing (Figure 17.6). Thus a wound may have prolonged inflammation due to factors associated with the original injury (such as contamination or electrosurgery), or it may become inflamed afterwards due to subsequent events (licking or chewing at stitches, or excessive motion/tension).

All wounds require a good blood supply in order to deliver macrophages to the wound and progress to the proliferative phase; this is important in terms of achieving normal wound healing.

Understanding these factors becomes very important when large surgical procedures are carried out or where healing is delayed and decisions have to be made regarding reconstruction.

Infection

Bacterial infection causes a prolonged inflammatory phase and therefore delayed development of the proliferation necessary to seal the wound. It can also cause problems even once the proliferative phase has started, as bacteria cause sufficient inflammation to result in lysis and collapse of the extracellular matrix, and the wound edges will start to separate.

Concurrent skin disease such as pyoderma, atopy or clipper rash will decrease the likelihood of normal wound healing, not only because the patient is more likely to lick and interfere with the wound but also because the wound is inflamed for longer. The higher bacterial count on the skin surface also increases the

Prolonged inflammation

- Infection in the wound.
- Pyoderma, concurrent skin disease or 'clipper rash'.
- Necrotic material.
- Foreign material.
- Self-trauma.
- Location trauma (e.g. elbow wounds).
- Underlying non-union fracture or osteomyelitis.
- Poor technique with diathermy or electrosurgery.
- Seroma or haematoma.

Specific local factors

- Sarcoma.
- Mast cell tumour.
- Inappropriate topical medicine.

Poor vascular supply

- Tension on the wound.
- Tight sutures.
- Poor bandaging technique.
- Poor surgical technique.
- Disruption of blood supply or bruising after trauma.
- Anatomical loss of blood supply (e.g. skin flaps).
- Physiological cutaneous vasoconstriction: hypotension, pain, fear, hypothermia.

Location of wound

- Areas of high movement.
- Areas or patients with poor subcutaneous tissue underneath the wound.
- Areas of high impact or compression (e.g. elbows).
- Areas of high tension.

General status

- Theoretical: hypoalbuminaemia, low zinc, cachexia.
- Endocrine disease: hyperadrenocorticism, hypothyroidism.
- Nutritional status.
- Immune status.
- A few rare congenital skin disorders.

17.6 Endogenous factors affecting healing of surgical skin wounds.

risk of contamination of the wound edges and subcutaneous tissues during the procedure. Some surgeons use adherent sterile incise drapes to try to reduce this risk by covering the skin surrounding the wound during surgery (e.g. for implant surgery such as total hip replacement). However, in one veterinary study of elective surgery on animals with no evidence of skin disease, there was no advantage in using incise drapes (Owen *et al.*, 2009). It is not known whether use of an incise drape would achieve a decreased incidence of postoperative wound infection where there is pre-existing skin disease and an increased endogenous bacterial count.

Appropriate antimicrobial protocols should be selected for perioperative use in procedures that have been classified as contaminated or dirty and this will reduce postoperative infection. However, clipping prior to anaesthesia, long surgical times or long anaesthetic times have been shown to increase the infection rates even in clean or clean–contaminated procedures.

Foreign material

Foreign bodies or persistent inflammatory or necrotic lesions underneath a wound will delay healing (Figure 17.7) An example is a draining cutaneous sinus secondary to migrating grass awns.

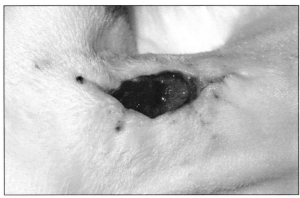

17.7 Granulating wound that had been sutured four times, but each time dehisced 10–14 days after repair. Underneath the granulation tissue was a sewing needle and thread. The wound healed uneventfully after foreign body removal. (© DM Anderson)

Vascular supply

Maintenance of the blood supply to the skin edges is very important in terms of achieving uneventful healing of surgical incisions. While surgeons are generally aware of the risks of loss of blood supply when generating a skin flap for reconstruction, more subtle reduction of blood flow is often overlooked. These subtle changes may compound other minor problems to result in wound breakdown.

Trauma and bruising to the skin may be an indication of multiple small thrombi compromising blood supply to the skin, or even a sign that the blood vessels to the skin have been avulsed. Allowing skin a few days to recover after trauma may be important in assessing what reconstructive procedure is appropriate in trauma patients.

Careful patient management during the anaesthesia, recovery and postoperative periods is also necessary to maintain good cutaneous perfusion. Hypotension, hypothermia, pain and fear are all important causes of reflex cutaneous vasoconstriction and this may persist for several days in some patients, especially during the first few days when a good blood supply is particularly important.

Nutritional status

Healing is delayed in animals with protein–calorie malnutrition, and weight loss is the single most important predictor of this condition.

- Animals that have major tissue trauma, burns, sepsis or systemic inflammatory conditions have an accelerated metabolic rate in response to the injury, which mobilizes wound repair mechanisms in the face of little nutritional intake. Eventually, there is protein–calorie malnutrition when the animal's intake can no longer match the nutritional drain of the accelerated metabolism.
- This is in contrast to animals that are chronically depleted nutritionally, such as in protein-losing disorders or starvation, where the metabolic rate is lowered and healing is slowed in order to conserve protein.
- Both of these circumstances can result in delayed wound healing secondary to inadequate nutrition.
- Wound healing in the cancer patient may also be compromised due to anorexia, cachexia or compromised organ function.

While nutritional supplementation of normal animals probably does not accelerate wound healing, it will make a difference to postoperative morbidity and mortality in animals that have documented weight loss or other contributory factors. Where large or complex surgeries are undertaken, attention to pre- and postoperative nutritional requirements is very important to support normal wound healing.

Immune status

Protein–calorie malnutrition causes depletion of the immune defence mechanisms within days. This increases the risk of infection even in low-risk surgeries and can result in sepsis due to cellular immunodeficiency. Thus in animals that are reluctant to eat postoperatively, the cascade of consequences may be devastating for the healing of the surgical incision.

The effects on healing in immunosuppressed patients are overcome if nutritional support is adequate. Thus feeding tubes and the use of high caloric density diets are important aspects of postoperative care.

Hypoproteinaemia may also delay healing, though in most veterinary studies there is no proven link between poor healing and low serum protein or albumin levels. What is probably more significant is the general metabolic effects of disease processes in animals with very low protein levels and it seems logical that these conditions should be addressed prior to surgery where possible, and that supportive measures, such as the use of feeding tubes, should be used to ensure adequate compensatory nutrition in the postoperative period.

Endocrine disease

In humans, diabetes mellitus is well known to cause significant impairment to wound healing, but this has not been documented in dogs and cats.

Hyperadrenocorticism causes delayed healing, but the biggest problem is weakening of scars with breakdown and remodelling of collagen, resulting in thinning of the linea alba and development of herniation. The initial phase of inflammation is also prolonged, as the inflammatory response is weak and the macrophages are unable to trigger the proliferative process quickly.

Hypothyroidism is well established as a cause of persistent surgical wound dehiscence, with delayed onset of granulation tissue and development of wound strength, but old surgical scars are not affected.

Data on risk factors for postoperative infection in the veterinary literature have produced conflicting results, showing endocrinopathy as a risk factor for infection in one study (Nicholson *et al.*, 2002) but not in another (Brown *et al.*, 1997).

Neoplasia

There is little published evidence that a residual tumour at the site of surgery results in an increased risk of dehiscence, but it is well recognized that certain tumours do cause delayed healing at the surgical or biopsy site. Mast cell tumours may cause delayed healing due to histamine release, which binds to histamine receptors on macrophages and inhibits fibroplasia. This causes an increased tendency for wound dehiscence associated with biopsy sites or incomplete excision.

In theory, administration of antihistamines during and after surgery should help to prevent this complication, but this has not been documented. These wounds may heal well when treated with corticosteroids, which would not normally be used to promote wound healing (see below).

Other tumours such as sarcomas or lymphoma may cause poor healing and these tumour types may be found upon biopsy of non-healing wounds.

Exogenous factors

Corticosteroids

Glucocorticoids stabilize cell membranes and inhibit inflammatory responses. This can result in delayed healing of surgical wounds, as the inflammatory phase is suppressed and the proliferative phase is unable to be triggered effectively. In theory, they may also cause an increased risk of infection, but this is not well documented in the veterinary literature.

The timing of corticosteroid therapy is critical. If therapy is started 3 days after the wound is created then it can be expected to proceed to normal healing with normal wound tensile strength at 7–10 days post-surgery. If the corticosteroid therapy is continued into the remodelling phase where the scar achieves full strength, some loss of strength may be expected with delayed remodelling, and scar weakness may be seen with widening and thinning of the scar. The dose rate used is also important: immunosuppressive doses cause much greater problems than lower anti-inflammatory or physiological dose rates.

In some circumstances it is not possible to stop corticosteroid therapy prior to surgery (e.g. patients with concurrent immune-mediated disease). In this case, it is possible to use vitamin A/zinc supplements to enable healing to progress successfully in the face of the corticosteroids. There are no veterinary products formulated for this use and clinical evidence is lacking, but there is some experimental evidence (Kaplan et al., 2004). Vitamin A should be given at a dose of 5000–20,000 IU once daily, although lower doses should be used in cats. Zinc is given at the dose rate recommended for zinc–responsive dermatitis. Zinc sulphate is used at 10 mg/kg/day and zinc methionine is used at 2 mg/kg/day. Supplementation in the presence of corticosteroid therapy may only be necessary for the first 10–14 days of healing. Pure vitamin A is teratogenic and carcinogenic for both patient and owner handling the capsules, and overdosing with zinc can cause gastrointestinal and hepatic toxicity.

Non-steroidal anti-inflammatory drugs (NSAIDs) do not have an adverse effect on healing either in the skin or in other tissues, though it would make sense for NSAIDs to be used with caution in surgical patients that have underlying gastrointestinal or renal disease (see Chapter 14).

Radiotherapy

Radiation has a significant negative effect on wound healing and the effects in inexperienced hands can be devastating. Radiotherapy interferes primarily with the proliferative phase of healing, so some centres will initiate the radiotherapy course with a single dose at the time of surgery and then not recommence until the wound is fully healed 2–3 weeks later.

Chemotherapy

Chemotherapeutic protocols do not necessarily directly affect wound healing, but side effects such as neutropenia, cachexia and protein malnutrition may be important. Chemotherapy agents are effective against tumours because they are effective against rapidly dividing neoplastic cells, but the surgical wound has a large number of dividing cells and these are also affected.

Most chemotherapy protocols in veterinary medicine use relatively low doses and the data found in human oncology studies may not be relevant to veterinary patients. Many of the drugs commonly used in veterinary oncology appear to be safe in the postoperative period (e.g. vincristine, vinblastine), but there is evidence that the heavy metal compounds (e.g. cisplatin, carboplatin) may significantly affect healing and they should be used with caution in surgical patients, particularly following gastrointestinal tract surgery. In the human literature, doxorubicin has been associated with increased risk of dehiscence after reconstructive surgery.

Complications of surgical wound healing

Delayed healing and dehiscence

Surgical wounds should no longer be inflamed or swollen by 72 hours after the surgery. The commonest cause of delayed healing is likely to be patient interference, with licking at stitches often being tolerated by owners as they perceive the animal to be 'cleaning the wound'. The most common causes of patient interference are inadequate analgesia, rough skin preparation (especially in sensitive areas such as perineal or peri-ocular skin) or tight skin sutures. Infection, bruising of the skin edges (due to rough tissue handling during surgery) and fluid accumulation (such as a seroma) will also cause prolonged inflammation.

As long as this inflammation is quickly limited, then in general the proliferative response is brisk and the sutures can be removed at 10–14 days after surgery. Wound dehiscence is seen when inflammation is not treated and the wound persists, with collagen lysis at the wound edges and failure to develop a fibrous scar. Most often, the skin edges are seen to be slightly reddened and they can be easily separated. The worst situation is where this failure to heal occurs in the deeper repaired structures, such as the body wall, and then there is a risk of dehiscence of the linea alba, which combined with the fragile skin repair can result in evisceration and death.

Prompt recognition of this failure of healing is important and abdominal incisions should be carefully checked for underlying hernias at suture removal.

Proliferation of a scar

Hyperproliferation of skin scars is rare in small animals; it is usually seen in horses (not ponies), which have a poor inflammatory response, and the development of chronic inactive granulation tissue is common. This results in large quantities of fibrous tissue laid down in the scar, creating a thickened appearance. Generally it is of cosmetic concern only.

Thinning of a scar

Sometimes an animal develops widening and thinning of old scars, especially where the underlying skin is stretched (e.g. ascites). Usually this is secondary to the stretching of the skin and remodelling of the collagen in the scar, but sometimes it occurs due to endocrine disease (see above).

'Suture sinus'

All suture materials are foreign bodies within the skin and as such trigger an inflammatory response, which will marginally delay healing.

Some suture materials are much less reactive than others (see Chapter 5). For example, subcutaneous sutures of polyglactin 910 will cause more suture reaction than poliglecaprone; and in surgical wounds that are contaminated or likely to be licked by the patient, or where there is pyoderma, polyglactin 910 may increase the inflammatory response and affect healing.

The reactivity of buried suture material will also affect the likelihood of infection associated with the suture material, particularly the knots.

Skin sutures may also play a role: braided nylon suture material, especially that which is stored on a reel and is not sterile, may cause a marked suture reaction and sinuses will form around the sutures where they enter the skin (Figure 17.8). The reaction around the passage of the suture through the tissues forms a tract, which starts to epithelialize and eventually triggers a foreign body reaction. Not only does this increase inflammation; it also increases irritation and the risk of self-trauma. These sinuses should resolve rapidly when the sutures are removed.

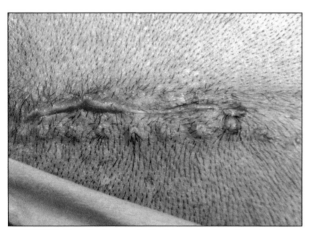

17.8 Surgical wounds that have been sutured using braided nylon stored on a reel are much more likely to form suture sinuses. There is a low-grade infection associated with each pass of the suture material through the skin and a tract forms which epithelializes. This is more likely to cause irritation and self-trauma, but this will resolve once the sutures have been removed. (© DM Anderson)

Low-grade contamination of the suture material and wound due to poor surgical preparation, poor aseptic technique or inadequate instrument sterilization may also result in 'suture sinuses'. The reaction associated with low-grade infection of a buried knot, particularly with braided material, results in an inflammatory response and delayed healing. Infection of the surgical wound after contaminated surgery, such as enterotomy, may be prevented by changing the instruments

and gloves prior to suturing the body wall and skin and using suture material that has not been used on the contaminated site.

Staples are usually less reactive and are less likely to be too tightly placed, but sometimes they are difficult to use.

Seroma formation

Careful apposition of the subcutaneous tissues also promotes healing of the incision. This achieves several objectives:

- Haemostasis
- Prevention of seroma formation
- Subcutaneous support for the skin (see earlier)
- Reduction of tension on skin edges (see below).

Seroma and haematoma formation underneath a surgical wound results in delayed healing due to the prolongation of inflammation in the area, an increase in tension on the skin edges (due to swelling) and fluid leakage through the skin. The end result in the wound is a longer period of inflammation and pain and delayed healing.

Where apposition of the subcutaneous tissues is difficult, drains may be used to allow removal of fluid. All types of drain will trigger a foreign body reaction, and the duration of drain placement has to be balanced against the inflammatory response to the drain itself.

Passive drains rely on gravity and capillary action to draw fluid out of the wound, whilst active drains have a mechanism that allows suction of fluid either continuously or intermittently, out of the wound.

Passive drains

The most common form of passive drain is a Penrose drain (Figure 17.9), which is a soft latex tube secured in the dead space and exited out through a small incision separate to the sutured surgical wound. The drain exit site should be placed at the lowest possible point, as it depends on gravity, and the drain should not be altered in any way as the volume exiting the wound depends on the surface area for capillary action.

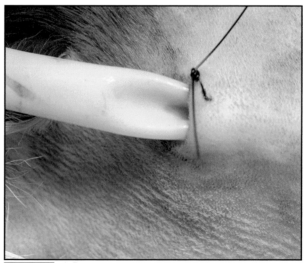

17.9 A Penrose drain is shown exiting the skin through a small stab incision and secured with a simple interrupted suture. (© DM Anderson)

Active drains

Active drains have rigid walls and are attached to some type of chamber to collect the aspirated fluid. The drain is placed through a separate stab incision and tunnelled under the skin into the dead space. The external end is attached to a bottle, which is under negative pressure, thus applying constant low level suction to the dead space and removing fluid as it accumulates. The skin is gently sucked on to the underlying tissues and seals quickly down (Figure 17.10).

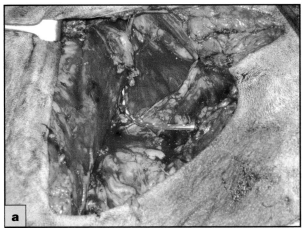

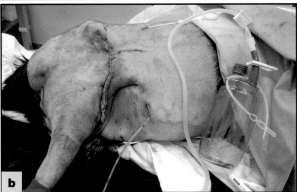

17.10 **(a)** A substantial wound resulting from the removal of a very large subcutaneous tumour in the inguinal fold with an active drain placed in the dead space prior to closure. **(b)** Wound following closure and skin sutures. Note there is a wound catheter placed dorsally to deliver local anaesthetic into the tissues as part of a balanced analgesia protocol. On the ventral aspect, the active drain is secured with a Chinese finger-strap suture and leads to a bottle, which is under negative pressure and applies continuous gentle suction to the drain. (© DM Anderson)

For further information and a full description on the use of surgical drains, the reader is referred to the *BSAVA Manual of Canine and Feline Wound Management and Reconstruction*.

Techniques to avoid complications in surgical wound healing

Good surgical technique is the most important aspect of ensuring normal healing of a surgical wound. Halsted's principles of surgery (see Chapter 21) – aseptic technique, haemostasis, atraumatic tissue handling, avoidance of foreign material, tissue apposition, management of tension – should be enough to ensure that the wound has a very short inflammatory phase and proliferation is underway within 24 hours. Postoperative management of the fresh sutured wound is also important, including:

- Allowing the wound to seal before it becomes contaminated
- Appropriate use of antibiotics
- Maintenance of vascular perfusion
- Ensuring appropriate skin tension
- Prevention of trauma and tension until the wound has tensile strength.

Wound sealing before contamination

At the end of surgery, the skin surrounding the wound is usually cleaned prior to recovery. It is important that the product used is non-irritant and that the surface of the incision itself is not cleaned.

- Sterile saline and sterile surgical swabs are used to wipe the surrounding skin clean and the sutures are not touched.
- Dilute skin antiseptics may be used to clean the skin, but not hydrogen peroxide solutions, which may only be suitable for removing blood or other fluid stains from the fur.

The wound is then covered with a light sterile dressing for 6–12 hours postoperatively. This allows the wound to seal and prevents bacterial contamination of the blood clot between the skin edges in the early postoperative period. Usually these dressings peel off within 48 hours, but by then the surface of the incision should be sealed with granulation tissue and epithelial cells.

There is some evidence to suggest that dressing surgical wounds with adhesive hydrocolloid dressings results in better and more organized healing. This may be particularly useful in areas where wound healing may be delayed due to location or contamination (e.g. perianal or wounds under tension).

Appropriate use of antibiotics

A standardized practice policy should be established to ensure that antibiotics are only given when appropriate (see Chapter 18).

- Where antibiotics are given, they should be chosen according to the likely nature of the bacteria involved.
- Antibiotics must be in the tissue fluid at therapeutic levels at the time of the first incision.
- Antibiotics given once the incision has been made, or postoperatively, do not make any difference to the incidence of postoperative infection. Thus, long-acting preparations are not suitable for perioperative use and intravenous or intramuscular preparations should be used in order to ensure that they are effective.

Vascular perfusion

Factors that may cause reflex cutaneous vasoconstriction, which compromises the vascular supply to the skin, include:

- Long complex reconstructive procedures, which can cause profound hypothermia due to exposure of large areas of prepared skin as well as heat loss through the exposed tissues
- Patients also dehydrate through the drying effect of the exposed tissues under the theatre lights and even covering these with saline-soaked swabs may not be sufficient to prevent dehydration and subsequent hypotension
- Poor anaesthetic technique may result in the appreciation of some pain
- In surgeries that involve large skin flaps, handling of the tissues can cause vasospasm directly. Reduced blood flow in the cold skin flap may result in thrombosis of vessels and ultimately loss of the distal part of the skin flap due to avascular necrosis (Figure 17.11).

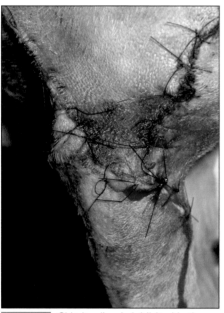

17.11 Skin healing is inhibited in the presence of infection, tension or inflammation, or where the blood supply is compromised. In this case, the tip of an axial pattern skin flap has been sutured on a place of increased mobility (the elbow) and this may have contributed to the necrosis seen here. (© DM Anderson)

Maintenance of vascular perfusion during and after surgery is important and may be aided by avoiding hypothermia, bruising, hypotension, stress, pain and fear. Many physiological responses cause decreased perfusion of the skin, both during surgery and postoperatively.

Good skin perfusion is essential for normal healing and subtle decreases from vasoconstriction may compound the poor perfusion due to wound tension, resulting in poor initiation of the healing process and ultimately in wound breakdown.

Skin tension

The normal rapid healing of a surgical wound occurs when there is accurate apposition of skin edges with appropriate sutures and no tension (see Figure 17.5). Tension reduces vascular perfusion to the edges of the skin and probably also results in repeated disruption of the granulation tissue as it forms between the skin edges. This prolongs the healing process and increases the risk of wound breakdown. This is often seen in the clinical situation with necrosis of the skin edges where there is tension or where three edges come together (Figures 17.12 and 17.13). Tension will also increase the risk of patient interference and pain.

Simple surgical techniques to relieve tension include releasing incisions, use of skin flaps and walking sutures. Pre-surgical planning is necessary to use these techniques successfully (see *BSAVA Manual of Canine and Feline Wound Management and Reconstruction*). Considerable experience is necessary for some techniques and the surgeon should always try to pre-plan the surgery.

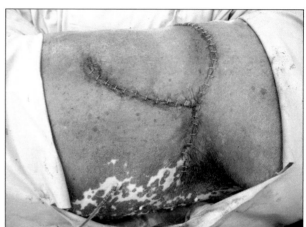

17.12 Large acute avulsion injury in a young Staffordshire Bull Terrier repaired using several strategies to promote primary surgical healing: (i) poliglecaprone subcuticular sutures take the tension on the skin (this is a non-reactive absorbable monofilament suture material and so should generate little risk of infection secondary to the contaminated wound, as well as stabilizing the wound edges over a wide mobile area); (ii) the 'at risk' triangle where the three lines of sutures meet is sutured with monofilament nylon (which is easier to place accurately and loosely, as well as less likely to cause vascular necrosis of the skin tip); (iii) staples are used as a non-reactive suture material for the majority of the repair (this also speeds up the end of what had already been a long surgery); (iv) a suction drain is visible exiting on the ventral aspect of the abdomen to prevent seroma formation. (© DM Anderson)

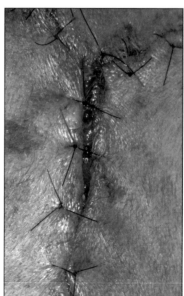

17.13 In this wound, the point at which the three edges come together is healing well, but there is too much tension on the lower part of the incision: there is prolonged swelling (as evidenced by the tight sutures) and the wound edges have separated. In this section, primary healing is not possible. (© DM Anderson)

Prevention of trauma and tension

All pet owners should be given written instructions regarding wound care, which should include restricted activity until the wound is healed. The owner should be quite clear that the animal must have its activity restricted until the veterinary surgeon deems it appropriate for normal activity to be resumed. The instruction sheet should specify that the animal should not jump up on to furniture, run up/down steps or run around the garden in between its short lead walks for toilet purposes. This is particularly important after midline coeliotomy incisions, but also applies to reconstructive procedures where activity increases the risk of seroma formation underneath the wound. The instruction sheet should also specify that the owners should inspect the wound twice daily for cardinal signs of inflammation such as heat, redness, swelling, increased pain or discharge, and should inform the owner when to seek veterinary attention.

Adequate postoperative instructions prevent the owner from ignoring the delicate time in the immediate postoperative period when simple management techniques may make all the difference.

Healing of other tissues

The gastrointestinal, urinary and reproductive tracts essentially heal in the same phases as the skin, but the healing is normally more rapid. The proliferation of enterocytes and urothelial cells starts almost immediately after wounding, but as these cells provide little mechanical strength the sutures hold the wound together for the first 3–4 days. Most visceral dehiscence occurs within 72–96 hours after the incision has been made.

Intestinal mucosa

Appositional repair is still the best technique in dogs and cats. Closure relies on the sutures for approximately 72 hours and thereafter the wound must heal by the normal process of proliferation of the stromal cells and formation of matrix.

Good healing of the intestinal mucosa relies on blood supply and luminal nutrition of enterocytes, which means that normal motility and early oral alimentation are important aspects of encouraging normal healing. Intestinal wounds rapidly develop strength and although there is lysis at the wound edges, the bursting strength of the upper gastrointestinal tract should be at least 75% that of normal tissue by the end of 14 days after wounding.

Epithelial mucosa

Epithelial surfaces usually have a rich blood supply and therefore will heal rapidly. The good blood supply also contributes to resistance against infection. This is combined with 30% more epithelial stem cells than epidermal surfaces and therefore epithelialization of defects is quicker.

Urothelium

Urothelium proliferates rapidly after wounding and the bladder in particular heals very quickly, achieving 100% of the strength of the normal tissue by 14 days. Urine leakage around ureteral or urethral tears will cause a marked proliferative response causing fibrosis and scarring or stricture. If the urine is diverted, epithelialization of defects is very rapid as long as the epithelial defect is not circumferential (i.e. there is longitudinal integrity).

References and further reading

Abrama F, Argiolas S, Pisani G, Vannozzi I and Miragliotta V (2008) Effect of a hydrocolloid dressing on first intention healing surgical wounds in the dog: a pilot study. *Australian Veterinary Journal* **86**, 95–99

Brown DC, Conzemius MG, Shofer F and Swann H (1997) Epidemiologic evaluation of postoperative wound infections in dogs and cats. *Journal of the American Veterinary Medical Association* **210**, 1302–1306

Harari J (1993) *Surgical Complications and Wound Healing in the Small Animal Practice*. WB Saunders, Philadelphia

Kaplan B, Gönül B, Dinçer S *et al.* (2004) Relationships between tensile strength, ascorbic acid, hydroxyproline, and zinc levels of rabbit full-thickness incision wound healing. *Surgery Today* **34**, 747–751

Laing EJ (1989) The Effect of antineoplastic agents on wound healing: guidelines for the combined use of surgery and chemotherapy. *Compendium Continuing Education* **11**, 136–143

McCaw D (1989) The effects of cancer and cancer therapies on wound healing. *Seminar in Veterinary Medicine and Surgery (Small Animal)* **4**, 181–286

Owen LJ, Gines JA, Knowles TG and Holt PE (2009) Efficacy of adhesive drapes in preventing bacterial contamination of clean canine surgical wounds. *Veterinary Surgery* **38**, 732–737

Nicholson M, Beal M, Shofer F and Brown DC (2002) Epidemiologic evaluation of postoperative wound infection in clean-contaminated wounds: a retrospective study of 239 dogs and cats. *Veterinary Surgery* **31**, 577–581

Swaim SF and Krahwinkel DJ (2006) *Wound Management*. WB Saunders, Philadelphia

Williams J and Moores A (2009) *BSAVA Manual of Canine and Feline Wound Management and Reconstruction, 2nd edn*. BSAVA, Gloucester

Surgical wound infection and antimicrobial prophylaxis

Chris Shales

Introduction

The term **antimicrobial** can be applied to any compound that inhibits or kills microorganisms. Strictly speaking, the term **antibiotic** should be reserved to describe natural compounds produced by organisms that kill or inhibit other organisms (usually bacteria), but the terms antimicrobial, antibiotic and antibacterial are often used interchangeably.

Antimicrobial prophylaxis (perioperative antibiosis) refers to the administration of antimicrobials in the period immediately before, during and potentially for a limited time after a surgical procedure (usually no more than 24 hours).

It is important to understand the difference between prophylactic and therapeutic antimicrobial use:

- **Prophylactic** antimicrobial use is the administration of antimicrobials in the absence of infection, with the aim of preventing it
- **Therapeutic** antimicrobial use is the use of antimicrobials to treat an established bacterial infection.

The aim of antimicrobial prophylaxis is to achieve an effective concentration of the antimicrobial agent in the tissues *before* bacterial contamination occurs and thereby reduce the number of contaminating bacteria to below the critical level required to cause an infection. **Prophylactic** antimicrobial use is only intended to encompass the time period of the procedure itself and approximately 3–6 hours following closure of the surgical wound (i.e. until a fibrin seal is formed). It is not intended to prevent postoperative contamination.

Therapeutic antimicrobial use is treatment of an established infection and requires the prescription of a course that extends beyond clinical cure. Therapy is based on identification and sensitivity testing of the causative organism.

Surgical site infections (SSIs) are defined as any infection occurring at the surgical site within 30 days, or 1 year if implants remain *in situ*.

Bacteria can be classified as Gram-positive or Gram-negative, and as aerobes, facultative anaerobes or obligate anaerobes (Figure 18.1). Gram staining can give an indication of likely susceptibility to therapy because the lipopolysaccharide coating around the cell wall of Gram-negative organisms renders them less permeable to many drugs. The mechanism of action of the drug can also affect whether organisms capable of anaerobic metabolism are susceptible.

Gram staining	Aerobes	Facultative anaerobes	Anaerobes
Gram-positive	*Staphylococcus* spp. *Streptococcus* spp.		
Gram-negative	*Pseudomonas aeruginosa*	*Enterobacter* spp. *Pasteurella* spp. *Klebsiella* spp. *Escherichia coli*	*Bacteroides* spp.

18.1 Examples of bacteria commonly isolated from SSI samples classified using Gram staining and their requirement for oxygen.

Wound infection

All surgical wounds are contaminated with bacteria, but not all become infected. A critical level of contamination is required before infection occurs, often quoted as approximately 10^5 organisms per gram of tissue or millilitre of fluid. This figure oversimplifies the situation since there are many factors involved in determining whether contamination of a wound will result in infection.

Bacterial contamination during a surgical procedure can originate from the flora of the animal itself (endogenous bacteria) or the environment or temporary skin contaminants (exogenous bacteria) (Figure 18.2).

Effective aseptic (Chapters 2 and 16) and operative (Chapter 21) techniques are essential to minimize the level of contamination and colonization of the tissues. There are a number of key factors for the surgeon when considering the potential for wound contamination and subsequent infection, including:

- Classification of surgical wounds
- Classification and incidence of surgical wound infections
- Factors that affect surgical wound infection (host

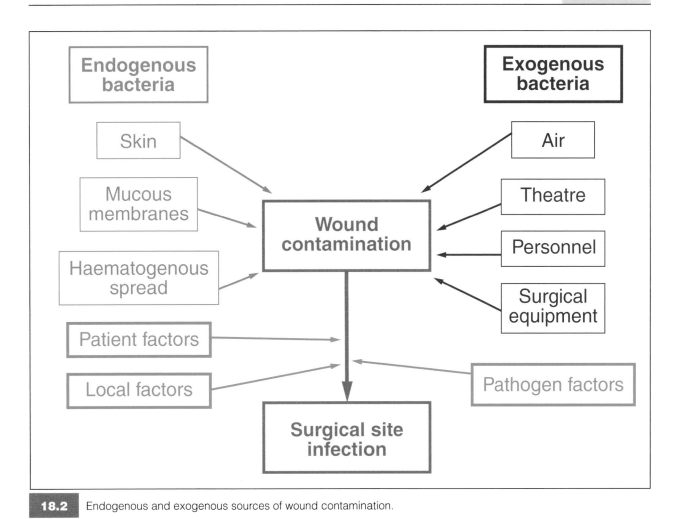

18.2 Endogenous and exogenous sources of wound contamination.

risk factors, surgical wound factors, pathogen factors)
- Prevention of surgical wound infection
- Antimicrobial drugs.

Classification of surgical wounds
Surgical wounds can be classified according to the level of bacterial contamination present at the time of the procedure (Figure 18.3). While this is simplistic, it can be a useful starting point when considering the appropriate prophylactic antimicrobial protocol and in decision-making regarding the prescription of post-operative antimicrobial therapy.

Classification of surgical wound infections
The United States Center for Disease Control and Prevention (CDC) has developed a standardized classification system for SSIs (Figure 18.4).

Incidence of surgical wound infection
The reported incidence of SSI varies roughly in accordance with the National Research Council (NRC) classification of the wound. Clean and clean–contaminated procedures are associated with an approximately 2–5% risk of postoperative infection; contaminated and dirty procedures are reported as having a 4.6–12% and 6.7–18.1% risk, respectively.

Surgical wound classification	Description
Clean	Non-traumatic elective procedure No entry into gastrointestinal, urogenital or respiratory tract No break in aseptic technique (e.g. elective uncomplicated cutaneous mass removal)
Clean–contaminated	Entry into a hollow viscus with no significant spillage (e.g. cystotomy, ovariohysterectomy) and no infection present (e.g. cystitis, cholecystitis); or a clean procedure following a minor break in aseptic technique
Contaminated	Fresh (<6–8 hours old) traumatic wounds Spillage from a contaminated viscus during surgery Entry into a hollow viscus in the presence of infection (e.g. cystitis, cholecysitis) Clean surgery following a major break in aseptic technique
Dirty	Infected surgical site (bacteria multiplying within tissue) Purulent discharge encountered Wound open and untreated for >6–8 hours

18.3 Four basic classifications of surgical wounds.

Superficial incisional SSI

- Within 30 days of surgery.
- Only skin or subcutaneous tissues of the incision itself.
- Purulent discharge, microorganisms isolated.
- One or more of the following present: pain; localized swelling; erythema; heat.

Deep incisional SSI

- Within 30 days of surgery or 1 year if implants present.
- Deep layers (muscle, fascia) of the incision.
- One or more of the following present: purulent discharge; infection does not involve an organ/space; spontaneous incision dehiscence or incision deliberately opened when fever present; presence of incision pain unless culture negative; abscess formation or other evidence of infection during further imaging, histopathology or re-operation.

Organ/space SSI

- Within 30 days of surgery or 1 year if implants present.
- Any area other than the incision that was opened or manipulated during the surgery.
- One or more of the following present: purulent discharge from drain placed in organ/space; microorganisms identified from samples; abscess or other evidence of infection evident on further imaging, histopathology or re-operation.
- Diagnosis by attending clinician.

18.4 CDC classification of surgical site infection (SSI).

Factors affecting surgical wound infection

Risk factors for SSI vary according to the study performed. Although some common factors are identified, the importance of some proposed risk factors is not clear. The following is a summary of the pertinent literature from both veterinary and human sources.

Host risk factors

Animals with systemic conditions or receiving medications that reduce the competence of their immune system are susceptible to chronic or recurrent infection and are candidates for antimicrobial prophylaxis, regardless of the assessment of the procedure itself.

Systemic diseases associated with an increased risk of infection in humans include diabetes mellitus, chronic renal failure, hepatic insufficiency and neoplasia. In veterinary patients, concurrent endocrinopathy has been associated with an eight-fold increase in the risk of infection (Nicholson *et al.*, 2002) but many of the other factors have failed to be recognized. The lack of subdivision of broad diagnoses such as endocrinopathy in veterinary studies and disagreement between some reported human and veterinary risk factors may reflect true interspecies differences or could result from the reduced power of the veterinary studies compared with those available in human medicine.

Additional factors that affect the animal as a whole and should be considered in relation to increased susceptibility to infection include: geriatric status; severe malnutrition; active infection elsewhere in the body; obesity; American Society of Anaesthesiologists' preoperative assessment score (ASA score) ≥3 (see Chapter 8); and being an entire male.

Surgical wound factors

Local factors that are or may be associated with increased risk of infection following surgery are given in Figure 18.5.

Factor	Comments	References
Clipping patient prior to induction	Skin reaction associated with clipping allows increased numbers of bacteria to grow on surface. Risk minimized if surgery occurs immediately after clipping (i.e. clipping immediately after induction). Minimizing damage to skin is also important (see Chapter 16)	Brown *et al.* (1997); Beal *et al.* (2000)
Inadequate skin preparation	Endogenous bacteria represent the most common surgical wound contaminants. Effective and sustained reduction in their numbers is a significant factor in reducing surgical infection rates (see Chapter 16)	
Length of general anaesthesia	Increased length of anaesthesia (independent of duration of surgical procedure) associated with increased risk of postoperative infection in veterinary patients undergoing clean or clean–contaminated procedures. After 60 minutes, each additional hour of anaesthesia increased infection risk by 30% for clean procedures	Beal *et al.* (2000); Nicholson *et al.* (2002); Eugster *et al.* (2004)
Length of surgical time	Surgical time identified as risk factor for infection in some studies. Procedures lasting 90 minutes are associated with a two-fold increase in risk compared with one lasting 60 minutes, with each additional hour of surgery doubling the risk	Brown *et al.* (1997); Nicholson *et al.* (2002); Eugster *et al.* (2004)
Areas of devitalized tissue (including excessive use of diathermy)	Compromised tissue represents an ideal growth substrate for microorganisms; requirement for debridement by macrophages hampers effective immune response to infection	
Seroma/haematoma formation	Provide excellent growth medium for microorganisms (particularly *Staphylococcus* spp.), exacerbated by poor activity of host immune response in fluid environment	
Foreign material	Any foreign material (e.g. implants, contamination by road debris following traffic accident) provides haven for microorganisms to evade host immune system and proliferate. Suture material (especially braided multifilament and particularly non-absorbable, such as silk) dramatically reduces number of contaminating bacteria required for infection to occur	
Wound classification	Classification of wound as dirty before procedure	Eugster *et al.* (2004)
Previous local radiotherapy	Surgery carried out on areas previously treated by radiotherapy associated with significant risk of postoperative infection	
Propofol	Use of propofol as induction agent reported to increase risk of surgical wound infection by factor of 3.8. Correct storage in refrigerated area and use of fresh vials as recommended by manufacturer likely to negate this potential problem	Heldmann *et al.* (1999)

18.5 Surgical wound factors for increased risk of infection.

Pathogen factors

The critical number of bacteria per gram of tissue required to cause an infection will vary depending on the local environment and the animal's ability to resist colonization, as discussed above. In addition to these considerations, the virulence and pathogenicity varies between bacteria species. For example:

- *Staphylococcus aureus* has a thick capsule that helps to resist phagocytosis
- Other bacteria (e.g. *Clostridium* spp.) release cytotoxic substances
- The lipopolysaccharide cell wall surrounding Gram-negative bacteria offers some protection from the immune system and penetration by antimicrobials and also forms toxic breakdown products when the cells die (endotoxins), all of which increase virulence compared with Gram-positive bacteria (Dunning, 2003).

The bacteria most frequently associated with small animal surgical wound contamination are endogenous skin flora, particularly *Staphylococcus pseudintermedius* and *S. aureus*. In cats, *Pasteurella multocida* is also a common endogenous organism and SSI isolate. *Escherichia coli* is relatively frequently cultured, due to its association with the urogenital and gastrointestinal systems in small animals. The majority of obligate anaerobes isolated from surgical wound infections are *Bacteroides* species (Dunning, 2003). Surgery carried out on different organ systems and areas within the animal will also risk contamination by organisms present as endogenous flora.

Prevention of surgical wound infection

Complete elimination of SSIs is an unrealistic goal and there will be a minimum level of infection that will occur regardless of the surgeon, facilities and level of care provided. Therefore, the aim must be to reduce the incidence of SSI to this minimal level. The reduction of SSI occurrence to this base level can only be achieved by a multi-layered approach to case and hospital management. Areas involved in achieving this goal are given in Figure 18.6 (see also Chapters 16 and 19).

Strict aseptic technique

This is one of the key areas in minimizing the SSI risk to patients (see Chapter 16). Aseptic technique is just as relevant for minimizing postoperative contamination of surgical wounds as it is for minimizing intraoperative contamination of the surgical site and, therefore, this should continue in the ward area. Preoperative and postoperative wound, drain and catheter management are important to reduce the risk of contamination outside the operating theatre:

- Every surgical wound should be covered with an adhesive dressing before leaving theatre, to provide protection from the hospital environment until the fibrin seal has formed
- Wet or soiled dressings must be replaced promptly to avoid strikethrough contamination
- Drains and catheters must be maintained with strict aseptic technique as they are risk factors for acquiring a nosocomial infection
- Good surgical technique is important in reducing the impact of the procedure on the local tissue environment.

Perioperative antimicrobial protocol

Strict adherence by all staff to a defined protocol will reduce SSI occurrence, but only in conjunction with the other factors. Reliance on antimicrobial use to make up for inadequate patient and hospital management is costly, ineffective and will lay the foundations for outbreaks of drug-resistant hospital-acquired infections.

Most of the studies in veterinary medicine on which assessment of risk factors and decisions regarding perioperative antimicrobial administration are based have been carried out on clean or clean–contaminated procedures. These are very broad categories and the inclusion of contaminated or even dirty procedures into an analysis would further increase the number of variables to the point where individual procedures within the categories would need to be assessed, as is happening in human medicine.

Surveillance

One member of the hospital team (a veterinary surgeon or nurse with an interest in infection control) should be appointed to the position of infection control practitioner (ICP). This person is required to take responsibility for ensuring thorough and regular monitoring of sterilization procedures, assessment and control of environmental contamination within the hospital, and monitoring of the incidence of SSI.

Area	Comments
Thorough patient assessment	Identification of host-associated risk factors and thorough planning of procedure to minimize anaesthetic and surgical time
Strict aseptic technique	Including theatre design, personnel clothing, patient preparation, instrument sterilization
Number of theatre personnel	Risk of SSI directly influenced by number of people in theatre
Perioperative antimicrobial protocol	Strict adherence by all staff to defined protocol to reduce risk of SSI
Surveillance	One member of hospital team appointed as infection control practitioner
Prompt discharge	Each additional day spent in intensive care increases risk of SSI. Prompt discharge to home environment reduces risk of hospital-acquired infection
Effective analgesia	Patients receiving effective pre-emptive multimodal analgesia will eat, heal, fight infection, allow nursing and be discharged more quickly and efficiently than those without adequate analgesia
Hand hygiene	Routine hand hygiene of appropriate standard between handling animals in the hospital

18.6 Means of reducing incidence of SSI.

Clinicians in the hospital must report SSIs to the ICP so that data can be collected regarding the severity, timing, causative organism, nature of the procedure, theatre used, etc. The data can be used to identify and address potential outbreaks of infection as they occur, to determine the appropriate perioperative antimicrobial protocol and also to reassure owners that every reasonable step has been taken to avoid infectious complications.

Antimicrobial drugs

Classification and mechanism of action

- A **bacteriostatic** compound is one that inhibits the growth of bacteria so that the animal can mount an effective immune response.
- A **bactericidal** compound is one which itself causes the death of the organism.

In reality, these two categories are not mutually exclusive, since the concentration of the antimicrobial will often determine whether it is bacteriostatic or bactericidal. The classification therefore depends on whether the dosing regime can achieve a suitable tissue concentration to be bactericidal before negatively affecting the treatment through drug toxicity, cost or practicality of dosing (Figure 18.7).

$$\frac{\text{Minimum bactericidal concentration (MBC)}}{\text{Minimum inhibitory concentration (MIC)}} \text{ } \mathbf{<4\text{--}6}$$

MBC = the minimum concentration that kills 99.9% of the organism
MIC = the minimum concentration that inhibits growth of the organism

Generally, bactericidal drugs have an MBC that is relatively similar to the MIC. Dosage regimes to achieve tissue concentrations of >6 times the MIC in order to achieve bactericidal activity (MBC) are not commonly recommended.

18.7 Bactericidal activity.

Antimicrobial classes

Beta-lactam antimicrobials

This group includes penicillin, penicillin derivatives and the cephalosporins. These compounds are not metabolized in the body but are excreted unchanged in the urine, at high concentration. Cephalosporins differ slightly in structure from the penicillins but all beta-lactams work by damaging bacterial cell wall production during growth, resulting in increased cell permeability and eventual osmotic lysis (isotonicity in the host is hypotonic to the bacteria). This mechanism of action renders the beta-lactams susceptible to reduced efficacy in hypertonic environments, when cell wall turnover is at a low level or when penetration into the cell wall is inhibited by pore size (e.g. Gram-negative bacteria).

Penicillin derivatives: Benzyl penicillin (**penicillin G**) has activity against Gram-positive cocci, most anaerobes and some of the more fastidious Gram-negative aerobes including *Haemophilus*, *Pasteurella* and some

Actinobacillus spp. Beta-lactamase is an enzyme that breaks down the beta-lactam ring and therefore affords bacterial resistance to the target beta-lactam antibiotic structure. Penicillin G is broken down by gastric acid and this, along with high levels of resistance among the beta-lactamase-producing *Staphylococcus* and *Bacteroides* spp., limits its use in a clinical situation.

Alterations in the spectrum of activity, improved absorption from the gastrointestinal tract and resistance to beta-lactamase have been achieved by synthetic modification of the basic penicillin G molecule. **Beta-lactamase-resistant penicillins** (e.g. dicloxacillin, meticillin, oxacillin) have improved activity against staphylococci but only fair activity against other Gram-positive organisms.

Ampicillin and **amoxicillin** add Gram-negative activity to the basic penicillin G spectrum of activity. Protection against beta-lactamase using clavulanic acid increases the activity of these compounds against organisms that have developed resistance by this method, but does not increase their spectrum of activity to include organisms with innate resistance such as *Pseudomonas* and *Enterobacter* spp.

A fourth class of penicillin-derived compounds is described as having an extended spectrum of activity. This class includes drugs such as **carbenicillin** and **ticarcillin**, which boast efficacy against *Pseudomonas* spp. and an enhanced efficacy against *Klebsiella* and *Proteus* spp. These compounds may be less effective than the other classes against anaerobes and are available in combination with clavulanic acid to impart beta-lactamase resistance.

Imipenem boasts one of the broadest spectrums of activity available, including *Pseudomonas* spp., and is extremely resistant to beta-lactamase-induced degradation. Whilst expensive and currently only available as an injectable preparation, it can be helpful when dealing with resistant infections, based on culture and sensitivity results, in the absence of viable alternatives. Imipenem is not effective against meticillin-resistant *Staphylococcus aureus* (MRSA).

Injectable depot preparations of penicillins are prepared as relatively insoluble compounds and the concentration reached in the body fluids is low and may not be efficacious. These long-acting preparations have no place in antimicrobial prophylaxis.

Cephalosporins: The cephalosporins are grouped in generations one to three, which can be used to give generalized information regarding their spectrum of activity. Cephalosporin resistance to beta-lactamase generally renders them more effective against *Staphylococcus* spp. than the penicillins, but the degree of resistance can vary between drugs of the same generation.

- First-generation cephalosporins (e.g. **cefalexin** and **cefazolin**) have a spectrum of activity similar to amoxicillin, i.e. they have activity against both Gram-positive and Gram-negative organisms, with some activity against anaerobes.
- Second-generation cephalosporins (e.g. **cefuroxime**) have a slightly narrower spectrum of activity but are more effective against *Enterobacter* spp., some *Proteus* spp., *Escherichia coli* and *Klebsiella* spp. Overall they are effective against Gram-positive organisms and have enhanced

Gram-negative activity when compared with the first generation but are considered relatively poor against anaerobic bacteria.

■ Third-generation cephalosporins (e.g. **ceftazidime**) have more activity than the other generations against Gram-negative bacteria but less against Gram-positive organisms (including *Staphylococcus* and *Streptococcus* spp.) and are considered poor against anaerobes. Their predominant advantage over previous generations is activity against the Gram-negative *Pseudomonas aeruginosa*, *Enterobacter* spp. and *Serratia*, but activity is not uniform across this generation and therefore each individual drug needs to be assessed for suitability.

Cefovecin is a third-generation cephalosporin that is highly protein bound and therefore has an extremely long elimination half-life. It has shown activity *in vitro* against *Staphylococcus*, *Pasteurella*, *Escherichia coli* and some anaerobic bacteria, but there is inherent resistance among *Pseudomonas*, *Enterococcus* spp. and *Bordetella bronchiseptica*. Fourth-generation cephalosporins follow the trend of increased efficacy against Gram-negative organisms and are also reported to have reduced potential to induce resistance. Unlike second- and third-generation cephalosporins, their increased activity against Gram-negative organisms has not been at the expense of Gram-positive organism sensitivity and they retain the characteristics of the first-generation in this regard. Their importance in human medicine largely precludes their use in animals at this time.

Aminoglycosides

These bactericidal antimicrobials prevent bacterial protein synthesis by inhibiting ribosomal function. By inhibiting protein synthesis they can reduce the production of beta-lactamase by bacteria and therefore act synergistically with beta-lactam antimicrobial agents. Examples include **gentamicin** and **amikacin**.

Aminoglycosides are very effective against Gram-negative bacteria, including *Pseudomonas* spp., and some Gram-positive organisms, including *Staphylococcus* spp. They have no activity against anaerobic organisms, due to the reliance on oxygen-driven active transport for uptake of the compound by the bacteria. They have activity against *Nocardia* and some atypical mycobacterial organisms.

Renal toxicity: Aminoglycoside-induced renal toxicity in the dog manifests initially as a reduced ability to produce concentrated urine and can progress to azotaemia as a result of inhibition of renal tubular cell function. Aminoglycosides can also inhibit renal prostaglandin synthesis, which leaves the kidney less able to maintain the glomerular filtration rate in response to changes in systemic blood pressure. For this reason, concurrent non-steroidal anti-inflammatory drug therapy is not advised.

Toxicity of aminoglycosides correlates to the trough concentrations reached between doses, whereas bactericidal efficacy is related to the peak concentration reached, independent of time spent at that concentration. Therefore maximum efficacy and minimal risk from toxicity are achieved by once rather than twice daily dosing.

Patients susceptible to changes in renal perfusion or suffering from increased susceptibility to nephrotoxicity should be treated with caution, or the aminoglycoside group avoided altogether. The risk of toxicity can be minimized by maintaining patient hydration, avoiding other nephrotoxic agents and once daily dosing. Concerns regarding the risks of toxicity limit the use of this class of antimicrobial agents.

Fluoroquinolones

This group of bactericidal antimicrobials inhibits DNA gyrase and therefore disables cell reproduction. They have poor activity against anaerobes, do not act effectively against *Streptococcus* or *Enterococcus* spp., but are considered effective against some other Gram-positive and many Gram-negative aerobes, including *Pseudomonas*.

Administration to very young animals is contraindicated due to the risks of cartilage metabolism disturbance and tooth discoloration. **Enrofloxacin** should be used with caution in cats, due to the reported risk of acute-onset blindness following administration. **Marbofloxacin** has a reduced risk of this toxic side effect.

The efficacy of this group is considered concentration dependent, though time spent above the minimum inhibitory concentration (MIC) may be important for some organisms.

Generally, resistance to fluoroquinolones has been relatively slow to appear among veterinary bacterial isolates. Unfortunately, low levels of plasmid-mediated resistance have been demonstrated in several organisms, including efflux of the drug from the organism (e.g. *Staphylococcus aureus*), decreased drug uptake due to reduced pore size (*Pseudomonas aeruginosa*) and cell wall structural alterations.

Potentiated sulphonamides

Trimethoprim/sulphonamide and related compounds inhibit the synthesis of folate, which is essential for bacterial cell survival. They are considered broad-spectrum bactericidal compounds with efficacy against Gram-positive, Gram-negative and anaerobic organisms, but they have no activity against *Pseudomonas* or *Enterococcus* spp. Resistance is relatively common, especially among *Staphylococcus* spp., due to altered drug penetration and target enzyme changes. Increasing and rapid development of resistance via plasmid transfer along with some potential toxic effects (e.g. immune-mediated polyarthritis) has resulted in reduced use of this group in recent years. Meticillin-resistant *S. aureus* is often sensitive to this drug.

Tetracyclines

These compounds bind reversibly with one of the ribosome units. Ribosomes are a key component of protein synthesis. Tetracyclines are considered bacteriostatic and have efficacy against Gram-negative and Gram-positive organisms, with many anaerobes also showing susceptibility. They have limited action against *Staphylococcus* spp. and none against *Enterococcus*, *Pseudomonas aeruginosa* or *Enterobacter* spp.

Metronidazole

This drug impairs microbial DNA synthesis following metabolism by the microorganism to its active component. It has activity against Gram-negative anaerobes and most Gram-positive anaerobes. High doses (up to 25 mg/kg orally q12h or 10 mg/kg slow i.v. q12h) have been associated with seizure activity. Administration can be associated with a poor appetite due to an unpleasant taste in the animal's mouth, even when administered intravenously.

Lincosamides

Lincosamides are generally considered bacteriostatic antimicrobials that inhibit ribosome function and therefore inhibit protein synthesis. They can be bactericidal, depending on the concentration reached and the susceptibility of the organism. Lincosamides have activity against Gram-positive cocci and many obligate anaerobic bacteria. Whilst resistance among *Staphylococcus* spp. is not uncommon, high concentrations can be useful for an infection caused by penicillin-resistant staphylococci. They achieve high concentrations in bone, bile, prostatic fluid and milk. Animals with hepatic or renal dysfunction should be treated with caution.

Macrolides

The spectrum of activity of **erythromycin** is similar to the penicillins (Gram-positive and anaerobes) and it can be used instead of penicillin. Macrolides inhibit protein synthesis by binding to a ribosome subunit. They are considered bacteriostatic or bactericidal, depending on the concentration of the drug and organism susceptibility. Erythromycin has intestinal prokinetic effects that can contribute to the nausea, vomiting and diarrhoea experienced by a high proportion of animals treated with this drug.

Antimicrobial failure and resistance

Resistance to antimicrobial agents can be inherent or acquired.

- **Inherent** resistance of an organism to a compound can be predicted (for example, the lack

of efficacy of aminoglycosides against anaerobic bacteria).
- **Acquired** resistance usually requires a spontaneous genetic mutation or acquisition of additional genetic material.

Spontaneous mutations are slow to occur and often result in multiple alterations that render the organism less virulent, or more susceptible to other antimicrobial compounds. Sustainable and effective resistance occurs most commonly and far more quickly through the transfer of genetic material between microorganisms in the form of plasmids (extra-chromosomal DNA molecules that can be transferred between organisms). DNA conferring resistance can also be attained by transduction, transformation and conjugation.

Plasmid-mediated resistance is especially common among Gram-negative bacteria but can be transferred between both Gram-negative and Gram-positive organisms. The transfer of a single plasmid can confer resistance against several antimicrobial groups.

Inappropriate dosing intervals or tissue concentrations close to the MIC (see Figure 18.7) both contribute to the increasing prevalence of resistant organisms within a population of bacteria by selectively eliminating only the most susceptible organisms (Gould, 1999). Successive populations then have a greater proportion of organisms with varying degrees of resistance (Figure 18.8), many of which will swap plasmid-mediated resistance mechanisms. In a similar way, polypharmacy should be avoided whenever possible, as any organisms remaining will contain genetic material conferring resistance to multiple antibiotic classes.

Rational approach to antimicrobial prophylaxis

Research carried out in human and veterinary hospitals suggests that strict adherence to a standard protocol for the selection and administration of prophylactic

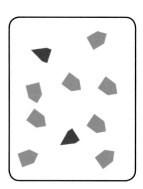

Mixed bacterial population

Resistant bacteria are more pointed and darker in colour but represent a minority of the population

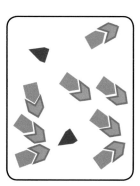

Antimicrobial selectively targets the susceptible proportion of the population

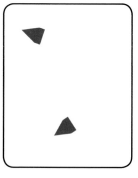

The remaining resistant bacteria are freed from the competition for resources

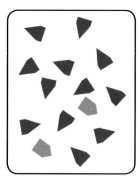

The population then becomes dominated by resistant bacteria whose numbers cannot be significantly reduced by the same antimicrobial agent

18.8 Selection pressure for antimicrobial resistance applied by the presence of the drug.

antimicrobials to surgical patients that will benefit from it significantly reduces the incidence of postoperative infection, reduces the selection pressure for resistant bacteria and allows the hospital to predict the costs involved (Brown *et al.*, 1997; Willemsen *et al.*, 2007). Despite this fact, multiple studies in the human literature suggest that compliance with prophylactic antimicrobial protocols remains poor, particularly relating to overuse during the postoperative period (Haydon *et al.*, 2010). Haphazard administration of different drugs at ineffective dose rates not only leaves individual animals open to infection; it also provides the ideal environment for the emergence of resistant strains of bacteria and is therefore likely to cost the hospital money in the long term.

The policy should provide not only standard dosages and a standard first-line choice of antimicrobial agent, but also clear guidelines on the assessment of each patient and procedure, taking into account the risk factors that have been discussed in this chapter. This assessment can then be used to decide whether antimicrobial prophylaxis is indicated and whether postoperative antimicrobial use is warranted.

During the selection process for the prophylactic antimicrobial agent, activity against the likely contaminants must be considered as well as the method of administration, the concentration required and the potential for toxic side effects. Most prophylactic antimicrobials are administered intravenously and take approximately 15–30 minutes to equilibrate with the tissue compartment. Despite lack of supportive evidence, the dosing interval is usually more frequent during the procedure than when the same drug is administered to the conscious patient, perhaps due to the diuresis usually present in patients undergoing surgery or the desire to maintain the concentration of time-dependent antimicrobials higher than the MIC until the wound is closed with a fibrin seal.

Clean procedures

Prophylactic antimicrobial administration is not warranted for short, clean procedures carried out on healthy tissue in an animal with a competent immune system, because the level of contamination should be low enough for the immune system to eliminate (Vasseur *et al.*, 1988; Brown *et al.*, 1997). Possible exceptions to this rule would be those procedures for which a surgical wound infection would be catastrophic, such as a total hip replacement or pacemaker implantation, where a permanent implant is used, or those clean surgeries where the surgical procedure is of a relatively long duration. In respect of the latter, 90 minutes is often given as the cut-off point, although this may be because it is the only time point that has been evaluated. Antimicrobial prophylaxis increases the proportion of resistant organisms within a hospital bacterial population and therefore administration should be justified in every case (Rubenstein *et al.*, 1994).

Clean–contaminated procedures

The human literature varies with regard to efficacy of antimicrobial prophylaxis for significantly reducing SSI rates for this category of surgery, depending on the procedure (Verschuur *et al.*, 2004; Skitarelić *et al.*, 2007). Whilst no prospective randomized controlled studies of this type exist in the veterinary literature, it is

likely that the influence of prophylactic antimicrobial administration in reducing SSI rates for clean–contaminated procedures would also be less than clear-cut. This may be because a wide variety of procedures, with a large range in the likelihood of contamination, are contained within this category. Decisions regarding the indication for antimicrobial prophylaxis should therefore include the potential number and virulence of organisms in the surgical site, in addition to host and local wound factors.

Contaminated procedures

The SSI rate for contaminated and dirty procedures is higher than for clean and clean–contaminated procedures. The presence of higher levels of contaminating organisms suggests that antimicrobial prophylaxis is warranted, although definitive study data are lacking.

Dirty procedures

The administration of an antimicrobial agent to these cases is classified as therapeutic and should therefore be based on culture and sensitivity results from representative samples (usually a wound-bed tissue sample following lavage). It is often appropriate to use empirically chosen drugs once the samples have been obtained, until results become available.

Resistance

The emergence of resistant strains also influences the rational approach to antimicrobial prophylaxis. Avoidance of over-prescribing antimicrobials has the potential to improve the efficacy of the commonly used compounds by reducing the selection pressure for ever-increasing proportions of resistant organisms within the population (Gould, 1999). The proportion of resistant bacteria within the population should then decline as their competitive advantage is reduced. In reality, this can be achieved by the responsible prescription of antimicrobial agents and following a few fundamental principles:

- Avoidance of unnecessary antimicrobial therapy (e.g. uncomplicated diarrhoea, upper respiratory tract infections, prolonged postoperative courses)
- Basing treatment of infection on culture and sensitivity results or, at the very least, thoughtful selection of a compound with activity against likely contaminants
- Use of an appropriate dosing interval and dosing towards the high end of the dose range to ensure a local tissue concentration above the MIC (unlikely with the majority of long-acting injections)
- Reserving the use of antimicrobials to which the incidence of resistance is known to be low for situations where their use to is specifically indicated by appropriate sensitivity results (e.g. fluoroquinolones)
- Strict adherence to a logical prophylactic antimicrobial protocol
- Selection of the antimicrobial agent based on the most likely contaminating bacteria whilst avoiding selection of highly engineered agents unless absolutely necessary
- Avoidance of postoperative antibiotic use unless an infection is confirmed.

Prophylactic antimicrobial protocol

The following protocol represents a logical approach to the administration of an antimicrobial agent where the presence of one or more risk factors has led the surgeon to consider that antimicrobial prophylaxis is appropriate.

Principles of surgical antimicrobial prophylaxis

These principles of surgical antimicrobial prophylaxis (perioperative antibiosis) are based on guidelines issued by the CDC.

- Use perioperative antimicrobials for procedures that are subject to risk of infection.
- Select a safe inexpensive bactericidal agent with a spectrum of activity against the organisms likely to cause SSIs in that patient population.
- Administer the antimicrobial compound such that bactericidal concentrations are present in the tissues at the time of skin incision.
- Maintain adequate tissue concentrations until the wound is closed and the fibrin seal formed (3–6 hours). Do not continue therapy beyond 24 hours.

Antimicrobial selection

For broad-spectrum bactericidal activity against likely pathogens, including efficacy against *Staphylococcus* and *Pasteurella* spp., amoxicillin/clavulanate, first-generation cephalosporins (e.g. cefazolin) and second-generation cephalosporins (e.g. cefuroxime) are common choices. Third-generation cephalosporins (e.g. ceftazidime) and fluoroquinolones (e.g. enrofloxacin) have too narrow a spectrum of activity to be considered appropriate. An exception would be surgery of the large intestine, where Gram-negative and anaerobic populations predominate and therefore a second-generation cephalosporin (e.g. cefuroxime) and metronidazole combined or other antimicrobials with equivalent activity could be considered.

Intravenous administration

The antimicrobial should be safe, cost-effective and rapidly distributed within the tissues. Intramuscular or subcutaneous administration routes are usually far slower to reach maximum levels in the tissue, may not reach the high tissue concentration that the intravenous route does and may require the dose to be given several hours before the induction of anaesthesia.

Timing: Intravenous administration should be as soon as is convenient following the induction of anaesthesia, whilst monitoring equipment is being placed and preparation of the surgical site is carried out.

Dose

The protocol should ensure that the dose administered is in the upper half of the therapeutic range to ensure that the MIC is reached at the operative site and to maximize efficacy (Figure 18.9).

Antimicrobial agent	Dose
Amoxicillin/clavulanate	20 mg/kg slow i.v.
Cefazolin (first-generation cephalosporin)	20–25 mg/kg slow i.v.
Cefuroxime (second-generation cephalosporin)	20–50 mg/kg slow i.v.

18.9   Prophylactic doses of antimicrobial agents.

Additional dosage: Evidence suggests that re-administration should occur within two half-lives of the antimicrobial agent. Generally if the procedure is likely to last longer than 3 hours, additional dosages of the prophylactic antimicrobial agent are administered following the initial dose (e.g. amoxicillin/clavulanate every 2 hours, or cefazolin up to 3–4 hours). The drug, route and quantity administered should be identical to that given at induction. Some surgeons will request administration every 90 minutes though the evidence for this requirement is lacking.

Prophylactic administration

The drug should remain at effective levels (above the MIC) until the fibrin seal has formed postoperatively (approximately 4–6 hours). Continuation of antimicrobial use for up to 24 hours may be performed when one or more risk factors for infection are present, though the evidence in favour of this is lacking. There is no evidence in the human or veterinary literature to support administration of perioperative antimicrobial agents beyond 24 hours postoperatively (Dunning, 2003).

Extension of use

Rates of SSI in humans who receive antimicrobials for 24 hours postoperatively are the same as those that receive a 5-day course and there is therefore currently no evidence to support the extension of prophylactic antimicrobial administration beyond the operative period (Dunning, 2003; Hedrick *et al.*, 2007). This includes those patients considered at increased risk of SSI during the preoperative assessment. In fact, in addition to needlessly adding to the cost of the procedure, inappropriate administration beyond 24 hours to this group of animals will significantly add to the selection pressure for resistant organisms within the hospital environment.

There is no evidence in the literature to support the continued use of antimicrobial agents until tubes or drains are removed postoperatively (Hedrick *et al.*, 2007*)*. In a study looking at cystostomy tubes, continuation of antimicrobial treatment did not prevent urinary tract infection and significantly increased the occurrence of resistant infections (Barsanti *et al.*, 1985). A more logical approach is to monitor these patients carefully and treat an infection if and when it occurs. Commonly, the onset of infection coincides with the possibility of removal of the tube or drain. The end of the tube can be submitted for culture, allowing selection of the most appropriate therapy, whilst adding to the likely success of treatment by removal of the foreign material. Furthermore, the bacteria present are more likely to be susceptible to the antibiotic selected while culture results are pending, as they have not previously been exposed to selection pressure from antimicrobial agents while the tube/drain was in position.

Therapeutic use of antimicrobial agents in the surgical patient

Dirty procedures

As discussed above, prophylactic antimicrobial agents used for clean, clean–contaminated or contaminated surgical procedures are either discontinued at the end of the procedure or a maximum of

24 hours postoperatively, depending on the surgeon's assessment of the risk factors.

Procedures classified as dirty are by definition either already infected or have sufficient numbers of bacteria at the surgical site that infection is inevitable. Whilst these do not count as SSIs for surveillance purposes, the considerations are similar concerning therapeutic rather than prophylactic antibiotic use. Treatment is based on culture results and continues for 2–3 days beyond the resolution of the disease, as assessed clinically or by repeated microbial testing when indicated.

Surgical site infection

Following the diagnosis of a SSI the main priorities should include:

- Cleaning the infected area
- Establishing drainage
- Gaining a representative sample for analysis
- Administration of appropriate systemic antimicrobial therapy
- Preventing further contamination of the wound or the hospital environment.

Cleaning the wound

Whilst some superficial incisional SSIs can be treated relatively conservatively, the appearance of purulent discharge from a wound is likely to result in a degree of dehiscence. In the absence of the natural establishment of drainage, the clinician may be required to remove sutures and partially open the wound to achieve the same result. Once opened, the area should be treated as an infected wound:

- Flushing with sterile Hartmann's solution is ideal since it is likely to be less damaging to the fibroblasts than 0.9% saline. Using a 20–30 ml syringe and a 19 gauge needle should provide approximately 8–10 psi for optimal lavage
- Dead tissue and foreign material should be removed (debridement), which can require a general anaesthetic. Tissue of questionable viability should be left in place to be removed at a later stage once it becomes clear that it is no longer viable. Adherent dressings may be required in the early stages as an aid to wound cleaning (see *BSAVA Manual of Canine and Feline Wound Management and Reconstruction*).

Some clinicians add antiseptic to lavage solutions and a few studies have suggested a slight benefit over saline. Chlorhexidine (0.05% or 1:40 dilution) can significantly reduce the contamination rate or the concentration of bacteria in the wound, compared with saline or saline with povidone–iodine (Popovitch and Nannos, 2000). However, the concentration of the agent must be strictly measured, due to the potential for toxicity to the granulation tissue, and should be used fresh as it tends to precipitate. The author does not routinely add antiseptics to lavage solutions due to the risk of toxicity and limited potential for significant benefit. There is no evidence to support the addition of antimicrobial agents to wound lavage solution during the management of wound contamination or infection.

Culture and sensitivity testing

It is essential to gain a sample of the pathogenic bacteria before commencing antibiotic therapy, as failure to do this can result in the use of an inappropriate agent and a considerable delay to successful treatment. The tissue or sample can be placed into a charcoal swab kit and submitted to the laboratory for both aerobic and anaerobic bacterial culture and sensitivity testing. A Gram stain will provide results more rapidly and will help to guide therapy.

Treating the infection

Interim treatment: Until the culture results are available, the infection should be treated with an empirically selected bactericidal broad-spectrum antimicrobial agent active against the likely contaminating organisms. Previous therapy needs to be taken into account and the response to therapy should be monitored carefully.

Antimicrobial choice: Adherence to a practice prophylactic antimicrobial protocol should make the usual prophylactic agent a suitable choice as a first-line broad-spectrum agent likely to be effective against the causative organism. Exceptions to this include SSIs that have developed despite recent administration of an antimicrobial, and those cases that have received ineffective courses of antimicrobial therapy. These cases may be more likely to be infected with a Gram-negative and/or resistant organism and may require choice of a novel agent.

Administration: Intravenous administration for the first 24 hours maximizes the potential for rapid efficacy of an appropriate agent and should be considered whenever possible. Progression of the infection or failure to show signs of improvement within 24–48 hours should stimulate a careful re-evaluation of the treatment, including the drug, dose and administration rate.

Interpretation of culture results: Interpretation of the culture results is important:

- A mixed or sparse growth is unlikely to represent the infectious agent and may indicate that the wound is not infected or poor sampling technique.
- Heavy growth of an isolate, particularly a pure heavy growth, is likely to be an accurate reflection of the causative agent and should therefore be acted upon.

Most SSIs, particularly orthopaedic SSIs, are due to a single organism. It should be remembered that the *in vitro* sensitivity results may not always accurately reflect the *in vivo* situation. Extended sensitivity profiles should be requested for multidrug-resistant organisms and the clinician should be able to discuss the treatment of the infection with the laboratory when appropriate.

Extension of systemic treatment: Treatment of infections with systemic antimicrobials should go on beyond the time taken to achieve clinical cure:

- Generally 2–3 days for soft tissue infections
- A minimum of 2 weeks for orthopaedic SSIs

involving the joint or bone (resulting in a total of 4–6 weeks of antibiotic therapy in many cases).

Increasing the dose of certain concentration-dependent antimicrobial agents can also increase their activity against resistant infections; for example, increasing the systemic dose of enrofloxacin to 20 mg/kg q24h in dogs with *Pseudomonas* infection can increase efficacy.

Topical therapy: Topical treatment can be helpful, particularly when dealing with resistant organisms. Topical antimicrobial therapy (e.g. gentamicin-impregnated collagen sponge or beads) can provide high concentrations of the drug at the site of infection, which would otherwise not be possible.

Antimicrobial dressings can also be a useful adjunct to therapy (e.g. silver- or honey-impregnated dressings) (see *BSAVA Manual of Canine and Feline Wound Management and Reconstruction*). The topical application of an antimicrobial agent without a vehicle for slow release (e.g. collagen sponge) is of questionable use, particularly in exudative wounds. Systemic administration of the drug will ensure that the exudate itself contains the agent, rather than relying on the compound moving into the tissues against the flow of fluid. Local administration also results in an initial high concentration that may be irritant or toxic.

Protection of the wound

Avoiding contamination of the area of the SSI from the environment (and *vice versa*) is an important part of treatment. Patients with suspected SSIs should be isolated and/or subject to barrier nursing until the infectious agent is identified. All animals with a confirmed resistant SSI must be isolated. Barrier nursing usually requires use of disposable aprons and gloves and allocation of equipment to that patient alone. There must be no transfer of bowls, stethoscopes, bedding or thermometers between animals without effective cleaning and preferably sterilization of these items.

References and further reading

Barsanti JA, Blue J and Edmunds J (1985) Urinary tract infection due to indwelling bladder catheters in dogs and cats. *Journal of the American Veterinary Medical Association* **187**, 384–388

Beal MW, Brown DC and Shofer FS (2000) The effects of perioperative hypothermia and the duration of anaesthesia on postoperative wound infection rate in clean wounds: a retrospective study. *Veterinary Surgery* **29**, 123–127

Boothe DM (2001a) Principles of antimicrobial therapy. In: *Small Animal Clinical Pharmacology and Therapeutics, 1st edn*, ed. DM Boothe, pp. 125–149. WB Saunders, Philadelphia

Boothe DM (2001b) Antimicrobial drugs. In: *Small Animal Clinical Pharmacology and Therapeutics, 1st edn*, ed. DM Boothe, pp. 150–173. WB Saunders, Philadelphia

Brown DC, Conzemius MG, Shofer F *et al.* (1997) Epidemiological evaluation of postoperative wound infections in dogs and cats. *Journal of the American Veterinary Medical Association* **210**, 1302–1306

Dunning D (2003) Surgical wound infection and the use of antimicrobials. In: *Textbook of Small Animal Surgery. 3rd edn*, ed. D Slatter, pp. 113–122. WB Saunders, Philadelphia

Eugster S, Schawalder P, Gaschen F *et al.* (2004) A prospective study of postoperative surgical site infections in dogs and cats. *Veterinary Surgery* **33**, 542–550

Gould I (1999) A review of the role of antibiotic polices in the control of antibiotic resistance. *Journal of Antimicrobial Chemotherapy* **43**, 459–465

Haydon TP, Presneill JJ and Robertson MS (2010) Antibiotic prophylaxis for cardiac surgery in Australia. *Medical Journal of Australia* **192**, 141–143

Hedrick TL, Smith PW, Gazoni LM *et al.* (2007) The appropriate use of antibiotics in surgery: a review of surgical infections. *Current Problems in Surgery* **44**, 635–675

Heldmann E, Brown DC and Shofer F (1999) The association of propofol usage with postoperative wound infection rate in clean wounds: a retrospective study. *Veterinary Surgery* **28**, 256–259

Nicholson M, Beal M, Shofer F *et al.* (2002) Epidemiologic evaluation of postoperative wound infection in clean contaminated wounds: a retrospective study of 239 dogs and cats. *Veterinary Surgery* **31**, 577–581

Popovitch CA and Nannos AJ (2000) Emergency management of open fractures and luxations. *Veterinary Clinics of North America: Small Animal Practice* **30**, 645–655

Ramsey I (2008) *Small Animal Formulary, 6th edn*. BSAVA Publications, Gloucester

Ramsey I (2011) *Small Animal Formulary, 7th edn*. (in press) BSAVA Publications, Gloucester

Rubenstein E, Findler G, Amit P *et al.* (1994) Perioperative prophylactic cefazolin in spinal surgery. *Journal of Bone and Joint Surgery – British Volume* **76**, 99–102

Skitarelić N, Morović M and Manestar D (2007) Antibiotic prophylaxis in clean-contaminated head and neck oncological surgery. *Journal of Cranio-Maxillofacial Surgery* **35**, 15–20

Vasseur PB, Levy J, Dowd E *et al.* (1988) Surgical wound infection rates in dogs and cats. Data from a teaching hospital. *Veterinary Surgery* **17**, 60–64

Verschuur HP, Wever W and van Benthem PP (2004) Antibiotic prophylaxis in clean and clean-contaminated ear surgery. *Cochrane Database of Systematic Reviews* **3**, CD003996

Weese JS (2008a) A review of multidrug resistant surgical site infections. *Veterinary Comparative Orthopaedics and Traumatology* **21**, 1–7

Weese JS (2008b) A review of post-operative infections in veterinary orthopaedic surgery. *Veterinary Comparative Orthopaedics and Traumatology* **21**, 99–105

Williams JM and Moores AL (2009) *BSAVA Manual of Canine and Feline Wound Management and Reconstruction*. BSAVA Publications, Gloucester.

Willemsen I, van den Broek R, Bijsterveldt T *et al.* (2007) A standardised protocol for perioperative antibiotic prophylaxis is associated with improvement of timing and reduction of costs. *Journal of Hospital Infection* **67**, 156–160

Hospital-acquired infection

Anette Loeffler

Introduction

Hospital-acquired infections (HAIs) or nosocomial infections (Greek: *nosokomeion* = hospital) are defined in human medicine as 'all clinically apparent infections that were not present or incubating in the patient prior to hospital admission'. They typically occur 48 hours or later after admission, within 3 days of discharge or within 30 days of an operation. HAIs also include infections that occur in hospital staff from pathogens acquired at work.

Of particular concern nowadays are HAIs caused by multidrug-resistant bacteria. These are linked to the frequent use of antimicrobials and antiseptics in human hospitals and multidrug-resistant organisms have also emerged in animal hospitals. If an unexpected or unusual series of HAI cases is recognized, they are referred to as outbreaks and require a prompt and rigorous search for a common source to reduce their impact. In humans, nosocomial infections lead to increases in morbidity and mortality and may prolong the length of stay in hospital. The associated financial burden for providers of human healthcare is substantial.

In veterinary medicine, nosocomial infections and outbreaks have been reported in small animal hospitals and practices and comprise a number of typical syndromes, such as catheter-site infections or diarrhoea. By definition, HAIs are unrelated to the original cause for admission or presentation to the veterinary facility. Thus, they can complicate treatment, be of considerable distress to owners and veterinary staff and potentially lead to complaints.

HAIs are occasionally referred to as 'nosocomial events' in order to highlight that the presence or absence of the infectious organism is rarely confirmed at the time of admission. In the context of this chapter, the term HAI will be applied to infections associated with both veterinary hospitals and veterinary practices and will also apply to the large caseload of animals seen as outpatients or admitted as day cases for minor procedures or routine surgery. For many cases of suspected HAI where clinical signs only develop after discharge, it is difficult to determine whether the infectious pathogen was acquired in the hospital or at home.

In line with the increasing antimicrobial resistance in human HAIs, multidrug-resistant bacteria have also emerged in veterinary facilities. The frequent use of antimicrobial drugs and antiseptics and disinfectants in veterinary hospitals puts selective pressure on colonizing and infecting microorganisms so that resistant organisms can proliferate and eventually evade antimicrobial prophylaxis or therapy. In equine hospitals, it has been shown that bacteria colonizing patients on admission are less resistant than those isolated from carrier sites following several days of hospitalization. Resistance patterns usually reflect the antimicrobial usage pattern of a country, region or, potentially, hospital. Similarly, at least for human hospitals, it has been shown that a restriction of certain antimicrobial classes or cyclical use have led to improvements in antimicrobial susceptibility, emphasizing the role of prescribing behaviour on the development of nosocomial infections.

Types of infection

Nosocomial infections often present as characteristic clinical syndromes. The most commonly reported are:

- Surgical site infections (SSIs)
- Intravenous catheter (and arterial line)-associated infections (Figure 19.1)
- Catheter-associated urinary tract infections
- Diarrhoea
- Pneumonia.

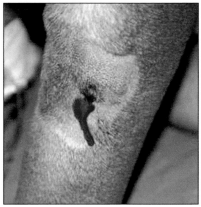

19.1 Suspected nosocomial infection at an intravenous catheter insertion site: haemorrhagic discharge with swelling and discoloration of the surrounding tissue. (Courtesy of S Baines).

The severity of HAI ranges from mild and transient to life-threatening diseases and fatal outcomes. Although the interaction between pathogen and host is complex, some HAIs may resolve rapidly without additional treatment (e.g. after removal of suture material), while others may require more intense treatment than the original presenting disease and lead to prolonged hospitalization and increased cost.

Typical clinical signs associated with individual syndromes are listed in Figure 19.2.

Some types of HAI may be related to certain groups of pathogens. For example, infections associated with urinary catheters often involve endogenous organisms such as *Escherichia coli*, possibly from faecal contamination, while skin commensals such as staphylococci are frequently isolated from SSIs. In general though, opportunistic pathogens may affect any site or organ as long as predisposing factors exist and the identity of the causative agent should be confirmed by microbiological culture.

While septicaemia is only rarely reported in the context of HAI, cases tend to be severe and more often fatal. Septicaemia may be catheter- or surgery-related even without clinical signs at the catheter insertion site or the surgical skin wound.

Pathogens

HAIs can be caused by viral, bacterial or fungal pathogens and, in a broader sense, by parasites (infestations). These can be introduced to the veterinary facilities by animals, their owners, veterinary staff or less commonly by fomites or live vectors.

Multidrug-resistant and zoonotic bacteria

In dogs and cats, HAIs with multidrug-resistant and zoonotic bacteria have received particular attention due to their potential impact on public health (Figure 19.3). Canine and feline infections with meticillin-resistant *Staphylococcus aureus* (MRSA), vancomycin-resistant enterococci (VRE), multidrug-resistant or extended-spectrum beta-lactamase (ESBL)-producing *Escherichia coli* and *Clostridium difficile* may require comprehensive owner education following extensive media coverage of their human counterparts.

In addition, less 'high-profile' organisms like coagulase-negative staphylococci or *Klebsiella* spp. may also be involved in HAIs. Coagulase-negative staphylococci are the most frequent bacteria associated with nosocomial bloodstream infections in people and the third most common pathogen in human HAI overall

Type of infection	Clinical signs	Potential predisposing factors
Intravenous catheter site infections	Inflammation, swelling, purulent or haemorrhagic discharge at insertion site; lymphadenopathy	■ Catheter in place for long duration ■ Poor technique ■ Inadequate skin preparation ■ Contaminated catheter ■ Type of connector ■ Number of disconnections ■ Biofilm-producing bacteria
Surgical site infections	Inflammation, swelling, purulent discharge at surgical site	See Chapter 18
Septicaemia	Varied; lethargy; tachycardia; tachypnoea; fever or hypothermia; leucocytosis or leucopenia	■ Catheter-associated infections ■ Infected wounds ■ Contaminated surgical sites ■ Other organ infections if severe or if in immunocompromised patients (see Chapter 11)
Urinary tract infections	Dysuria; inflammation; swelling around insertion site; haematuria	■ Poor hygiene ■ Poor technique ■ Oversized catheters ■ Catheter material ■ Biofilm-producing bacteria ■ Use of antimicrobial agents while catheter is in place
Respiratory tract infections	Dyspnoea; cough; fever; depression, especially after vomiting/regurgitation or intubation; leucocytosis	■ Aspiration of oropharyngeal contents during anaesthesia or in debilitated animals ■ Megaoesophagus ■ Nasogastric tubes ■ Bacteraemia ■ Inhalation of contaminated air ■ Assisted ventilation
Gastroenteritis	Diarrhoea; inappetence; (vomiting)	■ Antimicrobial therapy ■ Contaminated environment ■ Change in diet
Skin and underlying soft tissue infections, ectoparasite infestations	Inflammation, swelling, papules, pustules, crusts or pain around pre-existing wounds or on skin; scaling, crusting or alopecia affecting larger areas of skin	■ Spontaneous wounds ■ Chronic skin disease ■ Ectoparasite infestations
Fever of unknown origin	Fever	■ Infection with viral agents ■ Catheter site infections ■ *Clostridium difficile* colitis (in humans)

19.2 Syndromes typically associated with nosocomial infection in small animal patients.

Bacteria	Reference
Meticillin-resistant *Staphylococcus aureus* (MRSA)	Weese *et al.* (2006)
Coagulase-negative staphylococci	Sidhu *et al.* (2007)
Vancomycin-resistant enterococci (VRE)	van Belkum *et al.* (1996)
Salmonella typhimurium	Wright *et al.* (2005)
Multidrug-resistant *Escherichia coli*	Sidjabat *et al.* (2006)
Extended-spectrum beta-lactamase (ESBL) producing *E. coli*	Sanchez *et al.* (2002)
Klebsiella, Serratia, Proteus spp.	Glickman (1981)
Acinetobacter baumanii	Francey *et al.* (2000)
Pseudomonas aeruginosa	Fine and Tobias (2007)
Clostridium difficile	Kruth *et al.* (1989); Weese and Armstrong (2003)

19.3 Examples of multidrug-resistant bacteria that have been associated with nosocomial infection in dogs and cats.

(National Nosocomial Infections Surveillance System, Health Protection Agency). These bacteria are often highly drug-resistant commensals which are only harmful if the host is immunocompromised, or if they gain a selective advantage following antimicrobial therapy, or if invasive devices such as catheters facilitate their invasion of deeper tissues.

Viral, fungal and parasitic infections

Other more veterinary-specific diseases such as kennel cough, or infection with calicivirus or parvovirus, may be acquired in veterinary practices if infection control measures are inadequate.

Fungi that may be involved in HAIs include dermatophytes such as *Microsporum canis*, *Aspergillus* spp. and *Candida* spp. In human hospitals, fungal infections due to *Candida* spp. are typically reported in association with enteral tubes for nutritional support or where broad-spectrum antibiotics are used in severely immunocompromised patients. With continuous advances in veterinary care, such infections have to be considered in animal patients too, especially in those treated intensively.

Ectoparasites (e.g. *Cheyletiella* spp., *Sarcoptes scabiei* or fleas) may be transmitted to hospitalized animal patients either by direct contact or via environmental contamination, as many can persist in the environment for several days.

Sources of infection

Endogenous and exogenous infection

Patients may be infected by organisms originating from their own microflora if circumstances favour invasion (**endogenous infection**). This has been reported with catheter-associated or surgical site infections where colonizing bacteria are helped to bypass the body's natural defences. Alternatively, other hospitalized animals, veterinary staff or the environment can be the source of the infecting pathogen (**exogenous infection**).

Contact with carriers

Almost all MRSA isolates from canine and feline infections are genetically identical to MRSA clones dominant in human hospitals. This indicates that transmission occurred initially from humans to animals and that human carriers and people suffering from MRSA infection may be reservoirs and vectors for animal infection. In addition, many MRSA infections involve surgical sites or implants and may therefore have been acquired during or shortly after surgery. However, pet owners and the home environment may equally be sources of MRSA and even epidemiological typing of isolates is unlikely to reveal the source of infection.

Contaminated environments

Other nosocomial pathogens may also be carried by animals and people and shed into the environment with hair, skin squames, saliva, by aerosol or in faeces. Many microorganisms can persist in the practice environment for long periods, especially spore-forming organisms such as *Clostridium* spp. or *Aspergillus* spp. Staphylococci, including MRSA, can survive on dry surfaces for many months (Waagenvoort *et al.*, 2000) and *Pseudomonas* spp. can exist in moist or wet areas of the hospital, e.g. on water taps or in drains. Environmental reservoirs for nosocomial pathogens have been identified on items such as door handles, pens and computer keyboards as well as on medical equipment such as endoscopes, thermometers and laryngoscope handles. Genetically related MRSA and multidrug-resistant *Escherichia coli* isolates have been reported from animals and the hospital environment (Sanchez *et al.*, 2002; Loeffler *et al.*, 2005).

Incidence and risk factors

Nosocomial infections in humans affected about 7% of hospitalized patients in Europe in 2008 (European Centre for Disease Prevention and Control). Higher frequencies of up to 20% are reported from intensive care units, vascular and orthopaedic surgical wards. HAIs affecting surgical wounds, the urinary tract and the lower respiratory tract were the most frequent and SSIs accounted for around 15% of human HAIs. Surveillance to monitor the incidence of HAI is used to aid infection control programmes but surveillance systems require time and funding.

In veterinary medicine, the incidence of HAI is largely unknown. In one veterinary study, 3–6% of dogs and cats hospitalized in an ICU developed clinical signs of infection during their stay (Eugster *et al.*, 2004). In another, 82% of 38 veterinary teaching hospitals in North America reported outbreaks of nosocomial infection during the preceding 5 years (Benedict *et al.*, 2008). In the same survey, 19% of dogs and 16% of cats were thought to have been involved in a 'nosocomial event' but not all had been confirmed as infections.

The number of diagnostic procedures available and the treatment options for severely ill patients have grown substantially over the past two decades and, in parallel, owners' awareness and expectations have increased. Together, these factors have probably led to increased lengths of stay in veterinary hospitals and thus a rising number of HAIs in veterinary hospitals is likely. A recent study found that 23% of intravenous catheters yielded bacterial growth despite thorough cleansing of the insertion site (Jones *et al.*, 2009) while SSIs (Chapter 18) accounted for 46% of all animal HAIs in one survey (Murtaugh and Mason, 1989).

Surveillance

Surveillance is the responsibility of individual veterinary establishments and little is known about surveillance methods applicable to animal hospitals. In human hospitals, for example, the incidence of MRSA is measured in number of MRSA bacteraemia cases per non-MRSA *S. aureus* bacteraemia isolates, which is currently around 40% in UK hospitals. Although this figure does not inform on the number of MRSA infections overall, it has been identified as a good indicator for the MRSA burden in individual hospitals or healthcare trusts.

In veterinary medicine, MRSA infections are thought to occur infrequently compared with the number of other staphylococcal infections, but repeated courses of antimicrobial therapy, surgery and surgical implants and contact with human MRSA carriers have been shown to increase the risk of infection (Soares Magalhães *et al.*, 2010).

Risk factors

Although few data are published in the veterinary literature, risk factors for small animal HAIs (Figure 19.4) seem to mirror those documented in human hospitals (Boerlin *et al.*, 2001; Eugster *et al.*, 2004). Confirmed and proposed risk factors for individual clinical syndromes are summarized in Figure 19.2 and those for SSIs are detailed in Chapter 18.

By nature, veterinary hospitals are high-risk areas for exposure of animals to potential pathogens. However, exposure alone does not necessarily result in acquisition of the pathogen or disease. It was recently shown that 11 healthy dogs housed in kennels with either an MRSA-infected dog or with

MRSA carrier dogs remained MRSA-negative in a regularly cleaned environment (Loeffler *et al.*, 2010). On the other hand, veterinary hospitals will admit vulnerable patients and certain risk factors are directly linked to veterinary care (Figure 19.4). Recognition of such predisposing factors will help to implement appropriate preventive measures for each patient and thus limit occurrences.

While some risks, especially those related to hospital hygiene and transmission, can be minimized, those inherent to patients and treatment are more difficult to control. Furthermore, animal behaviour such as licking or soiling of catheters, wounds or bandages may present additional breaks in hygiene and predispose veterinary patients to HAI.

The presence of multidrug-resistant opportunistic bacteria either in the hospital environment or colonizing the patient may also contribute to the development of HAIs, as prophylactic antibiosis (where indicated) will be less effective. It is well documented that the widespread use of antimicrobials in humans and animals facilitates the development of resistant bacteria. In addition, antimicrobial therapy may suppress susceptible colonizing bacteria of the patient's microflora and allow resistant bacteria to persist and proliferate. Colonization with multidrug-resistant organisms prior to hospital admission or surgery has been identified as a risk factor for subsequent nosocomial infection with MRSA, *Escherichia coli* and enterococci (Wright *et al.*, 2005; Ogeer-Gyles *et al.*, 2006; Weese *et al.*, 2006).

Prevention

Fortunately, many HAIs can be prevented by simple and inexpensive measures. However, as some will continue to occur despite good infection control strategies, awareness and vigilance are required to minimize the risk of HAI for all patients (see Chapter 13).

Patient-related

- Age (e.g. neonates, very old animals).
- Underlying or concurrent disease (e.g. diabetes mellitus, pyoderma, neoplasia).
- Trauma (e.g. open wounds, burns).
- Carriage/colonization with multidrug-resistant bacteria prior to admission.

Treatment-related

- Prolonged, repeated or recent antimicrobial therapy.
- Immunosuppressive therapy.
- Surgery (especially contaminated or lengthy procedures; see also Chapter 18).
- Surgical implants.
- Invasive medical devices (e.g. catheters, drains, surgical implants).
- Long stay in hospital.

In-contact people

- Poor hand-washing compliance.
- Carriage/colonization of multidrug-resistant zoonotic pathogens.

Hospital environment

- Intensive care units.
- Environmental contamination due to inadequate practice hygiene.
- Inadequately processed medical equipment.
- Contaminated medicines or surgical materials.

19.4 Potential risk factors for nosocomial infection in dogs and cats.

PRACTICAL TIP

Any prevention strategy should focus on:

- Potential sources of infection
- Routes of transmission
- Recognition of susceptible hosts and their care.

In addition, the careful use of antimicrobial agents will be a key factor in preventing the emergence of multidrug-resistant bacteria in the hospital.

Microorganisms can only very rarely be hindered from entering the veterinary hospital. This may be the case with, for example, kennel cough or ectoparasites such as *Cheyletiella* spp. and fleas, which can be identified on admission through a thorough history taking and physical examination. A history of regular vaccinations in hospitalized animals will also contribute to the protection against some HAIs. The majority of potential pathogens, though, will enter the hospital *incognito* and the prevention of HAI needs to be based on the assumption that such organisms are present and to focus on interrupting the chain of transmission.

Hand hygiene

The single most effective measure in the prevention of HAI is good hand hygiene. This will help to reduce the exposure of patients to pathogens; it should include a correct hand-washing protocol and may be supported by the use of alcohol hand rub or gloves. Although hand hygiene is easy and inexpensive, poor compliance is common – as documented frequently in outbreak investigations of human HAI. Protective clothing such as masks, gowns, hats and shoe covers will also help to prevent HAI, but again compliance and their correct use need to be monitored for maximum benefit.

Environmental measures

Environmental infection control measures should include floors, furniture, medical and surgical equipment as well as consumables. One study showed that 18% of multidose-injection vials were contaminated with bacteria that could become a source of nosocomial septicaemia (Weese and Armstrong, 2003). Correct waste disposal is important, as most pathogens can survive in clinical waste such as dirty bandages or tissue.

A detailed discussion of infection control measures is beyond the scope of this chapter, but the principles of environmental practice hygiene should include:

- Training of staff
- Specification of what needs to be sanitized and how often
- Correct usage of cleaning and disinfecting agents according to the manufacturer's instructions
- Up-to-date documentation
- Monitoring of the effectiveness of hygiene measures.

The benefit of having one person coordinating and monitoring practice infection control strategies is well documented in human hospitals and recommended for veterinary facilities.

MRSA

Of particular concern for surgical patients may be the colonization of animals or in-contact humans (veterinary staff or owners) with MRSA. As for other staphylococci, MRSA can complicate SSIs and thus prolong healing and postoperative treatment. An occupational risk for MRSA carriage is now well documented for veterinary staff as for medical staff worldwide; and in the UK around 5–15% of veterinary staff are thought to carry MRSA nasally. Antimicrobial therapy, surgery and surgical implants have all been identified as risk factors for MRSA infection in dogs and cats. Contact with human MRSA carriers will also increase the risk of disease in animals, but staff screening for the prevention of MRSA infections is currently not recommended. A single nasal swab will only be 75% sensitive, and negative results may be false and can lead to complacency in hand hygiene practices or barrier precautions.

MRSA can be eliminated from carrier sites using topical antimicrobial agents, but this will only be successful as part of comprehensive control strategies. Instead, it should be assumed that any staff member or pet owner could be MRSA-positive, or carry other infectious organisms, and hand hygiene and barrier precautions should be implemented accordingly.

Host susceptibility

As the development of a HAI ultimately depends on the susceptibility of the host, any potential risk factors (as outlined above) must be identified promptly for each patient. With surgical patients automatically being at risk, particular care should be taken with all routes of transmission. In addition, all underlying or concurrent diseases that could predispose hospitalized patients to infection need to be addressed for ultimate support.

If outbreaks of contagious pathogens are recognized, the use of isolation facilities, restriction of elective admissions or closure of affected areas within the facility may be necessary until resolution to avoid new cases.

Practice strategies

In addition to these practical measures, the occurrence of HAI can be reduced by the following strategies:

- Regular staff training on the early recognition of clinical signs and potential causes of HAI. This includes awareness of contagious diseases (e.g. feline calicivirus infection, kennel cough), zoonoses (e.g. dermatophytosis, psittacosis) and newly emerging and imported diseases (e.g. leishmaniosis)
- Regular and critical review of infection control measures in order to maximize their benefit and cost-effectiveness. While such efforts may seem laborious, they will be helpful in the investigation and handling of HAI occurrences and will be useful to reduce litigation
- Conscientious use of antimicrobial drugs to reduce the development of the multidrug-resistant bacteria that are often involved in HAIs. This can be achieved by, for example, limiting the empirical use of antibiotics in favour of culture-based, targeted therapy and prudent use of antimicrobial prophylaxis for surgical procedures (see Chapter 18).

Examples of protocols and a compilation of best practices in infection control for small animal veterinary clinics have been published and can be adapted for any practice or hospital setting (Cherry, 2005; Anderson et al., 2008).

Investigation of occurrences

If problems are recognized or HAIs suspected within a hospital, prompt identification followed by elimination of the source of infection is essential to contain spread and avoid further cases or outbreaks. During these investigations, suspected cases need to be isolated and rigorous barrier precautions implemented. At the same time potential fomites need to be separated, cleaned and disinfected until the source has been identified and eliminated.

Awareness and identification of suspected cases

First of all, any 'nosocomial event' should be investigated and recorded even if an infectious process is not immediately apparent. This will include all clinical syndromes that may be associated with a HAI and all infectious processes that are unrelated to the reason for admission. Examples include overt inflammation at catheter insertion sites, or diarrhoea that develops after several days of hospitalization in an otherwise healthy patient admitted for orthopaedic surgery. Awareness of clinical signs and pathogens typically associated with HAIs will be helpful to any investigation, and suspected cases may be compared to surveillance records in order to identify related occurrences.

Identification of infectious pathogens

Correct identification of the causative pathogen will be fundamental for the successful management of the majority of individual patients, though for some cases of suspected HAI it may not be possible or practical to confirm an infectious agent, especially if they resolve rapidly or in mild cases where sampling would be invasive.

Laboratory identification of the causative organism should be performed for all suspected outbreaks or where an epidemiological link is suspected. Furthermore, as HAIs frequently involve multidrug-resistant bacteria, antibiosis alone may not be curative and environmental reservoirs must be prevented. For that reason, microbiological culture is likely to be cost-effective in the diagnosis of HAI, as ineffective empirical drugs can be avoided and recovery may be quicker. However, empirically chosen drugs may be used initially until the results of culture are known. Likewise, zoonotic pathogens need to be identified so that staff and clients can be informed accordingly.

Cytology and culture

An initial step to confirm the presence of an infectious process, particularly for superficial skin and wound infections or discharging deep tissue infections, can be cytology. It is cheap and quick to perform and will aid the choice of further sampling techniques. Samples of the affected tissue will then be submitted for culture (bacterial, fungal or possibly mycobacterial) and sensitivity testing. As many HAIs involve opportunistic bacteria, it may be difficult to evaluate the clinical relevance of the isolated organism. Therefore, it is particularly important to avoid contamination of the sample. Liaison with the microbiologist may be helpful to initiate additional cultures. The type of sample will depend on the clinical signs of the infection.

PRACTICAL TIPS

- For skin and wound infections, deep tissue samples submitted in plain containers or sterile saline may be required instead of surface swabs.
- For environmental sampling, swabs moistened in sterile saline and rolled over high-risk surface areas for 5–10 seconds should be suitable.
- For the purpose of screening for the presence of particular organisms, several samples can be pooled in order to reduce cost but sampling should include a wide range of hospital surfaces, medical equipment, hand-touch areas, remote areas where dust can settle and animal contact surfaces such as water bowls.

MRSA: Where repeated cases of MRSA infection are noted in animals, sampling of veterinary staff may be considered. However, as discussed above, screening for carriage needs to be handled with great care and may yield false-negative results.

- Swabbing should be performed on a strictly voluntary basis and results should be reported confidentially to the individual member of staff only.
- Consultation with the individual's GP is warranted in order to plan potential decolonization treatment if this is thought to be necessary.
- Decolonization of carrier sites with topical antimicrobial agents can be successful but long-term efficacy may be poor.
- As an occupational risk for MRSA carriage is now well documented in veterinary staff, it is important to search for other sources in the veterinary hospital to avoid re-colonization.

Recording and surveillance

Recording of suspected and confirmed cases of HAI is recommended to improve management and prevention of future cases. Surveillance or passive monitoring can include recording of:

- Frequencies of clinical syndromes, such as diarrhoea or coughing in hospitalized patients
- Catheter or surgical site problems in all patients, including outpatients
- Culture results of suspected HAIs.

Vigilance and communication between all staff and the person responsible for infection control are essential for good quality records. While catheter insertion or surgical site-related problems may be recognized and recorded readily as a suspected HAI, a hospital link may be less obvious in cases of respiratory or gastrointestinal disease or where signs developed after discharge. Records should be evaluated periodically and the results disseminated and discussed with the entire team. This will allow any necessary revisions of hygiene protocols, increase awareness and may also reduce the risk of contagious diseases to staff members.

Good owner communication is important to facilitate investigations into HAIs. Most people nowadays are aware of the risk of HAI when admitted to human hospitals. To minimize complaints, improve early identification after discharge and help treatment, owners should be made aware of the risk of HAI prior to leaving their animals in a veterinary hospital.

Conclusion

In conclusion, prevention of all HAIs is unrealistic, especially in view of the significant advances in veterinary diagnostics and disease management. However, an understanding of the clinical and epidemiological circumstances involved in HAIs and an open, proactive approach will help to reduce occurrences and support client confidence in hospital care.

References and further reading

Anderson M, Montgomery J, Weese JS and Prescott JF (2008) *Infection Prevention and Control Best Practices for Small Animal Veterinary Clinics*. Canadian Committee on Antibiotic Resistance http://www.wormsandgermsblog.com/uploads/file/CCAR%20Guidelines%20Final(2).pdf

Benedict KM, Morley PS and van Metre DC (2008) Characteristics of biosecurity and infection control programs at veterinary teaching hospitals. *Journal of the American Veterinary Medical Association* **233**, 767–773

Boerlin P, Eugster S, Gaschen F, Straub R and Schawalder P (2001) Transmission of opportunistic pathogens in a veterinary teaching hospital. *Veterinary Microbiology* **82**, 347–59

Cherry S (2005) A clean bill of health: practice hygiene. *In Practice* **27**, 548–551

Eugster S, Schawalder P, Gaschen F and Boerlin P (2004) A prospective study of postoperative surgical site infections in dogs and cats. *Veterinary Surgery* **33**, 542–550

Fine DM and Tobias AH (2007) Cardiovascular device infections in dogs: report of 8 cases and review of the literature. *Journal of Veterinary Internal Medicine* **21**, 1265–1271

Francey T, Gaschen F, Nicolet J and Burnens AP (2000) The role of *Acinetobacter baumannii* as a nosocomial pathogen for dogs and cats in an intensive care unit. *Journal of Veterinary Internal Medicine* **14**, 177–183

Glickman LT (1981) Veterinary nosocomial (hospital-acquired) *Klebsiella* infections. *Journal of the American Veterinary Medical Association* **179**, 1389–1393

Gregory S (2005) How good is your hand hygiene? *In Practice* **27**, 178–182

Johnson JA (2002) Nosocomial infections. *Veterinary Clinics of North America: Small Animal Practice* **32**, 1101–1126

Jones ID, Case AM, Stevens KB, Boag A and Rycroft AN (2009) Factors contributing to the contamination of peripheral intravenous catheters in dogs and cats. *Veterinary Record* **164**, 616–618

Kruth SA, Prescott JF, Welch MK and Brodsky MH (1989) Nosocomial diarrhoea associated with enterotoxigenic *Clostridium perfringens* infection in dogs. *Journal of the American Veterinary Medical Association* **195**, 331–334

Loeffler A, Boag AK, Sung J *et al.* (2005) Prevalence of methicillin-resistant *Staphylococcus aureus* among staff and pets in a small animal referral hospital in the UK. *Journal of Antimicrobial Chemotherapy* **56**, 692–697

Loeffler A, Pfeiffer DU, Lindsay JA, Soares-Magalhaes R and Lloyd DH (2010) Lack of transmission of methicillin-resistant *Staphylococcus aureus* (MRSA) between apparently healthy dogs in a rescue kennel. *Veterinary Microbiology* **141**, 178–181

Murtaugh RJ and Mason GD (1989) Antibiotic pressure and nosocomial disease. *Veterinary Clinics of North America: Small Animal Practice* **19**, 1259–1274

NNIS (1999) National Nosocomial Infections Surveillance (NNIS) System report. Data summary from January 1990–May 1999. *American Journal of Infection Control* **27**, 520–532

Ogeer-Gyles J, Mathews K, Weese JS, Prescott JF and Boerlin P (2006) Evaluation of catheter-associated urinary tract infections and multi-drug-resistant *Escherichia coli* isolates from the urine of dogs with indwelling urinary catheters. *Journal of the American Veterinary Medical Association* **229**, 1584–1590

Reynolds BS, Poulet H, Pingret JL *et al.* (2009) A nosocomial outbreak of feline calicivirus associated virulent systemic disease in France. *Journal of Feline Medicine and Surgery* **11**, 633–644

Sanchez S, McCrackin Stevenson MA, Hudson CR *et al.* (2002) Characterization of multidrug-resistant *Escherichia coli* isolates associated with nosocomial infections in dogs. *Clinical Microbiology* **40**, 3586–3595

Sidhu MS, Oppegaard H, Devor TP and Sørum H (2007) Persistence of multidrug-resistant *Staphylococcus haemolyticus* in an animal veterinary teaching hospital clinic. *Microbial Drug Resistance* **13**, 271–280

Sidjabat HE, Townsend KM, Lorentzen M *et al.* (2006) Emergence and spread of two distinct clonal groups of multidrug-resistant *Escherichia coli* in a veterinary teaching hospital in Australia. *Medical Microbiology* **55**, 1125–1134

Soares Magalhães RJ, Loeffler A, Lindsay J *et al.* (2010) Risk factors for methicillin-resistant *Staphylococcus aureus* (MRSA) infection in dogs and cats: a case-control study. *Veterinary Research* **41**, 55

van Belkum A, van den Braak N, Thomassen R *et al.* (1996) Vancomycin-resistant enterococci in cats and dogs. *Lancet* **348**, 1038–1039

Wagenvoort JHT, Sluijsmans W and Penders RJR (2000) Better environmental survival of outbreak vs. sporadic MRSA isolates. *Journal of Hospital Infection* **45**, 231–235

Weese JS and Armstrong J (2003) Outbreak of *Clostridium difficile*-associated disease in a small animal veterinary teaching hospital. *Journal of Veterinary Internal Medicine* **17**, 813–816

Weese JS, Dick H, Willey BM *et al.* (2006) Suspected transmission of methicillin-resistant *Staphylococcus aureus* between domestic pets and humans in veterinary clinics and in the household. *Veterinary Microbiology* **115**, 148–155

Weese JS, Rousseau J, Willey BM *et al.* (2006) Methicillin-resistant *Staphylococcus aureus* in horses at a veterinary teaching hospital: frequency, characterization, and association with clinical disease. *Journal of Veterinary Internal Medicine* **20**, 182–186

Wright JG, Tengelsen LA, Smith KE *et al.* (2005) Multidrug-resistant *Salmonella Typhimurium* in four animal facilities. *Emerging Infectious Diseases* **11**, 1235–1241

Haemostasis and blood component therapy

Gillian R. Gibson

Introduction

Haemostasis refers to the cessation of bleeding, which is achieved by a complex arrangement of balanced interactions between blood cells, the vasculature, plasma proteins and low molecular weight substances. A system of checks and balances ensures that, although a thrombus (clot) is formed and protected at the site of vessel damage to stop bleeding, vessel occlusion (thrombosis) is prevented. Haemostasis represents an equilibrium between the opposing processes of bleeding on the one hand and hypercoagulability and thrombosis on the other. Unbalanced or altered haemostasis most often tends towards haemorrhage, but when excessive thrombosis occurs it may cause significant disease.

As a general overview, bleeding following vascular injury must be stopped to prevent excessive blood loss.

Stages of haemostasis

There are three basic stages in haemostasis (Figure 20.1), which interact and overlap.

1. The first step (**primary haemostasis**) involves vasoconstriction and formation of a temporary platelet plug at the site of injury.

2. Activation and amplification of the coagulation cascade leads to the production of fibrin, an essential component of stable clot formation (**secondary haemostasis**).

3. The final stages (**tertiary haemostasis**) involve thrombus modifications, clot dissolution and vessel defect repair, to prevent vascular occlusion and to restore vascular integrity.

20.1 Stages in haemostasis.

Primary haemostasis and vascular integrity

Primary haemostasis refers to the process of vascular contraction, platelet adhesion and platelet aggregation to form the initial platelet plug at the site of vessel injury (Figure 20.2). Platelets, vascular endothelium and von Willebrand factor (vWf) are all essential components of this process.

Vascular integrity

A continuous monolayer of endothelial cells creates the inner lining of the vasculature (the endothelium). It functions as a semi-permeable barrier, allowing diffusion of gas across the membrane and controlling the passage of fluid and solutes. Blood cells and large molecular weight proteins are retained within the vascular compartment unless the endothelium is damaged. Endothelial cells have a role in inhibition of intravascular coagulation and regulation of haemostasis.

- When vascular damage occurs:
  - The endothelium is disrupted
  - Endothelial cells are activated
  - Haemostasis is initiated.
- Activated endothelial cells provide a surface for platelet adhesion, as well as expression of tissue factor (TF) and initiation of the coagulation cascade resulting in thrombin production.
- Vasoactive substances, including endothelin produced by damaged vascular endothelium, stimulate vasoconstriction and temporary reduction of blood flow to the site of injury.
- Reduced blood flow limits extravascular blood loss as well as slowing flow past the injury site, permitting platelet adhesion and activation of coagulation.

When in a non-activated state, the vascular endothelial cells exert antithrombotic properties to prevent the formation of occlusive thrombi on a normal, non-traumatized vessel wall.

Platelets

Circulating intravascular platelets adhere to the exposed collagen fibres of the vascular subendothelium after trauma (Figure 20.2a). These activated platelets:

- Undergo a shape change
- Secrete contents from their cytoplasmic granules (many of which amplify the activation of other platelets)
- Aggregate at the area of injury to form a temporary platelet plug, completing the process of primary haemostasis (Figure 20.2b).

Platelets are cytoplasmic fragments found in the blood, produced from megakaryocytes located primarily in the bone marrow. Megakaryocytopoiesis involves

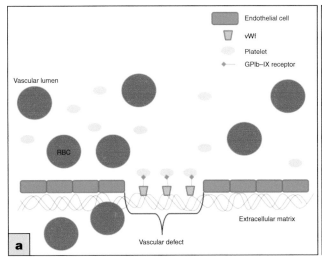

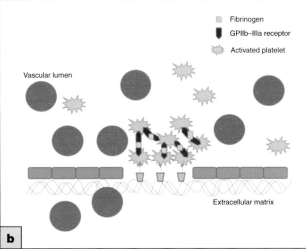

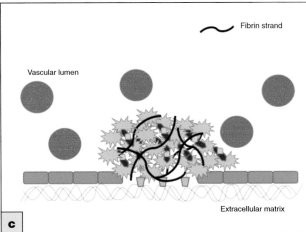

20.2 Primary haemostasis. **(a)** Platelet adhesion. Circulating platelets adhere to von Willebrand factor (vWf) bound to the exposed subendothelium (extracellular matrix) after the creation of a vascular defect. Note that red blood cells (RBCs) are able to pass through the defect, out of the vascular compartment (haemorrhage). **(b)** Platelet activation and aggregation. Activated platelets undergo a shape change, secrete granular contents and aggregate at the injury site to form a temporary platelet plug. Aggregation is enhanced by fibrinogen bridging between the GPIIb–IIIa receptors of adjacent platelets. **(c)** Stabilization of the platelet plug by fibrin and cessation of bleeding.

multiple divisions and lobulations of the progenitor cell nucleus without any cytoplasmic division. As the cytoplasm matures, it fragments to form platelets. Each megakaryocyte in the bone marrow is capable of producing thousands of platelets with a lifespan of approximately 5–7 days in dogs and less than this in cats.

The platelet membrane contains a variety of glycoproteins and phospholipids that are active participants in platelet activation, adhesion and coagulation, as well as numerous organelles and an extensive cytoskeleton.

1. Following activation, the platelet shape changes from a resting flat discoid structure to a spherical spiny shape with numerous filapodia extending from the membrane surface due to actin myofilaments in the cytoskeleton, increasing the surface area for thrombin generation, and activating an important surface receptor GPIIb–IIIa.
2. Following the platelet shape change, cytoplasmic secretory granules release their contents, some of which are platelet agonists (e.g. adenosine diphosphate (ADP), serotonin), contributing to further platelet aggregation. Other agonists, synthesized *de novo* by the activated platelet, include platelet-activating factor (PAF) and thromboxane A2 (TXA2).
3. The platelet plug forms through recruitment and activation of additional platelets, as well as increased cohesion of already adherent platelets. In general, combined agonist stimulation enhances the platelet response.

von Willebrand factor and fibrinogen: Platelet adhesion is facilitated by vWF (a multimeric glycoprotein, produced by megakaryocytes and endothelial cells) and fibrinogen, both bound to the subendothelium.

- Chains of dimers linked by disulphide bonds form multimers, which vary in molecular weight. The higher the molecular weight of the multimer, the more effective is its contribution to haemostasis.
- vWf is primarily constitutively secreted by the endothelial cells (small multimers), though a small proportion is stored in the alpha granules of platelets, and Weibel-Palade bodies in endothelial cells (large multimers).
- A variety of agents can stimulate release of vWf from the Weibel-Palade bodies, including histamine, thrombin, adrenaline, and 1-desamino-8-arginine vasopressin (DDAVP).
- When vWf is immobilized in the subendothelial collagen, it can bind to the platelet GPIb–IX receptor, facilitating platelets spreading across the exposed subendothelium (see Figure 20.2a).
- vWf and fibrinogen both enhance platelet aggregation by bridging between adjacent platelet GPIIb–IIIa receptors (see Figure 20.2b).
- Meanwhile, vWf bound to GPIb–IX platelet receptors and fibrin assists in stabilization of the temporary platelet plug.
- In the circulation, vWf is a carrier for coagulation Factor VIII. The non-covalent bond between vWf and Factor VIII is broken by thrombin, releasing Factor VIII for participation in coagulation initiated on the platelet surface.

Phospholipids and COX: Platelet membrane phospholipids include phosphatidyl serine (PS) and arachadonic acid (AA). PS, formerly referred to as platelet factor 3, is translocated to the membrane surface after platelet activation and accelerates the coagulation cascade. AA is released from the membrane phospholipids by the cleaving action of phospholipase.

Within the platelet, AA is metabolized to TXA2 via the cyclooxygenase (COX) pathway and through the action of thromboxane synthetase. TXA2 stimulates vasoconstriction and platelet aggregation; it is an important contributor to coagulation and hence an area to target when trying to prevent excessive platelet aggregation.

Some AA is metabolized to prostacyclin (PGI2), through COX and prostacyclin synthetase, which is a vasodilator and inhibits platelet function. Endothelial cells have higher levels of prostacyclin synthetase than platelets and consequently the major metabolite of AA in endothelial cells is PGI2.

COX-1 and COX-2: COX-1, a constitutively expressed form of COX, is present in platelets. Another form, COX-2, is found in many cell types, including endothelial cells, and is cytokine-inducible. It is due to this difference in enzyme pathways that COX-inhibiting drugs have their varied effects. Irreversible COX inhibitors, such as aspirin, result in inhibition of TXA2 production, consequently inhibiting platelet aggregation for the lifespan of the platelet. Non-aspirin non-steroidal anti-inflammatory drugs (NSAIDs) reversibly inhibit COX, therefore platelet inhibition is transient and mild. As platelets do not contain COX-2, COX-2 selective NSAIDs have no inhibitory effect on platelet aggregation.

Calcium: Platelet agonist receptors are transmembrane G proteins. Agonist–receptor binding triggers a constellation of inhibitory and stimulatory reactions, commonly mediated by an increase in free cytosolic calcium. Calcium-dependent processes lead to increased platelet adhesion and fibrinogen binding, as well as enhanced platelet aggregation. Therefore, drugs that are calcium-channel blockers (e.g. diltiazem, barbiturates) may prevent this increase in cytosolic calcium concentration and suppress platelet aggregation through this and other mechanisms.

Secondary haemostasis

The process of secondary haemostasis results in the stabilization of the initial platelet plug by fibrin, produced as an end product of the coagulation cascade.

The coagulation cascade consists of an amplifying series of enzymatic reactions, resulting in thrombin-mediated fibrin formation. It is the net of polymerized fibrin that stabilizes the platelet plug within 5–10 minutes of the initial vascular injury (see Figures 20.2c and 20.3).

Most steps in the cascade involve:

- An enzyme
- A substrate (fibrinogen, fibrin, or proenzyme form of coagulation factor)
- A cofactor (activated Factors V and VIII).

The reactions occur on a phospholipid surface, such as the membrane of platelets, leucocytes or endothelial cells, in the presence of free ionized calcium (Ca^{2+}).

Coagulation factors

Most coagulation factors and cofactors are produced by the liver and circulate in an inactivated form. Factors II, VII, IX and X are vitamin K dependent, requiring completion of a vitamin K-dependent carboxylation reaction in the liver to become functional.

Most factors are referred to by a number (Roman numeral) followed by the letter 'a' when they are activated (e.g. Factor VII or FVIIa).

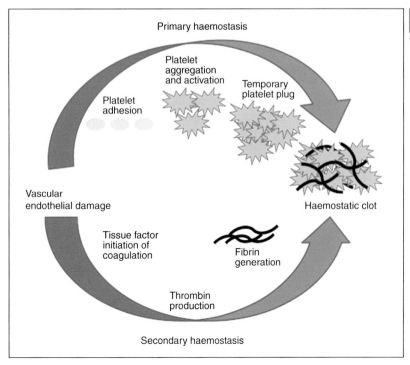

20.3 Primary and secondary haemostasis resulting in the formation of a stable clot.

Extrinsic and intrinsic coagulation pathways

Traditionally coagulation has been described as a series of enzymatic reactions divided into extrinsic and intrinsic pathways, each pathway having separate activators and sequential factor activation prior to meeting at the 'common' pathway, culminating in fibrin formation.

- The extrinsic pathway involves Factors III (TF) and VII.
- The intrinsic pathway is initiated by Factor XII activation, and includes Factors XI, IX and VIII (Figure 20.4).

However, it is now well recognized that:

- There are significant interactions between the intrinsic and extrinsic pathways
- There are essential interactions between coagulation factors and cell surfaces
- FXII does not have a role in the initiation of coagulation *in vivo*; rather, coagulation is initiated by TF expression and the extrinsic pathway.

Although the familiar coagulation model or Y diagram shown in Figure 20.4 is not a completely accurate model of modern understanding of physiological haemostasis, it is useful for understanding alterations to haemostasis and haemostatic testing currently available.

Coagulation as a cell-based process

More recently coagulation has been described as a cell-based process, recognizing that coagulation does not occur in the plasma (fluid) phase, but rather at membrane surfaces at the site of injury. The interaction of the coagulation factors with the altered membrane surface effectively draws together the important components for the enzymatic reactions required for rapid coagulation. These coagulation reactions are not supported when the cell is in its resting state. Once activated, the cell membrane surface undergoes a conformational procoagulant change, such as the expression of PS on the external surface.

- As described in primary haemostasis, vascular damage exposes the extracellular matrix, initiating vWf-mediated platelet adhesion and activation.
- With platelet activation, PS is exposed.
- Simultaneously, TF-bearing cells in the matrix bind Factor VII (in the presence of Ca^{2+}), forming the activated complex TF–FVIIa.
- This complex activates FX, which together with cofactor FVa generates a small amount of thrombin. TF–FVIIa also activates Factor IX, an example of where the 'extrinsic' pathway interacts to activate part of the 'intrinsic' pathway.

Thrombin

Thrombin (Factor IIa) drives amplification and progression of coagulation. It activates Factors XI and V on the platelet surface, as well as the platelets themselves.

- Thrombin cleaves vWf from FVIII, releasing vWf for platelet adhesion and aggregation, as well as activating Factor VIII.
- Factor XIa in turn activates FIX, which forms the 'tenase' complex, FIXa–FVIIIa–Ca, on the platelet surface and generates FXa.
- FXa rapidly binds to FVa, cleaving prothrombin to generate a burst of thrombin.
- Thrombin cleaves fibrinogen into soluble fibrin monomers, which are then polymerized into long fibres to stabilize the initial clot (see Figure 20.2c).
- Thrombin also activates Factor XIII, which serves to stabilize the fibrin clot by cross-linking the fibrin fibres.
- Thrombin activation of Factors V and VIII provides positive feedback on the intrinsic and common pathways through Factor XIa, and forms activated protein C (APC).
- APC provides some inhibition of coagulation via inactivation of Factors Va and VIIIa, as well as by promoting fibrinolysis.

20.4 A simplified coagulation cascade.

Factor deficiencies

Animals with an intrinsic pathway factor deficiency may experience bleeding despite having a normal extrinsic pathway, and *vice versa*. For example, animals with Factor VIII or IX deficiency (haemophilia A or B, respectively) experience spontaneous bleeding despite an intact extrinsic coagulation pathway. Similarly Factor VII deficiency (extrinsic pathway) is associated with bleeding, despite having a normal intrinsic pathway. These examples help to illustrate how the pathways are simultaneously occurring processes with significant interactions.

Tertiary haemostasis

Fibrinolysis is the degradation of the fibrin clot by fibrinolytic enzymes, primarily plasmin.

- During coagulation, plasminogen (the inactive zymogen) binds to the forming fibrin.
- Stimulated endothelial cells release tissue plasminogen activator (t-PA), which works on the bound fibrin–plasminogen complex to release plasmin.
- Plasmin cleaves fibrinogen, and soluble and cross-linked fibrin, each yielding different degradation products (Figure 20.5).
  - Fibrinogen and soluble fibrin are degraded to fibrin(ogen) degradation products (FDPs).
  - Cross-linked fibrin yields cross-linked fibrin degradation products and D-dimers.

Inhibitors of coagulation

There are several mechanisms for inhibiting and localizing coagulation to the site of injury.

- Endothelial cells release ADPase and prostacyclin, both of which inhibit platelet activation and aggregation.

- The natural flow of blood effectively dilutes the local concentration of coagulation factors present at the site of tissue damage, thereby limiting fibrin production.
- TF pathway inhibitor, mostly bound to endothelial surfaces, down-regulates the TF–FVIIa–FXa complex, preventing additional thrombin generation.
- Endothelial cell surface thrombomodulin binds thrombin, leading to activation of protein C. APC, with cofactor protein S, inhibits activation of both Factors V and VIII, decreasing thrombin production and subsequent fibrin generation.
- Antithrombin III (AT III) inhibits thrombin and inactivates Factors XIIa, XIa, IXa and Xa, and less effectively VIIa. AT III is activated by heparin and/or heparin-like glycosaminoglycans in the endothelial wall.

There are also inhibitors of fibrinolysis, including antiplasmin (which binds plasma free plasmin) and plasminogen activator inhibitors 1 and 2. Although other inhibitors have been described their discussion is beyond the scope of this chapter.

Pathophysiology of altered haemostasis

Imbalances of haemostasis most often result in haemorrhage, but equally significantly may cause thrombosis. Understanding the consequences of failure of different parts of the haemostatic system (vascular integrity, platelet plug formation, fibrin clot formation and fibrinolysis) helps direct the investigation, identification and appropriate therapy of the haemostatic disorder.

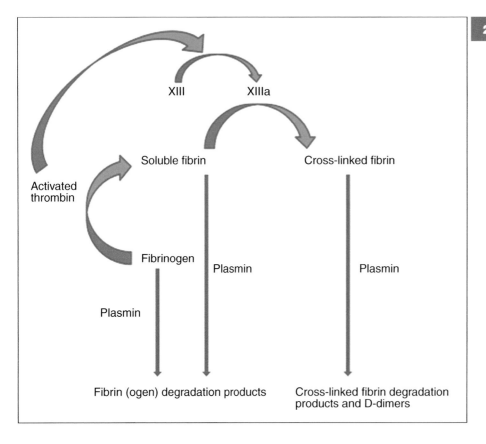

20.5 Fibrinolysis.

Vascular disease

The intact blood vessel wall is the primary barrier to bleeding. Disruption of vascular integrity may occur as a result of variety of disease processes or trauma. The degree and appearance of haemorrhage varies depending on the size and location of the affected vessel.

Vessel damage may be caused by surgery, trauma or vascular anomalies, as well as neoplastic, inflammatory and granulomatous diseases leading to vascular wall infiltration and erosion. The clinical signs of vasculitis-associated disorders are diverse, but the vascular consequences may lead to areas of ischaemia as well as haemorrhage.

- Increased vascular permeability seen with vasculitis may affect blood vessels of any size in any part of the body.
- The inflammation may be focal or widespread in association with toxic, infectious, immune-mediated, inflammatory and neoplastic disorders.
- Inflammatory cell deposition in or surrounding the vessel wall contributes to vascular necrosis and exposure of subendothelial collagen, perpetuating inflammation and activating coagulation.

Alterations in the collagen and connective tissue of the vascular or perivascular tissues as a consequence of acquired or, more rarely, congenital disorders may result in a vasculopathy manifested by increased tendency to bruise after only minor trauma (e.g. animals with diabetes mellitus or Cushing's syndrome).

Disorders of primary haemostasis

Primary haemostatic disorders result in failure of the formation of a functional platelet plug due to either a quantitative defect in platelets (**thrombocytopenia**) or a qualitative platelet function defect (**thrombocytopathia**).

Characteristic clinical signs include petechiae (pinpoint haemorrhages) and ecchymoses (larger bruises), which are usually visible on mucosal surfaces such as oral, nasal and urogenital mucosa, on lesser haired areas of skin (pinnae, ventral abdominal/inguinal region), or identified during an ophthalmological examination (hyphaema or retinal haemorrhage).

- In addition to superficial bruising, bleeding from mucosal surfaces may result in epistaxis, gastrointestinal haemorrhage (melaena, haematemesis, haematochezia), oral bleeding, vaginal bleeding, haematuria or excessive bleeding after surgery or venepuncture (though these signs may also be recognized with disorders of secondary haemostasis).
- Neurological abnormalities, such as depression, seizures, ataxia or central blindness, may accompany cerebral bleeding.
- In situations of extensive external haemorrhage, clinical signs of blood loss anaemia (pallor, lethargy, weakness, collapse) may develop.

Quantitative platelet defects

Thrombocytopenia is a consequence of inadequate platelet production, increased platelet consumption or destruction, sequestration or excess loss.

Platelet production defects may be accompanied by other cytopenias due to:

- Infectious diseases (e.g. ehrlichiosis, feline leukaemia virus (FeLV), feline immunodeficiency virus (FIV), *Rickettsia rickettsii*, parvovirus)
- Drug and toxin exposure (e.g. chemotherapeutic drugs, beta-lactam antibiotics, sulfadiazine, oestrogen compounds, NSAIDs, griseofulvin, methimazole/carbimazole)
- Primary bone marrow disorders (myelodysplastic syndromes, megakaryoblastic leukaemia, dysthrombopoiesis, marrow panhypoplasia or pure megakaryocytic hypoplasia).

One of the most common causes of thrombocytopenia in the dog and cat is immune-mediated destruction, which may be primary idiopathic or secondary associated with drug exposure, infectious diseases, neoplasia, immune-mediated diseases and disseminated intravascular coagulation (DIC).

- Increased platelet activation and removal from the circulation seen with some drugs (e.g. heparin) or infectious agents, foreign surface activation (e.g. indwelling intravenous or arterial catheters), vasculitis, severe burn injuries, venomous snake bites, or blood loss at multiple sites leading to significant platelet consumption can lead to moderate to severe thrombocytopenia.
- Widespread endothelial damage and activation of coagulation and accelerated platelet consumption may result in significant thrombocytopenia (e.g. DIC).

Hypersplenism: Platelet sequestration occurs as a normal physiological process in the spleen (primarily) as well as the liver and bone marrow to some degree. Abnormal sequestration of platelets in the spleen in a pathological condition called hypersplenism may reduce the circulating platelet pool by as much as 90%, and may be accompanied by additional cytopenias.

Qualitative platelet defects

There are numerous acquired and hereditary causes of qualitative platelet defects. Animals with these disorders demonstrate clinical signs of a primary haemostatic condition, but have a normal platelet count.

von Willebrand's disease: The most commonly encountered hereditary cause of platelet function disorders in dogs is von Willebrand's disease (vWD), which has been described in over 50 breeds of dog, but is rare in cats. It is inherited as an autosomal trait, likely to be a recessive disorder in some breeds, and as a dominant disorder with variable penetrance in others. It is classified into three types: quantitative deficiencies of vWf are classified as either Type 1 or Type 3, depending on the severity of the deficiency, and qualitative deficiencies of vWf are classified as Type 2 (Figure 20.6).

- **Type 1** vWD is most common, reported in many breeds of dog, and results from a deficiency in functional vWf. The severity of bleeding is not only

Type classification	vWf level	Haemorrhagic tendency	Breeds
Type 1 vWD	Reduced vWf:Ag levels	Variable. Increased bleeding associated with surgery or post-trauma. Spontaneous bleeding occasionally	Dobermann; Airedale Terrier; German Shepherd Dog; Shetland Sheepdog; Standard Poodle; and other breeds
Type 2 vWD	Reduced concentration of high molecular weight vWf multimers	Severe	German Shorthaired Pointer; German Wirehaired Pointer
Type 3 vWD	Completely or almost completely absent	Severe (most severe of all three types)	Scottish Terrier; Chesapeake Bay Retriever; Dutch Kooiker; Shetland Sheepdog; and other breeds

20.6 Type classification of canine von Willebrand's disease (vWD). vWF:Ag=von Willebrand factor antigen.

dependent on the vWf level, but also on the breed. For example, Dobermanns (a breed typical for Type 1 vWD) exhibit bleeding more frequently than Airedale Terriers with the same disease.

- Dogs with **Type 2** disease have low concentrations or absence of the high molecular weight vWf multimers and have more severe clinical signs than those with Type 1 disease.
- Dogs with **Type 3** vWD have almost no detectable vWf, resulting in a severe bleeding disorder.

Interestingly, dogs with vWD do not commonly have petechiae.

Other hereditary conditions: Uncommon inherited platelet function disorders have been reported in cats (Chediak Higashi syndrome in Persians, vWD in a Himalayan cat) and many breeds of dog (Otter Hound, Great Pyrenees, Basset Hound, Spitz, Grey Collie, American Cocker Spaniel).

Acquired conditions: Conditions associated with acquired thrombocytopathia include uraemia, platelet-inhibitory drug administration (including but not limited to aspirin and other NSAIDs, verapamil, barbiturates, dextran and hydroxyethyl starch, heparin, cephalothin and sulphonamide antibiotics), hepatic dysfunction, antiplatelet antibodies, infectious diseases (e.g. *Ehrlichia canis*, FeLV, *Yersinia pestis*), dysproteinaemias, neoplasia and feline dietary arachidonate deficiency.

Acquired vWD has been associated with lymphoproliferative and myeloproliferative diseases and monoclonal gammopathies in humans, but it is not well characterized in dogs.

Disorders of secondary haemostasis

Typical clinical signs of a secondary haemostatic defect include haematoma formation, haemarthrosis, haemoptysis, bleeding into body cavities (pleural and peritoneal spaces) and extensive bruising. Whereas hereditary coagulopathies usually involve a single-factor deficiency, dogs or cats with acquired coagulopathies have reduced levels of multiple coagulation factors.

Acquired coagulopathies

Vitamin K deficiency or antagonism: Any condition causing a deficiency in vitamin K may lead to a coagulopathy. Several clotting factors (II, VII, IX and X) are dependent on vitamin K as a cofactor for an essential

carboxylation reaction required for effective calcium binding during clot formation. Adequate levels are maintained by intestinal absorption of dietary vitamin K as well as vitamin K produced by bacteria in the ileum and colon. In the hepatocyte, vitamin K is reduced to its active form by the enzyme vitamin K reductase, where it serves as a cofactor for vitamin K-dependent carboxylase (Figure 20.7). During the carboxylation reaction it is oxidized to vitamin K epoxide, requiring reduction by the enzyme vitamin K epoxide reductase to 'recycle' back to vitamin K.

Vitamin K deficiency can be a result of:

- Impaired intestinal absorption or hepatic recycling of vitamin K
- Impaired fat absorption
- Reduction in gut flora (oral antibiotic administration)
- Vitamin K antagonist ingestion (anticoagulant rodenticide, e.g. warfarin).

Many gastrointestinal, hepatic and pancreatic disorders have been associated with vitamin K-responsive coagulopathies (e.g. infiltrative bowel diseases, exocrine pancreatic insufficiency, cholestasis, biliary obstruction).

Anticoagulant rodenticides irreversibly block the activity of the recycling enzyme *vitamin K epoxide reductase*, preventing regeneration of vitamin K, and depletion of functional vitamin K–dependent coagulation factors.

Liver disease: As most of the coagulation factors are produced in the liver, animals with hepatic dysfunction (e.g. portosystemic vascular anomaly, cholestatic disorders, hepatic necrosis, neoplasia) may have associated bleeding tendencies. Although spontaneous bleeding rarely occurs, these animals are at an increased risk for bleeding following an invasive procedure such as biopsy or surgery. Other mechanisms of liver disease associated coagulopathies include platelet dysfunction, DIC, vitamin K deficiency (see above) and impaired hepatic clearance of activated clotting factors, plasminogen and FDPs.

Angiostrongylus vasorum infection: This helminth parasite may be associated with primary or secondary haemostatic abnormalities, which may not become apparent until significant tissue trauma (injury, surgery) is induced. Although there have been endemic pockets in Wales, Ireland and Southern England, the

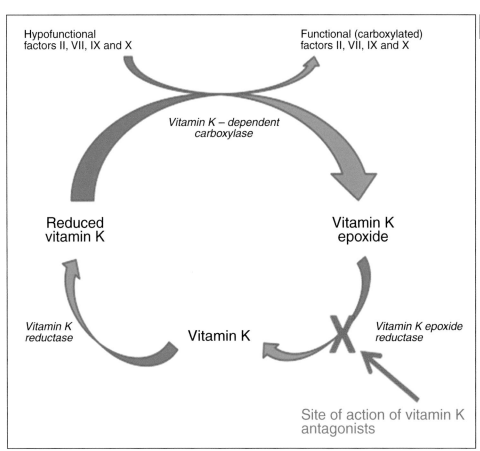

Hypofunctional factors II, VII, IX and X

Functional (carboxylated) factors II, VII, IX and X

Vitamin K – dependent carboxylase

Reduced vitamin K

Vitamin K epoxide

Vitamin K reductase

Vitamin K

Vitamin K epoxide reductase

Site of action of vitamin K antagonists

geographical range of the parasite is expanding. Haemostatic abnormalities described are variable and have included thrombocytopenia, prolongation of pro-thrombin time (PT) and/or activated partial thrombo-plastin time (aPTT), or prolonged buccal mucosal bleeding time (BMBT), but some affected dogs with clinical evidence of haemorrhagic tendencies have not had any coagulation parameter abnormality. The exact mechanism of coagulopathy associated with *Angio-strongylus vasorum* infection has not been identified, though it is suggested that a chronic form of DIC may occur.

Disseminated intravascular coagulation: The term DIC is used to describe a secondary disease pro-cess where uncontrolled coagulation and fibrinolysis are triggered by a variety of primary disorders. Haemostatic equilibrium is disrupted due to continu-ous activation of coagulation, leading to consumption of coagulation factors, coagulation inhibitors and inhibitors of fibrinolysis.

Animals may present with signs of haemorrhage and/or thrombosis. Coagulation testing often reveals a hypercoagulable profile, followed by hypocoagulabilty as the disease progresses. Coagulation activation, due to endothelial damage, tissue damage or platelet acti-vation, may accompany a vast array of primary disease processes, including sepsis, heatstroke, burns, pan-creatitis, trauma, immune-mediated haemolytic anae-mia, viral infections and neoplasia.

Clinical signs of DIC are highly variable and may include spontaneous haemorrhage and simultaneous or developing thrombotic signs (organ failure), though in some cases no outward signs may be apparent at the time of diagnosis via coagulation testing.

DIC is a life-threatening disorder, secondary to a critical illness, and should be assessed in at-risk surgical patients or those with overt clinical signs of haemorrhage and/or thrombosis. Early, aggressive therapeutic intervention may help to reduce significant morbidity and mortality associated with DIC.

Dilutional coagulopathy: In the emergency patient with acute major blood loss, treatment to restore vas-cular volume is essential. However, if a large volume of fluids lacking in platelets and coagulation factors is administered (e.g. crystalloids, colloids, stored whole blood, packed red blood cells), a dilutional coagulo-pathy may develop and contribute to persistent blood loss. Correction of the coagulopathy requires admin-istration of coagulation factors, fibrinogen and/or platelets, achieved by the use of appropriate blood components (see Blood component therapy below).

Inherited coagulopathies

Although it is expected that animals with hereditary coagulopathies will present with signs of bleeding at a young age (e.g. teething, bruising after minimal trauma, bleeding from injection sites or following rou-tine neutering procedures), some mild forms may not become apparent until adulthood. Therefore, a level of suspicion for a hereditary coagulopathy should still be maintained even if the animal has undergone a prior surgical procedure without any evidence of sig-nificant haemorrhage.

Haemophilia: Haemophilia is an X-linked recessive disorder identified in many animal species, including dogs and cats, caused by a deficiency in either Factor VIII (haemophilia A) or Factor IX (haemophilia B). Males are either normal or affected, whereas females may be homozygous normal, heterozygous carriers, or rarely homozygous affected.

The disorder has been reported in numerous dog breeds, with a high prevalence of haemophilia A noted in German Shepherd Dogs. Many canine breed groups encourage haemophilia screening, and if screening tests are abnormal, specific factor analysis should be pursued to characterize the disorder. The severity of bleeding in affected animals varies from mild to severe, possibly fatal haemorrhage. Carriers are not always easily identified by coagulation testing (screening tests or specific factor analysis), and pedigree analysis may be required. Molecular diagnostic techniques to identify carrier females are being developed.

Autosomal factor deficiencies: Unlike X-linked disorders, autosomal factor deficiencies are likely to affect male and female animals with equal frequency. There are several factor deficiencies reported in veterinary medicine, including Factors I (fibrinogen), II (prothrombin), VII, X, XI and XII. The clinical severity varies depending on the factor involved (Figure 20.8).

Disorders of fibrinolysis

Excessive fibrinolysis
Conditions leading to a deficiency or abnormality in fibrinogen function (congenital), reduced clearance of tissue plasminogen activator (t-PA) (e.g. liver disease), or administration of fibrinolytic drugs (e.g. streptokinase) may all result in clot dissolution and significant haemorrhage.

Thrombotic disorders
Excessive inhibition of fibrinolysis may result in thrombosis. Vascular endothelial injury, blood stasis and hypercoagulability are the main ingredients for thrombus formation. The clinical signs exhibited by animals depend on the location of the thrombi and the effect on the organ with obstructed blood flow.

Many disease processes are associated with thrombotic complications through a variety of mechanisms,

including cardiac disease, neoplasia, protein-losing diseases (e.g. AT III), endocrine disorders (hyperadrenocorticism, diabetes mellitus, hypothyroidism), immune-mediated disease (immune-mediated haemolytic anaemia, systemic lupus erythematosus), pancreatitis and systemic inflammatory disorders.

Clinical findings (such as acute respiratory distress with pulmonary thromboembolism or acute-onset paraplegia, cold distal extremeties, or lack of femoral pulses with aortic thromboembolism) will often raise suspicion for thromboembolism, which may be confirmed by non-invasive or invasive imaging techniques.

Assessment of haemostasis in the surgical patient

Thorough routine presurgical assessment should include consideration of the patient's coagulation ability. Careful review of the patient history, physical examination and initial pre-anaesthetic blood tests may provide information as to the aetiology of, or identify risk factors for, haemostatic disorders requiring further investigation, even in the absence of clinical signs of haemorrhage or thrombosis.

Questions, answered by review of the patient's medical record or owner interview, that may alert the surgeon to the possibility of a coagulation disorder are listed in Figure 20.9.

Patients with an identified increased risk for bleeding, or with clinical evidence of a coagulopathy, require further diagnostic investigation. The purpose of coagulation testing is to characterize the nature and cause of the coagulopathy before proceeding with invasive diagnostic or therapeutic procedures. Drug therapy likely to be associated with a coagulopathy should be discontinued if possible. In some emergency situations it may not be possible to complete the laboratory evaluation of haemostasis or allow time for drug withdrawal prior to surgery; however, some rapid in-house testing may give a preliminary diagnosis and assist selection of specific and supportive therapies.

Factor deficiency	Clinical signs	Breeds affected
Factor I (fibrinogen)	Haemorrhagic tendency due to inadequate platelet aggregation and clot formation	Bernese Mountain Dog; Lhasa Apso; Vizsla; collies; Bichon Frise
Factor II (prothrombin)	Moderate to severe bleeding tendency	Boxer; Otter Hound; English Cocker Spaniel
Factor VII	Mild bleeding tendency	Beagle; Alaskan Malamute; Miniature Schnauzer; Boxer; Bulldog; many other dog breeds; cats
Factor X	Homozygous affected animals: severe bleeding, usually fatal at birth. Heterozygous animals: variable bleeding tendency (asymptomatic to severe)	American Cocker Spaniel; Jack Russell Terrier; mixed-breed dogs; cats
Factor XI	Bleeding tendency variable, usually mild – severity increases with concurrent stress on haemostatic system (e.g. surgery)	English Springer Spaniel; Kerry Blue Terrier; Great Pyrenees; Weimaraner
Factor XII	Not associated with clinical bleeding	Miniature and Standard Poodle; Shar Pei; German Shorthaired Pointer; cats
Multiple factor deficiencies: Carboxylase deficiency leading to vitamin K-dependent factor deficiency	Severe or fatal bleeding episodes in clinically affected animals	Devon Rex cat

20.8 Inherited coagulation factor deficiencies reported in the dog and cat.

- Is the animal receiving any medication that may affect the haemostatic system (aspirin, warfarin analogues, other NSAIDs)?
- Any possible exposure to anticoagulant toxins (rodenticides)?
- Any excessive or unexpected bleeding or bruising following no or minimal trauma (vaccination, venepuncture, teething, epistaxis, haematuria, melaena)? If so, at what age?
- Any excessive or unexpected bleeding or bruising following previous surgical procedures?
- Any history of travel; and, if so, to what parts of the country/world (infectious disease exposure)?
- If the patient's breed is associated with a bleeding disorder, have any studies of the patient's coagulation status been performed? Is there any information known about bleeding in related animals (e.g. vWD)?
- Has the animal ever received a blood product transfusion?
- Is *Angiostrongylus vasorum* infection a risk for this patient?

20.9 The possibility of a coagulaton disorder may be explored by asking the owner questions and reviewing the patient's medical record.

In all cases of postoperative haemorrhage, inadequate local surgical haemostasis (e.g. slipped ligature, inadvertent vessel damage) should be ruled out prior to completing exhaustive laboratory coagulation testing. Repeated surgical intervention may be necessary and should be performed without detrimental delay to the patient. Traumatic haemorrhage (long bone fracture, vascular avulsion) may similarly require prompt surgical attention.

If a systemic bleeding disorder is suspected, the pattern of haemorrhage evident from the history and physical examination may help to identify the disorder as either a primary or secondary haemostatic defect.

Figure 20.10 details the different coagulation testing abnormalities that are commonly encountered, and the likely disorder or cause of bleeding. Thorough evaluation of haemostasis in a bleeding patient, or a patient at risk for haemorrhage, gives the veterinary surgeon essential information enabling provision of appropriate therapy and restoration of normal haemostatic mechanisms.

Primary haemostasis tests

Platelet count

An anticoagulated (usually EDTA) whole blood sample is obtained for determination of platelet number (frequently included in a complete haemogram), performed by an automated analyser. A blood smear, made from a drop of anticoagulated blood, should be prepared for review.

- The normal platelet count for dogs and cats is approximately $150{-}450 \times 10^9/l$.
- Lower platelet counts may be normal in certain breeds, such as Cavalier King Charles Spaniels (normal function may be found with platelet numbers of $50 \times 10^9/l$) and Greyhounds (normal function may be found with platelet numbers of $110{-}130 \times 10^9/l$), but thrombocytopenia in dogs of these breeds may also be pathological and cannot be excluded on the basis of breed alone.
- Spuriously low platelet counts may occur with:
  - Traumatic venepuncture leading to platelet clumping (activation of haemostasis)
  - Inadequate recognition of large platelets by automatic analyser
  - Sample ageing (*in vitro* aggregation)
  - Cold agglutinins
  - In some cases, anticoagulant-induced clumping.

It is imperative to examine the blood film to confirm or disprove thrombocytopenia.

Estimation of platelet number: An estimation of platelet number can be obtained by calculating the average number of platelets counted in the red cell monolayer on 5–10 high-power fields (hpf). An adequate number of platelets would be 8–12/hpf, as each platelet noted on this magnification approximates $15{-}20 \times 10^9/l$.

Platelets	BMBT	aPTT (or ACT)	PT	FDP	Interpretation	Other comments
↓	↑	N	N	N	Thrombocytopenia	
N	↑	N	N	N	Thrombocytopathia von Willebrand's disease (vWD)	If vWD accompanied by concurrent Factor VIII deficiency, may have slightly prolonged aPTT
N	N	↑	N	N	Intrinsic pathway disorder: Haemophilia A (Factor VIII) Haemophilia B (Factor IX) Factor XI deficiency Factor XII deficiency	Factor XII deficiency may be identified by coagulation testing, but is not associated with any bleeding tendency in the animal
N	N	N	↑	N	Extrinsic pathway disorder: Factor VII deficiency Early rodenticide toxicity Vitamin K deficiency/antagonism	
N	N	↑	↑	N or ↑	Common pathway or multiple factor deficiency: Rodenticide toxicity Vitamin K deficiency/antagonism Liver disease	In some cases of rodenticide toxicity with significant haemorrhage, platelet counts may be decreased
↓	↑	↑	↑	↑	Disseminated intravascular coagulation Hepatic failure	Variable patterns may result with these conditions
N	N or ↑	↑	↑	N	Hypofibrinogenaemia Dysfibrinogenaemia	Fibrinogen levels decreased

20.10 Interpretation of coagulation tests. ACT = activated clotting time; aPTT = activated partial thromboplastin time; BMBT = buccal mucosal bleeding time; FDP = fibrin(ogen) degradation products; N = normal; PT = prothrombin time.

Platelet clumping: Examination of the feathered edge of the blood smear may identify platelet clumps, which although they cannot be used to estimate platelet quantity, may suggest that the platelet count has been artefactually lowered due to their presence. Resampling is advised if there is significant platelet clumping affecting the ability to quantify platelets accurately. In some cases, replacing EDTA anticoagulant with sodium citrate may overcome anticoagulant-induced clumping.

Platelet size and volume: In addition to platelet number, platelet size should be noted. The mean platelet volume (MPV) may be provided by the automated analyser. Elevated MPV tends to suggest the presence of larger, more functional platelets as a consequence of stimulated thrombopoiesis. Visibly enlarged platelets may also be noted on a blood smear. Cavalier King Charles Spaniels are known to have giant platelets (macrothrombocytosis) without any functional significance.

Platelet function: Spontaneous bleeding is more likely to occur in patients whose platelet count is below $25–50 \times 10^9$/l. However, primary haemostatic defects can sometimes be noted in those animals with only mild thrombocytopenia ($75–100 \times 10^9$/l), questioning the functional integrity of those platelets. An assessment of platelet function that can be performed in the clinic is the BMBT (see below). This test is indicated in animals with normal (or elevated) platelet counts in which there is clinical suspicion of a primary haemostatic disorder. It is expected that thrombocytopenic patients will have prolonged bleeding times and as such the BMBT would be unnecessary.

Further investigations

Discovery of significant thrombocytopenia warrants further investigation to ascertain the underlying cause and, if possible, correction prior to proceeding with surgery.

Drug-induced thrombocytopenia:

- If a drug-induced thrombocytopenia is suspected (and any drug should be considered a potential cause), the drug should be discontinued for approximately 2–6 days and the platelet count rechecked.
- If the platelet count normalizes, the drug should not be used in the patient again and caution and close monitoring of the platelet count should be taken if initiating therapy with a related drug of the same class.
- If the patient's condition does not allow for discontinuation of the drug, further investigation should include a full haematology, biochemistry and urinalysis (if not already performed) to exclude or identify other diseases.

Other cytopenias: As thrombocytopenia may accompany other cytopenias, a complete white blood cell count and differential count, as well as red cell mass and morphology evaluation, are imperative. Biochemical and urine abnormalities may aid in directing investigation towards one of the many possible causes of thrombocytopenia. Evaluation of other coagulation parameters helps to rule in or out secondary haemostatic disorders (e.g. DIC).

Bone marrow aspiration: If the coagulation profile is normal, bone marrow aspiration and/or biopsy is recommended, especially if multiple cytopenias are noted on haematology, or if leukaemia, multiple myeloma or any myeloproliferative disorder is suspected. Survey thoracic and abdominal radiographs and/or ultrasonography to identify occult neoplasia may be considered, as well as testing for infectious disease where relevant.

Bone marrow aspirate cytology or histopathological review of core biopsy samples provides useful prognostic information. The samples must be evaluated with a concurrent circulating blood sample, to correlate bone marrow findings with peripheral cell morphology and numbers. Most cases of immune-mediated thrombocytopenia will have hyperplasia of the megakaryocytes, which offers a better prognosis than bone marrow findings of megakaryocytic hypoplasia. These procedures are unlikely to cause significant bleeding even in severely thrombocytopenic animals.

Buccal mucosal bleeding time

The BMBT test is the only test routinely available to the veterinary practitioner as an *in vivo* assessment of primary haemostasis. This test may be helpful for the identification of a primary haemostatic defect when the platelet count is adequate, and is unnecessary in thrombocytopenic patients. It is recommended to use this as a screening test preoperatively in dog breeds predisposed to vWD, as well as dogs living in *Angiostrongylus vasorum* endemic regions.

The procedure is performed by making a small superficial cut in the buccal mucosa, using an automated spring-loaded device (Technique 20.1). The platelet plug formed during primary haemostasis will normally be sufficient to stop the bleeding. The bleeding device produces a cut which is standardized (depth and length) as necessary for reproducible results, and has a permanently retracting blade designed for single use. The time from when the incision is made until bleeding ceases is recorded.

The BMBT is the time recorded from the start to finish of bleeding, which for dogs should be <4 minutes and cats <2.5 minutes.

TECHNIQUE 20.1
The buccal mucosal bleeding time (BMBT) test

1 The patient is restrained in lateral recumbency, and may require sedation for the test.

2 A length of roll gauze is tied around the maxilla, folding the non-dependent lip outwards to expose the maxillary buccal mucosal surface.

➤

3 The gauze is used to hold the lip in place as well as provide vessel congestion (without causing patient discomfort), and tied above the nose as if securing an endotracheal tube.

4 The incision site should be free of visible vessels and ideally allow blood to flow away from the incision towards the mouth.

5 The safety tab is carefully removed from the bleeding device before resting the casing on the incision site, applying gentle pressure.

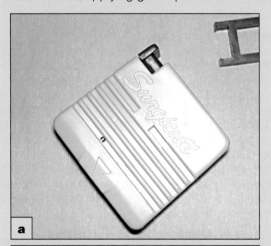

(a) Bleeding time device. **(b)** Inner workings of bleeding time device demonstrating spring-loaded retractable blade.

6 The trigger is depressed, creating the incision(s); timing begins; and the device is removed from the mucosa.

7 Excess blood is gently blotted, taking great care not to touch the incision or forming platelet plug.

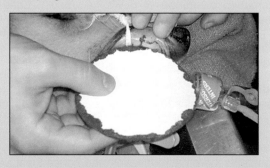

8 The test (and timing) is complete once bleeding from the incision stops.

PRACTICAL TIPS

- Prolongation of the BMBT occurs in patients with vWD, congenital and acquired platelet function defects, or immune-mediated vasculitis syndromes, as well as severe thrombocytopenia.
- Animals with disorders involving coagulation factors, such as haemophilia or vitamin K antagonism, are not expected to have an abnormal BMBT.

von Willebrand factor

The BMBT offers a screening test for disorders of primary haemostasis, such as vWD. Specific quantitative and qualitative tests of vWf are available, as well as genetic testing for some breeds.

A quantitative measurement of vWf in the patient compared with a pooled plasma sample from healthy dogs is offered by von Willebrand factor antigen (vWf:Ag) assays. Due to the variability in trait expression, the factor level alone cannot be used to predict which dogs with reduced vWf will have impaired haemostasis, as not all dogs with decreased vWf exhibit increased bleeding tendencies. However, if an animal has a documented decrease in vWf:Ag, appropriate preparations and precautions should be taken if surgical intervention is required, especially if the vWf:Ag level is <35%.

The results are reported as a percentage of normal, with interpretative ranges in three categories: normal, borderline and vWD. Sampling for vWf:Ag most often requires separation and freezing of plasma obtained from sodium citrate anticoagulated whole blood. The vWf:Ag level may be affected by sample haemolysis (reduced), tissue trauma (increased), sample collection and processing methods, as well as by hormones and daily fluctuations. As a result, when screening for vWD yields a borderline vWf:Ag level, repeat testing is recommended. The reference laboratory should be contacted for specific submission requirements prior to sampling.

Genetic tests have been developed that can detect vWf gene mutations in some dog breeds, and have been used in conjunction with vWf:Ag levels to identify normal or carrier animals.

Other platelet function tests

Platelet aggregometers and the PFA-100 analyser are used in some research and specialist laboratories to assess *in vitro* platelet adhesion, aggregation and secretion. Patient whole blood samples must be assayed within hours, which limits test availability.

Secondary haemostasis tests

Coagulation tests are available for use in-clinic or at reference laboratories and typically identify abnormalities in the intrinsic, extrinsic or common pathways. All coagulation tests require careful sample handling and atraumatic venepuncture. Most tests utilize sodium citrate anticoagulated whole blood. If testing is delayed (e.g. sending the sample to a reference laboratory) separation of the plasma from the red cells and freezing the plasma portion immediately after collection may improve sample quality and test reliability. The manufacturer or laboratory should be consulted for test-specific sampling requirements.

Activated clotting time

The activated clotting time (ACT) provides a screening test of the intrinsic and common pathways and is available as a point-of-care test by both manual and automated methods. The manufacturer's recommendations for test procedure and interpretation should be used for the automated analyser method.

The following description refers only to the manual tube ACT method. Diseases or conditions associated with prolonged ACT are similar to those for prolonged aPTT (see below) and are noted in Figure 20.10, though the ACT is generally less sensitive than the aPTT.

1. A diatomaceous earth (contact activator) vacuum sampling tube warmed to 37°C is required.
2. Blood is collected directly into the tube using vacuum draw, as transferring samples obtained with a needle and syringe affects the reliability of the test.
3. The first few drops of blood are discarded before attaching the ACT test tube.
4. Once blood is collected and mixed with the activator, timing of the test commences, after which the tube is incubated at 37°C for 60 seconds.
5. The tube is gently rotated every 5–10 seconds while being monitored for clot development, at which time the test and timing are complete.
6. Normal result (manual method) for dogs is <110 seconds, and for cats is <75 seconds.

Activated partial thromboplastin time

The aPTT (APTT, PTT) is another screening test of the intrinsic and common pathways, assessed by a point-of-care automated analyser method or via coagulometers in a reference laboratory. Method-specific sampling and species-specific reference ranges should be used to interpret test results (seconds) and ideally species-, age- and breed-matched control samples should be assayed for comparison. Diseases or conditions associated with prolonged aPTT are noted in Figure 20.10. The test is relatively insensitive and prolongation of aPTT may suggest either >70% reduction in a single factor, or less marked reductions in multiple factors.

Prothrombin time

The PT provides a screening test of the extrinsic and common pathways. Sampling guidelines supplied by the manufacturer or reference laboratory (similar to those for aPTT) and result interpretation should be followed.

Diseases or conditions causing prolongation of PT are listed in Figure 20.10. As Factor VII has a very short half-life, and its functionality is dependent on vitamin K carboxylation, PT may be affected earlier than aPTT in circumstances of vitamin K deficiency or antagonism.

If the ACT or the aPTT is prolonged, assessment of the PT will help to differentiate between an intrinsic and common pathway defect, and a combined coagulopathy involving several coagulation factors. If a hereditary factor deficiency is suspected based on breed and coagulation test results, specific factor analysis is required for confirmation.

Coagulation tests may be used to identify disorders of haemostasis, as well as for monitoring response to therapy. When using anticoagulant therapy: aPTT is used to monitor response to heparin; and PT for monitoring patients receiving warfarin. Similarly repeating coagulation tests for animals receiving coagulation factor replacement (typically via fresh frozen plasma therapy, or whole blood transfusion) or vitamin K supplementation may be useful to confirm efficacy of therapy.

Thromboelastography

Thromboelastography (TEG) is a global test assessing all phases of coagulation. It requires use of a specialized instrument that is becoming increasingly popular in university and referral practices, and assesses the time to clot formation, clot development, and overall clot strength on samples of fresh or citrate anticoagulated whole blood. Information provided by TEG allows identification of both hypo- and hypercoagulable disorders and it is useful for monitoring the response to therapy (e.g. heparin, clopidogrel, warfarin, transfusion therapy). Its usefulness and clinical relevance are currently limited by its availability.

Coagulation inhibitors

Functional assays of AT III activity are available and are useful for evaluating patient anticoagulant ability. Reduced AT III activity may be a result of decreased production (e.g. liver disease), increased hepatic clearance of AT III complexes (consumptive coagulopathy, heparin therapy), or increased loss (e.g. protein-losing nephropathy).

Other anticoagulants may be in circulation and can contribute to abnormalities detected on routine coagulation tests. Abnormal inhibition of coagulation may be suspected when mixing patient and species-matched control plasma fails to correct the coagulation abnormality *in vitro*.

Fibrinolysis

Fibrin/fibrinogen degradation products

During the process of soluble fibrin and fibrinogen degradation by plasmin, FDPs are generated (see Figure 20.5). An elevated serum or plasma FDP level is indicative of increased fibrinolysis (localized or DIC, internal haemorrhage), increased fibrinogenolysis, or decreased clearance of FDPs (reduced hepatic or renal function). Increased FDPs may also prolong PT, aPTT, ACT and platelet function tests due to their competition with fibrinogen along many routes of the coagulation pathway and platelet binding sites.

D-dimers

Insoluble cross-linked fibrin is degraded by plasmin to yield cross-linked FDPs and D-dimers (see Figure 20.5). Whereas increased FDPs indicates increased fibrinolysis, increased plasma D-dimers represents increased formation and consequent degradation of cross-linked fibrin (activation of coagulation and fibrinolysis).

Increased D-dimers may occur as a result of thromboembolic disease or DIC, as well as recent surgery, trauma, infection, internal haemorrhage, liver disease, or neoplasia. D-dimer measurement is tending to replace FDP assessment in clinical practice in dogs, but current test methods do not appear to provide reliable results or information in cats.

Blood component therapy

Blood products are used to treat a variety of conditions, including those associated with anaemia, haemostatic disorders, sepsis, DIC and specific factor deficiencies.

Indications

Red blood cell products

Red blood cell (RBC) products provide the recipient with an additional red cell mass, thereby increasing the oxygen-carrying capacity of the blood and improving oxygen delivery to peripheral tissues. There is not a precise packed cell volume (PCV) below which a transfusion is required, although any patient with a PCV <20% should be considered a potential candidate. Some animals with peracute blood loss and hypovolaemia may benefit from RBC transfusions at a higher PCV, as their PCV will predictably fall following fluid resuscitation with non-blood-containing fluids. The decision to transfuse red cells is therefore based on several factors, including the haemoglobin concentration (or PCV), onset of anaemia (acute *versus* chronic), presence of ongoing losses and, most importantly, the clinical signs of the patient. Tachypnoea, tachycardia, bounding peripheral pulses, collapse, lethargy and weakness are all signs that would prompt the consideration of an RBC transfusion. Haemoglobin-based oxygen carriers, such as Oxyglobin when available, have also been successfully used in both dogs and cats.

Plasma products

Plasma products are a source of coagulation factors and various plasma proteins, and deficiencies of these factors or selected proteins are an indication for their use. Plasma products are most beneficial to patients with inherited or acquired coagulopathies. The benefit of a plasma transfusion to a hypoproteinaemic patient is limited – the half-life of albumin is very short and with protein-losing diseases many units of plasma would be required to correct the albumin deficit. Different formulae and calculations exist for calculating a patient's albumin deficit. A conservative estimate guideline is that 45 ml of plasma/kg would be required to raise the serum albumin level by 10 g/l if there were no ongoing losses. For example, a 20 kg dog would require at least 900 ml of plasma (4–5 units) to raise the serum albumin level from 10 g/l to 20 g/l.

Understanding and defining the needs of the patient enables the veterinary surgeon to select the most appropriate therapies (Figure 20.11), many of which include isolated blood components to permit specific replacement therapy. Specific replacement therapy permits a smaller volume transfusion and helps to prevent consequences potentially associated with volume overload in both the euvolaemic and hypovolaemic transfusion recipient.

Types of blood product

Blood collection yields fresh whole blood. Whole blood can either be stored or separated into packed red blood cells (PRBCs), fresh plasma, stored plasma or platelet-rich plasma concentrates (Figure 20.12).

Blood component processing requires variable-speed temperature-controlled centrifuges for most of the products described. The precise centrifugation protocol used is dependent on the centrifuge and the component being isolated.

Condition	Fresh whole blood (FWB)	Stored whole blood (SWB)	Packed red blood cells (PRBCs)	Platelet-rich plasma/platelet concentration (PRP/PC)	Fresh frozen plasma (FFP)	Cryoprecipitate
Anaemia	Acceptable	Acceptable	Best	No benefit	No benefit	No benefit
Thrombocytopenia Thrombocytopathia	Acceptable	Supportive care if anaemic and hypoproteinaemic	Supportive care if anaemic	Best	Supportive care if hypoproteinaemic or concurrent coagulopathy	No benefit
von Willebrand's disease Haemophilia A (Factor VIII)	Acceptable	Supportive care if anaemic and hypoproteinaemic, but does not provide required clotting factors	Supportive care if anaemic, but does not provide clotting factors	No benefit	Acceptable	Best
Coagulopathy	Acceptable	Supportive care if anaemic and hypoproteinaemic, but does not provide clotting factors	Supportive care if anaemic, but does not provide clotting factors	No benefit	Best	Little benefit for most coagulopathies – limited to Factors VIII, XIII, vWf, fibrinogen and fibronectin

20.11 Patient condition and therapeutic blood product choice. vWF = von Willebrand factor.

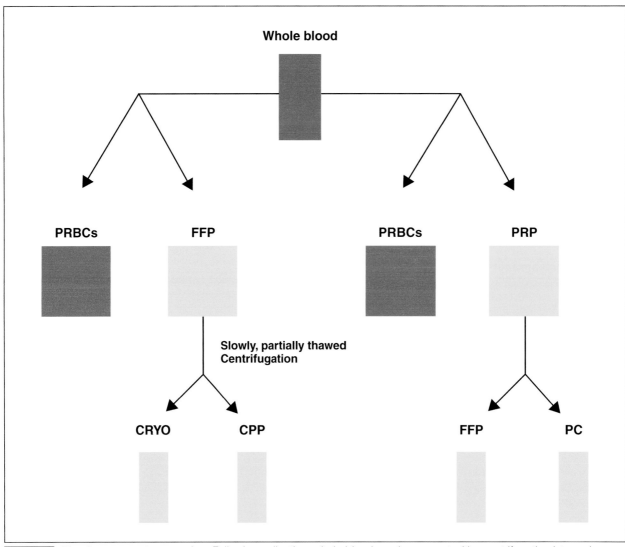

20.12 Blood component processing. Following collection, whole blood can be separated by centrifugation into various compound products, based on different centrifugation speeds and time. CPP = cryoprecipitate-poor plasma; CRYO = cryoprecipitate; FFP= fresh frozen plasma; PC = platelet concentration; PRBCs = packed red blood cells; PRP = platelet-rich plasma.

PRACTICAL TIPS

- Closed collection systems with integral tubing for component transfer prevent microbial contamination. The tubing should be sealed prior to unit storage.
- If blood is collected into open systems it should be used immediately, or refrigerated and administered within 24 hours.

Red cell products

Fresh whole blood: Fresh whole blood (FWB) is collected following strict aseptic technique. It is not refrigerated and used within 8 hours of collection. All blood components (RBCs, platelets, labile and stable coagulation factors, plasma proteins) are present and functional. FWB is most commonly used in private veterinary practices; however, if components were always available, the administration of FWB would be restricted to anaemic patients with concurrent haemostatic defects.

Stored whole blood: FWB not used within 8 hours of collection may be stored in a refrigerator at 1–6°C for approximately 28 or 35 days (anticoagulant dependent). The unit is then reclassified as stored whole blood (SWB), which differs from FWB only by the absence of functional labile clotting factors and platelets. When available, SWB may be useful in anaemic animals with concurrent hypoproteinaemia.

Packed red blood cells: PRBCs are separated from the plasma by centrifugation. The PRBC unit provides the same red cell properties as a unit of whole blood. PRBC transfusion is indicated in severely anaemic animals to provide additional oxygen-carrying support. The PCV of the unit is greater than that of whole blood and is usually in the range of 70–80%, with the volume yield dependent on the donor haematocrit. PRBCs may be stored at 4°C for 20 days, with an extension to 35 days if preservative solution is added. PRBC transfusion provides the oxygen-carrying capacity of a full unit of blood within a reduced volume (minus plasma portion), helping to prevent adverse consequences that may result from volume overload in a euvolaemic patient.

Plasma products

Fresh frozen plasma: Fresh frozen plasma (FFP) is separated from PRBCs and frozen within 8 hours of collection, preserving the labile coagulation Factors V and VIII as well as all other coagulation factors and plasma proteins. Plasma that is refrozen after thawing, or prepared and frozen later than 8 hours after collection, loses its labile coagulation factors. FFP is indicated for use in animals with acquired or inherited coagulopathies (inherited factor deficiencies, vitamin K deficiency, DIC, severe liver disease) and may be used prophylactically in surgical patients with known coagulopathies or at the time of active bleeding. As FFP contains other plasma proteins, it may be used in animals with hypoproteinaemia; however, large volumes and repeated transfusions are required to produce a clinically significant and sustained improvement. FFP may be stored for up to 1 year when frozen below −20°C.

Stored frozen plasma: Stored frozen plasma (SFP) is FFP >1 year of age, plasma not frozen quickly enough to protect labile factors, or FFP that has been thawed and refrozen without opening the bag. Many useful clotting factors and anti-inflammatory proteins will have been lost, but SFP can be used for colloidal support (hypoproteinaemia) and may still provide some vitamin K-dependent factors. SFP may be stored frozen at −20°C for 5 years from the date of collection.

Platelet-rich plasma and platelet concentration: Platelet-rich plasma (PRP) and platelet concentration (PC) may be prepared from FWB, but these products are some of the most challenging to prepare due to the delicate nature of platelets. To enhance survival and function of the platelets in the resulting product, extreme care and attention must be given to the unit during all phases of handling. FWB is centrifuged on a 'light' spin (reduced centrifugation time and speed). PRP is separated from the PRBCs and may be administered to the recipient, stored, or further processed into PC and FFP.

PRP and PC may be stored at 20–24°C, with gentle agitation, for 5 days when collected using a closed system. Due to the higher storage temperature than other blood products, platelet products are more susceptible to bacterial contamination and should be used within 4 hours of collection if collected in an open system. They are used when there is uncontrollable, severe or life-threatening bleeding (e.g. intracranial haemorrhage) associated with thrombocytopenia/pathia, but the difficulties associated with their production often results in the use of more readily available FWB. A novel lyophilized PC product has been recently introduced in the United States and is currently being used in a multicentre clinical trial.

Cryoprecipitate and Cryo-poor plasma: Preparation of cryoprecipitate (Cryo) provides a source of concentrated vWf, Factor VIII, Factor XIII, fibrinogen and fibronectin from a unit of FFP. Cryo can be prepared from FFP within 12 months of collection. A unit of FFP is slowly thawed until only approximately 10% of the plasma remains frozen, and then centrifuged according to protocol. The Cryo-poor plasma (CPP),

or the cryosupernatant, is harvested, leaving behind the Cryo in a small volume of plasma (10–15 ml). The CPP contains many clotting factors (including vitamin K-dependent Factors II, VII, IX and X), as well as other anticoagulant and fibrinolytic factors, albumin and globulin. The Cryo and remaining CPP are immediately refrozen and should be used within 1 year of original collection. The administration of desmopressin (DDAVP) 30–120 minutes prior to donation will increase the amount of vWf in the donor FFP and increase Cryo yield.

Cryo is used in the management of patients with bleeding due to deficiency or dysfunction of Factor VIII (haemophilia A), vWf or fibrinogen. It should be the first choice transfusion product for a euvolaemic patient with significant vWf deficiency undergoing a non-emergency surgical procedure, as it will supply the necessary factors in a small volume transfusion. CPP may be used for other coagulopathies not requiring supplementation of the Cryo components or hypoproteinaemia. A novel lyophilized canine Cryo product has been introduced in the United States.

Haemoglobin-based oxygen carriers

Oxyglobin (OPK Biotech, Cambridge, MA) is a sterile solution of purified polymerized bovine haemoglobin that increases plasma haemoglobin concentration, shifting the majority of the oxygen content of the blood to the plasma (see also Chapters 9 and 10). It has been approved for use in dogs for the treatment of anaemia, regardless of cause, and has been successfully used in cats (off-licence). Oxyglobin provides a suitable alternative to PRBCs for temporarily increasing the oxygen-carrying capacity of the blood (lasting approximately 24 hours in the circulation) and may be less immunogenic than PRBCs when initially treating a dog with immune-mediated haemolytic anaemia. Oxyglobin should be administered with care, monitoring for evidence of circulatory overload and possible development of pulmonary oedema and/or pleural effusion as a consequence of its colloidal volume-expanding properties. Recently the manufacturer of Oxyglobin ceased production, and it is unclear if it will return to the market.

Collection, storage and administration of blood

Donors

Canine donors: Canine donors should be healthy, well tempered, large-breed dogs weighing at least 25 kg and between 1 and 8 years of age. They should receive routine veterinary preventive healthcare, including vaccination according to practice protocols and no medications at the time of donation, with the exception of flea preventive, routine worming medication, or heartworm preventive (location specific). It is preferable to use dogs that will remain still with minimal restraint during the blood collection procedure, avoiding sedation and the possible consequences of its use. Any dog that has previously received a transfusion is unsuitable as a donor.

Pre-donation tests for canine donors include determination of blood type (DEA 1 – see below), yearly haematology and general biochemistry profiles, as well as screening for infectious diseases endemic to their region or to a geographical location where they have previously lived. Infectious diseases of concern, which have the potential to be transmitted by blood transfusion, include *Babesia* spp., *Leishmania* spp., *Ehrlichia* spp., *Anaplasma* spp., *Neorickettsia* spp., *Brucella canis, Trypanosoma cruzi, Bartonella vinsonii* and haemotropic mycoplasmal organisms. Excluding dogs that have travelled outside the UK currently prevents the need for exhaustive infectious disease testing the UK, but infectious disease prevalence may increase with global pet travel and climate change.

Feline donors: Feline donors should be healthy, clinically well, cats between 1 and 8 years of age, receiving routine veterinary preventive healthcare. They should weigh at least 4 kg. Unlike canine donors, cats usually require sedation for the donation. Given the problems with naturally occurring alloantibodies in cats (see Feline blood types below) it is essential that all feline donors, as well as recipients, be blood typed to prevent mismatched transfusions. To assess the donor's general health, haematology, serum biochemistry and infectious disease screening for FeLV, FIV and feline haemotropic mycoplasmas (PCR) are evaluated each year. Cats with positive infectious disease screening results should be excluded from the donor pool. Furthermore, to maintain a negative infectious disease status, active donor cats should be confined to living indoors to avoid exposure to infectious diseases.

Screening healthy donor cats for *Bartonella* spp., *Cytauxzoon felis, Ehrlichia* spp., *Anaplasma* spp. and *Neorickettsia* spp. may be considered. Controversy remains over testing donor cats for feline coronavirus, as many clinically well cats have positive titres yet never develop clinical feline infectious peritonitis (FIP) and transmission of clinical disease via blood transfusion has not yet been documented. Similarly, *Toxoplasma gondii* screening antigen, antibody or DNA tests are not recommended, as healthy cats may have positive test results, which are not necessarily a concern for the safety of the blood transfusion.

Blood types
RBC types are determined by species-specific inherited antigens present on the cell surface. The frequency of canine and feline blood types varies with geographical location and breed. Blood-type incompatibility is observed clinically as transfusion reactions or neonatal isoerythrolysis, the occurrence and severity of which is variable between individuals and species.

Canine blood types: The dog erythrocyte antigen (DEA) nomenclature is most commonly used to describe canine blood types. Although at least a dozen antigens have been identified, typing antisera for only six of these is currently available: DEA 1.1, 1.2, 3, 4, 5 and 7.

- For each DEA group except DEA 1, a dog may be positive or negative.
- The DEA 1 group has at least two subtypes: DEA 1.1 and 1.2.
- A third subtype, DEA 1.3, has been described but it has not been extensively evaluated.
- A dog may be positive for only one of these DEA 1 subtypes, or it may be negative for all three.

The relevance of blood type is related to its antigenic potential. The most antigenic blood type is DEA 1.1.

- There are no naturally occurring alloantibodies against DEA 1.1. As such, most dogs will not experience a severe transfusion reaction if they receive DEA 1.1-incompatible blood on their first transfusion.
- However, sensitization will occur in DEA 1.1-negative dogs receiving DEA 1.1-positive cells, producing antibodies that can cause an acute haemolytic transfusion reaction after repeated antigen exposure (e.g. a second transfusion with DEA 1.1-positive blood). Production of antibodies after red cell antigen sensitization may occur as early as 4 days after transfusion.

Blood typing is based on an agglutination reaction using polyclonal or monoclonal antibodies.

- Agglutination in the presence of these antibodies identifies the presence of the particular red cell antigen (positive).
- Lack of haemoagglutination indicates that the dog is negative for the test antigen.

As DEA 1.1 is the most antigenic blood type, the DEA 1.1 status of both the donor and recipient are determined prior to transfusion.

> **PRACTICAL TIP**
>
> As a general rule:
>
> - DEA 1.1-negative dogs should only receive DEA 1.1-negative blood
> - DEA 1.1-positive dogs may receive either DEA 1.1-negative or DEA 1.1-positive blood.

DEA 1.1 testing can be performed by a variety of reference laboratory and in-house methods. Typing for antigens other than DEA 1.1 requires the use of polyclonal antisera, available from only a few specialized blood service laboratories, and is generally not required.

To prevent false-positive or undeterminable results, autoagglutination must be ruled out prior to typing. In-saline autoagglutination may sometimes be overcome by washing the cells. If agglutination persists, thereby preventing typing, or in any situation where the results are unclear or testing is not immediately available, the recipient is considered to be DEA 1.1-negative and should only receive DEA 1.1-negative blood until a blood sample may be retyped. In some cases, typing results yield a mixed field reaction, suggesting the presence of more than one type of RBC (e.g. after recent transfusion), or a weak positive result (possibly DEA 1.2-positive), or a false-negative result (severely anaemic dog).

Feline blood types: Blood groups in cats are described by the A–B system, which includes three blood types: A, B and AB. The blood types are inherited as a simple dominant trait, with A being dominant over B.

- Genotypically **type A** cats are either homozygous *a/a* or heterozygous *a/b*.
- **Type B** cats are homozygous *b/b*.
- **AB** is a rare blood type in which a third allele is present at the same locus, permitting expression of both A and B antigens.

Typing of cats prior to transfusion is imperative. Cats have naturally occurring alloantibodies present in their plasma, which are isoagglutinins against the RBC antigen they lack. These antibodies are found in all type A and B cats after 2 months of age; their formation does not require prior exposure through transfusion or pregnancy; and they may cause a potentially fatal immediate transfusion reaction as well as neonatal isoerythrolysis. Therefore, **all donor and recipient cats** must be blood typed prior to transfusion, even in an emergency situation.

Blood typing can be performed by several methods, indicating agglutination in the presence of A or B cells, determining the blood type as type A, B or AB. If using an in-house card test kit, it is advisable to confirm B or AB typing results by a second method, such as a gel card (reference laboratory), back typing, or cross-matching (major and minor), prior to transfusion. Autoagglutination must be excluded prior to typing, and false results may occur in anaemic and diseased cats.

If type A blood is administered to a type B cat, the risk of a transfusion reaction is greatest, as anti-A antibodies induce rapid intravascular haemolysis (with complement activation) of the donor RBCs. The signs of an acute haemolytic transfusion reaction may occur after the cat has received as little as 1 ml of type A blood, and may be fatal. Clinical signs of such a reaction include depression, agitation, bradycardia, apnoea, hypopnoea, vocalization, salivation, urination, defecation and possibly in later stages tachycardia, tachypnoea, haemolysis and haemoglobinuria.

If type B blood is administered to a type A cat, the transfusion reaction is significant but often less than severe, resulting in accelerated destruction of the RBCs (extravascular haemolysis).

PRACTICAL TIPS

- Type A cats must only receive type A blood.
- Type B cats must only receive type B blood.

Type AB cats do not have either alloantibody. The rarer AB cat should ideally receive type AB blood, but when that is not available type A blood is the next best choice.

- The anti-B alloantibodies present in a type A cat may induce a mild transfusion reaction when administered to a type AB cat.
- The anti-A alloantibodies of type B cats would likely cause a moderate to significant transfusion reaction if administered to a type AB cat.
- In a situation where a type A donor is to be used for a type AB recipient, it would be advisable to remove the donor plasma and transfuse only washed RBCs to try to avoid incompability.

Neonatal isoerythrolysis: The presence of naturally occurring alloantibodies may cause neonatal isoerythrolysis in type A and AB kittens born to a type B queen, due to the ingestion of colostral anti-A alloantibodies in the first few days of life. Within hours to days of colostrum ingestion, clinical signs of red cell haemolysis become apparent, including anaemia, haemoglobinaemia, jaundice, haemoglobinuria and in some cases death. Neonatal isoerythrolysis may be prevented by only mating type B queens with type B toms, or by removal and foster nursing of at-risk kittens for the first 2–3 days of life.

Type B prevalence in cat breeds: Breeds with a documented increased prevalence of type B compared with the non-pedigree cat population include: British Shorthair, Devon Rex, Persian, Somali, Abyssinian, Himalayan, Birman and Scottish Fold. Siamese have been reported as 100% type A. Previous prevalence reports from the US and UK have suggested that the majority of domestic non-pedigree cats are type A (>90%), but recent studies indicate that the prevalence of type B is increasing.

Cross-matching

Cross-matching determines the serological compatibility between the patient and donor RBCs, detecting sensitization to different red cell antigens. Cross-matching in dogs should be performed when:

- The recipient has been previously transfused more than 4 days prior (even if it received DEA 1.1-negative blood)
- There has been a history of a transfusion reaction
- The recipient's transfusion history is unknown.

A recent study has shown that pregnancy does not appear to sensitize dogs to RBC antigens (Blaise *et al.*, 2009). Therefore, previously pregnant dogs can be donors; and if these dogs were to require a transfusion, no cross-match would be required on first transfusion as for other transfusion naive dogs. If the patient receives a transfusion and 4–5 days elapse, cross-matching must be repeated as the recipient may no longer be compatible with the same donors.

PRACTICAL TIPS

- The major cross-match is an assessment of the compatibility (as assessed by agglutination) between the donor RBCs and patient plasma/serum.
- The minor cross-match assesses the interaction between the donor plasma/serum and patient RBCs.

Minor cross-match incompatibilities are less frequently the cause of haemolytic transfusion reactions and are mostly of concern when large volumes of plasma are to be administered. Patient autoagglutination or haemolysis may result in incompatibility and a control should be run with the patient RBCs and patient serum.

Ideally cats should be cross-matched prior to the first transfusion, even when using a compatible type donor as assessed by currently available A–B blood group system typing methods. A recently detected novel red cell antigen (*Mik*), different from the A–B system, caused cross-match incompatibility in a type A cat and raised concern that there may also be transfusion reactions as a consequence of naturally occurring alloantibodies directed towards yet unidentified feline red cell antigens (Weinstein *et al.*, 2007). Additional *Mik* antigen-negative cats have since been identified following investigation of haemolytic transfusion reactions after first-time transfusion with group system A–B-compatible blood. If the donor or recipient blood type is unknown, or if the cat has been previously transfused, a cross-match must be performed (Technique 20.2).

Despite using blood products from a cross-matched compatible donor, it is still possible for a patient to experience a haemolytic or non-haemolytic transfusion reaction, and recipient monitoring during and after administration of the product is essential.

TECHNIQUE 20.2
Feline in-house cross-match procedure

This method is simple and can be performed rapidly.

1 Collect blood into an EDTA tube from the recipient and donor.

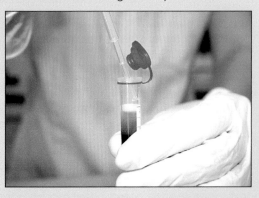

2 Centrifuge the samples (1000 g for 60 seconds) to settle the red blood cells.

3 Remove the supernatant plasma and transfer it to a clean labelled glass or plastic tube.

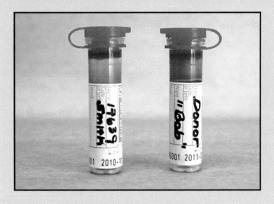

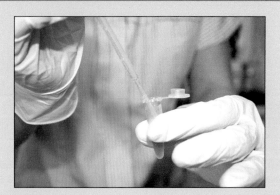

4 For each donor, prepare three slides labelled 'Major', 'Minor' and 'Recipient control'.

5 Place 1 drop of red blood cells and 2 drops of plasma on to each slide according to the following:

- Major cross-match = donor red blood cells + recipient plasma
- Minor cross-match = recipient red blood cells + donor plasma
- Recipient control = recipient red blood cells + recipient plasma.

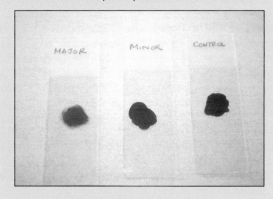

6 Gently rock the slides to mix the plasma and red blood cells.

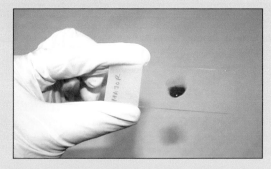

7 Examine for haemagglutination after 1–5 minutes:

- Presence of agglutination is indicative of incompatibility
- Recipient control agglutination will invalidate results.

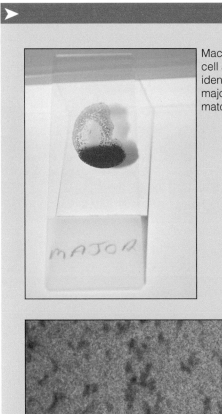

Macroscopic red cell agglutination identified on major cross-match.

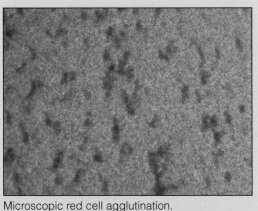

Microscopic red cell agglutination.

Blood collection systems

All whole blood collection should take place in an aseptic manner and should use an appropriate anticoagulant.

Anticoagulants: The anticoagulant solutions most often used are:

- ACD (acid–citrate–dextrose)
- CPD (citrate–phosphate–dextrose)
- CPDA-1 (citrate–phosphate–dextrose–adenine).

CPD and CPDA-1 are most commonly used in commercially available closed collection systems. The volume of anticoagulant used and product storage time varies depending on the composition of the anti-coagulant, addition of a preservative solution and the collection method.

PRACTICAL TIPS

- ACD is used at a ratio of 1 ml of anticoagulant to 7–9 ml of blood.
- CPD and CPDA-1 are typically used in a ratio of 1 ml of anticoagulant to 7 ml of blood.

Use of other anticoagulants (e.g. sodium citrate, heparin) is not recommended.

Open and closed collection systems: Whole blood may be collected using a closed or open collection system.

- A **closed system** is one in which the only exposure of the collection bag or its contents to air prior to administration is when the needle is uncapped to perform venepuncture during collection. Examples of a closed system are commercially available 450 ml blood collection bags containing 63 ml of CPD/CPDA-1 anticoagulant with an attached 16 gauge needle used in dogs weighing >25 kg. Multi-bag systems with empty transfer satellite bags and red cell preservative may be used for component processing.
- Any system in which there is one or more additional sites of potential bacterial contamination during blood collection or processing is by definition an **open system**. All blood products collected in an open system must be administered within 4 hours, or used within 24 hours if stored in a refrigerator (1–6°C). Collection using syringes or empty bags with added anticoagulant, as used in cats and for other small volume collections, is classified as an open system.

Collection volume: The volume of blood that may be collected safely from canine and feline donors is approximately 20% of their blood volume, every 3–4 weeks. A recommended volume limit is 18 ml/kg for dogs and 10–12 ml/kg for cats. Most volunteer donor schemes using client-owned pets as donors extend the donation interval to every 8 weeks.

Assessment before donation

Prior to every donation, information on the donor animal is reviewed and a brief questionnaire is completed by the owner. The age and general good health of the donor and date of last donation are confirmed. Results of a full physical examination and PCV or haemoglobin concentration are assessed and recorded in the donor file.

Collection procedure

The jugular vein is the recommended venepuncture site in both dogs and cats, due to its size and accessibility.

PRACTICAL TIPS

- To avoid cell damage or excessive activation of coagulation factors, collection should be performed with a rapid uninterrupted single stick.
- Strict aseptic technique and use of sterile equipment will minimize the possibility of bacterial contamination.
- All donors must be closely monitored during blood collection by assessing their mucous membrane colour, pulse rate and quality, and respiratory rate and effort. If any concerns develop, the donation should be discontinued.

Most dogs are able to donate without the use of sedation, and it is preferable to train a donor to the procedure. Placing the dog in lateral recumbency on a soft blanket on a table facilitates comfortable restraint (for donor and veterinary personnel) for the 10 minutes required for blood collection. It also allows adequate digital pressure to be applied to the venepuncture site for haemostasis whilst the animal maintains a recumbent position post-donation.

Whole blood collection using a blood bag: Collection of whole blood from dogs using a commercial blood bag (Technique 20.3) may be accomplished via gravity alone, but use of a specialized vacuum chamber, to which suction is applied, may decrease the donation time and therefore the amount of time the donor must be restrained.

TECHNIQUE 20.3
Canine whole-blood collection procedure

1 Clip hair over the jugular groove and apply EMLA cream. This is usually completed at the time of the health check, prior to the donor being placed on the donation table.

2 Restrain the animal securely and comfortably (lateral recumbency on the table is recommended).

3 Prepare the site of venepuncture aseptically.

4 Apply pressure at the thoracic inlet to raise the jugular vein and facilitate palpation and visualization of the vessel. Avoid contamination of the venepuncture site.

5 Use the guarded haemostat or clamp provided with the blood collection bag on the donor tubing to prevent air from entering the bag when the needle is exposed.

6 Place the bag on the scale and set the weight to zero.

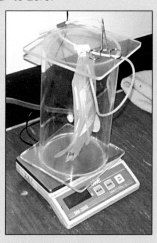

- If using a vacuum chamber, the bag is suspended inside the chamber from the clip on the chamber lid, with the donor tubing and needle outside the chamber (seated in a small notch at the top). The whole apparatus is set on the scale and the weight is set to zero. The vacuum seal is tested and suction turned off prior to venepuncture.

7 Remove the needle cap and perform venepuncture using the 16 gauge needle attached to the collection bag. Remove the clamp or the haemostat. If no flashback is seen in the donor tubing, check for any occlusion in the donor tubing and the needle placement.

8 The bag should be positioned lower than the donor to aid gravitational flow.

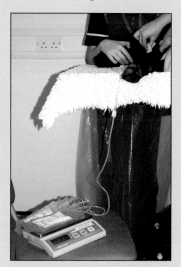

- If using vacuum-assisted collection, the suction may be turned on at a recommended vacuum pressure of 6.5–24 kPa (50–180 mmHg).

9 Periodically invert the bag (gently) to mix blood and anticoagulant (not required with vacuum-assisted collection).

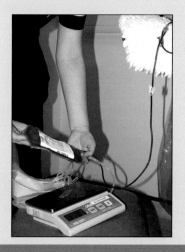

10 A gram scale is used to monitor the weight of the bag during collection, to ensure that an adequate and not excessive amount of blood is collected to preserve the appropriate anticoagulant to blood ratio.

11 When the bag is full (405–495 ml blood = 426–521 g weight), turn off the suction (if used), clamp the donor tubing, remove the needle from the jugular vein and apply pressure to the venepuncture site to prevent haematoma formation.

12 *Allow the tubing to refill with anticoagulated blood and clamp the distal (needle) end with a hand sealer clip or heat sealer.

13 Clamp the entire length of the tubing in 10 cm segments to be used for subsequent cross-matches.

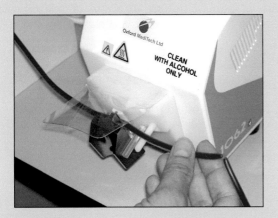

14 Label the bag with product type, donor identification, date of collection, date of expiration, donor blood type, donor PCV (or haematocrit or haemoglobin) and phlebotomist identification. Type prior to use and storage.

*If using a multi-bag system for blood component preparation, steps 12–14 may be replaced by the processing procedure (centrifugation, plasma extraction).

TECHNIQUE 20.4
Blood collection via syringe

1 Syringes for collection should be prefilled with an appropriate anticoagulant (1 ml CPDA-1 per 7 ml blood). Cats usually require sedation: commonly used protocols include combinations of midazolam and ketamine intravenously, or isoflurane/oxygen administered by mask.

2 An intravenous catheter is placed in the cephalic vein of the feline donor, either before (preferably) or after sedation, for the purpose of administering intravenous fluids after the blood donation.

3 Follow steps 1–4 in Technique 20.3 (Canine whole blood collection). The feline donor is restrained in sternal recumbency, with the forelimbs over the edge of the table and the head raised.

4 Perform venepuncture. Without removing the needle, fill each syringe in turn. If an over-the-needle catheter is used, remove the stylet following venepuncture and advance the catheter into the vein. Attach an extension set and fill each syringe in turn.

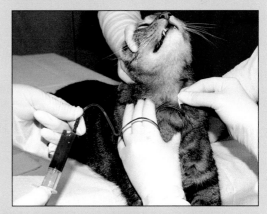

5 Invert the syringe several times (gently) after collection to mix the blood and anticoagulant.

6 After collection, remove the needle from the jugular vein and apply pressure to the venepuncture site to prevent haematoma formation.

Whole blood collection using a syringe: This open method allows collection of smaller volumes of blood, or collection of blood when sterile collection bags are not available (Technique 20.4).

PRACTICAL TIPS

- **For dogs**: 18 gauge needle, 19 gauge butterfly catheter, or 18 gauge over-the-needle intravenous catheter is required.
- **For cats**: typically a 19 or 21 gauge butterfly catheter is used.

After donation

- Dogs are offered food and water following donation. Activity should be restricted to lead walks only for the next 24 hours.
- Cats should have an intravenous catheter placed as part of the donation procedure for provision of fluid replacement in the form of intravenous replacement crystalloid solution at 30 ml/kg over approximately 3 hours following donation.
- The donor must be closely observed during recovery from sedation/anaesthesia and may be offered food and water once fully awake.

Storage

Red cell products: Red cell products should be stored in a refrigerator maintained at 1–6°C, in an upright position to help to maximize red cell survival, permitting gas exchange and RBC metabolism and preserving red cell membrane integrity. The shelf life of the product is based on the anticoagulant preservative solution used in collection. Specialized blood storage refrigerators with built-in temperature alarms are available, or a dedicated regular household refrigerator with low in-and-out traffic may be used. A refrigerator thermometer should be checked daily to ensure appropriate storage conditions.

Plasma products: Almost all of the plasma products are stored frozen at –20°C or below. Regular household freezers may suffice, but the temperature can vary depending on the section of the freezer used. The temperature should be checked daily using a thermometer, and opening and closing of the freezer should be minimized.

- When initially freezing the plasma, an elastic band should be placed around the bag, which is removed once frozen. This creates a 'waist' in the bag. Disappearance of this 'waist' during storage suggests that the unit has thawed and refrozen, signifying compromise of storage conditions and plasma quality.
- The entire plasma bag should be enclosed in a sealed plastic bag, which remains in place during plasma thawing to protect the injection ports from contamination.
- The frozen plasma unit is vulnerable to cracking if dropped, and should be handled with care.

Labelling: All blood products should be labelled with product type, donor identification, donor blood type, date of collection and date of expiration.

Blood product administration

Blood products are usually administered intravenously, but may also be given via an intraosseous route if required (e.g. kittens, puppies). They should *not* be given intraperitoneally.

An in-line blood filter (170–260 μm) is required for all blood products (including plasma) and is incorporated in standard blood infusion sets. Paediatric filters with reduced dead space or microaggregate filters of 18–40 μm are useful for infusing smaller volumes of products and blood collected in syringes.

- Stored red cell products do not need to be warmed prior to use, unless they are being given to neonates or very small animals.
- Plasma products are gently thawed in a warm water bath prior to administration.
- Packed red cells stored without preservative may be resuspended in or co-administered with 100 ml physiological saline to decrease their viscosity.

Volume: The amount of blood product to be administered depends on the specific product, desired effect and patient's response.

A general rule of thumb is that 2 ml of transfused whole blood/kg recipient bodyweight will raise the PCV by 1%. Most patients will receive between 10 and 22 ml/kg, and a suggested formula to calculate the amount of whole blood required for transfusion is:

Volume (ml) =   [85 (dog) or 60 (cat)] × bodyweight (kg)
                × [(desired PCV – actual PCV)/donor PCV]

For PRBC or FFP the average volume for infusion is 6–12 ml/kg.

When administering plasma products to treat a coagulopathy, reassessment of the coagulation parameters (usually PT and/or aPTT) for improvement offers guidance as to the success of the therapy.

Cryoprecipitate transfusion is an effective way of providing a concentrated amount of vWf to dogs with vWD in a very small volume of plasma. Each unit of Cryo is prepared from 450 ml of FWB, separated into approximately 200 ml of FFP, and eventually concentrated into a plasma volume (unit) of 10–15 ml. The recommended dose of Cryo is 1 unit/15 kg.

Rate of administration: The rate of administration depends on the cardiovascular status of the recipient.

- In general, the rate should only be 0.25–1.0 ml/kg per hour for the first 20 minutes.
- If well tolerated, the rate may then be increased to deliver the remaining product within 4 hours.
- In an animal with an increased risk of volume overload (cardiovascular disease, impaired renal function) the rate of administration should not exceed 3–4 ml/kg/hour.

If it is likely to take more than 4 hours to deliver the desired volume, the product may be divided so that a portion remains refrigerated for later use.

An animal should not receive food or medications during a transfusion, and the only fluid that may be administered through the same catheter is 0.9% saline.

Monitoring: Visual inspection of the product is necessary, especially when using stored red cells or plasma. Discoloration of the red cells (brown, purple) or the suspension fluid or the presence of clots may indicate bacterial contamination, haemolysis, or other storage lesions. Plasma bags must be examined for evidence of thawing and refreezing, and cracking and tearing of the bag.

The following parameters should be measured prior to the transfusion (as baseline) and then every 15–30 minutes during and 1, 12 and 24 hours after transfusion:

- Attitude
- Rectal temperature
- Pulse rate and quality
- Respiratory rate and character
- Mucous membrane colour and capillary refill time.

PCV and total protein should be assessed at a reasonable time interval following transfusion. Plasma and urine discoloration (e.g. icterus, haematuria) should be noted whenever patient blood samples are obtained or urine is passed during or following transfusion. To encourage diligent recording during the transfusion, it is helpful to design a transfusion monitoring sheet (Figure 20.13), with time points and monitoring parameters noted. Careful monitoring will allow for prompt recognition and treatment of transfusion reactions as well as evaluation of transfusion efficacy.

Oxyglobin: Oxyglobin may be administered via a routine intravenous giving set and does not require use of an in-line filter.

- The labelled dose for a normovolaemic dog is 10–30 ml/kg to be given at a rate of ≤10 ml/kg/h, but many dogs require much lower administration rates.
- Off-label use in cats, based on reports of clinical experience, suggests a total daily dose of 10–15 ml/kg. Cats have been found to be more susceptible to volume overload, and the rate of administration suggested is no greater than 1–2 ml/kg/hour, reduced even further in euvolaemic patients to 2–3 ml/hour.

Complications of blood administration

Any undesired side effect noted as a consequence of a blood product transfusion is considered a **transfusion reaction**. The frequency and severity of reported transfusion reactions is variable. The types of transfusion reactions recognized may be classified as immunological (haemolytic or non-haemolytic) and non-immunological, as well as acute or delayed.

Immunological transfusion reactions

Acute haemolytic reactions: The most concerning type of transfusion reaction is an acute haemolytic reaction with intravascular haemolysis. These are antigen-antibody, type II hypersensitivity reactions. This type of reaction is seen in type B cats receiving type A blood as well DEA 1.1-negative dogs sensitized to DEA 1.1 upon repeated exposure, amongst other scenarios. Clinical signs may include fever, tachycardia, dyspnoea, muscle tremors, vomiting, weakness, collapse, haemoglobinaemia and haemoglobinuria

---

PRODUCT: PRBC   FFP   FWB   SWB   Cat blood

Date administered:_____   Date donated:_____

Recipient _____   Donor

Name:_____   Name:_____

Case number: _____   Donor number: _____

Blood type: _____   Blood type: _____

Body weight: _____   PCV/TS: _____

                                                 Volume: _____

MONITORING FLOW CHART

	Time	Flow rate	T	P	R	Pulse quality	mm/CRT	PCV*	TS*	Plasma* colour	Urine Colour
Pre-trans											

Start Time:_____

15 min								X	X	X	
30 min								X	X	X	
60 min								X	X	X	
Post-trans											
6-12 hours post											

Finish Time:_____

* Note: or at other times as specified by clinician, i.e. if suspect transfusion reaction

Comments: _____

_____

TRANSFUSION RATE GUIDELINES:

Initial infusion in a stable patient at 0.25–1 ml/kg for first 15–20 min
If no reaction noted then rate can increase to deliver remaining product over 4–6 hours, not to exceed 10ml/kg/h

20.13   Example of a blood transfusion monitoring sheet.

potentially leading to shock, DIC, renal damage and in some cases death.

- Treatment for an acute haemolytic transfusion reaction involves immediate discontinuation of the transfusion, and treatment of the clinical signs of shock, including fluid therapy.
- Antihistamines and corticosteroids may be administered (Figure 20.14).
- Aggressive fluid therapy may be required and patients should be carefully monitored for the development of fluid overload (measure central venous pressure, heart rate, lung auscultation).
- Blood pressure and urine output should be monitored as hypotension may follow, and the use of pressor agents and diuretics may be necessary (low-dose dopamine infusion, furosemide).

Febrile non-haemolytic reactions: Febrile non-haemolytic transfusion reactions and reactions to blood contaminated with bacteria may have similar signs, with the development of a significant fever during or shortly after the transfusion.

- The donor and recipient blood type should be confirmed and a cross-match performed.
- The product type, date of expiration, volume and rate of administration should be confirmed.
- A sample of donor and recipient blood should be examined for evidence of haemolysis and saved for Gram-stain examination, microbial culture and further infectious disease screening if needed.
- Broad-spectrum intravenous antibiotic administration should be initiated if bacterial contamination is suspected (e.g. cephalosporin, amoxicillin/clavulanate, fluoroquinolone), and adjustments to the therapeutic choice made on the basis of the antibiogram results once available.
- As DIC and renal failure may occur, monitoring the animal's coagulation profile, urea, creatinine and electrolytes is advisable.

Delayed haemolytic reaction: A delayed haemolytic reaction with extravascular haemolysis may be recognized 2–21 days post-transfusion with similar but less severe signs to an acute haemolytic reaction (± bilirubinaemia/bilirubinuria). Jaundice, anorexia, pyrexia and a declining PCV may be noted. This type of reaction less frequently requires intervention other than antipyretic administration. If the decline in red cells affects the patient, a cross-match must be performed prior to any subsequent transfusions.

Non-haemolytic immunological reactions: Non-haemolytic immunological reactions are those of acute type I hypersensitivity reactions (allergic or anaphylactic), most often mediated by IgE and mast cells. They have a range of clinical signs, including urticaria, pruritis, erythema, oedema, vomiting and dyspnoea (pulmonary oedema).

- If this type of reaction occurs, the transfusion should be discontinued and the patient examined for evidence of haemolysis and shock.
- Antihistamines and corticosteroid medication (see Figure 20.14) may be required.
- If the reaction subsides, the transfusion may be restarted at 25–50% of the previous rate.
- If there is evidence of anaphylactic or anaphylactoid reaction or shock, adrenaline, intravenous fluids, antihistamines, H_2 blockers (cimetidine, ranitidine), colloids, dopamine and aminophylline may also be administered in addition to the above treatment measures as needed (see Figure 20.14).

Reactions to leucocytes and platelets may occur, manifested by a febrile non-haemolytic transfusion reaction, which may last up to 20 hours after the transfusion. These are recognized as an increase in body temperature by >1°C without an obvious underlying cause.

Other delayed immune-mediated transfusion reactions that may occur include post-transfusion purpura (thrombocytopenia noted within the first week after blood transfusion), neonatal isoerythrolysis and immunosuppression of the recipient.

Drug group	Drug	Dosage and route of administration
Corticosteroid	Dexamethasone	Dogs and cats: 0.5–1.0 mg/kg i.v., i.m.
Antihistamine	Diphenhydramine	Dogs and cats: 1.0–2.0 mg/kg i.m.
	Chlorphenamine	Dogs (small to medium): 2.5–5.0 mg i.m. q12h Dogs (medium to large): 5.0–10.0 mg i.m. q12h Cats: 2–5 mg/cat i.m. or slow i.v. Maximum recommend dose in both dogs and cats: 0.5 mg/kg q12h
H_2 blocker	Cimetidine	Dogs: 5.0–10.0 mg/kg i.v. [a], i.m., orally q8h Cats: 2.5–5.0 mg/kg i.v. [a], i.m., orally q12h
	Ranitidine	Dogs: 2.0 mg/kg i.v. [a], s.c., orally q8–12h Cats: 2.5 mg/kg i.v. [a] q12h or 2 mg/kg/day i.v. constant rate infusion
Other	Furosemide	1.0–4.0 mg/kg i.v. q8–12h or as needed
	Dopamine	2.0–5.0 µg/kg/min i.v. constant rate infusion
	Calcium gluconate 10%	50.0–150 mg/kg i.v. [a] slowly to effect
	Adrenaline	Low dose: 10.0–20.0 µg/kg i.v. High dose: 100.0–200.0 µg/kg i.v.

20.14 Drugs commonly used in the management of transfusion reactions. [a] When administered by intravenous route, these drugs should be diluted and administered slowly.

Non-immunological transfusion reactions

A large number of non-immunological transfusion reactions have been described.

- Anaphylactoid reactions, which often result from too rapid an infusion rate, tend to subside after discontinuation of the transfusion or reduction of the infusion rate.
- Circulatory overload requiring diuretic therapy may occur in any patient receiving an excessive volume of blood products, or those with cardiac or renal disease.
- Hypocalcaemia as a consequence of citrate intoxication is identified most commonly following administration of large volumes of plasma or whole blood, and patients with impaired liver function are at greatest risk. Clinical signs of hypocalcaemia (vomiting, muscle tremors, tetany, electrocardiogram changes) may be resolved with the supplementation of calcium gluconate (Figure 20.14).
- Other recognized non-immunological reactions include polycythaemia and hyperproteinaemia, hypothermia, coagulopathy, thrombosis, microbial contamination, hyperammonaemia, hypophosphataemia, hyperkalaemia, acidosis, pre-transfusion (*in vitro*) haemolysis, haemosiderosis, air embolus, and infectious disease transmission.

Preventive measures necessary to minimize the risk of transfusion reactions include appropriate donor screening, collection, preparation, storage and administration of products. Adherence to standard protocols helps to ensure safety and efficacy of transfusions in practice.

References and further reading

Blais MC, Rozanski EA, Hale AS, Shaw SP and Cotter SM (2009) Lack of evidence of pregnancy-induced alloantibodies in dogs. *Journal of Veterinary Internal Medicine* **23**, 462–465

Boudreaux MK (2000) Acquired platelet dysfunction. In: *Schalm's Veterinary Hematology, 5th edn*, ed. BF Feldman, JG Zinkl and NC Jain, pp. 496–500. Lippincott Williams and Wilkins, Philadelphia

Brainard BM, Meredith CP, Callan MB *et al.* (2007) Changes in platelet function, hemostasis, and prostaglandin expression after treatment with nonsteroidal ani-inflammatory drugs with various cyclooxygenase selectivities in dogs. *American Journal of Veterinary Research* **68**, 251–257

Brooks M (2000) Transfusion of plasma and plasma derivatives. In: *Schalm's Veterinary Hematology, 5th edn*, ed. BF Feldman, JG Zinkl and NC Jain, pp. 838–843. Lippincott Williams and Wilkins, Philadelphia

Brooks MB and Catalfamo JL (2009) Platelet dysfunction. In: Kirk's Current Veterinary Therapy XIV, ed. JD Bonagura and DC Twedt, pp. 292–297. Saunders Elsevier, St Louis

Bücheler J and Giger U (1993) Alloantibodies against A and B blood types in cats. *Veterinary Immunology and Immunopathology* **38**, 283–295

Callan MB (2000) Red blood cell transfusions in the dog and cat. In: *Schalm's Veterinary Hematology, 5th edn*, ed. BF Feldman, JG Zinkl and NC Jain, pp. 833–837. Lippincott Williams and Wilkins, Philadelphia

Callan MB and Giger UG (2002) Effect of desmopressin acetate administration on primary hemostasis in Doberman Pinschers with type-1 von Willebrand disease as assessed by a point-of-care instrument. *American Journal of Veterinary Research* **63**, 1700–1706

Carr AP, Nibblett BM and Panciera DL (2009) Von Willebrand's disease and other hereditary coagulopathies. In: *Kirk's Current Veterinary Therapy XIV*, ed. JD Bonagura and DC Twedt, pp. 277–280. Saunders Elsevier, St Louis

Center SA (1996) Pathophysiology of liver disease: normal and abnormal function. In: *Strombeck's Small Animal Gastroenterology*, ed. WG Guilford, SA Center, DR Strombeck, DA Williams and DJ Meyer, pp. 553–632. WB Saunders, Philadelphia

Day and Kohn (2011) *BSAVA Manual of Canine and Feline Haematology and Transfusion Medicine, 2nd edn*. BSAVA, Gloucester.

Feldman B (2000) Blood transfusion guidelines. In: *Kirk's Current Veterinary Therapy XIII: Small Animal Practice*, ed. JD Bonagura, pp. 400–403. WB Saunders, Philadelphia

Forcada Y, Guitian J and Gibson G (2007) Frequencies of feline blood types at a referral hospital in the south east of England. *Journal of Small Animal Practice* **48**, 570–573

Gentry PA (2000) Platelet biology. In: *Schalm's Veterinary Hematology, 5th edn*, ed. BF Feldman, JG Zinkl and NC Jain, pp. 459–466. Lippincott Williams and Wilkins, Philadelphia

Gentry PA and Nyarko K (2000) Platelet lipids and prostaglandins. In: *Schalm's Veterinary Hematology, 5th edn*, ed. BF Feldman, JG Zinkl and NC Jain, pp. 453–458. Lippincott Williams and Wilkins, Philadelphia

Giger U (2000) Blood typing and crossmatching to ensure compatible transfusions. In: *Kirk's Current Veterinary Therapy XIII: Small Animal Practice*, ed. JD Bonagura, pp. 396–399. WB Saunders, Philadelphia

Giger U and Blais MC (2005) Ensuring blood compatibility: update on canine typing and crossmatching. *Proceedings American College of Veterinary Internal Medicine* 2005, pp. 721–723

Griot-Wenk ME, Callan MB, Casal ML *et al.* (1996) Blood type AB in the feline AB blood group system. *American Journal of Veterinary Research* **57**, 1438–1442

Griot-Wenk ME and Giger U (1995) Feline transfusion medicine: blood types and their clinical importance. *Veterinary Clinics of North America: Small Animal Practice* **25**, 1305–1322

Hale AS (1995) Canine blood groups and their importance in veterinary transfusion medicine. *Veterinary Clinics of North America: Small Animal Practice* **25**, 1323–1332

Harrell KA and Kristensen AT (1995) Canine transfusion reactions and their management. *Veterinary Clinics of North America:Small Animal Practice* **25**, 1333–1364

Hohenhaus A (2000) Transfusion reactions. In: *Schalm's Veterinary Hematology, 5th edn*, ed. BF Feldman, JG Zinkl and NC Jain, pp. 864–868. Lippincott Williams and Wilkins, Philadelphia

Hohenhaus AE (2000) Blood banking and transfusion medicine. In: *Textbook of Veterinary Internal Medicine, Diseases of the Dog and Cat, 5th edn*, ed. SJ Ettinger and EC Feldman, pp. 348–356. WB Saunders, Philadelphia

Johnstone IB (2000) Coagulation inhibitors. In: *Schalm's Veterinary Hematology, 5th edn*, ed. BF Feldman, JG Zinkl and NC Jain, pp. 538–543. Lippincott Williams and Wilkins, Philadelphia

Kristensen AT and Feldman BF (1995) General principles of small animal blood component administration. *Veterinary Clinics of North America: Small Animal Practice* **25**: 1277–1290

Licari LG and Kovacic JP (2009) Thrombin physiology and pathophysiology. *Journal of Veterinary Emergency and Critical Care* **19**, 11–22

Neel JA, Birkenheuer AJ and Grindem CB (2009) Thrombocytopenia. In: *Kirk's Current Veterinary Therapy XIV*, ed JD Bonagura and DC Twedt, pp. 281–287. Saunders Elsevier, St Louis

Prittie JE (2003) Triggers for use, optimal dosing, and problems associated with red cell transfusions. *Veterinary Clinics of North America: Small Animal Practice* **33**, 1261–1275

Rudloff E and Kirby R (2009) Disseminated intravascular coagulation: diagnosis and management. In: *Kirk's Current Veterinary Therapy XIV*, ed. JD Bonagura and DC Twedt, pp. 287–291. Saunders Elsevier, St Louis

Schneider A (1995) Blood components: collection, processing and storage. *Veterinary Clinics of North America: Small Animal Practice* **25**, 1245–1261.

Schneider A (2000) Principles of blood collection and processing. In: *Schalm's Veterinary Hematology, 5th edn*, ed. BF Feldman, JG Zinkl and NC Jain, pp. 827–832. Lippincott Williams and Wilkins, Philadelphia

Smith SA (2009) The cell-based model of coagulation. *Journal of Veterinary Emergency and Critical Care* **19**, 3–10

Stockham SL and Scott MA (2002) Haemostasis. In: *Fundamentals of Veterinary Clinical Pathology*, pp. 155–225. Blackwell Publishing, Ames, Iowa

Tablin F (2000) Platelet structure and function. In: *Schalm's Veterinary Hematology, 5th edn*, ed. BF Feldman, JG Zinkl and NC Jain, pp. 448–452. Lippincott Williams and Wilkins, Philadelphia

Tocci LJ and Ewing PJ (2009) Increasing patient safety in veterinary transfusion medicine: an overview of pretransfusion testing. *Journal of Veterinary Emergency and Critical Care* **19**, 66–83

Wardrop KJ, Reine N, Birkenheuer A *et al.* (2005) Canine and feline blood donor screening for infectious disease. *Journal of Veterinary Internal Medicine* **19**, 135–142

Weinstein NM, Blais MC, Harris K *et al.* (2007) A newly recognized blood group in domestic shorthair cats: the *Mik* red cell antigen. *Journal of Veterinary Internal Medicine* **21**, 287–292

Principles of operative technique

21

Geraldine B. Hunt

Introduction

Almost 90 years after his death, Halsted's principles (Figure 21.1) remain one of the most important creeds for the surgeon. Many of Halsted's principles are tangible and easily recognized. The importance of asepsis is stressed by everyone practising surgery (although not always adhered to as diligently as it should be). Haemostasis (or the lack thereof) is readily evident and demands attention before each surgery is completed and the patient discharged from hospital. Most surgeons understand the need to minimize dead space and take measures to close it.

- Strict asepsis during preparation and surgery.
- Good haemostasis to improve visibility and limit infection and dead space.
- Minimize tissue trauma.
- Good surgical judgement ensuring elimination of dead space and adequate removal of material.
- Minimize surgery time through knowledge of anatomy and technique.
- Correct use of instruments and materials.

21.1 Halsted's Principles of Surgery.

Some of Halsted's principles, however, are less tangible and require experience, a lot of practice and seeing the consequences of breaking them before surgeons can confidently observe them. For instance, what does it mean to minimize tissue trauma? How, exactly, does a surgeon handle tissues 'gently'? How can surgery time be minimized when the surgeon is trying to be careful and thorough?

This chapter aims to highlight the most important principles of surgery that have an impact on outcome. It will also provide practical hints as to how better to follow Halsted's principles. More information on instruments can be found in Chapter 4.

Incision and excision of tissue

Using a scalpel

The scalpel is used for sharp incisions where the plane of tissue to be cut is known and identified, and the likelihood of damaging adjacent structures is minimal. In general, tissues that are incised with the scalpel are collagen-rich and poorly vascular. The scalpel is also used to make small stab incisions through tough layers such as the linea alba, submucosa of the stomach and the bladder wall. The scalpel should not be used for extensive subcutaneous exploration, or anatomical-style dissection to tease tissues apart for greater visualization. A variety of scalpel handles and scalpel blades are available for different purposes.

PRACTICAL TIPS

- The larger blades (e.g. No. 10) are generally used to make long straight skin incisions.
- The smaller blades (e.g. No. 15) are useful for thinner skin, curving incisions and those that need to follow contours, such as on the feet or the face.
- Small pointed blades (e.g. No. 11) are used to make stab incisions or for sharp dissection in restricted areas such as joints.

Stab incisions

When making a stab incision, the layer of tissue to be incised should be immobilized with forceps or stay sutures, and pulled taut to avoid it moving away from the blade. It should also be elevated from underlying structures that could be damaged by the blade, such as abdominal viscera when puncturing the linea alba or the far wall of a hollow viscus.

Straight and contoured skin incisions

For straight skin incisions with a larger blade, the scalpel is held in the palm of the hand with the forefinger stabilizing it, guiding it and modulating the amount of pressure. This facilitates use of the belly of the blade (Figure 21.2).

For a contoured skin incision, or one made with a smaller blade, the scalpel is best held in a pencil grip, which facilitates using the tip of the blade (Figure 21.3). The skin should always be immobilized by the thumb and forefinger of the non-dominant hand, to ensure that it does not slide away or bunch up as the scalpel passes, which would lead to a ragged incision or one that slices obliquely through the skin, increasing postoperative inflammation and discharge (Figure 21.4).

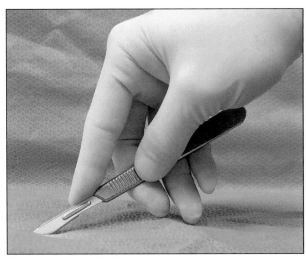

21.2 Correct instrument handling for a larger blade (No. 10). Note how the belly of the blade is applied to the surface to be cut.

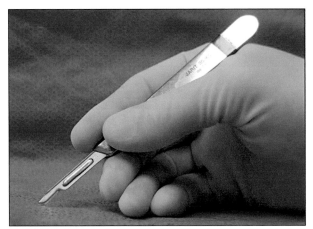

21.3 Correct instrument handling for a smaller blade (No. 15). This allows more precise application of the tip of the blade and the cutting edge directly behind it.

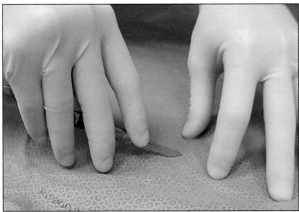

21.4 Demonstration of the correct technique for making a skin incision. The skin is stretched and stabilized with the non-dominant hand, allowing the blade to incise cleanly.

Using scissors

Scissors are used for either sharp or blunt dissection. While it is important to ensure that structures are not accidentally cut, blunt dissection should be reserved mainly to identify tissue planes for sharp dissection or diathermy. Tearing tissues apart with blunt dissection

is more traumatic than sharp dissection, less controllable and may lead to poorer surgical exposure. The exception is when dividing fatty tissues with thin-walled vessels, in which haemostasis can be achieved by tearing because the torn vessels then retract and close spontaneously.

Sharp dissection using scissors is facilitated by first establishing a tissue plane with haemostats or dissecting forceps. The blades of the scissors are then passed on either side of the tissue plane and the blade farthest from the surgeon is elevated until it can be seen through the tissue plane, thus ensuring that no large vessels, nerves or other vital structures are at risk. The tissue is cut and alternating dissection and incision continued.

PRACTICAL TIP

This process can be hastened by the surgeon and assistant working as a team, with the surgeon establishing the plane of dissection and stabilizing the tissue to be incised, and the assistant cutting with scissors after first applying cautery or haemoclips if indicated (Figure 21.5).

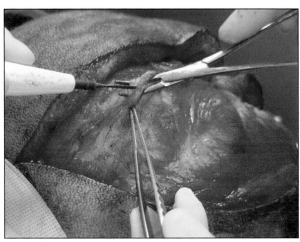

21.5 Coordination between surgeon and assistant when dividing tissue planes. The plane of dissection is established by the surgeon and the tissues are elevated prior to being separated by the assistant (in this case with diathermy).

Scissors should be held with the thumb in one ring and the third finger in the other ring, thereby allowing the first two fingers to direct and stabilize the instrument (Figure 21.6).

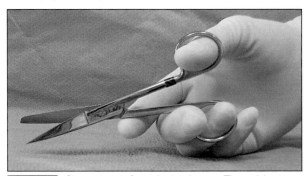

21.6 Correct use of surgical scissors. These blunt-sharp pointed scissors are used for cutting suture material.

Establishing planes of dissection

Most structures that require dissection comprise different tissue planes that either make up the layer itself, or attach it to surrounding structures.

Dissecting structures from the surrounding connective tissues is best achieved by careful identification, isolation and division of tissue layers one at a time. Dissection should proceed parallel to delicate structures known to be present in the area, such as blood vessels, nerves, ureters or other organs.

Plane-by-plane dissection requires good visualization, surgical lighting, retraction and suction. Delicate dissection is facilitated by atraumatic forceps such as DeBakeys (Figure 21.7), right-angled dissecting forceps such as Lahey (Figure 21.8) and a fine open-ended suction cannula (the internal cannula of a small Poole suction tip works well).

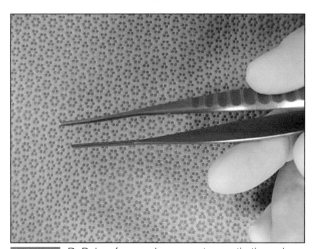

21.7 DeBakey forceps have an atraumatic tip and are designed for handling delicate tissues such as blood vessels.

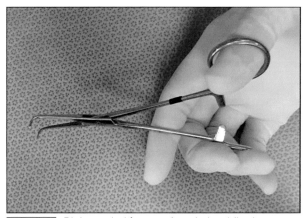

21.8 Right-angled forceps (e.g. Lahey bile duct forceps) are useful for establishing planes of tissue dissection and stabilizing the tissue plane for division with scissors or diathermy.

- A plane of dissection should be established using blunt forceps.
- Blunt dissection proceeds long enough to pass the forceps beneath the tissue plane and elevate it away from deeper structures (Figure 21.9), enabling vessels to be identified, or confirming that the tissue layer can be safely incised with blunt tipped scissors such as Metzenbaums.
- If vessels can be seen passing through the tissue

layer, they are dissected and clamped with haemostats and ligated, coagulated with diathermy or clamped with titanium clips (e.g. Hemoclips) before division (pre-emptive haemostasis).
- Blunt dissection is resumed until the next tissue plane is identified and dealt with similarly. If there is good coordination between the surgeon and assistant this process proceeds rapidly, even with intricate surgeries such as mediastinal mass removal.

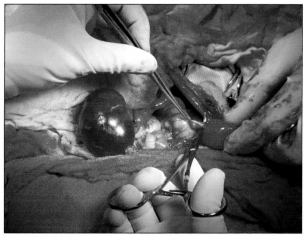

21.9 Use of atraumatic forceps and right-angled forceps to isolate vessels prior to ligation during nephrectomy.

Blunt dissection of fragile tissues, such as loose connective tissue, the liver and the prostate gland, can be performed with a fine-ended suction cannula such as the interior Poole sheath (as described above).

- The cannula is used to stretch and divide the tissues while applying suction that keeps the surgical field free of blood.
- The suction cannula can be applied directly to a bleeding point and diathermy directed though the cannula itself for focused haemostasis.
- The suction cannula can also be used to stabilize tissues for sharp dissection by an assistant.

Haemostasis

Good haemostasis is Halsted's second principle of surgery. Although the consequences of profuse haemorrhage following damage to a large blood vessel are understandably feared by surgeons, and discussed with clients, effective haemostasis is taken for granted during most surgical procedures. Many small blood vessels are cut during even routine surgical procedures and a minority require intervention. Vessel retraction, platelet plugging and physiological coagulation usually occur promptly (see Chapter 20) and therefore it is usually only the larger, visible vessels that require ligation. However, surgeons should realize that there are numerous potential sources of blood loss if coagulation is impaired for some reason. Ongoing bleeding in a patient with a coagulopathy may not just occur from obvious surgical sites, but in the form of a slow ooze from all damaged surfaces, including those that have simply been handled during the procedure.

Different methods of haemostasis

If bleeding does not stop within a few seconds of tissue damage, and unless it is obviously life-threatening, a number of steps are usually taken for haemostasis (Figure 21.10), depending on the size of the blood vessel, the amount of haemorrhage that is occurring and the need for maintaining a clear visual field.

- Digital pressure.
- Haemostats.
- Packing with surgical swabs.
- Lavage with saline.
- Ligatures.
- Topical haemostatic agents.
- Tourniquets.
- Other methods (clips, lasers, tissue fusion, diathermy).

21.10 Methods of haemostasis.

Digital pressure

Digital pressure stems the flow while enough platelets accumulate to form a plug, or a stable clot forms. Pressure should be applied for at least 60 seconds in cases of minor haemorrhage and up to 5 minutes for more serious haemorrhage. Haemostasis may be assisted by first applying surgical swabs (sponges) to the site, providing a scaffold upon which the blood clot can form. Digital pressure is recommended as a first strategy for bleeding even from large arteries and can be effective in facilitating haemostasis even in large vessels such as the pulmonary artery.

Haemostats

If simple digital pressure is ineffective, the bleeding point may be identified and a haemostat applied. The haemostat crushes the tissues releasing tissue thromboplastin that further stimulates coagulation. The haemostats are left in position for at least 5 minutes, at which stage they may be released and, in many instances, haemorrhage will not recur. Alternatively, the surgeon may choose to apply a ligature to the bleeding vessel (see below).

Surgical swabs

If the bleeding point is deep within the tissues, within a body cavity, or in close proximity to a structure that might be damaged by haemostats, such as the facial nerve during total ear canal ablation or the ureter during ovariohysterectomy, further pressure may be applied by packing the cavity tightly with surgical swabs.

- Swabs are packed on top of one another and held in position until blood stops oozing through the fabric. This indicates that active haemorrhage has stopped and coagulation is (hopefully) taking place. This manoeuvre may also buy the surgeon some time to ask for additional equipment such as vascular forceps, allow the assistants to relax for a few moments, or simply enable the surgeon to reorganize their thoughts.
- Packing can be used for single bleeding points, or generalized bleeding from viscera such as the liver.
- The packing is left in place for at least 5–10 minutes. It is helpful to use a clock or stopwatch, as time passes slowly under these circumstances.
- After an appropriate duration, the packing is removed piece by piece. The last swab is removed carefully to avoid dislodging blood clots.

Bleeding may either have ceased, or slowed enough to enable visualization for application of a haemostat or suture.

Lavage with saline

If haemorrhage continues in a body cavity or confined space, it can be difficult to identify the exact point of bleeding. Saline lavage to remove blood clots and clear the field, then flooding the area and looking down through the saline pool, can be helpful for lifting adjacent flimsy tissues away from the bleeding point. Ongoing haemorrhage into a saline pool appears as a tendril of blood rising like chimney smoke from the bleeding point, allowing careful application of thumb forceps or a haemostat. Pressure and other physical effects of the saline, such as the cold temperature, will also sometimes stop the bleeding (examples of this include surgery of the nasal cavity, liver and slow oozing from other intra-abdominal or intrathoracic sites). However, saline used in body cavities is usually warmed to avoid promoting patient hypothermia.

Ligatures

Ligatures are used for discrete bleeding points that are unlikely to stop of their own accord, or where it is feared they may resume bleeding following surgery.

The size of suture material and pattern used are dependent on the size of the patient, blood vessel, and amount of perivascular tissue that must be crushed to achieve occlusion of the vessel. The length of time the suture material maintains its strength is not as important as the ability of the surgeon to tie a secure, tight knot.

- Small subcutaneous vessels, or vessels such as the ovarian artery or testicular artery in cats or small dogs, can be ligated using a simple square knot.
- Wider pedicles or vessels should be ligated using a surgeon's knot or a sliding knot to crush the tissues better and avoid slippage of the ligature while securing the second throw.
- Binding knots such as the Miller's knot, or modified Miller's knot, involve passing the suture around the pedicle twice before tying, producing leverage and enabling greater pressure to be applied.

Transfixing sutures: Transfixing sutures pass through the structure to be ligated before being wrapped around the outside and tied again. This serves to reduce the risk of the ligature slipping off the end of the pedicle and facilitates maintenance of inward pressure. The figure-of-8 suture is a form of transfixion suture.

Transfixion sutures are appropriate for closed castration, particularly in large dogs, where slippage of the vessels within the tunica vaginalis might otherwise occur. They may also be applied to flat surfaces, such as the liver, lung or a perforated blood vessel where complete occlusion of the lumen is not desirable. The suture is passed carefully across the defect in a cruciate or horizontal mattress pattern and provides haemostasis as a result of closing the defect.

Haemostatic sutures may also be 'stented' by passing them through a piece of Teflon felt (pledget), muscle, or fat, which then provides a wider zone of pressure on the bleeding point when the suture is tightened.

Topical haemostatic agents

Haemostasis may also be facilitated by application of natural or synthetic substances. The astringent properties of the 'styptic pencil' cause tissues to shrink, thereby closing small blood vessels. Astringents are not commonly used intraoperatively, but a variety of other products are available to assist with coagulation.

Native tissue: Application of native tissue to a bleeding point brings tissue thromboplastin as well as providing a scaffold for blood clotting. Fat, omentum and exposed muscle can be used.

Fibrin glue: Processed natural products include fibrin glue, which produces a clot in its own right. Fibrin glue is made up of fibrinogen and thrombin. The fibrinogen and thrombin are injected through one nozzle into the site of a vessel tear. Thrombin acts as an enzyme and converts the fibrinogen into fibrin in 10–60 seconds. The newly converted fibrin acts as a tissue adhesive. This glue has been used for repairing dural tears, bronchial fistulas and for achieving haemostasis after spleen and liver trauma. It is also employed in 'no sutures' corneal grafting.

Other processed products: The following products can be applied directly to the site:

- Surgicel (Johnson & Johnson), or oxidized cellulose polymer (polyanhydroglucoronic acid), is an acidic material that reacts with blood, forming a reddish-brown pseudoclot that stops the bleeding. Furthermore, it has bactericidal activity against more than 20 bacterial species and is absorbable. Because it is formed into a fabric, it can be used to 'bind' the bleeding site
- Gelfoam (Pharmacia & Upjohn), in the form of purified pork skin gelatine USP granules, is able to absorb and hold many times its weight of blood and other fluids within its interstices
- Lyostypt (B Braun) is purified collagen fleece and causes platelet adhesion and Factor XII activation. It is reported to achieve haemostasis faster than other products and be absorbed more readily
- Bone wax (B Braun) is made of beeswax with a softening agent (petroleum jelly). It stops bone bleeding by physically occluding the bleeding points.

Haemostasis may also be augmented with the application of cold or ice-cold saline and topical vasoconstrictors such as phenylephrine.

Tourniquets

If serious haemorrhage is predicted and cannot be avoided by meticulous dissection and ligation, the surgeon may choose to occlude circulation to the body part prophylactically. This is most commonly achieved by the application of a tourniquet. Tourniquets are easily applied to the limbs. Commercial tourniquets are available, or they can be fashioned from conforming bandages or rubber drains. A tourniquet may also be combined with an Esmarch bandage to exsanguinate the limb to provide a completely bloodless field.

Tourniquets should be able to exert sufficient force to occlude arterial flow and distribute the pressure over a wide area, rather than concentrate it. Use of a narrow tourniquet increases the risk of pressure damage to underlying structures such as nerves.

PRACTICAL TIPS

- Tourniquets are most effective when applied above the elbow or stifle, where the large vessels can be compressed against the bone.
- Application at the level of the tibia or antebrachium can also be effective.
- It is difficult to achieve adequate occlusion with application below the carpus or tarsus as the complex bony anatomy makes compression of all vessels unlikely.
- Tourniquets should only be applied for short periods of time (<90 minutes). Longer applications will result in more postoperative inflammation.

Patients with tourniquets should always be identified in a way that ensures that the tourniquet is not accidentally left in place. A piece of adherent tape applied to the forehead is one mechanism, with the anaesthetist being responsible for ensuring that the tape, tourniquet and tube are all removed during recovery.

Other methods

Haemostasis may be achieved using titanium or polypropylene clips. It may also be achieved using lasers, tissue fusion (e.g. Ligasure; Valley Lab), diathermy, or a combination thereof (e.g. Force Triad; Valley Lab).

Diathermy: Diathermy (electrocautery) units produce heat at the surgical site. Different electrical waveforms produce different tissue effects.

- A **constant** waveform produces heat very rapidly, enabling the surgeon to vaporize or cut tissue with minimal coagulation.
- An **intermittent** waveform produces less heat and, instead of vaporizing tissue, produces a coagulum.

'Blended currents' are modifications of the cycle that produce better cutting or haemostasis.

- **Bipolar diathermy** passes current between two tines of a forceps handpiece, allowing very precise application of heat since only the tissue grasped is included in the electrical circuit. This is good for restricted areas close to sensitive structures such as nerves. Because the return function is performed by one tine of the forceps, no patient return electrode is needed and therefore there are no issues with patient positioning or skin impedance. Bipolar diathermy is more effective than monopolar in a wet surgical field.
- The most commonly used form of diathermy is **monopolar**, in which the diathermy pencil/blade is the active electrode and the return electrode is a plate or patch applied to the patient's skin remote to the surgical site. The current passes through the patient as it completes the circuit from the active electrode to the patient return electrode. Care

must be taken to reduce the risk of current shorting to another site and producing an electrical burn. Monopolar diathermy may be used by applying the tip of the handpiece to the tissue or by applying the tip to an instrument, e.g. haemostats attached to a vessel (conductive diathermy).

Electrosurgical cutting divides tissue with electric sparks that focus intense heat at the surgical site. This is most effective when the surgeon holds the electrode a little way from the tissue, rather than trying to use the diathermy pen like a scalpel blade. Electrosurgical units are also available that use radiofrequency ablation, producing very rapid and precise cutting similar to that obtained with a laser.

Care and handling of tissue

Primum non nocere (above all else, do no harm). This Hippocratic principle is commendable, but of course impossible when surgery is performed. However, minimization of harm is essential to achieving reliable, safe and comfortable outcomes for patients. Returning to Halsted's principles, minimizing tissue trauma through gentle tissue handling should always be a primary goal (Figure 21.11).

- Avoid excessive blunt dissection.
- Avoid excessive traction.
- Handle tissues only when absolutely necessary.
- Separate only those tissue planes necessary for visualization or excision.
- Avoid repeated changes in retractor position.
- Do not allow retractors to tear or stretch tissue excessively.
- Keep tissues moist with the regular application of saline.
- Avoid exposure to irritant or inflammatory substances (e.g. talc, lint, urine, bile or intestinal contents).
- Use appropriate instruments.

21.11 Aims for tissue handling.

Using surgical instruments and materials

There are many instruments available to the surgeon, some of which have been developed for very specific uses. Most surgeons use a small number of key instruments during the course of everyday practice and the design and roles of many of these are described and illustrated in Chapter 4.

Forceps

Forceps come in different styles, depending on the purpose for which they are being used and the tissues upon which they are being used.

- Thumb forceps are used like pincers, with the surgeon controlling the locking action.
- Locking forceps, like haemostats or atraumatic forceps, are self-retaining.

Thumb forceps: Thumb forceps should be held in a pencil grip, which allows them to function as an extension of the fingers. Novice surgeons have a tendency to hold them in the palm, such as when they are used to retract tissues for anatomical dissection. When held like this, they function as an extension of the wrist,

reducing fatigue by allowing the muscles of the forearm to exert traction. This is not an appropriate use during soft tissue surgery, as the tissues are retracted in other ways.

- Thumb forceps should be held between the thumb and forefinger, using the second finger to stabilize and guide them (Figure 21.12).
- They should be gripped so that the surgeon's fingers are far enough back not to limit visibility of the tissues being grasped.
- The grasp should be precise, on the layer of tissue the surgeon wishes to cut or suture, and the forceps should be used to retract or manipulate that specific tissue layer into appropriate alignment.

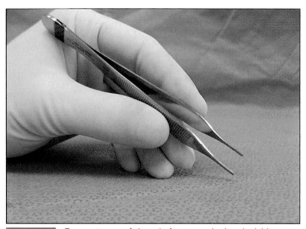

21.12 Correct use of thumb forceps, being held in a pencil grip as an extension of the fingers.

Examples include grasping the linea alba and drawing it medially, allowing the subcutaneous tissue to retract so that the fibrous tissue of the linea alba itself can be identified and a needle passed through it confidently. Another example is grasping across the cut edge of an intestinal incision and rolling the forceps so that the serosal surface is visible (thereby inverting the mucosa) to enable placement of a slightly oblique suture that engages the submucosa without incorporating too much mucosa and allow apposition of the serosal surface without eversion of the mucosa.

- **Toothed forceps** (rat-tooth, Adson, Brown–Adson) are designed to grasp the tissue and prevent it sliding between the jaws. While the use of toothed forceps might seem to be overly traumatic, it is preferable to using blunt forceps and having to reapply them as they lose their grip.
- Sturdy toothed forceps should also be used to retract collagen-rich tissues where some force is required.
- **Atraumatic forceps** such as DeBakey forceps (see Figure 21.7) are indicated for friable or fragile tissues such as the liver, lung or blood vessels, where perforation will result in leakage of air or fluid. These forceps are used for grasping and tissue manipulation but are not appropriate for tissue retraction.

Locking forceps: In instances where prolonged tissue retraction is required, locking forceps are indicated.

- **Allis** and **Littlewood forceps** have a saw-toothed edge that holds tissues well. However, they exert a crushing force and are only used on collagen-dense tissues such as the linea alba. Allis forceps should never be used on skin or bowel, where tissue necrosis could lead to postoperative complications, unless the tissue to which they have been applied is later excised.
- **Babcock forceps** are similar in design to Allis forceps, but possess a flat cross-hatched surface designed to indent tissues without crushing them (Figure 21.13). Babcocks are the forceps of choice for delicate structures and can be used with the bowel, lung and liver.

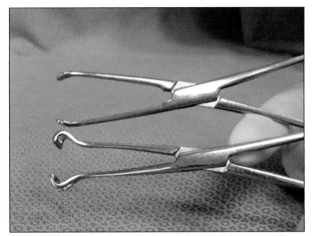

21.13 Allis (top) and Babcock (bottom) forceps. Allis forceps have a saw-toothed edge designed for grasping and retracting collagen-rich tissues. They cause crushing of the tissue edge and should not be used for the skin. Babcock forceps have a non-crushing tip designed for delicate tissues.

Locking forceps should never be used across a skin edge. If skin retraction is required, skin hooks or stay sutures should be applied to the subdermal or subcutaneous layer, rather than the skin edge itself. Further examples of atraumatic forceps are the Cooley and Satinsky (designed for blood vessels) and the Doyen bowel forceps.

Retractors

Retractors may be hand-held or self-retaining and their design is dependent on the tissues or region in which they are to be used (see Chapter 4). Retractors may have a blade or tines, with sharp or blunt points. Pointed retractors may have a single or multiple points.

Hand-held retractors: Hand-held retractors are designed to be used by an assistant. Their advantage is that they are quick and easy to reposition, affording instantaneous flexibility.

- The Army–Navy and Senn retractors are double-ended and can therefore be reversed when the requirement for retraction changes.
- The pointed tines of the Senn or Mathieu retractor might be used for skin retraction and the retractor reversed to use the flat blade in the deeper tissues where nerves or vessels might be damaged (Figure 21.14). Examples include retraction for tracheal surgery, or total ear canal ablation.

- The Army–Navy retractor has two lipped blades of different sizes, with the longer blade used in the deeper tissues.
- Most retraction of intra-abdominal organs is performed using flat, blade-style retractors such as the malleable ribbon retractor (Figure 21.15).
- The Allison lung retractor (Figure 21.16) consists of a handle and an ovoid retraction surface of multiple wires. It is also very useful in the abdomen due to its broad shape and reduced tendency to slide off the tissues.

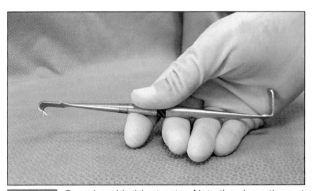

21.14 Senn hand-held retractor. Note the sharp tines at one end and the blade at the other end, allowing the retractor to be reversed for different purposes.

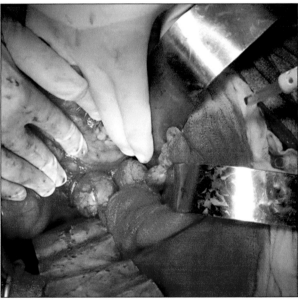

21.15 Malleable ribbon retractors. A number of retractors are being used in the abdominal cavity to expose an adrenal gland tumour. Note that the malleable retractors allow the assistants to keep their hands out of the surgical field and therefore use of retractors is preferable to fingers for the same purpose.

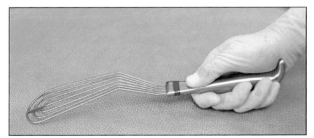

21.16 Allison lung retractor. A flat-bladed hand-held retractor is useful for retracting abdominal viscera as well as the lung or heart.

Abdominal and thoracic organs should be protected by saline-soaked swabs when retraction is performed. Swabs should always be counted in and out of the abdomen or thorax.

Self-retaining retractors: Self-retaining retractors have the advantage that they do not require someone to hold them and therefore they free up the assistant for other duties, such as suctioning or cutting sutures. Self-retaining retractors usually engage the soft tissues with sharp or blunt tines.

Disadvantages include tissue trauma as a result of the tines, and the fact that retraction usually only occurs in one plane. The box joint and handles of the retractor may also interfere with visualization or manipulation of the surgical site.

■ Self-retaining retractors are most often used in the limbs, or for approaches to the neck, where lateral retraction is most important. The Gelpi (sharp-pointed) (Figure 21.17) and Weitlaner (sharp- or blunt-pointed) (Figure 21.18) are most commonly used.
■ Gelpi retractors are also useful for sternotomies, as their single, sharp tips can be engaged in the cartilage between the sternebrae, providing secure retraction with minimal risk of the retractors slipping cranially or caudally.
■ Self-retaining retractors are also used commonly in the abdomen (Balfour; Figure 21.19) and thorax (Finochietto; Figure 21.20).

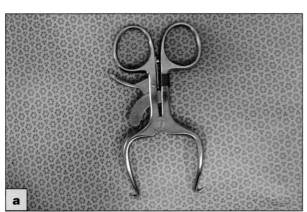

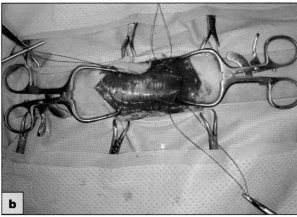

21.17 **(a)** Gelpi self-retaining retractor. The sharp tips engage the tissue with little risk of slipping, but can tear the tissues if too much retraction is applied.
(b) Gelpi retractors being used in the neck during surgery for a collapsing trachea.

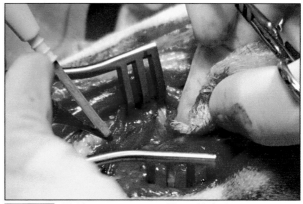

21.18 Weitlaner retractors with multiple tines to distribute pressure over a greater area. The tines can be either sharp or blunt.

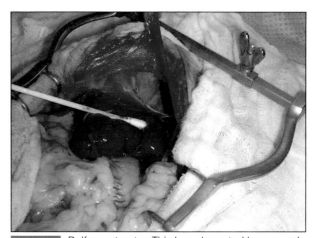

21.19 Balfour retractor. This has elongated hoops and is useful for retraction of soft tissues where the blades do not need to engage the tissue (i.e. when there is little chance of slippage).

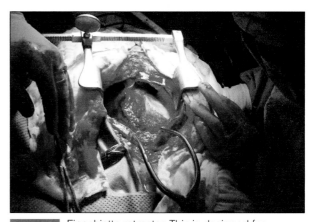

21.20 Finochietto retractor. This is designed for thoracic retraction. The blades are ridged to engage the tissues better. In areas where slippage is likely, the Gelpi retractor is often used as well.

The Lone Star is a self-retaining retractor system composed of retractor rings and elastic stays. It is a flexible adjustable system that provides optimal exposure and access to the operative area, as it has the ability to adapt rapidly to changes in the field with minimal effort as the procedure progresses. The Lone Star is particularly useful for perineal surgery, where retraction in a variety of directions is required, along with 360-degree access to the surgical site.

Stay sutures

Stay sutures are used in situations where hand-held or self-retaining retractors are not appropriate. In some instances, the tissues are too fragile to use surgical instruments (e.g. mediastinum, bladder wall) (Figure 21.21). In other situations, the surgeon is working within a body cavity or in a confined area where retractors would be too bulky. Stay sutures can also be customized for the particular application and placed in a variety of positions, retracting in various directions and providing flexibility that may not be achievable with conventional retractors.

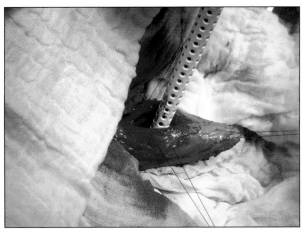

21.21   Use of stay sutures in the bladder wall. Note how the abdominal contents are protected from contamination and kept moist with saline-soaked laparotomy swabs. Note also the multi-holed Poole suction cannula.

- Stay sutures are placed carefully, so as to not damage the tissue.
- They may be passed through once or twice, depending on whether additional holding capacity is required.
- In some instances, they are placed in a mattress fashion to improve holding capacity.
- The two ends of the stay suture are usually grasped in a haemostat. The haemostat may then be held by a surgical assistant, allowed to fall to the side (with the weight of the instrument providing traction), or clamped to drapes around the incision to maintain retraction.
- Sometimes it is appropriate to place stay sutures between two body parts and tie the suture for the period of time over which retraction is required. One such instance is creation of a pericardial cradle, where the edges of the incised pericardium are sutured to the tissues of the thoracic wall or adjacent drapes during heart surgery.

Stay suture material should be synthetic and monofilament to cause less tissue drag. It should be sufficiently thick to reduce the risk of cutting through the tissues. Needles should be round-bodied with a tapered point (see Chapter 5) to avoid creating a tear in the tissue that might later enlarge when traction is applied to the suture.

Moist saline-soaked swabs

Saline-soaked swabs are used:

- To keep tissues moist
- To protect tissues from retractor blades

- To absorb blood and body fluids
- To blot the wound to keep it clear of blood while the surgeon is working
- For packing when haemostasis is required.

They should be moistened by applying saline to the swab, rather than by dunking the swab in the saline bowl. If swabs are soaked and then wrung out, the saline should be discarded as it will contain large amounts of lint.

The surgeon or assistant should always keep count of the number of swabs opened and make sure that the count matches before the surgical wound is closed, as retained swabs have been reported in many locations, including the thoracic and abdominal cavities, lumen of the stomach, airway and soft tissues following fracture repair or major soft tissue reconstruction.

Wound lavage

Wound lavage is beneficial for a number of reasons. It is used after lengthy procedures or those in which contamination is known to be present.

- Vigorous lavage using warm sterile saline dislodges bacteria, lint from surgical swabs, talc from surgical gloves, blood clots, intestinal contents, urine and other foreign or irritant material.
- Repeated flooding of the site with saline, followed by suction, can be used to confirm whether haemorrhage is still occurring or there is ongoing air leakage following a lung lobectomy or biopsy, or biliary tract surgery.

Lavage is most beneficial when appropriate volumes of saline are used (dilution effect), with physical dislodgement of debris by application of hydrostatic pressure, in a pulsatile way. It is important to remove all lavage fluid with suction, as fluid in the wound impairs the normal immune response.

Surgical suction

The use of surgical suction:

- Enables the surgical site to be cleared of blood to improve visualization
- Allows retrieval of saline (used to flush away blood and debris, moisten tissues and identify bleeding points)
- Permits suctioning of aerosolized gases liberated during diathermy.

Suction units should be designed specifically for surgical application so that they:

- Do not create too much noise
- Do not exert forces capable of damaging soft tissues
- Have a mechanism for retrieving suctioned fluid in a sealed reservoir.

Cannulae used for suction vary from rigid tubes with a single end-point to flexible multi-holed tubes. They may be disposable or reusable.

- Rigid straight (Frazier) cannulae with end-holes are used for suction of blood or other body fluids from a fairly rigid surface such as a joint, or taut tissue plane, and improve visualization.

- Rigid cannulae may also have a flared end with multiple holes (Yankauer) that reduces the risk of sucking soft tissues into the lumen. They were originally designed for oral suction but are useful for other flexible soft tissue sites (retroperitoneum, perineum).
- Rigid sleeves with multiple side holes, usually surrounding a rigid interior cannula (Poole), are used to remove large amounts of fluid from body cavities. The multiple holes reduce the risk of omentum or membranous mediastinum occluding the cannula (see Figure 21.21).

Surgical lighting

Surgery cannot be performed safely if the surgeon cannot see the surgical site. Ideally, an operating room should be equipped with at least two ceiling-mounted lights capable of being focused on the surgical site (see also Chapter 1).

- The lights should not emit too much heat, should not cast shadows and should allow accurate interpretation of colours.
- Either sterilized light-handle covers or sterile handles should be available so that the surgeon can control the light.
- The two lights should have articulated attachments that allow them to be directed towards the patient at virtually any angle and should be capable of moving independently:
  - One light is used as a 'primary' light, usually centred above the surgeon
  - The other is a 'secondary' light that is directed in at an angle and often moved during the course of the surgery.

The surgeon or assistant should take note of changes in lighting during the procedure and ensure that the lights are positioned so as to avoid them being obscured by the surgeon or assistant. This is especially important when working in body cavities. Some time should be taken at each stage of the surgical procedure to ensure that the lighting is optimal. Poor visualization during surgery is often the result of poor light position.

Head lights

Intraoperative illumination may also be achieved with surgical head lights. These are mandatory for microsurgery and delicate procedures in very restricted surgical fields. A large variety of head lights is available, with different options for the head piece, type of illumination and integration with operating loupes. It takes a while to become accustomed to using loupes and head lights, so surgeons planning to purchase this equipment should trial different products and ensure that they feel comfortable before purchasing.

Closure of tissue planes

Closure of tissue planes has the following goals:

- Immediate restoration of function (muscle bellies, pleural space)
- Eliminate risk of displacement of contents (abdominal wall, hollow organs)
- Elimination of dead space
- Haemostasis (particularly in the subcutis)
- Relief of tension on other layers
- Restoration of epithelial coverage.

The number of layers and types of suture pattern should be chosen to fulfil the above goals in a timely fashion without excessive tissue handling and without leaving inappropriately large amounts of suture material in the wound. It is not always necessary to close every tissue plane that was incised, and some individual tissue planes may be combined for closure.

Closure of tissue planes should ideally not impede normal movement of the tissues (gliding of tendons, independent action of muscles).

PRACTICAL TIPS

- 'Tacking' or 'walking sutures' that may be used to eliminate dead space or stretch skin should be planned carefully, with consideration for the relative positions of the layers when the patient becomes ambulatory.
- Closing a mobile layer to a more fixed independent layer with tacking sutures may actually be more painful, create more inflammation and have a higher risk of failure if excessive traction develops because the natural position of the tissues was misjudged during closure.

Dead space and drains

All surgeons are aware of the importance of minimizing dead space. This can be often achieved by placing additional layers of suture, for example, in the inguinal region of male dogs. Failure to close the fatty layer dorsal to the prepuce following laparotomy can lead to haematoma formation, severe swelling and seroma. In this instance, where infection is not present, it is most appropriate to avoid the problem by incorporating that layer in a subcutaneous suture, rather than placing a drain.

PRACTICAL TIP

Drains should be reserved for:

- Wounds that are infected or severely contaminated
- Wounds in which discharge due to tissue necrosis is anticipated
- Wounds in which all the fluid cannot be removed during the surgical procedure
- Wounds that cannot be closed by simple suturing of tissue planes.

If a drain is placed in a clean wound with residual dead space, it should be a closed system, attached to some form of suction reservoir. The drain should remain in place until a constant low volume of fluid is draining. (For further information on types of drain, see Chapter 17.) An alternative to drain placement in clean wounds is to use soft padded bandages to press the skin against the underlying tissues, thereby discouraging subcutaneous fluid formation.

Placement of sutures in tissue
Sutures are used to:

- Close tissue planes
- Re-appose vital structures
- Retract tissues with minimal handling
- Stabilize and exteriorize tissue and organs.

Needle-holders
Regardless of their purpose, the vast majority of sutures are placed using needle-holders (see also Chapter 4).

Needle-holders, like scissors, are held in the palm of the hand, with the thumb in one ring and the second or third finger in the other. This leaves the first finger free to stabilize and guide the instrument. Sometimes it is helpful to hold the needle-holder in the palm with the fingers and thumb wrapped around the outside of the rings, especially if the needle has to be reversed or driven in an unusual direction. When held this way, it is usually necessary to change the grip to release the needle and clamp it again for the next pass.

The needle should be clamped firmly in the jaws of the needle-holder to avoid it rocking or slipping (Figure 21.22).

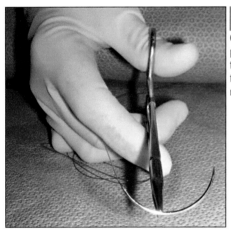

21.22 Correct placement of the needle in the jaws of the needle-holder.

PRACTICAL TIPS

- The needle should be clamped at the tip of the jaws, rather than halfway down. This ensures that the needle can be presented to the tissue plane being sutured without having to push the jaws into the tissues first.
- The needle is usually clamped about one-third of the way from the eye (or where the suture is attached), i.e. two-thirds of the distance from the point. This leaves a long enough portion of needle for it to be driven through the tissue and grasped on the other side, while avoiding leverage and rocking of the needle in the jaws of the needle-holder if it is held too close to the suture end.
- When passing the needle through tough collagen-rich tissue, the needle may be grasped closer to the point.

Orientation and rotation: The needle is usually positioned at right angles to the jaws of the needle-holder, but the orientation can be changed when working at awkward angles. Tilting the needle so that the tip

advances ahead of the needle-holder is useful when working in tight spaces. In extreme instances, the needle can be held parallel to the needle-holder, and the needle advanced with vertical rather than lateral motion. Regardless of the orientation, the needle should always be rotated through the tissues, and the rotation continued as the needle is withdrawn from the other side, thus ensuring that the needle travels in the direction of its curve.

Retraction and visualization: When suturing a tissue plane, the plane should be identified and retracted or advanced away from the surrounding tissues using forceps. Placing some tension on the tissue plane will facilitate penetration with the needle and avoid tissue tenting or folding. The tip of the needle should be visualized emerging on the other side to ensure that no other tissues are engaged.

A good example is grasping the subcutis and retracting it away from the skin edge when suturing it. This is preferable to attempting to engage the subcutis by scooping it from beneath the everted skin, which often leads to accidental perforation of the skin or inclusion of the dermis, leading to skin indentation. Retraction and visualization of the linea alba likewise avoids the risk of incorporating the subcutis and possibly missing the linea alba altogether.

Suturing angle: When considering the angle at which to suture a tissue plane, it should be remembered that suturing is most comfortably undertaken towards the surgeon or towards the non-dominant hand. Right-handed surgeons thus find it more comfortable suturing from right to left.

Palm position: Suturing is also more comfortable with the palm pointing downwards rather than upwards (Figure 21.23). When it is necessary to reverse the suture (e.g. at the end of a continuous suture when creating a loop on one side of the incision), the needle is reversed in the needle-holder and the surgeon changes their grip so that the hand covers the needle-holder and thus is oriented palm down. The palm-down position is also beneficial when working in a tight space, as the instrument can be oriented through a wider range of angles, rather than having the surgeon's hand interfere with laying the needle-holder or haemostats flat against the patient.

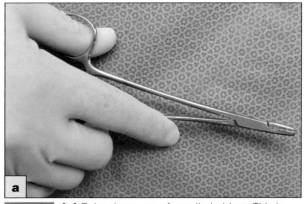

21.23 **(a)** Palm-down use of needle-holders. This is more comfortable and allows the hand to move in a more natural direction than using the instrument with the palm facing upwards. (continues) ▶

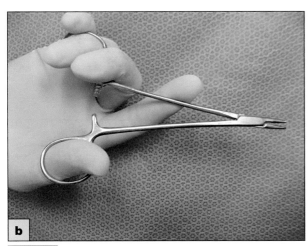

21.23 (continued) **(b)** Holding needle-holders with the palm upwards. While sometimes unavoidable, this allows for less range of movement and feels more awkward.

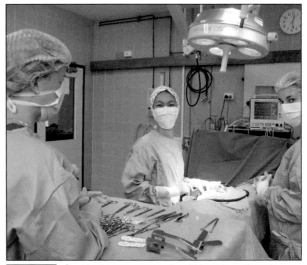

21.24 Surgical instruments should be placed on the table in an orderly fashion and maintained in this order wherever possible. The instruments should be cleaned by the assistant each time they are returned to the table.

The surgical assistant

The surgical assistant plays a very important role during the surgery and effective utilization of the assistant contributes greatly to a successful outcome. The role of the assistant includes:

- Managing the surgical table and passing instruments
- Assisting with surgical retraction and haemostasis
- Ensuring that diagnostic samples are not lost
- Keeping count of surgical swabs
- Running a continuous suture and cutting sutures.

Effective engagement of the surgical assistant ensures that the surgery proceeds efficiently and with minimal interruption.

The surgical assistant must be well trained in operating room conduct and must adhere to aseptic technique. To ensure good teamwork, the surgeon should take time to explain what is expected of the surgical assistant and discuss the surgical plan. It is important for the surgical assistant to be familiar with each procedure so that they can participate actively in the surgery. Understanding the sequence of events in the surgical procedure will allow the assistant to ensure that instruments are available and are presented to the surgeon in an orderly fashion. The surgical assistant should be familiar with the name and intended use of the surgical instruments so as to anticipate the surgeon's next step.

Surgical table

Keeping the surgical table organized is a very important task (Figure 21.24). Much time can be wasted looking for instruments on a disorganized surgical table. During complicated procedures, it is extremely important that the assistant pays attention to the surgical table to ensure that the requested instruments are available immediately. A disorganized table can also lead to injuries or a break in aseptic technique if scalpel blades and needles are left unattended. Where possible, the assistant should clean blood and tissue from the instruments before the surgeon requires them again. The surgical assistant should also try to avoid distractions, such as non-surgical conversation.

Retraction

The surgical assistant is vital in providing retraction during the surgical procedure. The importance of excellent visualization cannot be underestimated and the assistant should be utilized to guarantee that this is achieved. The assistant should understand normal anatomy and be careful not to traumatize the organs being retracted.

When holding a retractor, the assistant's attention must be focused on the patient. Turning around to take something from the surgical table, or from another technician, will cause the retractor to move, which may cause a delay if the retractor then needs to be repositioned, or could even cause damage to the patient.

Samples

The assistant should ensure that all samples collected during the surgery are placed in the appropriate containers and labelled. This may require liaison with another technician, or the assistant to put the clearly marked samples safely aside for processing once the operation is completed. The assistant should establish a system to ensure that samples are not forgotten or inadvertently thrown away.

Involvement of the assistant

The surgical assistant is an important addition to the surgical team and it is important to engage them actively in the procedure. By training the surgical assistant in instrument recognition and handling along with aseptic techniques and relevant anatomy, it is possible to achieve increased efficiency and decreased surgical time and intraoperative complications.

As well as utilizing their assistant properly, surgeons should also be mindful of allowing them time to relax, especially when they are holding retractors for long periods of time (Figure 21.25). The surgeon should also foster an environment where all participants are committed to ensuring the best outcome for the patient. On occasions, the assistant might make observations or have suggestions, and they should be allowed to voice respectfully any concerns that might arise during the procedure.

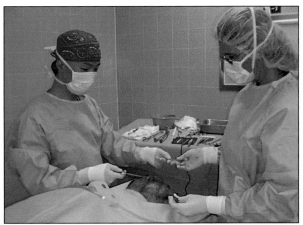

21.25 The assistant should be actively engaged in the surgery, trying to anticipate the surgeon's requirements for the next stage, whether it be retraction or passing something from the instrument table.

Minimizing operative time

Some surgeons are fast and some are slow. Fast surgeons can be sloppy, while slow surgeons can be meticulous. It is possible to be too fast, but being slow is far more common.

Sacrificing attention to detail in a quest for speed is clearly not in the patient's best interests, but extending surgical time by becoming fixated on details that are not really important to the final outcome can also be detrimental, because:

- Increased surgical time leads to a higher infection rate
- Tissues dry out
- There is more opportunity for tissue handling (which in itself causes trauma)
- There is more bacterial contamination from the environment
- The patient is subjected to a longer anaesthetic with greater risk of hypotension, hypothermia and dehydration.

So how can a surgeon minimize operative time and still be diligent? Faster surgery comes with time and experience, but in watching novice surgeons it becomes evident that a small number of basic mistakes have the greatest role in prolonging surgical time (Figure 21.26).

Simple principles for veterinary surgeons to reduce the amount of time spent in surgery and improve patient outcomes are given in Figure 21.27.

- **Poor positioning on the operating table**. This may confound the surgical approach, as the normal anatomical landmarks may not be evident, or the relationship between structures may be distorted.
- **Poor understanding of local anatomy**, in particular the associations between structures and the best way to identify blood vessels and nerves. This leads to excessive time spent dissecting the area, relocating retractors, lavaging, suctioning and trying to decide what to do next.
- **Fear of cutting the wrong thing**. In trying to avoid damaging something important, surgeons often tease and manipulate tissue for extended intervals until it gives way. This is time-consuming and usually results in more tissue trauma than simply proceeding with sharp dissection. It may also limit the surgical exposure, compromising visualization or the ability to manipulate instruments at the site.
- **Poor retraction** due to not using the assistant or retractors properly. This impedes visualization and makes it difficult to make timely decisions and proceed with the different steps of the procedure.
- **Keeping an untidy instrument table**. A lot of time can be wasted trying to find the correct instrument, clean it, or untangle it from everything else on the table.
- **Not establishing adequate haemostasis** and making repeated attempts to clamp or cauterize bleeding points without adequate visualization.

21.26 Common mistakes that prolong surgical time.

- Develop a surgical plan preoperatively.
- Make sure that the person positioning the patient on the table knows exactly what is required for the given procedure and confirms it with the surgeon if anything is unclear.
- Review the important anatomy and be confident of knowing the origins, attachments and relationships of important structures to one another. If necessary, bring an illustration into the room and refer to it.
- Practise skills in identifying and dividing tissue planes.
- Use the surgical assistant.
- If needing to cut something that cannot clearly be identified, consider the risks in the context of structures known to inhabit the area. For example, cutting a small sensory nerve going to the skin will have much less impact than cutting a motor nerve going to the triceps muscle. Cutting a peripheral artery, while spectacular, is not likely to result in any permanent damage to the patient, but cutting the nerve running next to it might. Identify the structures that the unidentified tissue is going to: if it attaches to the skin it is probably safe to proceed; if it is entering the mass that is about to be removed and not exiting again, it will have to be cut at some point anyway.
- If nervous or flustered, take time out. If the bleeding points cannot be easily identified, try digital pressure or packing for a few minutes. Use the time to tidy the instrument table. Let the assistant relax. Reposition the lights. Clean gloves and instruments with sterile saline. Think back through the surgical plan. Take a few deep breaths. Enjoy yourself.

21.27 Simple principles for veterinary surgeons to reduce the amount of time spent in surgery and improve patient outcomes.

Suture patterns and surgical knots

Thomas Sissener

Introduction

The selection of an appropriate suture pattern is important to the successful outcome of surgery. The surgeon's aim is to choose a suture pattern that will close the incision and give maximum mechanical support with minimal tissue reaction. Halsted's surgical principles are as applicable during the closure of the incision as they are to its opening. Using the correct suture pattern will help to restore anatomical alignment of tissues, obliterate dead space, minimize tissue trauma and preserve blood supply to the tissues.

Perhaps the most vital component of the correct suture pattern is the surgical knot. Tying a secure knot will provide an anchor for the pattern to stay intact and perform its intended purpose. This chapter will review many of the common suture patterns used in small animal surgery and provide a basis for the rational selection of patterns for particular wounds, as well as discussing the importance of knot selection and tying techniques.

Classification of patterns

A large number of suture patterns have been described for use in veterinary surgery. They are typically classified with regard to the following:

- Placement in either a continuous or interrupted fashion
- Effect on anatomical alignment of tissue (i.e. appositional, inverting, or everting)

- One-layer *versus* two-layer closure patterns
- Effect on tension (e.g. tension-relieving sutures)
- Anatomical location of the sutures (e.g. subcuticular, skin).

These categories help in understanding how the choice of the suture pattern will affect the closure of a particular wound. These choices may also directly affect the length of surgery and the healing process.

Interrupted *versus* continuous patterns

Both interrupted and continuous patterns have arguments for and against them (Figure 22.1). Many novice surgeons may be more comfortable with the use of simple interrupted closures, but studies have demonstrated that a simple continuous suture pattern can be just as effective in closing a variety of surgical incisions.

Simple interrupted sutures

- Simple interrupted sutures are easy to place and result in apposition of tissues, unless excessive tension is applied (which results in mild inversion).
- Since each individual suture is tied with a knot, failure of one suture does not necessarily lead to disruption of the entire suture line.
- However, this results in more knots and more suture material within the wound, potentially resulting in more inflammatory reaction to foreign material and an increased risk of infection.

Type of pattern	Advantages	Disadvantages
Interrupted	- Allows precise adjustment of tension at each point along the wound to spread forces along the margins - Failure of one knot may not cause entire suture line to fail	- Poor economy of suture material - More knots, therefore more suture material left in wound
Continuous	- Relatively airtight and fluid-tight - Faster than interrupted lines - Better economy of suture material - Less suture material left in wound - Distributes tension evenly over length of closure	- May cause purse-string-like effect and result in stricture in smaller viscus - Failure of anchoring knot may cause unravelling of entire suture line

22.1 Factors to consider with continuous and interrupted suture patterns.

Continuous sutures

- A continuous suture pattern is a fast and effective method of closing an incision.
- The suture material is continuous throughout closure with only a knot at either end, decreasing the amount of foreign material in the wound.
- However, if either knot becomes undone, the whole suture line can fail.
- The simple continuous suture pattern is considered relatively resistant to leakage of fluid and gas, and tension forces are distributed more evenly along the suture line.
- Use of a continuous suture pattern closure in intestinal surgery has been shown to have no increased risk of dehiscence when compared with simple interrupted closure (Weisman *et al.*, 1999) and in some cases, such as tracheal anastomosis, the simple continuous pattern has been shown to be better (Demetriou *et al.*, 2006).

As with all suture patterns, successful closure using a continuous pattern relies on the correct selection of suture material, secure knot tying and proper identification and incorporation of holding-layer tissues. Gentle handling of the tissues and suture material itself are also important.

Applications

Linea alba: The failure of a continuous abdominal closure suture pattern is usually due to surgeon error in not placing the sutures correctly in the strength-holding layer (fascia) or problems with the knot, not with the suture pattern itself. Therefore, as long as care is taken to include the linea alba and external rectus sheath, and attention is paid to the knot tying, suture selection and correct placement, simple continuous closure of the linea alba is faster and more efficient than simple interrupted closure.

Deep incisions: Due to the difficulty of placing sutures and tying knots in deep locations, a continuous suture pattern is often easiest for closure of incisions such as those for diaphragmatic hernia repair and incisional gastropexy.

Intestinal anastomosis: Both simple continuous and simple interrupted suture patterns will typically prevent leakage after closure of healthy intestinal tissue as long as the submucosa is included and the suture spacing is not too far apart. Leakage following intestinal anastomosis typically occurs at the mesenteric surface, so particular care must be taken at this location, where visualization during suture placement is more difficult. Closure of intestinal anastomosis using a simple continuous appositional suture can be achieved, but it is suggested that using two packets of suture may be preferable, one for each side that meet in the middle at the antimesenteric surface. This may help in preventing a 'bottleneck' narrowing or stricture at the lumen that may result from using one packet of suture.

Gingival and larger skin flaps: Interrupted suture patterns are indicated for closure of gingival flaps and larger skin flaps. Failure or necrosis of part of the flap may result in unravelling of the whole suture line rather than a local area if a continuous pattern is used.

Appositional, inverting and everting patterns

- Appositional sutures bring the tissue edges into close approximation, with the tissue edges in contact as they were before incision.
- Inverting suture patterns result in the tissue edges turning away from the surgeon (e.g. into the lumen of a hollow viscus organ).
- Everting suture patterns turn the tissue edges outwards and toward the surgeon.

Appositional sutures

There has been a shift towards the use of appositional suture patterns over recent years. This is in part due to studies that document at least equivalent if not superior healing compared with the more traditional inverting patterns that were used in closing hollow viscera. The erroneous belief that serosa-to-serosa contact was needed to provide a fluid-tight seal is no longer justified, and bringing tissues into correct anatomical alignment (one of Halsted's principles) can in fact speed up the healing process and potentially result in a reduced incidence of stricture (Radasch *et al.*, 1990; Kirpensteijn *et al.*, 2001).

Closure of enterotomies or enterectomies can be achieved with either simple interrupted or simple continuous appositional sutures to avoid inversion and potential narrowing of the intestinal lumen. Appositional suture patterns are also very useful in closure of fascial planes, skin, muscle, and tendons. The exception may be in areas of tension, where some types of tension-relieving suture pattern may result in slight tissue eversion.

Inverting sutures

Inverting suture patterns turn the edges of the incision away from the surgeon and inwards, apposing the outermost layers of the incision against each other. They have traditionally been used to close hollow viscera such as the gastrointestinal tract, bladder and uterus. Inversion results in the individual layers of the tissue at the incision edges not being apposed, which may compromise primary healing and delay deposition of an early fluid-tight fibrin seal across the mucosa at the incision site.

It is now known that an interrupted appositional pattern provides mechanical bursting strength equal to a continuous inverting pattern in bladder closure without narrowing the luminal space (Radasch *et al.*, 1990). This is less important in viscera with a larger diameter and inverting patterns may still be used in procedures such as gastric invagination to address questionably viable gastric wall tissue during gastric dilatation–volvulus (GDV) surgery. Skin does not heal well when inverted.

Everting sutures

Everting suture patterns result in the tissue edges puckering out towards the surgeon. They should be avoided in visceral surgery because this may increase the risk of adhesions. For this reason, they are primarily used in skin as an aid to dissipate tension along the skin closure line, though their tendency to evert is not ideal for closure of skin. Avoiding skin tension by using other methods of managing tension or by using reconstructive techniques to mobilize additional tissue is preferable to fighting against tension with tension-relieving skin sutures. Everting patterns are used to achieve endothelium-to-endothelium contact when closing incisions in blood vessels and the heart, to avoid thrombus formation on exposed collagen.

One- *versus* two-layer patterns

Suture patterns may also be described with regard to their usefulness in closing multiple layers of tissues. Some patterns can partially close an incision (like the simple continuous pattern) and therefore a two-layer closure would consist of closing the remaining layer(s) on top, such as may be used to close a gastrotomy incision, with one suture line in the mucosa and submucosa and one in the seromuscular layer. Other patterns may require that all the tissue layers are engaged to be properly applied in the first layer (e.g. the Gambee suture pattern), on top of which a second inverting pattern may be used to complete a two-layer closure.

Tension-relieving sutures

There are relatively few indications for these types of sutures. Quilled sutures use additional surgical implant material and are therefore restricted to the skin only. Preferably, all tension should be borne by the stronger subdermal tissues of the wound so that there is minimal or no tension on the skin sutures themselves. Relief of tension along a suture line is best accomplished by good apposition and tension sutures in the deeper fascial holding layers rather than skin.

Suture patterns

Appositional sutures

Simple interrupted

This is the most basic of all suture patterns, and possibly the most commonly used.

1. To start the pattern, the needle is introduced 2–5 mm away from the tissue edge. For a right-handed surgeon this is usually from the top edge of the incision if the closure is horizontal, or from the right edge if it is vertical.
2. The wrist is turned with the curve of the needle to penetrate the far tissue at the same distance (typically 2–5 mm) from the edge. If a larger gap exists between the tissues, the needle can be grasped after passing through the first tissue edge and then reintroduced at the same level through the other tissue edge.
3. The knot is then tied and left offset so that it does not rest on the incision (Figure 22.2).
4. The ends are cut, typically leaving 2–3 mm 'tags', but this depends on the selection of suture material. For skin, the ends of the suture are typically cut longer to allow easy suture removal.

Interrupted intradermal (buried knot)

Irritation of the superficial tissues from knots on subcuticular and subcutaneous tissues may lead to licking and self-trauma. In addition, burying the knot in a subcutaneous closure can lead to a better cosmetic appearance. The interrupted intradermal pattern is essentially an upside-down simple interrupted suture.

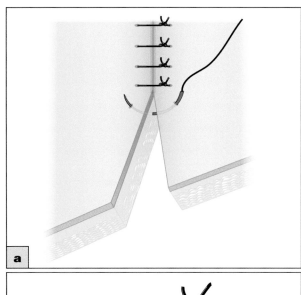

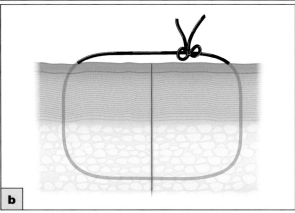

22.2 **(a)** Simple interrupted suture pattern. **(b)** The appearance of the knot relative to the incision.

1. Instead of starting from the far edge, the suture is started from the near edge and from deep within the incision. The needle exits just under the skin and crosses the incision to enter at the same level just under the skin, curving the needle to exit deep in the incision again.
2. When the knot is tied, care is taken to have the needle and tag end on the same side of the loop being pulled down to bury the knot (Figure 22.3).

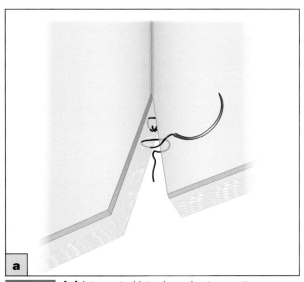

22.3 **(a)** Interrupted intradermal suture pattern. (continues) ▶

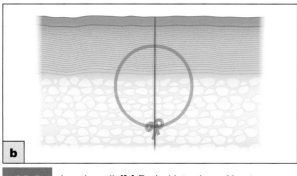

22.3 (continued) **(b)** Buried intradermal knot.

Interrupted cruciate

The interrupted cruciate (or figure-of-eight) pattern is essentially two linked simple interrupted sutures tied with one knot. This decreases the number of knots and increases the speed of placement over simple interrupted sutures. It can also help to spread localized tension better than simple interrupted sutures. It is a reasonable alternative for surgeons who want a speedier closure but remain uncomfortable with continuous patterns.

The pattern is placed in an identical way to a simple interrupted pattern, but instead of tying after the first suture is placed, a second simple interrupted suture is placed next to the first with even spacing (3–5 mm) and the tag and needle end are then tied (Figure 22.4). Care must be taken to cut both loops of suture prior to removal to avoid dragging pieces of suture material that have been exposed to the external environment back through the wound.

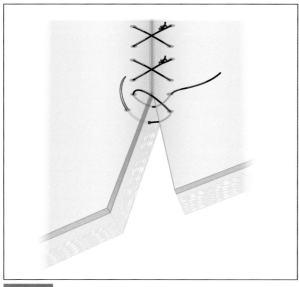

22.4 Interrupted cruciate suture pattern.

Gambee

The Gambee suture is a specialized pattern used primarily for the closure of intestine to prevent excessive eversion of intestinal mucosa, which can be a challenge during closure. This suture is not commonly used in small animal surgery as it is difficult to place accurately.

1. This suture is very similar to a simple interrupted suture and starts with a bite through the serosa into the mucosa and lumen, but the needle is

returned through the mucosa and into the muscularis before crossing the incision at the same level into the opposite side muscularis and out of the mucosa.
2. The needle is then reintroduced from the lumen through the mucosa and remaining tissue levels to exit the serosa (Figure 22.5).
3. The knot is then tied as for a simple interrupted suture.

The modified Gambee suture is placed similarly, but does not penetrate the visceral lumen.

An alternative interrupted suture pattern known as the Poth and Gold crushing suture can also be used for intestinal closure. It is placed similarly to a simple interrupted suture but tightened to the point that it cuts through the serosa and muscularis to tighten on the submucosal layer, which is the suture holding layer.

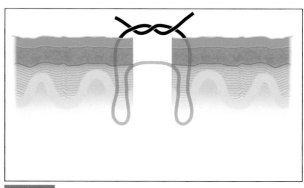

22.5 Gambee suture.

Simple continuous

The simple continuous suture pattern is started with a simple interrupted suture, but only the end without the needle (the 'tag' end) is cut. Taking an appropriately spaced and adjacent bite with the needle perpendicular to the incision then continues this pattern. The result is suture material that advances diagonally across the incision but perpendicularly below it (Figure 22.6a). The suture line is ended by tying the last loop of suture exterior to the tissues to the single strand attached to the needle.

A simple continuous **running suture** is a simple continuous suture where the suture material advances diagonally both across the incision and below it (Figure 22.6b).

Continuous intradermal

The continuous intradermal pattern is often used to provide apposition of skin and remove tension from the skin sutures. An absorbable suture material is typically used and most surgeons will utilize a continuous pattern like the continuous intradermal to close the superficial subcutaneous tissues. Studies have shown that a buried continuous subcuticular suture may result in a better cosmetic appearance to the skin after canine ovariohysterectomy at the time of re-examination.

1. The pattern starts with a buried knot (see Figure 22.3) and only the tag end is cut.
2. The suture material at the needle end is then advanced forward in the dermis or subcuticular tissue *parallel* to the long axis of the incision.

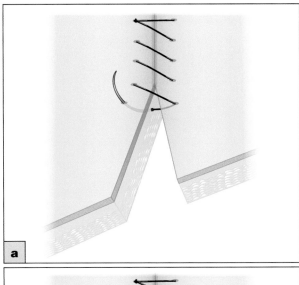

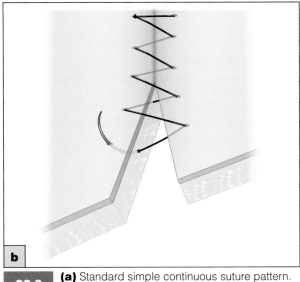

22.6 **(a)** Standard simple continuous suture pattern.
(b) Running simple continuous suture pattern.

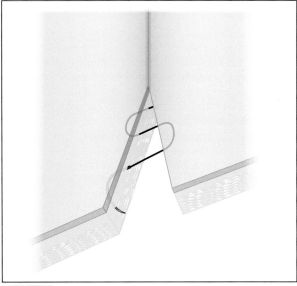

22.7 Continuous intradermal (mattress) suture pattern.

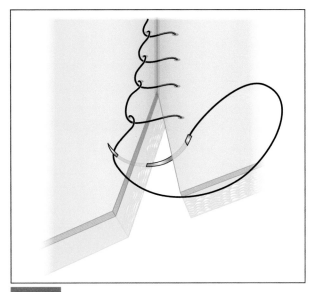

22.8 Ford interlocking suture pattern.

3. In order to achieve a straight and neat line closure, it is important that the needle and suture material enter at the same tissue level on the opposing side of the incision that it exited on the other side (Figure 22.7).
4. The suture line is completed with a buried knot using the last loop of suture material and the single strand attached to the needle.

A continuous subcutaneous suture pattern is a continuous version of the interrupted intradermal suture where the bites run *perpendicular* to the skin edge rather than parallel to it.

Ford interlocking
The Ford interlocking suture ('blanket stitch') is a continuous suture pattern that provides some of the advantages of an interrupted pattern by partially 'locking' each suture in place as the pattern progresses and having each suture loop cross the wound perpendicular to the cut edge.

The pattern is very similar to a simple continuous pattern and starts the same way, but as the suture line progresses the needle end is placed through the opposing side loop, resulting in the locking of the loop (Figure 22.8).

The continuous nature of the suture means that the closure is more rapid than simple interrupted patterns and it distributes tension better. Wound edges may also be better apposed, because the bites cross the surgical wound perpendicular to it. The locking feature means that the line is less likely to be completely disrupted as a result of self-trauma by the patient.

This suture pattern is not economical with suture material and can be more time-consuming to remove than simple interrupted or continuous sutures, since each suture loop must be cut individually to avoid pulling suture material that has been exposed to the external environment through the wound.

Inverting sutures
Lembert
The Lembert pattern is similar to the vertical mattress pattern and is used to close hollow viscera in either an interrupted or continuous fashion. The needle should not penetrate into the lumen, but should penetrate the submucosa. Since the important holding layer is the submucosa, the surgeon should ensure that this layer

is engaged, even if this means occasionally entering the lumen.

1. The pattern starts by introducing the needle into the serosal surface 8–10 mm away from the incision, penetrating down through the submucosa and following the curve of the needle, exiting about 3–4 mm from the incision edge on the same side as it entered.
2. The needle then crosses the incision *perpendicularly* and enters the serosa 3–4 mm away from the edge, penetrating down to the submucosal level and following the curve of the needle to exit again about 8–10 mm away (Figure 22.9).
3. As the suture is tightened, it inverts the tissues.

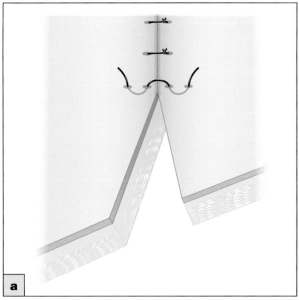

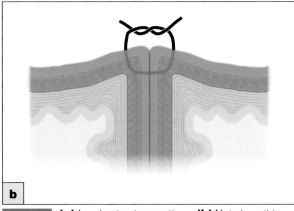

22.9 (a) Lembert suture pattern. (b) Note how this suture inverts the tissues.

In the continuous version, the suture bites are placed *perpendicular* to the incision (which differentiates this pattern from the Cushing and Connell, below).

Halsted
The Halsted pattern is a variation of the Lembert, and is essentially two Lembert sutures placed side by side with the ends knotted (Figure 22.10). Just as two linked simple interrupted sutures make a horizontal mattress suture, so two linked Lembert sutures make a Halsted suture. This produces an interrupted inverting pattern.

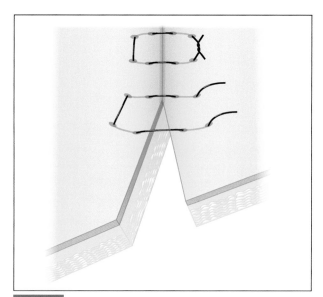

22.10 Halsted suture pattern.

Connell and Cushing
These two similar continuous patterns are perhaps the most widely used inverting patterns to close hollow viscera. The patterns are almost identical, except for the fact that the Connell pattern penetrates through the mucosa into the lumen, whereas the Cushing pattern does not. A good way to remember the difference between these two is that the word 'Connell' contains an 'l' for 'lumen'.

1. The pattern typically starts with a simple interrupted or Lembert suture with a knot at one end of the incision.
2. The needle is then advanced *parallel* to the incision, introducing it through the serosa and into the muscularis and submucosa tissues for a Cushing pattern and into the lumen for the Connell pattern.
3. The needle is passed parallel to the incision along the curve of the needle by a slight twisting of the wrist until it exits the serosa again.
4. The suture is brought to the other side of the incision and reintroduced into the serosa on that side directly across from the exit point on the other side. The suture should cross the incision perpendicularly.
5. The suture is then continued similarly down the line.
6. When the suture material is pulled taut, the incision inverts (Figure 22.11) .
7. The suture pattern is ended in the same fashion as other continuous patterns, by tying the needle end to the last loop.

Utrecht pattern
This pattern is very similar to the Cushing pattern and is primarily used for closing the uterus during Caesarean section. The rationale is that inversion of the uterine tissue may help to decrease the incidence of abdominal adhesions, though there may not be any inherent advantages over the more common Cushing pattern.

The pattern starts with a simple interrupted, Lembert, or buried knot suture and then proceeds similarly to the Cushing pattern except that the needle is advanced at an angle of 30–45 degrees to the incision instead of parallel to it, resulting in a 'herring bone' type pattern on closure (Figure 22.12).

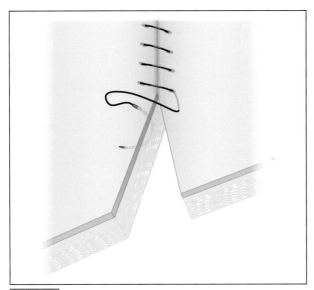

22.11 Cushing suture pattern.

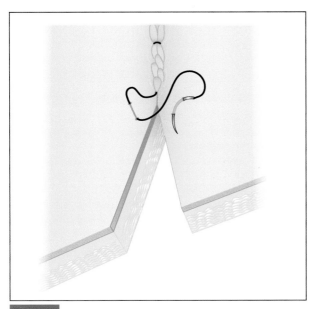

22.12 Utrecht suture pattern.

Parker–Kerr oversew

This pattern is recommended for closing the stump of a hollow viscus and will invert the edges back into the stump.

1. It utilizes the haemostat used temporarily to hold the stump closed by suturing over it with a Cushing pattern.
2. The haemostat is then slowly withdrawn from under the Cushing pattern and as the suture is tightened the edges invert.
3. A second layer consisting of a Lembert pattern is then used to oversew the stump (Figure 22.13) and the needle end is tied to the tag end left at the start of the Cushing pattern.

Clinically there are few applications for this pattern and it is not commonly used, due to concerns about excessive tissue inversion and stump abscesses. Modified versions of the oversew technique have

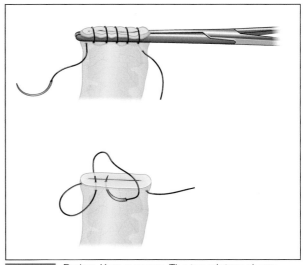

22.13 Parker–Kerr oversew. The top picture shows suturing over the haemostat with a Cushing pattern while the bottom shows the Lembert oversew.

been used to lend additional closure security to some procedures, such as partial lung lobectomy. These modifications consist of using interrupted horizontal mattress sutures through the parenchyma, and especially the bronchus, followed by a simple continuous pattern oversew on the resected edge.

Purse-string

Indications for use of the purse-string suture pattern are closure of visceral stumps and securing percutaneous tubes that enter a viscus (e.g. gastrostomy, enterostomy and cystostomy tubes).

1. This pattern is a circular variation of the Lembert pattern. Equal bites are taken around the circumference of the stump, hollow viscus or planned '-ostomy' site until the suture needle ends up back at the beginning.
2. The suture is typically pre-placed before the tube is inserted, to avoid compromising the tube lumen or suture material trapping the tube in place making removal difficult.
3. The suture is tightened around the placed '-ostomy' tube and the ends are tied to each other to secure a seal around the tube (Figure 22.14).

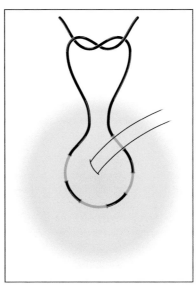

22.14

Purse-string suture.

For closing a hollow viscus, the edges may need to be rolled inwards with an instrument as the suture is tightened to achieve mucosal inversion and a fluid-tight seal.

Everting sutures

Horizontal mattress

1. The horizontal mattress suture pattern uses two parallel and equidistant passes of suture material across the incision, resulting in an eccentrically placed knot on the side of the incision line.
2. The first simple interrupted suture crosses the incision line and the second simple interrupted suture is started from the far side and comes back towards the surgeon (Figure 22.15).
3. The pull of the suture as it is tightened places pressure over a broad area away from the incision edge, thus making it less likely to tear through the tissue edges.

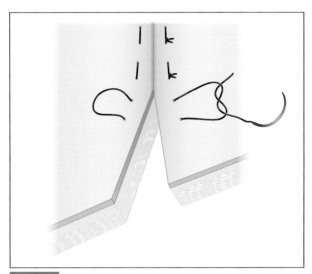

22.15 Horizontal mattress suture pattern.

Concerns that pressure from the suture strand running parallel with the wound edge may reduce the cutaneous blood flow to the wound edge between the two suture loops are not substantiated by laser Doppler flowmetry studies (Sagi *et al.*, 2008). More tension on the suture will result in further eversion of the tissues. The pattern can also be performed as a continuous horizontal mattress pattern and is then started with a simple interrupted suture, as for most continuous patterns.

Tension-relieving sutures

Vertical mattress
This interrupted suture pattern is also primarily used in the skin or fascia to dissipate tension along a suture line.

1. It is started by inserting the needle 8–10 mm away from the skin edge and passing it down into the underlying tissues, across the incision line to exit at about the same distance (8–10 mm) on the far side.
2. The needle is then reintroduced on the far side at the same level, perpendicular to where it exited,

but only 3–4 mm from the incision edge.
3. It then crosses the incision line again and exits 3–4 mm from the edge and at the same perpendicular level where it was first introduced (Figure 22.16).
4. A knot is then tied after appropriate tension has been placed on the suture material.

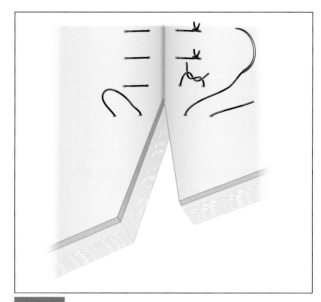

22.16 Vertical mattress suture pattern.

Near and far patterns
These two patterns are slight modifications of the vertical mattress pattern, where the suture is passed above the wound twice, and are also used in areas of tension. They are the result of passing the needle through the tissues in a different order than the vertical mattress, therefore resulting in a knot that lies above the incision rather than one eccentrically placed to one side (Figure 22.17).

These patterns can be used for closure of deeper tissue layers and can be useful reconstruction procedures where tension along the wound can be challenging. They are also occasionally used to close smaller flat tendons, since they resist tension well because all suture passes are in the same vertical plane.

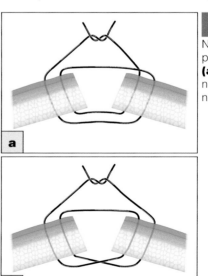

22.17
Near and far patterns. **(a)** Far-far-near-near. **(b)** Far-near-near-far.

Quilled

A quilled suture pattern is typically used in combination with a simple interrupted closure to support the closure in areas of tension. A quill is defined as material used to distribute the tension from the suture along a greater surface area. Suitable materials for a quill include small diameter rolled gauze or intravenous tubing. A vertical mattress suture can be used to ensnare the quill on both ends of the incision along the closure line (Figure 22.18) or small 10–15 mm pieces of intravenous fluid tubing can be cut and horizontal mattress sutures placed directly through the tubing on either side of the incision (Figure 22.19). The knot ends up on top of one of the quills. Some surgeons prefer to pass the suture material through the lumen of the quill.

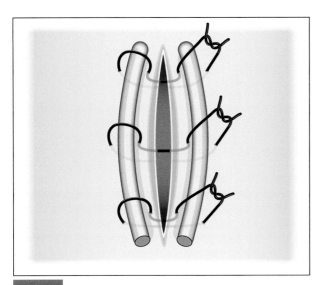

22.18   Quilled vertical mattress sutures.

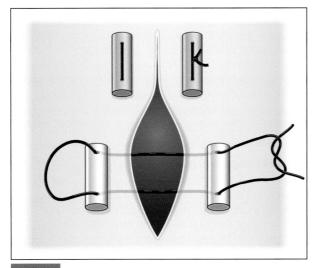

22.19   Quilled horizontal mattress sutures.

Double butterfly

This more recently described interrupted pattern has been used with success in closing areas of tension during oncological reconstruction procedures. It requires less force to close a given distance under tension than either simple interrupted or horizontal mattress suture patterns, resulting in a reduced risk

of ischaemic necrosis, dehiscence and suture pull-out (Austin and Henderson, 2006). It is most useful in deeper tissues to reduce tension on the skin.

1. The pattern is started by introduction of the needle into the deeper tissues parallel along the wound edge and exiting further up the incision.
2. The needle and suture cross the incision and take a bite along the opposite edge horizontal to the incision, then cross the incision to come back to the near edge with a similar bite.
3. The incision is crossed one last time and another horizontal bite of the tissues is taken.
4. This results in a figure-of-eight pattern within the deeper tissues and horizontal to the skin edges (Figure 22.20).

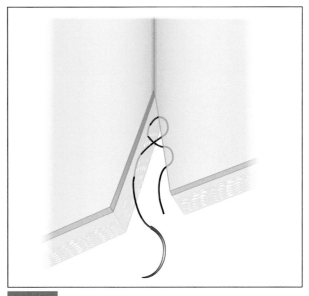

22.20   Double butterfly suture pattern.

'Walking' sutures

Walking sutures are buried knot sutures placed in the undermined subcutaneous tissues, anchoring them to the underlying fascia. They are tied under tension, pulling ('walking') the subcutaneous tissues forward to the anchoring point, often resulting in a small visible dimple in the overlying skin. The suture should not penetrate the skin itself. If rows of walking sutures are placed, they are typically placed in staggered lines, like the bricks in a wall, to avoid compromise of local blood vessels. By tightening the underlying fascia, the tension is taken off the skin closure.

This is an extremely useful closure technique, particularly when combined with skin undermining. The placement of walking sutures is preferred to the use of stents or quilled skin sutures where possible. Furthermore, drawing the edges of a large skin wound together using stay sutures to overcome wound tension and facilitate placement of subdermal sutures is preferable to all the above-mentioned types of tension-relieving sutures.

Modified Mayo/'vest over pants'

This is a specialized pattern mostly used for imbrication or tightening of retinacular fascia tissue during surgical management of cranial cruciate ligament rupture, patella luxation, or abdominal herniorrhaphy. It results in tissue overlap instead of tissue apposition, thus tightening the tissues on the side of application. Although very effective for this purpose, it has few other applications as it does not provide direct apposition of tissue layers.

This interrupted suture pattern resembles horizontal mattress sutures and is placed similarly apart from the direction of bites in the second side of the wound to be penetrated (i.e. bites in both sides of the wound are placed superficial to deep, rather than being reversed in the second side as for a horizontal mattress suture) (Figure 22.21).

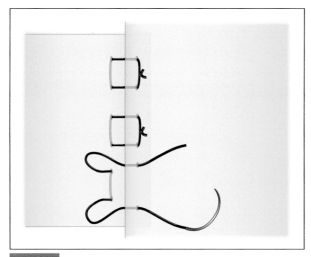

22.21   Modified Mayo suture pattern.

Suture patterns for tendon repair
These are reviewed and illustrated in the *BSAVA Manual of Canine and Feline Musculoskeletal Disorders.*

Rational pattern selection for particular wound closures

The surgeon does not need a large arsenal of suture patterns to close most of the wounds and incisions encountered daily. For the majority of wound closures, simple interrupted, buried knot simple interrupted, simple continuous and perhaps cruciate or Ford interlocking patterns will suffice.

The key elements to successful closure are recognizing the tissue holding layer, making sure that this is engaged by the suture, and ensuring that there is minimal tension on the skin closure. The holding layers are typically fibrous tissues such as the subdermal tissue of skin, fascia over muscle, tendons and ligaments, and the submucosa in the viscera. Closure of layers such as the subcutaneous tissues and fat may affect the cosmetic appearance of the wound and reduce the risk of developing a seroma or haematoma, but will have minimal contribution to the strength of the overall wound itself.

Selection factors
Factors to consider when selecting a suture pattern include:

- Length of the incision
- Location of the incision
- Shape of the wound
- Thickness and tendency for tissue layers to separate
- Closures resulting in a seal
- Tightness of suture patterns
- Species
- Patient disposition
- Need for fast closure
- Surgeon preference.

Figure 22.22 summarizes common uses for the many suture patterns; Figure 22.23 suggests suture patterns to be used for commonly encountered incision closures.

Length of incision
Intestinal biopsy incisions are usually closed with simple interrupted one-layer appositional sutures as they are not long incisions. Longer incisions such as those resulting from transposition of axial pattern flaps are typically closed with continuous suture patterns to increase speed.

Location of incision
Deep incisions or wound closures such as those of a diaphragmatic rupture are often closed with a continuous pattern, because multiple interrupted knots can be difficult to tie deep within the abdomen.

Shape of the wound
Some wounds may be straight lines, while others are curved or consist of wound edges that are of differing lengths. Continuous suture patterns work best on relatively straight or gently curving incisions. Interrupted sutures will more easily allow correction of wound edge alignment in awkwardly shaped wounds and compensation between wound edges of differing lengths.

Thickness and separation tendency
Some viscera may lend themselves more easily to two-layer closures. A gastrotomy incision generally separates into two distinct layers (mucosa and submucosa together; and muscularis and serosa together), which can be closed using two-layer closure techniques. Most bladder surgery occurs in patients with chronic disease and thickened bladder walls and two distinct layers are often apparent after cystotomy as above. A normal bladder has very thin walls and a single layer closure is preferred.

Closures resulting in a seal
It is imperative that closure of some tissues should result in an air-tight or fluid-tight seal to avoid leakage of luminal contents. Gastrointestinal and urogenital tract surgery requires selection of suture patterns that ensure an adequate seal is formed to prevent significant postoperative complications. A good seal is often achieved by well placed appositional suture patterns.

Tightness of suture pattern
Skin sutures should be placed more loosely than in other layers during closure as this will allow for postoperative swelling. Failure to do this will result in local ischaemia, bruising and patient discomfort. Although skin tension is best avoided by appropriate closure of deeper tissues or use of reconstructive techniques, some wound types may require tension-relieving sutures.

Suture pattern	Useful features	Common uses
Simple interrupted (see Figure 22.2)	Anatomical apposition of layers. Failure of knot does not result in failure of suture line. Simple to perform	Skin, subcutaneous tissues, fascia, linea alba, enterotomies, intestinal anastomosis, stomach, urinary tract, blood vessels, nerves
Buried knot or interrupted intradermal (see Figure 22.3)	Good cosmetic closure. Knot protected from self-trauma and irritation	Intradermal skin closure, walking sutures
Interrupted cruciate (see Figure 22.4)	Increased speed over simple interrupted; fewer knots. Spreads localized tension	Skin, linea alba (to small extent)
Gambee (see Figure 22.5)	Prevents excessive eversion of intestinal mucosa. Less susceptibility to wicking out intestinal contents	Intestinal enterotomies or anastomosis
Simple continuous (see Figure 22.6)	Relatively quick. Provides good air- and fluid-tight seal. Less suture material in wound	Skin, subcutaneous tissues, fascia, muscle, linea alba, enterotomies, intestinal anastomosis, stomach, urinary tract, uterus, diaphragmatic hernias, incisional gastropexies, tracheal anastomosis
Continuous intradermal (see Figure 22.7)	Good apposition of skin. Decreases some skin tension. Better cosmetic appearance. No suture removal in fractious patients	Subcutaneous or intradermal tissues
Ford interlocking (see Figure 22.8)	'Locks' in place to help prevent unravelling. Continuous pattern to increase speed of placement	Skin
Lembert (see Figure 22.9)	Does not penetrate lumen of bowel. Can be interrupted or continuous	Hollow viscus, imbrication of fascia, oversewing Cushing's for Parker–Kerr
Halsted (see Figure 22.10)	Interrupted pattern of two side-by-side Lembert sutures. Faster than interrupted Lembert	Hollow viscus
Connell and Cushing (see Figure 22.11)	Less inversion than Lembert. Connell does not penetrate lumen	Hollow viscus
Utrecht (see Figure 22.12)	Decreased abdominal adhesions to uterus	Closure of uterus after Caesarean section
Parker–Kerr oversew (see Figure 22.13)	Inverts mucosa on closure of stumps of viscera	Closing stumps of hollow viscus
Purse-string (Figure 22.14)	Provides secure seal around tubes	Closing stumps of hollow viscus, securing tubes within organs
Horizontal mattress (see Figure 22.15)	Relieves tension. Resists pull-out through tissues	Skin, subcutaneous tissues, fascia, muscle, flat tendons and ligaments
Vertical mattress (see Figure 22.16)	Relieves tension. May be stronger than horizontal mattress and result in less eversion	Skin, subcutaneous tissues, fascia
Near and far patterns (see Figure 22.17)	Relieves tension. Allows closure in deeper layers	Skin, subcutaneous tissues, fascia
Quilled (see Figures 22.18 and 22.19)	Relieves tension. Less direct pressure on tissue surface	Skin
Double butterfly (see Figure 22.20)	Relieves tension. Allows closure in deeper layers	Skin, subcutaneous tissues
'Walking' sutures	Relieves tension. Allows closure in deeper layers. Advances skin to decrease tension on skin closure	Subcutaneous tissues, fascia
Modified Mayo (see Figure 22.21)	Provides overlap and results in imbrication of tissues	Retinacular fascia during stifle surgery

22.22 Common indications for various suture patterns.

Type of procedure	Commonly used suture patterns
Skin closure	Apposition: simple interrupted, interrupted cruciate, simple continuous, Ford interlocking Tension relief: horizontal mattress, vertical mattress, near and far patterns, quilled sutures
Subcutaneous closure	Interrupted intradermal, simple interrupted, simple continuous, continuous intradermal, horizontal mattress, near and far patterns, double butterfly, walking sutures
Fascial closure, linea alba	Simple interrupted, simple continuous, interrupted cruciate, Lembert, horizontal mattress, near and far patterns, modified Mayo
Bladder	Simple interrupted, simple continuous, Connell, Cushing, Lembert, Halsted
Stomach	Simple interrupted, simple continuous, Lembert, Halsted, Connell, Cushing
Intestine	Simple interrupted, simple continuous, Gambee, Poth and Gold crushing
Uterus	Simple interrupted, simple continuous, Lembert, Halsted, Connell, Cushing, Utrecht
Diaphragm	Simple continuous, Ford interlocking

22.23 Suture patterns for different procedures.

Temporary closure of eyelids over a proptosed globe is a good indication for use of quilled sutures. This closure technique takes the strain off the tissues on the eyelid and makes removal easier. Care must be taken to ensure that the suture bites are partial thickness, since full penetration of suture material may lead to rubbing of the cornea and result in corneal ulcers.

Species

Cats have different skin thickness from dogs and therefore some suture patterns, such as the continuous intradermal, may be more difficult to place. Good subcutaneous apposition in cats can often be achieved with a simple continuous suture line.

Patient disposition

Fractious patients, or those not likely to be re-examined for suture removal, will benefit from selection of an intradermal closure without skin sutures.

Need for fast closure

Patients with a critical illness or where intraoperative problems or anaesthetic-related complications are encountered will benefit from reduced time in the theatre. Continuous suture patterns can decrease surgical time and this may make a difference in the recovery of critically ill patients.

Although often more stable, patients with major reconstructive procedures or large linea alba closures would also benefit from reduced surgical time using continuous suture patterns.

Surgeon preference

The surgeon's comfort with certain suture patterns may also affect selection. Several patterns may achieve a similar closure but it is important that the surgeon feels confident in the pattern that is selected.

Knot tying

Correct knot tying is essential to the success of a suture pattern and closure of an incision. It is typically the knot that fails and not the suture material. Poorly tied knots may result in incisional dehiscence and resulting complications.

A knot is defined as two throws on top of each other and can take various forms, such as a square knot, granny knot, surgeon's knot and half hitch. Multiple square knots provide the most reliable anchor for a suture pattern or ligature.

The biggest factors that contribute to knot security are:

- Type of suture material
- Length of cut ends ('tags')
- Structure of the knot itself
- The tension at which the knot is tied.

As a general rule, multifilament suture materials have better knot security than monofilament suture materials. Correct tensioning of the knot is important but, to avoid strangulating tissues, tension should not be excessive. This is particularly important with skin sutures, as excessive tension can cause irritation and discomfort leading to self-trauma of the sutures.

Types of knot

The type of knot formed during tying largely depends on the surgeon's technique.

- Square knots are produced by reversing direction on each successive throw and maintaining even tension.
- Failure to reverse the direction will result in a granny knot.
- Failure to tighten a square knot with even tension will result in a slip knot.

Square knot

This knot is the most important to be familiar with and is used to anchor the majority of suture patterns and ligatures. The knot is started with a simple knot with one throw and the direction is reversed during each successive throw. Even tension with both strands parallel to the plane of the knot will ensure that it locks in place correctly (Figure 22.24a).

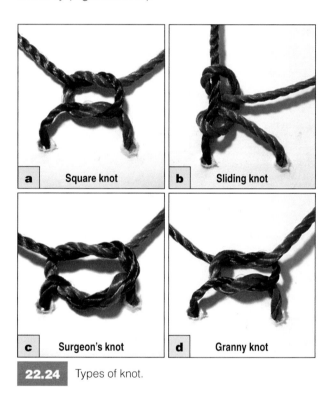

| a | Square knot | b | Sliding knot |
| c | Surgeon's knot | d | Granny knot |

22.24   Types of knot.

Slip knot (sliding knot)

The sliding knot is the same as a square knot except that even tension is not kept on the strands: one strand is held with more upwards pressure. This results in a knot that can slide down to tighten, but equally can loosen easily unless it is either converted to a square knot or has square knots thrown over it to secure the initial knot (Figure 22.24b).

Surgeon's knot

The surgeon's knot is similar to a square knot except that the first knot has one strand passed over the instrument or finger twice, thus creating a larger coefficient of friction and temporarily keeping the first throw snug while a second standard square knot throw is placed on top (Figure 22.24c). Due to the asymmetrical nature of the first knot, the surgeon's knot should always be followed by a square knot to ensure security.

This knot can be used to the surgeon's advantage in securing pedicles or areas under light tension. The use of a surgeon's knot with catgut is not recommended, due to the material's tendency to fray with the increased tension. Several square knots over the initial surgeon's knot will help to keep it secure. Surgeons should aim to become proficient with both the sliding knot and the surgeon's knot.

Granny knot

A granny knot results from failing to reverse direction each time a simple throw is made while tying a square knot (Figure 22.24d). For many types of sutures, this is not as secure as a square knot and is not recommended (Rosin and Robinson, 1989).

Chinese finger-trap

The Chinese finger-trap is a series of knots tied along a tube to secure the tube to the skin. As tension is placed by pulling on the tube, the finger-trap tightens and prevents removal.

This series of knots is started by a simple interrupted suture in the skin near the exit of the tube, leaving both tag ends long. The suture material is passed criss-cross along the tube to each side, with a single or double throw, or a square knot or surgeon's knot placed on each side to indent slightly but not occlude the tube. This is repeated at intervals of 0.5–1 cm at least five or six times, until it is finished with a knot containing multiple throws for security (Figure 22.25).

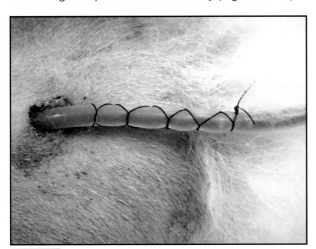

22.25   A Chinese finger-trap suture used to secure an active suction drain.

Aberdeen knot

The Aberdeen knot is made of multiple half hitches and is used to end continuous suture pattern lines. It is quick to tie and allows the resulting knot to be easily buried.

The knot is produced by passing a loop derived from the single tag at the end in a looped fashion through the loop (Figure 22.26a), then drawing this resulting loop down tight and repeating the steps multiple, typically four to six, times. The knot is ended by placing the single strand completely through the loop and drawing it tight (Figure 22.26b). The single strand (still with the needle on) can be introduced through the incision and out 0.5–1 cm away, and as it is tightened the knot becomes buried. The buried strand only contains one tag rather than the typical three from the end of a continuous line.

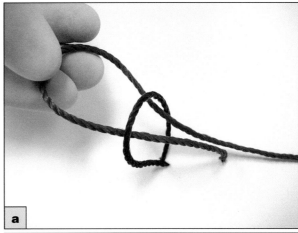

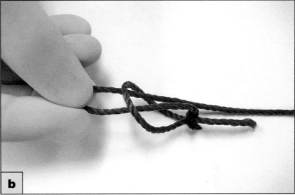

22.26   **(a)** Starting an Aberdeen knot. **(b)** Continuing the Aberdeen knot.

Methods of knot tying

Hand tying

There are two methods of hand tying: either one-handed or two-handed.

- Two-handed tying produces the most reliable results in obtaining consistent square knots (Technique 22.1), but can be difficult in deep areas like the abdomen of deep-chested dogs.
- The one-handed technique requires more dexterity, but is more adaptable to deeper areas and can be quicker to tie (Technique 22.2). It also allows tension to be maintained on the material while tying, but is more wasteful of suture material.

An instrument, such as a pair of scissors, can be held in the free hand while performing the one-handed technique, whereas both hands are needed with two-hand tying. Both techniques require practice to ensure that clinical application provides reliable knot security.

Instrument tying

This is the easiest way to tie a knot and is useful in almost all situations. Instrument tying uses less suture material than hand tying, but it may not provide the tactile feel during tying that hand tying does. Despite this, most surgeons are very comfortable with instrument ties and they can be used in almost all situations (Technique 22.3). Of the three techniques, this is the most important to be comfortable with, although mastery of all three methods will give the surgeon the ability to tie knots in all clinical situations.

TECHNIQUE 22.1
Two-handed square knot for right-handed surgeons

1 Drape one end of the suture material around the left index finger, with the finger extended 'like a gun'.

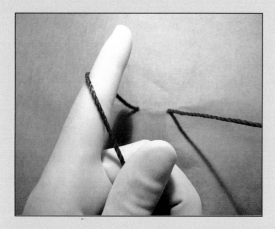

2 Bring the other end of the suture material across the first suture line, using the right hand (out of picture).

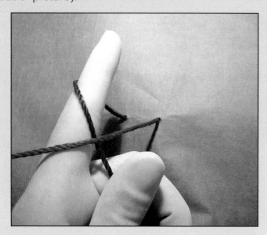

3 Using the left index finger, wrap it under the first line to grab the second line, pulling it through the loop.

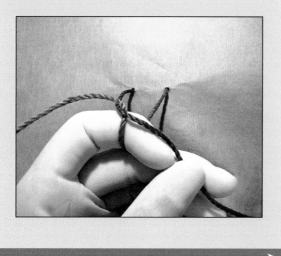

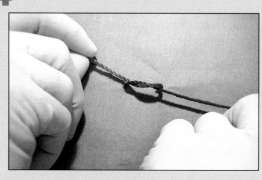

4 The first throw is completed.

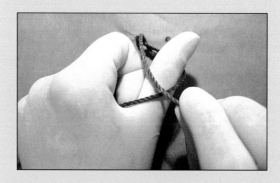

5 With the first suture arm running over the left thumb and through the palm of the left hand, place the left thumb through the loop formed by draping the second suture arm over it.

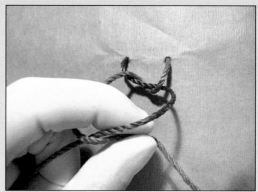

6 Bring the index finger to the thumb and grasp the second suture, pulling it through the loop to complete a square knot.

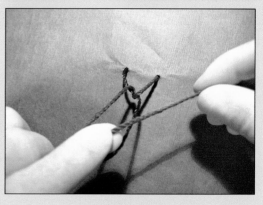

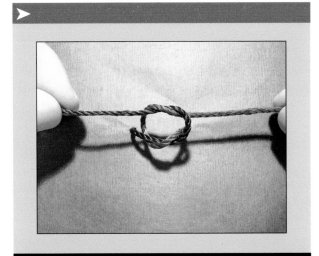

TECHNIQUE 22.2
One-handed square knot for right-handed surgeons

1 Drape the right end of the suture material across the palm side of the fingers of the right hand, securing the suture between thumb and index finger.

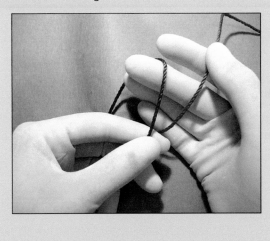

2 Drape the left end of the suture material over the middle finger.

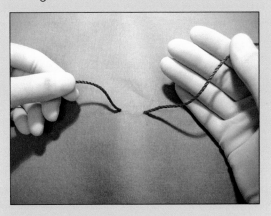

3 Using the middle finger to go over the left suture end, catch the right suture with the nail tip of the finger.

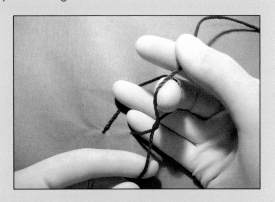

4 Pull the right suture end through.

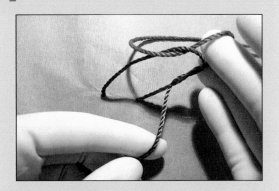

5 The first throw is completed.

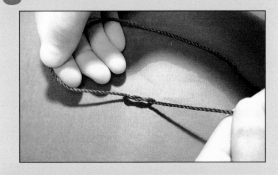

6 Run the left end of the suture over the index and middle finger of the right hand.

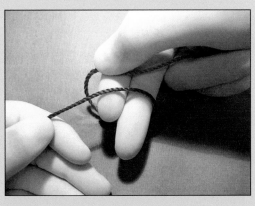

7 Go over the suture to catch the right suture next to it.

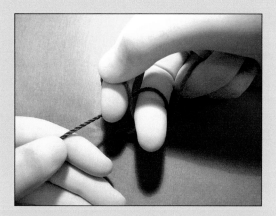

8 Pull it through to complete the square knot.

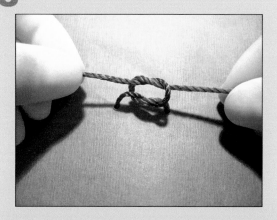

TECHNIQUE 22.3
Instrument tie for right-handed surgeons

1 Holding the needle end in the left hand (instrument in the right), throw one loop of suture over the instrument and grab the other 'tag' end of the suture with the instrument and pull it through the loop.

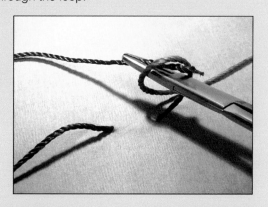

2 Tighten the throw by pulling hands apart with even tension flat to the surface to prevent a sliding knot.

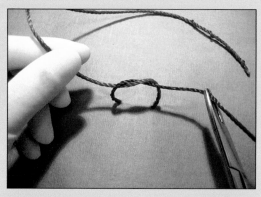

3 Release the end of the suture with the instrument; loop another throw around the needle-holder and grab the tag end, pulling it through again.

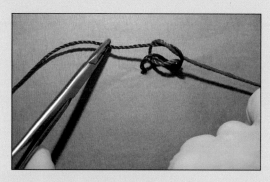

4 The hands should tighten the throw as with the first, but should be moving in the opposite direction from the first throw.

5 Successive throws are then placed similarly.

References and further reading

Austin BR and Henderson RA (2006) Buried tension sutures: force-tension comparisons of pulley, double butterfly, mattress, and simple interrupted suture patterns. *Veterinary Surgery* **35**, 43–48

Demetriou JL, Hughes R and Sissener TR (2006) Pullout strength for three suture patterns used for tracheal anastomosis. *Veterinary Surgery* **35**, 278–283

Kirpensteijn J, Maarscalkerweerd RJ, van der Gaag I, Kooistra HS and van Sluijs FJ (2001) Comparison of three closure methods and two absorbable suture materials for closure of jejunal enterotomy incisions in healthy dogs. *Veterinary Quarterly* **23**, 67–70

Radasch RM, Merkley DF, Wilson JW and Barstad RD (1990) Cystotomy closure: a comparison of the strength of appositional and inverting suture patterns. *Veterinary Surgery* **19**, 283–288

Rosin E and Robinson GM (1989) Knot security of suture materials. *Veterinary Surgery* **18**, 269–273

Sagi HC, Papp S and Dipasquale T (2008) The effect of suture pattern and tension on cutaneous blood flow as assessed by laser Doppler flowmetry in a pig model. *Journal of Orthopaedic Trauma* **22**, 171–175

Weismann DL, Smeak DD, Birchard SJ and Zweigart SL (1999) Comparison of a continuous suture pattern with a simple interrupted pattern for enteric closure in dogs and cats; 83 cases (1991–1997). *Journal of the American Veterinary Medical Association* **214**, 1507–1510

Index